BSAVA Manual of
Avian Practice
A Foundation Manual

Editors:

John Chitty
BVetMed CertZooMed CBiol MSB MRCVS
Anton Vets,
Unit 11, Anton Mill Road, Andover,
Hampshire SP10 2NJ, UK

Deborah Monks
BVSc (Hons) CertZooMed, FACVSc (Avian Health) DipECZM
Brisbane Birds and Exotics Veterinary Service,
191 Cornwall Street, Greenslopes,
Queensland 4120, Australia

Published by:

British Small Animal Veterinary Association
Woodrow House, 1 Telford Way,
Waterwells Business Park, Quedgeley,
Gloucester GL2 2AB

A Company Limited by Guarantee in England
Registered Company No. 2837793
Registered as a Charity

Titles in the BSAVA Manuals series:

For further information on these and all BSAVA publications,
please visit our website: **www.bsava.com**

Contents

Quick reference guides

CD Contents

Contributors

Mike Cannon BVSc MANZCVS (Avian Health) GradDipEd
Cannon and Ball Veterinary Surgeons, 461 Crown Street, West Wollongong, New South Wales 2500, Australia

John Chitty BVetMed CertZooMed CBiol MSB MRCVS
Anton Vets, Unit 11, Anton Mill Road, Andover, Hampshire SP10 2NJ, UK

Lorenzo Crosta MedVet PhD DipECZM (Zoo Health Management) GP Cert (Exotic Animal Practice)
Veterinari Montevecchia, Via Como, 5 - 23874 Montevecchia (LC), Italy

Stefka Curd DVM DipECZM (Avian)
Weidgasse 13, 5304 Endingen, Switzerland

Bob Doneley BVSc FANZCVS (Avian Medicine) CMAVA
Veterinary Medical Centre, Building 8156, Main Drive, University of Queensland, Gatton 4343, Queensland, Australia

Kevin Eatwell BVSc(Hons) DZooMed (Reptilian) DipECZM (Hereptology and Small Mammals) MRCVS
Royal (Dick) School of Veterinary Studies, Hospital for Small Animals, Easter Bush Veterinary Centre,
Roslin, Midlothian EH25 9RG, UK

M. Scott Echols DVM DipABVP (Avian Practice)
Echols Veterinary Services, Salt Lake City, Utah 84121, USA and The Medical Center for Birds, 3805 Main Street,
Oakley, California 94561, USA

Brett Gartrell BVSc PhD MANZCVS (Avian Health)
Wildbase, Institute of Veterinary, Animal and Biomedical Sciences, Massey University, Tennent Drive,
Palmerston North 4442, New Zealand

Stacey Gelis BSc BVSc (Hons) MANZCVS (Avian Health)
Melbourne Bird Veterinary Clinic, 1 George Street, Scoresby, Victoria 3179, Australia

James M. Harris OAM BS DVM FRSPH
Mayfair Veterinary Clinic, 2 Russell Crescent, Sandy Bay, Tasmania 7005, Australia

Jean-Michel Hatt Dr.med.vet DipACZM DipECZM (Avian)
Clinic for Zoo Animals, Exotic Pets and Wildlife, Vetsuisse Faculty, University of Zurich, Winterthurerstrasse 260,
CH-8057, Zurich, Switzerland

Craig Hunt BVetMed CertSAM DZooMed (Reptilian) MRCVS
Chine House Veterinary Hospital, Sileby Hall, Cossington Road, Sileby, Loughborough, Leicestershire LE12 7RS, UK

Alan Jones BVetMed MRCVS
64 Deans Close, Stoke Poges, Buckinghamshire SL2 4JX, UK

Richard Jones VSc MSc MRCVS
Avian Vet Services, Gauntlet Birds of Prey Centre, Manchester Road, Knutsford, Cheshire WA16 0SX, UK

Alistair Lawrie BVMS (Hons) FRCVS
The Lawrie Veterinary Group, 25 Griffiths Street, Falkirk FK1 5QY, UK

Amber Lee BVSc
VCA South Shore (Weymouth), 595 Columbian Street, South Weymouth, Massachusetts 02190, USA

Angela M. Lennox DVM DipABVP (Avian and Exotic Companion Mammal) DipECZM (Small Mammal)
Avian and Exotic Animal Clinic, 9330 Waldemar Road, Indianapolis, Indiana 46268, USA

Michael Lierz Dr.med.vet DZooMed DipECZM (WPH) DipECPVS
Clinic for Birds, Reptiles, Amphibians and Fish, Justus-Liebig University Giessen, Frankfurter Street 91–93,
35392 Giessen, Germany

Alessandro Melillo DVM SPACS
Clinica Veterinaria OMNIAVET, Rome, Italy

Deborah Monks BVSc(Hons) CertZooMed FACVSc (Avian Health) DipECZM
Brisbane Birds and Exotics Veterinary Service, 191 Cornwall Street, Greenslopes, Queensland 4120, Australia

Andrés Montesinos LV MS PhD CertExoticMed AVEPA
Centro Veterinario Los Sauces, C/Santa Engracia 63, 28010 Madrid, Spain

Michael Pees DVM DipECZM (Avian and Herpetology)
Clinic for Birds and Reptiles, University of Leipzig An den Tierkliniken 17, 04103 Leipzig, Germany

Aidan Raftery MVB CertZooMed CBiol MRSB MRCVS
Avian and Exotic Animal Clinic, 221 Upper Chorlton Road, Manchester M16 0DE, UK

Alex Rosenwax BVSC MANZCVS (Avian Health)
Bird and Exotics Veterinarian, Green Square, 1 Hunter Street, Waterloo, New South Wales 2017, Australia

Peter Sandmeier DVM DipECZM (Avian)
Kleintier- und Vogelpraxis, Tafernstrasse 11b, 5405 Baden-Daettwil, Switzerland

Petra Schnitzer Med Vet DipECZM (Avian) GP Cert (Exotic Animal Practice)
Exotic Vet South Tyrol, Dorf-Tirol (BZ), Italy

Brian L. Speer DVM DipABVP (Avian Practice) DipECZM (Avian)
The Medical Center for Birds, 3805 Main Street, Oakley, California 94561, USA

Brian Stockdale BVM&S MRCVS
Ivy Cottage, 9 Meadow Lane, Loughborough LE11 1JU, UK

Thomas N. Tully Jr DVM MS DipABVP (Avian) DipECZM (Avian)
Department of Veterinary Clinical Sciences, Louisiana State University, Skip Bertman Drive, Baton Rouge,
Louisiana 70803, USA

Yvonne van Zeeland DVM MVR PhD DipECZM (Avian and Small Mammal) CPBC
Division of Zoological Medicine, Department of Clinical Sciences of Companion Animals, Faculty of Veterinary Medicine,
Utrecht University, Yalelaan 108, 3584 CM Utrecht, The Netherlands

David Williams MA MEd VetMD PhD DipECAWBM CertVOphthal CertWEL FHEA FRSB FRCVS
Department of Clinical Veterinary Medicine, University of Cambridge, Madingley Road, Cambridge CB3 0ES, UK

Elisa Wüst
Clinic for Birds, Reptiles, Amphibians and Fish, Justus-Liebig University Giessen, Frankfurter Street 91–93,
35392 Giessen, Germany

Petra Zsivanovits DVM DipECZM (Avian)
Tieraerztliche Praxis fuer Vogelmedizin, Wiesenweg 2–8, 23812 Wahlstedt, Germany

Foreword

The *BSAVA Manual of Avian Practice* will be a useful addition to the successful set of BSAVA Foundation Manuals. Whilst the BSAVA Manual series has two in-depth specialist avian manuals, this new title is intended for general practitioners who need to know about the avian patients that present to their general practice and who do not have access to specialized knowledge or equipment. It should also appeal veterinary students, as well as technicians and nurses, who either see very few birds or would like to develop a special interest in this area.

The avian manuals have evolved and improved over the years – for instance, colour illustration is now easy to provide (compared with 20 years ago) and the illustrations in this manual are excellent. Quick Reference Guides are a useful innovation to guide the clinician, especially those with limited time. There are many basic techniques which are described very well and, as a true sign of the times, there is an accompanying set of video clips that enhance the written descriptions.

To accomplish all this, the editors – John Chitty and Deborah Monks – have picked a truly international set of authors who all have immense practical experience with birds of many different families and can all write with authority. The groups of birds covered are those seen most commonly in general practice: parrots and their relatives, birds of prey (eagles, hawks, falcons and owls) and Passeriformes (including Mynah birds, finches and canaries). If required, a greater depth of information is presented in the current specialized manuals, namely the *BSAVA Manual of Psittacine Birds* and the *BSAVA Manual of Raptors, Pigeons and Passerine Birds*.

This book will be successful as it fills an otherwise unoccupied niche and will be widely read and appreciated. The authors and editors, as well as the BSAVA, are to be congratulated on producing this excellent manual.

Nigel Harcourt Brown
BVSc DipECAMS FRCVS

Preface

There are many texts available on avian medicine at present, and with two already published by the BSAVA, the question begs to be asked why produce another one?

The answer is surprisingly simple – available texts highlight, quite correctly, what is possible and the ideal standards of current avian practice. However, this is not always practical and for general practitioners who lack specialized equipment, yet need to see birds on an occasional basis (or who would like to embark on a career in avian medicine), such standards can be off-putting. In the UK, the presence of avian species and their needs in the RCVS list of Day 1 Competencies highlights the need to provide material to help the non-specialized avian veterinary surgeon. To aid in this, in this manual we have concentrated on the species more commonly seen in practice – parrots, passerines and raptors.

As editors, our approach was simple: we asked authors to write the chapters from the perspective of their current experience and knowledge, yet utilizing the tools they had when first starting in practice. However, new technologies and specialized techniques cannot be ignored, so the authors have alluded to those where appropriate. More advanced knowledge can be found in the companion volumes to this title, namely the *BSAVA Manual of Psittacine Birds* and the *BSAVA Manual of Raptors, Pigeons and Passerine Birds*.

The BSAVA Manual of Avian Practice consists of two parts. The first section provides an overview of biology, husbandry, anatomy and nutrition, along with clinical techniques such as radiography and anaesthesia. The second section of the manual focuses on clinical presentations. Clinical signs in birds are rarely, if ever, pathognomonic and these chapters provide a logical approach to the more common presentations seen by practitioners. The exception is the chapter on infectious diseases, where the emphasis is on recognition and specific pathogen testing, as well as prevention and control of the spread of disease.

We are extremely grateful to all the authors for their invaluable contributions, as well as to the Woodrow House publishing team for their help and support during the production of the *BSAVA Manual of Avian Practice*. We would also like to thank our families for their forbearance and patience during the writing and editing of the book.

Finally, we would like to dedicate this book to the memory of Andrew Thwaites who will never be far from our thoughts, and to the arrival of Cole Bullingham whose birthday nearly waited for that of this manual.

John Chitty and Deborah Monks
December 2017

Species guide

Stacey Gelis

Disclaimer:

The following information, particularly the comments relating to the behavioural characteristics of particular species and sexes, are of a general nature and are meant as a guide only. As with all animals, there are always exceptions and individual birds need to be assessed on their own characteristics and clinical signs, regardless of species or gender

If birds are to lead full and enriched lives in a captive environment, it is important that keepers understand how each species has adapted to, and interacts with, its natural environment. This will enable keepers to meet the physical and psychological needs of the birds in their care.

Equally, veterinary surgeons (veterinarians) require an understanding of each species and its unique characteristics to help optimize their ability to treat avian patients. This chapter is aimed at providing some basic information on a variety of avian species commonly presented in clinical practice. This information will encourage the general practice veterinary surgeon to approach and deal with these species with confidence.

Psittaciformes

Macaws

Natural history

The macaws are a group of small to large Neotropical parrots characterized by bare facial patches of varying sizes and long tails, which are as long as or longer than the body. They comprise several of the most enigmatic species of parrot, including the Blue and Gold Macaw (Figure 1.1) and the Hyacinth Macaw. Species vary in size from the 30 cm long Noble Macaw to the largest Green-winged and Hyacinth Macaws (95–100 cm). They originate from South and Central America and Mexico.

Macaws are sexually monomorphic and the young resemble the adults; the larger species reach sexual maturity at 2–5 years.

Characteristics and considerations for captivity

Their size and bold colours make the large macaws extremely desirable as pet birds worldwide. However,

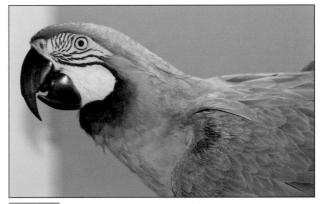

1.1 Blue and Gold Macaw.

they require a lot of attention if they are to be kept successfully in the domestic situation. They can be destructive, noisy and intimidate unprepared owners. These factors, combined with their large size, make a bird that is very demanding in its needs. Macaws require a keeper with lots of time, patience and ingenuity if they are not to develop behavioural problems. They have a reasonable talking ability, but are generally not as proficient as Grey Parrots or some Amazon species.

Macaws can exhibit undesirable behaviours such as biting or screaming in response to inappropriate environmental and owner-induced stimuli. The Scarlet Macaw in particular and, to a lesser extent, the Military and Great Green Macaws have a reputation for these behaviours. These behaviours, whilst undesirable in a captive environment, form one method of communication within the wild flock. Generally speaking, the Blue and Gold and Hyacinth Macaws tend to be the gentler specimens. However, every individual is different and it is imperative that a keeper learns to read the body language of the birds in their care to avoid unpleasant interactions.

The smaller 'mini' macaws are more like conures in their behaviour; some have higher pitched disruptive screams than the larger species. The smaller species often sleep in hollows at night, and providing a roosting nest may give them more security. However, nests may need to be removed if the birds display undesirable sexual behaviour in captivity, particularly females. An alternative may be to provide a covered perch, such as a box with no bottom. This provides roosting security whilst the lack of substrate inhibits nest preparation.

Diet

In the wild, most macaws consume a variety of wild fruits, seeds, nuts and, inadvertently, insects; some species actively seek protein in the form of water snails, fish in drying ponds, lizards and even carrion. Like many parrots, macaws are opportunists. However, some are more specialist feeders, such as the Hyacinth Macaw, which eats predominantly palm nuts and in general shuns fruit.

Amazon parrots

Natural history

Amazons are medium- to large-sized stocky parrots represented by about 30 species belonging to the genus *Amazona*. They originate from Central and South America, Mexico and the Caribbean. Amazons inhabit a wide range of environments from dry savannah to scrub forest and rainforest. Amazons are primarily green-bodied birds; individual species are distinguished by their facial, head and neck colours and wing markings. Figure 1.2 lists the body lengths and bodyweights of several species of Amazon parrots. Males tend to be larger and heavier than the females.

Most Amazon parrots are sexually monomorphic, but there are some exceptions. The White-fronted Amazon male has a larger area of red feathering on the lores and surrounding the eye than the female. The male also has red alulae and primary coverts on the wing; these are green in the female. The male Yucatan Amazon has a white forehead and forecrown, which is mostly dull blue in the female. In addition, the extent of the red coloration of the periophthalmic and cheek feathering on the male's face and primary coverts on the wing is much reduced or absent in the female.

Some of the Caribbean species are threatened with extinction in the wild and are the subject of conservation programmes.

Anatomically, Amazon parrots lack a uropygial gland, gall bladder and caeca.

Characteristics and considerations for captivity

Amazons are intelligent, long-lived (40–60 years) and playful. However, males in particular can become aggressive when reproductively active, particularly human-imprinted birds kept in isolation. This can also occur in breeding pairs, where males will often bully their females and where misplaced aggression can result in severe trauma to the female. In particular, species from the Yellow-headed Amazon complex and Cuban, Tucumán, Red-browed and Red-lored Amazons are prone to exhibiting these behaviours and need to be closely monitored and appropriately housed to allow the female some form of seclusion or escape.

Many of the commonly kept Amazon species have outgoing personalities and, as with most parrots, are less likely to bond with a single person if family interactions are shared amongst people in the household.

Several species are known for their talking ability, including Double Yellow-headed, Yellow-naped and Blue-fronted Amazons.

The Mealy Amazon is amongst the most docile and gentle of Amazons.

Amazons are great chewers and can be destructive to vegetation and household furniture. These species need to be kept active if obesity and related health problems are to be avoided.

Diet

Wild Amazon parrots feed on a wide variety of foodstuffs including fruits, berries, seeds, nuts, leaf buds and blossoms, mostly procured from the upper canopy. Sometimes insects are included.

Amazons are not generally fussy eaters, and many species are prone to obesity in captivity due to their sedentary lifestyles; they do well on high-protein, low-energy diets. Ideal captive diets are based on pellets rather than seeds and supplemented with vegetables, pulses, sprouts and fruits and an abundance of forage items. Birds should be monitored for obesity.

Cockatoos

Natural history

Cockatoos (family Cacatuidae) comprise 21 species found in Australia, Indonesia, New Guinea, the Solomon Islands and the Philippines. They are mostly medium to large birds (with the exception of the Cockatiel, which is discussed later) and are characterized by curved beaks, erectile crests and a lack of any bright green or blue colour in their plumage (Figure 1.3). Some inhabit arid and semi-arid open woodlands whilst others are true rainforest species.

Their diet in the wild consists of seeds, nuts, roots, berries, leaf buds and some insects. Some species have adapted as specialist feeders, such as the Glossy Black Cockatoo, which feeds specifically on the seeds of *Casuarina* and *Allocasuarina* trees, whilst other species are opportunist generalist feeders. Flocking behaviour is common in several species of cockatoos, such as the Galah and the Red-tailed Black Cockatoo.

Cockatoos nest mostly in open-topped hollow logs and lay between one and four eggs. Incubation lasts 22–31 days and weaning can take a considerable length of time, up to 6 months in Palm Cockatoos.

Characteristics and considerations for captivity

The larger cockatoo species can be destructive and noisy. In some species, feather destructive disorder, screaming and biting are common, reflecting a fault in how individuals have been raised and kept rather than

Species	Body length (cm)	Bodyweight (g)
Orange-winged	31–33	300–470
Blue-fronted	37	400
Yellow-crowned	35–38	400–460
Double Yellow-headed	35–38	480–600
Yellow-naped	35–37	375–480
Red-lored	32–35	315–485
White-fronted	23–26	200–230
Mealy	38–41	540–700
Saint Vincent	40	580–700
Imperial	48	<900

1.2 Body length and bodyweight ranges of several species of Amazon parrots.

1.3

(a) Sulphur-crested Cockatoo.
(b) Palm Cockatoo.

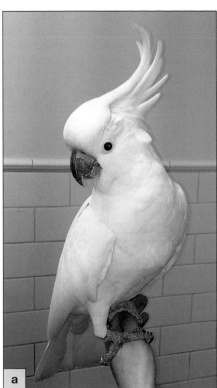

a

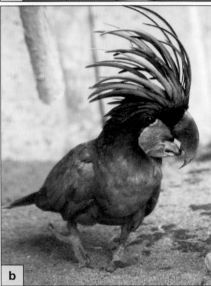

b

a fault with the bird. It must be remembered that cockatoos, like most parrots, are highly social birds which, in the wild, would constantly interact with flockmates throughout the day. Cockatoos should not be left alone for long periods of time.

- Sulphur-crested Cockatoos (see Figure 1.3a) can bite and be very noisy, but with appropriate care can be very rewarding pet birds.
- Galahs can make good pets, but require ongoing positive reinforcement to avoid the development of undesirable behaviours. Like Major Mitchell's Cockatoos, these birds have an increased propensity to remember aversive events associated with specific people.
- Corellas tend to be highly strung birds, very active, and can quickly develop inappropriate behaviours if not appropriately stimulated.
- Moluccan Cockatoos are extremely affectionate and so are very popular. However, they are also prone to

feather destructive disorder and can also be very noisy when their behavioural, emotional and psychological needs are not met.
- Of the black cockatoos, Red-tailed Black Cockatoo males tend to make the best pets. They are very affectionate, amenable to handling and seldom bite. However, they are noisy birds.

Diet
Cockatoos are primarily seed-eaters in the wild. However, in captivity, all-seed diets have led to obesity, lipomas, fatty liver disease and atherosclerosis. Galahs and Umbrella Cockatoos are particularly prone to obesity. These birds do much better on a pellet-based diet, supplemented with vegetables, sprouts, legumes and some fruit. High-fat seeds and domestic nuts should be avoided when feeding the Galah in particular.

Browse (branches containing leaves, bark, flowers and nuts) is an essential addition for most species to avoid boredom and undesirable behaviours.

The Black and Palm Cockatoos (see Figure 1.3b) have adapted to a slightly higher fat diet and the addition of some nuts and sunflower seeds may be given to supplement the standard recommended diet as described above. Some species, such as the Yellow-tailed Black Cockatoo and Gang-gang Cockatoo have an appetite for live insects and will even take animal protein (e.g. mice) at times, particularly when breeding.

Conures
Natural history
Conures are a large group of small- to medium-sized long-tailed Neotropical parakeets from South and Central America and the Caribbean islands. They range in size from the smallest *Pyrrhura* species (21 cm) to the Patagonian Conure (45 cm). Many, such as the Blue-crowned and Red-masked Conures, inhabit dry woodland whilst others, such as the Golden and Painted Conures, inhabit lowland rainforests. They generally live in pairs or small flocks although some, such as the Patagonian Conure, form large flocks.

In most species, nesting occurs in pairs in hollow logs, but the Patagonian Conure nests communally, digging burrows into sandstone or limestone cliff faces. Clutch sizes vary from three to eight eggs. The female incubates the eggs for 22–26 days. Young fledge 7–8 weeks after hatching.

Characteristics and considerations for captivity
Conures are very popular pet birds. The brightly coloured Sun (Figure 1.4) and Jenday Conures are highly desirable. Of the two, Jenday Conures usually make the better pets as they have a very sweet nature, are very sociable and bond well with people. They are also slightly less noisy than Sun Conures.

The Patagonian Conure is the largest of the conures and is a highly sociable bird. Hand-reared birds can make excellent pets and they are extremely intelligent. However, their gregarious nature means that they require lots of attention, otherwise they will vocalize loudly for long periods.

The smaller *Pyrrhura* conures are energetic and have the strong personality and character of a larger parrot but are quieter, less destructive and less likely to dominate an owner. The Rose-crowned Conure typically has the most amenable temperament and is

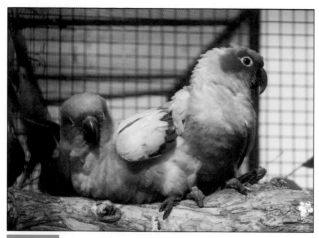

1.4   Sun Conures mating.

less likely to be territorial or to bite when in breeding condition – a characteristic which is typical of the Crimson-bellied (Figure 1.5a), Pearly and Blue-throated Conures. Painted Conures (Figure 1.5b) can be flighty, but once calmed down make good pets, although they are not common. Low (2013) reported that parent-reared *Pyrrhura* conures bought 3 weeks after leaving the nest and weaned are more independent and less likely to exhibit undesirable behaviours than hand-raised birds. Conures in general have limited speech capability.

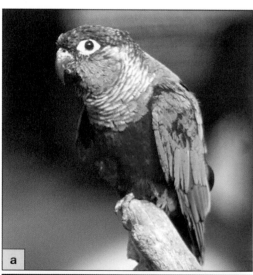

a

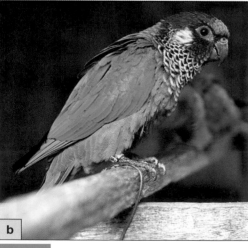

b

1.5   **(a)** Crimson-bellied Conure. **(b)** Painted Conure.

Diet

Conures eat a varied diet in the wild consisting of seeds, fruits, berries, vegetable matter and insects. In captivity they should be fed a pellet, vegetable and fruit diet, with occasional seeds and fresh browse.

Small parrots: Cockatiels, Budgerigars and lovebirds

Natural history

Cockatiels and Budgerigars ('Budgies') come from the drier interior areas of Australia and are highly nomadic in search of seeds and water. Their physiology is adapted to life in an environment of climatic extremes, producing a high number of offspring in quick succession when conditions are right, and suffering large losses during droughts. Budgerigars in particular form huge flocks after periods of good food availability. Budgerigars feed on the seeds of grasses and herbaceous plants; Cockatiels take advantage of grains, fruits and berries in addition to seeds. Both species nest in tree hollows and lay clutches of four to six eggs which are incubated for 18–21 days. Young fledge in 4–5 weeks and are independent 3 weeks later.

The nine species of lovebirds are African in origin; the Grey-headed Lovebird is indigenous to Madagascar (hence the synonym 'Madagascar Lovebird'). Lovebirds also inhabit dry woodland areas, and are sociable birds forming large noisy flocks, particularly at good food sources. The commonest species are monomorphic, but the Madagascar, Abyssinian and Red-faced Lovebirds are sexually dimorphic.

Lovebirds nest in crevices in cliffs and buildings, in weaver nests, tree hollows and arboreal termite mounds. Lovebirds tear strips of leaves and use these to line the nest. In captivity most species will readily nest in nest boxes, but require palm fronds or grasses for stripping.

They lay three to six white eggs that are incubated by both sexes for 21–23 days. Chicks fledge 6 weeks after hatching and are independent 2–3 weeks later.

Characteristics and considerations for captivity

Budgerigars and Cockatiels are perhaps the two most popular of all pet birds. Budgerigars come in an almost endless variety of colours and have very simple husbandry requirements, appearing to be equally content as single cage birds (as long as they experience appropriate regular human interaction) or as pairs or a group in an aviary. They are not noisy and some develop an extensive human vocabulary, although they do have a squeaky voice that can be hard to decipher at times. Budgerigars exhibit few behavioural problems. They are also easily bred in captivity.

Cockatiels are hardy, sociable and relatively undemanding pets with few of the behavioural problems encountered with larger parrots. They can form strong bonds with their owners. A common issue in captive females is a propensity for unrestricted egg laying, which can lead to health problems. Cockatiels can also be quite vocal and learn to mimic sounds and words.

Lovebirds were more popularly kept in the past, but have fallen out of favour. Some make great pets, but they have a reputation for being aggressive (particularly females, which are the dominant sex) and some have feather destructive and self-mutilation problems. The Peach-faced and Black-masked

Lovebirds can also be noisy. Lovebirds prefer to roost in nests at night. Although they are highly sociable, the notion that these birds must be kept as pairs or else they will pine away and die is a myth, and individual birds can lead healthy and enriched lives so long as they are provided with adequate human interaction and environmental enrichment.

Lories and lorikeets

Natural history

There are approximately 55 species of lories (Figure 1.6) and lorikeets, which originate from Indonesia, New Guinea, Australia and the South Pacific. They frequent forests and woodlands and are common visitors to gardens. They feed primarily upon nectar, pollen, fruits, lerp, scale and also some insects; unlike other parrots, seeds are only an occasional dietary item of most lorikeets. They often fly great distances following the flowering patterns of the plants upon which they feed. In other words, they eat high-energy diets but in turn expend a lot of energy in search of their food.

Lories and lorikeets form pairs to breed but in some species breeding pairs may also form loose colonies and breed in hollows in the same or neighbouring trees. Most species lay two eggs in a clutch and incubation lasts 23–26 days. Young birds fledge 7–9 weeks after hatching and reach independence quickly. They are opportunistic breeders and may nest year-round when conditions are favourable.

Anatomically, their brush tongues, thin-walled ventriculus and short overall intestinal tract reflect an adaptation to a high-liquid, high-sugar and low-protein diet.

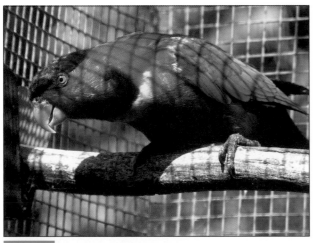

1.6   Yellow-bibbed Lory.

Characteristics and considerations for captivity

Lorikeets are by nature energetic extroverts that can be loud and aggressive, particularly when overstimulated or in breeding condition. Larger species are affectionate, playful, intelligent and inquisitive but, because of their diet and loose droppings, they are messy birds. Some species are extremely noisy and the sound can be harsh. Several are also excellent mimics of sounds and words, particularly those in the *Lorius* genus (e.g. Chattering and Black-capped Lories). Smaller species are less noisy and, in general, less affectionate and playful than the larger species. Their mimicking ability is also much reduced.

Appropriate housing and good hygiene are critical with these birds because of the high fluid content of their droppings. Enclosures and their surrounds need to be easily cleaned on a regular basis, to prevent the discarded food and droppings, which are flicked around the cage, becoming a source of bacterial or fungal infection.

These birds are particularly active and require frequent mental stimulation so environmental enrichment is an important part of successful husbandry. Browse from non-toxic plants and safe bird toys are important, as are novel food items. Positive reinforcement training is also an important part of successfully keeping these birds as pets.

Diet

This is an area of ongoing research but in general lorikeets have a poorly muscled ventriculus as an adaptation to a nectar, pollen and fruit-based diet.

There are many species of lories and lorikeets, which have all adapted to differing ecosystems. Generally they can be classified as nectarivores or omnivorous nectarivores (the latter of which opportunistically eat insects, leaves, bark, seeds and even animal protein).

In captivity, the diet of most species should be based on a limited amount of good-quality commercially produced liquid diet or nectar, a variety of fresh fruit and vegetables and a limited amount of dry powdered or pelleted food. Many retailers and some aviculturists have tried to feed these birds on a dry-based diet for convenience and because it produces a firmer dropping. However, apart from some of the Australian species, most species fare poorly on these diets. The lorikeet gastrointestinal tract is based on rapid transit of high-sugar, low-nutrient density food in a highly liquid environment, hence the reliance on liquid nectar and fruits and vegetables. Fruit or vegetables can be pureed and added to the wet mix several times a week for individuals that will not voluntarily eat them.

It should be noted that many nectars will spoil if left in warm conditions for hours and this can predispose to bacterial and fungal infections. Therefore, wet mixes should only be fed in small amounts that will be eaten within 1–2 hours, particularly during warm weather. These can be fed twice daily if necessary. In addition, *ad libitum* access to high-sugar nectars can lead to obesity and excessive behavioural stimulation. Foods of lower energy density such as vegetables, greens, fruits and branches from flowering plants need to be made available at other times throughout the day.

Some rarer species such as Musschenbroek's and Iris Lorikeets require seeds as a significant part of their daily diet.

Other psittacine groups

Natural history

African Grey Parrots are a subspecies of Grey Parrots from central Africa and are one of the best known cage birds worldwide. The Timneh African Grey is the other smaller, slightly darker subspecies of Grey Parrot from West Africa.

Greys roost communally in large numbers and continue to vocalize well after sunset. Sexual maturity is reached at 3–4 years of age.

The *Poicephalus* species are small- to medium-sized, short-tailed and stocky African endemic parrots. Some of the better-known species are the Senegal

Parrot, Jardine's Parrot, Red-bellied Parrot and Meyer's Parrot. Their small size and voices make them suitable for keepers with limited space. They can screech but, unlike some cockatoos, do not tend to do this for extended periods. They are fearless birds, often standing up to other birds much larger than themselves. Their strong pair-bonding means that they often bond to a single person within a family. Females in particular may be consistently aggressive towards their keepers if not exposed to positive reinforcement training on a regular basis. If a trust bond is broken between bird and owner, it can be difficult to rectify. Females can also be highly aggressive towards each other. On the other hand, well trained birds can be gentle and affectionate and can engage in entertaining behaviours.

There are two species of caiques, the Black-capped and the White-bellied. Both are found in South America, with the former found north of the Amazon River and the latter found to the south. They inhabit lowland forests, preferring the clearings and edges. They live in the forest canopy in small groups, using their loud calls for communication between flockmates and other groups of caiques. They are not particularly large at 23 cm in length and weigh approximately 130–170 g. Sexual maturity is reached at 3 years of age.

Eclectus Parrots (Figure 1.7) are medium to large stocky parrots (31–37 cm in length; weight 400–600 g) native to tropical and subtropical lowland forests of New Guinea, Indonesia, Australia and the Solomon Islands. There are 7–10 subspecies, which vary slightly in colour and size, but the males in all species are predominantly emerald green whilst the females are red with various shades of blue or purple. They have a unique social breeding structure amongst parrots: one breeding female may be attended to and mated by several males; the clutch size is two white eggs, which may be fertilized by different males, and incubation lasts 28–30 days. All the males in the group assist in feeding the chicks during the approximately 80-day rearing period. Females may spend up to 9 months a year in their breeding log. Some males may also tend to a second female.

There are several species of Australian parrots and parakeets that are commonly kept as avicultural birds. These include the genera *Neophema*, *Psephotus* and *Polytelis*, rosellas and Australian Ringnecks, King and Red-winged Parakeets and the New Zealand parakeets ('Kākāriki'). These birds inhabit the open woodlands, grasslands and rainforests of Australasia including New Zealand, New Guinea and the surrounding islands. They are primarily seed-eating birds, which also feed on native fruits, buds, shoots, nuts and occasionally insects. They nest in hollow logs. Reproductive information is summarized in Figure 1.8.

The Asiatic parakeets of the genus *Psittacula* are graceful, tightly feathered long-tailed parakeets, which are primarily green in colour with varying colours of the head and a ring behind the head. They include one of the most popular avicultural subjects, the Indian Ringnecked Parakeet, which is now available in an array of colours rivalling the Budgerigar. Other species, such as the Malayan Long-tailed and Emerald-collared Parakeet, are quite rare in aviculture. Asiatic parakeets tend to breed in pairs, although colony breeding has been successfully carried out with the Derbyan Parakeet and Malabar Parakeet. Unlike lories and conures, pair bonding is not strong in these species and the female is the dominant sex.

Genus	Clutch size	Incubation period (days)	Fledging (days)	Independence (weeks)
Rosellas	4–6+	18–21	35	2–4
Neophema	3–6+	18–25	28–35	2
Psephotus	4–6+	18–21	32–34	2
Polytelis, Alisterus, Aprosmictus	4–5	20–22	35	3
Australian ringnecks	4–6	19–22	34–39	3–4
Cyanoramphus	4–9	19–21	35–40	2–3

1.8 Reproductive statistics of Australian and New Zealand parakeets.

Characteristics and considerations for captivity

Greys are well known for their intelligence and ability to mimic. They are sensitive, social birds that prefer a quieter environment; however, environmental stimulation is essential. In inappropriate environments they can become fearful and engage in feather destructive behaviour. Improper socialization can also result in them becoming one-person birds.

Caiques are extremely active, acrobatic and highly entertaining parrots, similar to lorikeets in their activity levels. Consequently, they require lots of attention, environmental enrichment and positive reinforcement. They do form strong bonds with people and can emit loud calls at times, and their bites can be painful. They are not particularly good talkers. As with several other Neotropical parrots, caiques frequently lie on their backs and 'play dead'. They often run around rather than fly.

Eclectus Parrots (see Figure 1.7) are stunningly dimorphic and intelligent and generally quiet birds. However, they can still vocalize loudly on occasion and have reasonably good talking abilities. The unique fine

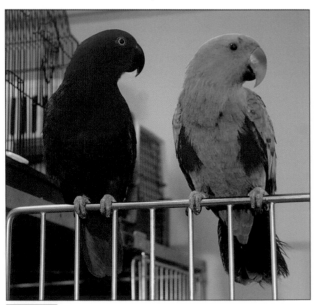

1.7 Pair of Eclectus Parrots (male on the right).

feather structure of their head and neck gives the impression of hairs rather than feathers. They are a female-dominant species and consequently some females may exhibit undesirable behaviours if appropriate training and positive reinforcement practices are not introduced at an early age. Feather destructive disorder is also not uncommon with this species, in part due to the difficulty of replicating the ecology and natural social structure of this species in captivity. In the wild, Eclectus Parrots are polyandrous (i.e. multiple males mate with one female) and polygynandrous (both sexes have multiple partners).

The Australasian parrots and parakeets are more commonly kept as aviary birds and the development of numerous colour mutations has cemented their popularity (Figure 1.9). In general, however, they make only fair pet birds. Some species can become quite aggressive towards their keepers (e.g. rosellas) and they tend to be flighty and do not seek direct human contact to the same extent as the South American species. Their talking abilities are also not as well developed. Kākārikis are an exception, often making good pet birds. They like to dig and bathe and should be kept in a cool environment (below 35°C).

The Asiatic parakeets have traditionally been kept as aviary birds, but as their popularity has increased so has their role as pet birds. Alexandrine Parakeets make great pets, whereas Indian Ringnecked Parakeets are more variable in temperament with some individuals losing their tameness soon after weaning, especially if not handled regularly. Malabar (Figure 1.10) and Derbyan Parakeets often remain tame after hand-rearing, whereas Moustached and Plum-headed Parakeets are more likely to revert to less desirable behaviours unless considerable effort is expended to provide positive reinforcement training.

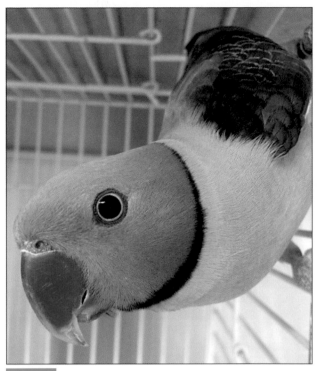

1.10   Male Malabar Parakeet.

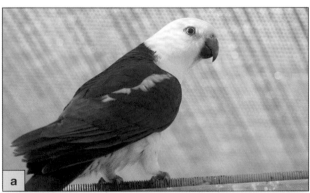

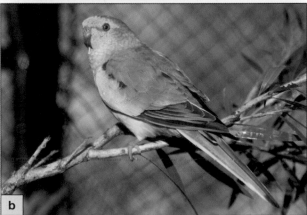

1.9   **(a)** Male Australian King Parrot (blue mutation).
(b) Male Turquoise Parrot.

Diet

Grey Parrots appear to be relatively more susceptible to disorders of calcium metabolism than many other species and benefit from artificial full-spectrum lighting where access to direct sunlight is not possible. They eat seeds, fruits and figs in the wild. In captivity they are fussy eaters and will quickly selectively feed on a seed-only diet if given the chance. They benefit from a balanced pellet-based diet where their calcium and vitamin D3 requirements can be successfully met.

Caiques eat fruits, berries and seeds in the forest canopy in the wild and will eat a wide variety of foodstuffs in captivity.

Eclectus Parrots feed on fruits, figs, nuts, flowers, buds and some seeds in the wild.

The Australian parrots and parakeets have traditionally been kept on seed-based diets supplemented with various green foods, vegetables and fruits. Pelleted diets can be substituted for most or all of the seed component of the diet, particularly in non-breeding birds, but as always birds need to be taught to feed on such food items.

Passeriformes

Mynahs

Natural history

Mynahs are a group of medium-sized passerine birds with strong feet belonging to the family Sturnidae, in the tribe Sturninae (mynahs and starlings). They originate from Asia and New Guinea. Some, such as the Common Mynah, have become well established as feral species in many countries around the world. They generally measure 23–29 cm in length. Mynahs in general are vocal, territorial birds, especially when breeding.

This group includes the larger *Gracula* or Common Hill Mynahs (Figure 1.11), characterized by their black

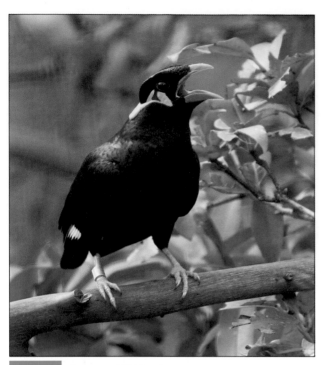

1.11 Common Hill Mynah.

Due to their rarity, Bali Mynahs are mainly kept as aviary birds with the aim of breeding. Some individuals are prone to feather destructive disorder in captivity. This behaviour can be self-inflicted or directed towards other birds, including young in the nest. The neck and head areas seem to be most commonly affected.

Diet
Mynahs are prone to haemochromatosis and so they should be fed a low-iron diet based on low-iron softbill pellets (preferably less than 100 ppm iron), chopped fruit and vegetables. Insects are important additions for breeding birds that are feeding chicks.

Birds fed diets based on dog kibble are at a higher risk of developing iron-storage disease, and citrus fruits should also be avoided in birds with pre-existing iron-storage disease or fed diets of unknown iron content.

Canaries and finches
Natural history
The generic term 'finch' applies to a broad range of predominantly seed-eating small passerines with conical bills. Included in this group are birds in the families Fringillidae (true finches), Emberizidae (buntings and sparrows), Estrildidae (waxbills, grassfinches, munias and mannikins), Ploceidae (weavers) and Viduanae (whydahs/widow birds) (Figure 1.12).

Canaries and finches come from across the world and most of the more commonly kept species are open grassland seed-eaters with varying degrees of insect consumption, which increases during breeding. Nests vary from open cups to closed globular nests and are usually constructed from grasses, twigs or leaves in vegetation, although some utilize small tree hollows and some weaver nests are intricately woven. Most species nest in pairs but some *Viduanae* spp. are parasitic on estrildid finches. Figure 1.13 gives more reproductive data on the various finch taxa.

Characteristics and considerations for captivity
The best known finch is the Domestic Canary, which is valued for its singing abilities.

The Zebra Finch is another commonly kept finch because it is so easily bred in captivity, is inexpensive and is relatively hardy. The gaudily coloured Gouldian Finch is also extremely popular because of its visual appeal and ease of breeding, although it is not as

bodies and yellow facial wattles. These birds are forest canopy dwellers and tend to hop around. By contrast, most of the other species in this group spend time walking on the ground in a characteristic manner with exaggerated head movements and long strides.

One species, the Bali or Rothschild's Mynah, is critically endangered in the wild and is the subject of a captive breeding and reintroduction programme.

Most mynahs breed in tree hollows where three to five light blue/green eggs (sometimes spotted) are laid on a nest constructed from soft twigs and leaves. Incubation lasts 14–16 days, fledging occurs at 28 days after hatching and young are chased away by their parents anywhere from 7–17 days post-fledging. Mynahs can live to over 20 years of age.

Characteristics and considerations for captivity
Hill Mynahs are popular as pet birds principally due to their mimicry talents. Many are hand-reared specifically for this purpose. All will learn to mimic sounds and some, but not all, are excellent mimics of human speech.

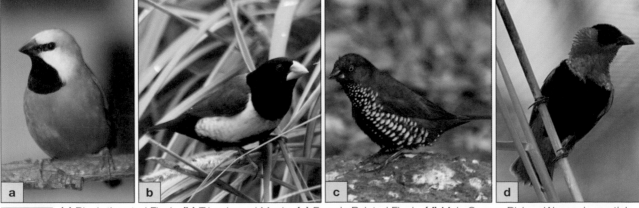

1.12 **(a)** Black-throated Finch. **(b)** Tri-coloured Munia. **(c)** Female Painted Finch. **(d)** Male Orange Bishop Weaver in nuptial plumage.

Family	Nest type	Clutch size	Incubation (days)	Fledging (days after hatching)
Fringillidae	Cup	2–4	12–14	16–18
Emberizidae	Cup	2–4	12–14	16–18
Estrildidae	Domed	2–6	12–15	20–24
Ploceidae	Woven/domed; elaborate	2–6	12–14	18–22 (Bishops 14–16)
Viduidae	Parasitize nests of waxbills and finches	1–4	10–11	20–22

1.13 Reproductive data of common finches.

hardy as some other finches. The Bengalese Mannikin is an entirely domesticated species from Asia which does not exist in the wild but is rather derived from various mannikin species. Because of its domesticity it is often used as a foster breeder for other, harder to breed species.

Finches in general are usually kept as aviary birds or as ornamental birds in cages in houses. Occasionally, hand-raised finches become available as pets. Although not as expressive or interactive as psittacine birds, these birds make close companions as pets due to their social behaviour in the wild and are suitable for those who like a quieter, smaller avian companion.

Diet
Most finches are primarily seed-eaters and there are seed mixes available for different types of seed-eaters (e.g. canary mix, waxbill mix). These should be supplemented with vegetable matter such as leafy greens (both domestic produce and weeds) and seeding grasses. Some species such as Parrotfinches also eat fruit. Many of the more insectivorous species also benefit from live food such as mealworms, maggots and small crickets, but these are seldom necessary for survival; rather, they are used for breeding these birds. Manufactured 'soft-food mixes' with higher protein content and added vitamins and minerals are often provided and the more domesticated species take these readily. The provision of soluble and insoluble grits is also beneficial to many of these birds.

More recently, some manufacturers have produced extruded crumbles for finches that are nutritionally more balanced than seed diets, but the birds need to be taught to eat these foods and they are perhaps more suitable as a dietary base for pet birds (rather than aviary birds), as they can be more closely monitored for acceptance. If these extruded diets are used it is still important to supplement them with green food as mentioned above. However, insoluble grits are not required with pelleted diets.

Miscellaneous: softbills

Natural history
The term 'softbill' is a loose category that includes birds whose diets are not based on seeds and include frugivores, nectarivores, insectivores and even some carnivores. Species commonly kept include: Asiatic species (e.g. Pekin Robins, White-rumped Shama, thrushes, bulbuls, hornbills and bluebirds); African species (e.g. starlings, hornbills, turacos and barbets); and South American species (e.g. toucans, tanagers and honeycreepers). This is obviously a diverse group of birds that occupy a wide range of habitats and have differing social, nesting and feeding systems in place.

Characteristics and considerations for captivity
These birds are mostly kept as avicultural subjects for their colour, activity or unusual behaviour. Some are highly sociable in colonies of their own kind, for example, Metallic Starlings and oropendolas (*Psarocolius* spp.), whilst others are highly territorial and need to be kept in their own aviaries (e.g. toucans and hornbills). Some can be tamed as pet birds, but several of the larger species can be aggressive towards their owners. Owners need to bear in mind that the nature of the food fed, and hence the droppings produced, by many of these birds means that optimal hygiene practices are essential if diseases are to be avoided.

Diet
Softbills are generally fed a commercial softbill pellet supplemented with fruit and vegetables (both often chopped), insects, nectar and meat-based supplements, depending on the requirements of individual species. Low dietary iron content is critical for some species, such as toucans and birds of paradise, if the onset of haemochromatosis is to be avoided. Specially formulated low-iron softbill pellets are available for these species. Some of the larger hornbills also require some whole prey items such as mice, rats and day-old chicks, whilst other species are mainly frugivorous.

Raptors

Hawks

Natural history
The Harris' Hawk (Figure 1.14) is a medium to large diurnal, non-migratory *Buteo* hawk whose natural distribution is from southwestern USA through Central to South America, although escapee birds have been

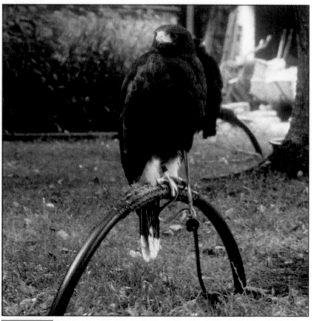

1.14 Harris' Hawk. (© John Chitty)

seen in Western Europe including the UK. It is a bird from arid and patchy woodland at lowland to mid-elevation habitats and is unique amongst raptors in that it often hunts in small groups, with parties of five forming the most successful hunting groups. Single birds hunt smaller prey. They can hunt either from a stationary perch or on the wing and feed on small mammals, as well as reptiles and birds up to the size of night herons. Typical of most raptors, females tend to be larger than males. They breed in pairs or in groups of up to seven individuals including both adults and juveniles.

Figure 1.15 compares the characteristics of three of the most common hawk falconry species found around the world: the Harris' Hawk, the Red-tailed Hawk and the Northern Goshawk.

Characteristic	Harris' Hawk	Red-tailed Hawk	Northern Goshawk
Body length (cm)	46–59	45–65	46–69
Wingspan (cm)	103–120	105–145	89–127
Bodyweight (g)	F: 760–1600 M: 540–850	F: 900–2000 M: 690–1300	F: 820–2200 M: 500–1200
Distribution	Southwestern USA, South America	North America, Canada, West Indies	Europe, Asia, North America
Wild diet	Mammals, birds, lizards, large insects Often hunts in groups	Small mammals (rodents), also birds, reptiles	Birds, small mammals
Other features	Easily trained; sociable	Common in USA; easily trained	Often prey from a perch Are equally successful at hunting mammals and birds

1.15 Characteristics of selected hawk species. F = female; M = male.

Characteristics and considerations for captivity

The Harris' Hawk is considered a 'beginner's bird' in falconry circles because of its temperament and overall falconry ability; it is one of the best hunters of rabbits and hares, as well as game birds. It is also easily bred in captivity and so is readily available. It is relatively easy to train compared to Merlins and Goshawks.

Harris' Hawks require mental stimulation, particularly when kept on their own, and are prone to screaming, particularly if bored. Improperly cared for and poorly trained birds can develop behavioural pathologies similar to the larger parrots. In the wild, they engage in 'back stacking', where birds may perch on each other's backs when perching spots are limited.

Red-tailed Hawks are popular in falconry worldwide; a perched Red-tailed Hawk will hunt prey flushed by a dog or by the falconer.

Diet

A wide and varied diet of whole prey items, including rats, mice and day-old chicks, should be provided, although these species do prefer small mammals. Lean meat-based diets are usually inadequate. Food items should not be fed *ad libitum* – this may lead to selective feeding on one prey type resulting in nutritional issues and/or obesity. Vitamin and mineral supplementation is not required if a variety of whole prey items are fed. Prey should be sourced from reputable, disease-free sources and be suitably prepared; blast frozen day-old chicks preserve the nutritional content and prevent bacterial spoilage far more effectively than freezing prey in domestic freezers. Frozen prey should not be kept for more than 3 months. Commercially harvested prey items should be free of medications and be euthanased by non-injectable chemical methods.

Falcons

Natural history

There are approximately 37 species of falcons in the genus *Falco* (Figure 1.16), distributed worldwide. These birds have thin tapered wings, perfectly suited to their hunting habit of flying high then diving at great speed ('stooping') at 140–200 km/h to snatch their prey. The Peregrine Falcon (Figure 1.16a) is the fastest of all birds. Some species, including the kestrel, hunt by hovering. Prey items may include birds, mammals,

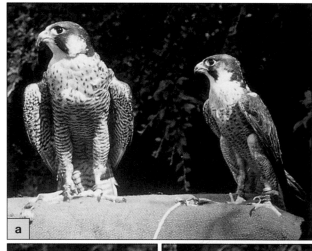

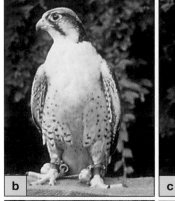

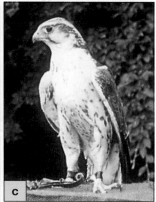

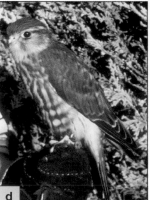

1.16 (a) Peregrine Falcon. The female (left) is larger than the male. (b) Lanner Falcon. (c) Saker Falcon. (d) Merlin. (© John Chitty)

reptiles and insects, with the dietary composition often correlated with predator size. The Gyrfalcon is the largest of the *Falco* genus, with females reaching a body length of 65 cm and a weight of 2.1 kg. By contrast, the male Merlin (Figure 1.16d) may be as small as 24 cm in body length and weigh as little as 165 g. The characteristics of several falcon species are listed in Figure 1.17.

Most species are sexually monomorphic, but males are a third smaller than females. Sexual maturity is reached at 2–3 years. Pairs may nest on cliff edges (e.g. Peregrines and Gyrfalcons), hollow logs, disused stick nests of other birds (e.g. Saker Falcons; Figure 1.16c) and even building ledges. Clutches average two to four eggs and incubation takes 29–35 days. On average, only 1.5 Peregrine chicks fledge per nest (White, 1994). Chicks fledge in 42–56 days and chicks remain dependent on their parents for 2–4 months post-fledging.

Falcons can live for up to 20 years in captivity.

Characteristics and considerations for captivity

Falcons are one of the most popular birds used for falconry. Peregrines are popular with experienced falconers due to their speed and agility, but can be aggressive when in breeding condition. Gyrfalcons are the largest and most highly prized of falcons. They are endurance athletes, chasing prey over many kilometres, and so are often fitted with radiotransmitters so they can be tracked.

Falcons are prone to pododermatitis ('bumblefoot') primarily due to a lack of exercise and hence reduced blood flow to the feet. Incorrect perching can compound these problems. Block perches for tethered birds should have a rough surface made of artificial turf or similar and the bird's feet should be checked every 2–3 weeks. Keeping birds in aviaries after their initial training period may also help prevent this problem, as will regular flying.

Intersex aggression is often seen in Merlins with the females attacking their mates, often fatally. These birds need to be carefully monitored during the breeding season.

Diet

Falcons are best fed whole prey items including day-old chicks and quail, supplemented with rats and mice, although they do prefer avian prey items. Pigeons are best avoided as, although freezing for 1 month may preclude transmission of trichomonad infections, it will not kill *Mycoplasma* or herpesvirus infections.

Eagles

Natural history

Eagles are large powerful birds of prey of which there are approximately 60 species worldwide. Most originate from Eurasia and Africa (e.g. the African Fish Eagle; Figure 1.18) with the remaining few living in Central and South America, Australia, the USA and Canada.

They range in size from the South Nicobar Serpent Eagle (40 cm, 450 g) up to the Steller's Sea Eagle (90 cm, 6.7 kg) and the Philippine Eagle (100 cm, 6.35 kg). Wingspans can reach up to 218.5 cm in the White-tailed Eagle. Females are typically larger than males.

Eagles have strong heavy beaks, muscular legs and powerful talons. Their large eyes give them the visual acuity to see prey at a substantial distance. They are often the apex aerial predators in their environment and may predate upon mammals, birds, reptiles and fish, depending on the individual species and the environment in which they live. Most species grab their prey without stopping and tear them apart upon landing on a perch or ledge. However, some species are carrion-eaters and so eat their prey on the ground. Smaller species may also feed on insects.

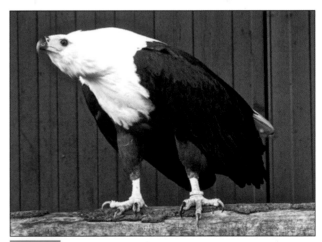

1.18 African Fish Eagle.

Characteristic	Lanner Falcon	Peregrine Falcon	Saker Falcon	Gyrfalcon
Size (cm)	35–50	36–58	47–55	48–65
Wingspan (cm)	90–110	74–120	105–129	110–160
Bodyweight (g)	F: 700–900 M: 500–600	F: 900–1500 M: 400–800	F: 970–1300 M: 730–990	F: 1180–2100 M: 805–1350
Distribution	Africa, Middle East, Mediterranean	Worldwide	Eastern Europe, Asia, North Africa	Colder parts of North America, Europe
Wild diet	Mostly birds (pigeons, quail); occasionally mammals, reptiles, insects	Mid-sized birds (pigeons); occasionally small mammals, reptiles, insects	Mid-sized diurnal rodents; occasionally birds	Ptarmigans, hares, rabbits, geese, ducks
Hunting method	Hunts horizontally	Dives from great height	Hunts horizontally close to ground	Shallow stoops and zig zags
Other comments	May hunt cooperatively in pairs	Fast flight, susceptible to injuries Territorial when nesting Hybrids common in falconry	Endangered Hybrids with Lanners and Gyrfalcons common in falconry	White and dark morphs exist Dislikes warmer temperatures Prone to aspergillosis

1.17 Characteristics of selected falcon species. F = female; M = male.

Eagles are strong flyers and soarers and are often found in open plains and mountains, although several species inhabit woodlands and forests. They can be found in deserts and semi-deserts, tropical forests, upper montane and coastal habitats.

They nest in pairs and are usually highly territorial. Their nests, known as eyries, are usually situated in large trees or cliffs, although some birds will nest on the ground. They usually lay one to three eggs at intervals of 2–6 days. Often the older chick will kill its younger siblings ('cainism') as a means of dominating the food supply. Incubation takes 35–51 days and is primarily undertaken by the female in most species. Juvenile birds often remain with their parents until the next breeding season.

It may take 4–5 years for birds to reach sexual maturity and in some species it can take up to 10 years before full adult coloration is achieved. The larger eagles can live to 25–30 years in the wild and up to 48 years in captivity. The smaller species such as Booted Eagles may live only for 12 years.

Characteristics and considerations for captivity

Eagles are intelligent powerful birds and their captive care, as either falconry birds or aviary birds, should only be undertaken by those with considerable raptor experience who have fully researched the species that they plan to obtain.

Mature human-imprinted eagles in particular can be very aggressive towards humans, associating people as both food providers and potential mates. Both scenarios can be fraught with danger. Handlers need to be aware that eagles' talons can cause a lot of damage, so experience in handling must be acquired before these birds are purchased. Eagles are easily stressed when moved and need to be closely watched after purchase.

Most eagles are not compatible with other species of birds or mammals. However, a mix of similarly sized eagle species of the same sex can be successfully exhibited on occasions. In aviary situations birds should be fed and watered through feeding drawers (or equivalent) and provision should be made to lock birds away if keepers need to enter the enclosure. Alternatively, easily accessible escape routes for the keeper should be available.

The Golden Eagle has a long tradition in falconry. It has even been used by Mongolians and Kazakhs to hunt wolves.

Diet

Eagles should be fed large whole prey items; in some countries commercially available manufactured raptor diets are available and are used to supplement whole foods.

Eagles do not need to be fed every day and larger species may be fed 4 days a week, with fasting days in between.

Owls

Natural history

There are 220–225 species of owls, found across all climate zones in all continents except Antarctica. Contrary to popular belief, not all owls are nocturnal; there are several crepuscular and diurnal species.

Owls range in size from the diminutive Elf Owl (31 g and 13.5 cm) up to the largest owl, the Great Grey Owl

(83 cm), and the heaviest owls, the Eurasian Eagle Owl (Figure 1.19) and Blakiston's Fish Owl, in which females can weigh up to 4.5 kg. Therefore, the information provided here is of a general nature and many species-specific variations occur.

Owls are characterized by their flat faces and forward-looking eyes, which give them binocular stereoscopic vision and excellent night vision. They have an unmatched hearing acuity assisted by the presence of facial discs: the circular arrangement of feathers directs sounds from varying distances to their asymmetrically positioned ears. The nocturnal hunters have a serrated outer rim to their flight feathers, making their flight noiseless.

Captive Eurasian Eagle Owls have escaped into the wild and are believed to form the basis of the wild birds found in the UK.

Owls typically nest in hollow logs, rock crevices or tunnels and lay on average three to four white eggs at 1–3 day intervals. However, some species such as Barn Owls and Snowy Owls can lay much larger clutches.

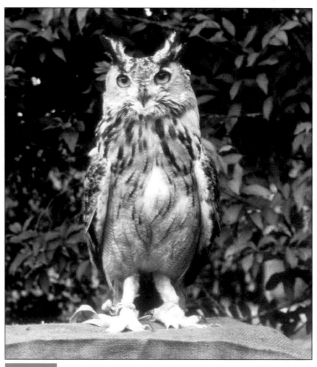

1.19   Eurasian Eagle Owl. (© John Chitty)

Characteristics and considerations for captivity

Owls generally adapt well to captivity and most species will readily go to nest. However, some species can become very aggressive towards people when they are breeding, particularly if imprinted upon humans. Care must be exercised when handling owls as their talons and beaks are very sharp. They also require regular exercise and their accommodation should allow for this.

Barn owls are commonly kept as they breed readily in captivity. However, they can be inactive, nervous and shy birds, quite messy to feed and require frequent interaction and positive reinforcement if they are to remain tame and trained. They can also be quite noisy, particularly at night.

Keeping the larger owls, such as the Eurasian Eagle Owl, requires a huge commitment to provide the training, exercise and behavioural enrichment which are required to keep these birds healthy in captivity. They can also be dangerous because of their size and strength. However, they are rarely used in hunting; they are most frequently kept as display or even 'pet' birds. They are easy to breed in captivity and birds are usually very easy to obtain.

Owls can be relatively long-lived, many species living 20–30 years and up to 60 years for Eurasian Eagle Owls in captivity.

Diet

Owls are primarily carnivorous and will eat whole prey items, regurgitating the indigestible fur and bones, the 'cast'. Most owls prefer rodents and other smaller mammals and, to a lesser extent, birds. Some species eat insects and others eat fish.

In captivity, they should be fed a range of whole prey items (e.g. mice, rats and day-old chicks) and insects, appropriate to their size. This is often done via feeding drawers or feeding chutes so that the birds do not associate food with people. Birds should be monitored for obesity.

References and further reading

Arent LR (2007) *Raptors in Captivity: Guidelines for Care and Management*. Hancock House, Surrey

Bird DM and Bildstein KL (2007) *Raptor Research and Management Techniques*. Hancock House, Surrey

Bockheim G and Congdon S (2001) *The Sturnidae Husbandry Manual and Resource Guide*. Disney Animal Kingdom, Lake Buena Vista

Chitty J and Lierz M (2008) *Manual of Raptors, Pigeons and Passerine Birds*. BSAVA Publications, Gloucester

Christides L and Boles WE (2008) *Systematics and Taxonomy of Australian Birds*. CSIRO Publishing, Melbourne

Collar NJ (1997) Family Psittacidae (Parrots). In: *Handbook of Birds of The World. Vol 4. Sandgrouse to Cuckoos*, ed. J del Hoyo, A Elliott and J Sargatal, pp. 280–477. Lynx Edicions, Barcelona

Connors N and Conners E (2005) *A Guide to Black Cockatoos as Pet and Aviary Birds*. ABK Publications, Burleigh

Coutteel P (2011) Passerine bird medicine. In: *Proceedings of the 11th European AAV Conference, Madrid*, pp. 270–284

Crissey SD, Ward AM, Block SE *et al*. (2000) Hepatic iron accumulation over time in European starlings (*Sturnus vulgaris*) fed two levels of iron. *Journal of Zoo and Wildlife Medicine* **31(4)**, 491–496

Davis KJ (2012) *Turacos in Aviculture*. Birdhouse Publications, Cresswell

Dorrestein GM (2005) Passerine and softbill medicine and surgery. In: *Proceedings of the 8th European AAV Conference & 6th Scientific ECAMS Meeting, Arles*, pp. 409–424

Foreshaw JM and Cooper WT (1989) *Parrots of the World, 3rd edn*. Lansdowne Press, Melbourne

Fox NC and Chick J (2007) *Falconry in the United Kingdom: An audit of the Current Position Prepared by the Hawk Board*. Hawk Board Publications, Malborough

Galama W, King C and Brouwer K (2001) *Hornbill Management and Husbandry Guidelines*. EAZA Hornbill TAG, Amsterdam, pp. 14–16

Garner JP, Meehan CL, Famula TR *et al*. (2006) Genetic, environmental and neighbor effects on the severity of stereotypies and feather picking in orange-winged Amazon parrots (*Amazona amazonica*): an epidemiological study. *Applied Animal Behaviour Science* **96(1–2)**, 153–168

Gelis S (2011) A review of the nutrition of lories and lorikeets. In: *Proceedings of the Association of Avian Veterinarians Australian Committee, Canberra*, pp. 87–103

Heinsohn R (2008) Ecology and evolution of the enigmatic eclectus parrot (*Eclectus roratus*). *Journal of Avian Medicine and Surgery* **22(2)**, 146–150

Heinsohn R and Legge S (2003) Breeding biology of the reverse-dichromatic, co-operative parrot *Eclectus roratus*. *Journal of Zoology* **259**, 197–208

Holland G (2007) *Encyclopedia of Aviculture*. Hancock House Publishers, Surrey

Jones MP, Chitty J and Ford S (2011) Raptor medicine and management. In: *Proceedings of the 11th European AAV Conference, Madrid*, pp. 462–475

Jones R (2011) *Salmonella typhimurium* infection as a cause of mortality and morbidity in captive bred falcon chicks in the UK. In: *Proceedings of the 11th European AAV Conference, Madrid*, pp. 171–172

Jordan R (2003) *A Guide to Macaws as Pet and Aviary Birds*. ABK Publications, Burleigh

Joseph L, Toon A, Schirtzinger EE *et al*. (2012) A revised nomenclature and classification for family-group taxa of parrots (Psittaciformes). *Zootaxa* **3205**, 26–40

Kingston R (2010) *The Finch...a Breeder's Companion*. Indruss Productions, Torbanlea

Konig C and Weick F (2008) *Owls of the World, 2nd edn*. Christopher Helm Publications, London

Low R (1998) *Hancock House Encyclopedia of the Lories*. Hancock House, Surrey

Low R (2013) *Pyrrhura Parakeets (Conures): Aviculture, Natural History, Conservation*. Insignis Publications, Mansfield

Meehan CL, Millam TR and Mench JA (2003) Foraging opportunity and increased physical complexity both prevent and reduce psychogenic feather picking by young amazon parrots. *Applied Animal Behaviour Science* **80(1)**, 71–85

Morris PJ, Avgeris SE and Baumgartner RE (1989) Haemochromatosis in a greater Indian hill mynah (*Gracula religiosa*): case report and review of the literature. *Journal of the Association of Avian Veterinarians* **3(2)**, 87–92

Parry-Jones J (2012) *Falconry: Care, Captive Breeding and Conservation*. David and Charles, Newton Abbot

Phalen DN, Olsen G and Ba KR (2005) Diagnosis, prevention and treatment of iron storage disease using the European starling as a model. In: *Proceedings of the 8th European AAV Conference, Arles*, pp. 136–140

Redig PT and Cruz-Martinez L (2009) Raptors. In: *Handbook of Avian Medicine, 2nd edn*, ed. TN Tully, GM Dorrestein and AK Jones, pp. 209–242. Saunders Elsevier, Philadelphia

Rowley I (1997) Family Cacatuidae (Cockatoos). In: *Handbook of Birds of The World. Vol 4. Sandgrouse to Cuckoos*, ed. J del Hoyo, A Elliott and J Sargatal, pp. 246–279. Lynx Edicions, Barcelona

Samour J (2006) Management of raptors In: *Clinical Avian Medicine Volume 2*, ed. G Harrison and T Lightfoot, pp. 915–956. Spix Publishing, Palm Beach

Samour J and Naldo JL (2005) Causes of morbidity and mortality in captive falcons in Saudi Arabia. *Proceedings of the 8th European AAV Conference, Arles*, pp. 85–91

Shephard M (1989) *Aviculture in Australia: Keeping and Breeding Aviary Birds*. Black Cockatoo Press, Melbourne

Sheppard C and Dierenfeld E (2002) Iron storage disease in birds: speculation on etiology and implications for captive husbandry. *Journal of Avian Medicine and Surgery* **16(3)**, 192–197

Taylor MR (2000) Natural history, behaviour and captive management of the palm cockatoo *Probosciger aterrimus* in North America. *International Zoo Yearbook* **37**, 61–69

Turner DA (1997) Family Musophagidae (Turacos). In: *Handbook of Birds of The World. Vol 4. Sandgrouse to Cuckoos*, ed. J del Hoyo, A Elliott and J Sargatal, pp. 480–507. Lynx Edicions, Barcelona

Vincent M (2007) The preliminary studies of wild toco toucans (*Rhampastos toco*) – a keeper's experience in the field. *Ratel* **34(3)**, 8

Webster JD (2007) Skeletal characters and the systematics of estrildid finches (Aves: Estrildidae). In: *Proceedings of the Indiana Academy of Science* **116(1)**, pp. 90–107

White CM (1994) Family Falconidae. In: *Handbook of Birds of the World. Vol 2. New World Vultures to Guinea Fowl*, ed. J del Hoyo, A Elliott and J Sargatal, pp. 216–275. Lynx Edicions, Barcelona

Willette M, Ponder J, Cruz-Martinez L *et al*. (2009) Management of selected bacterial and parasitic conditions of raptors. *Veterinary Clinics of North America: Exotic Animal Practice* **12(3)**, 491–517

Specialist organizations and useful contacts

Avibase – the world bird database
www.avibase.bsc-eoc.org

Anatomy and physiology

Peter Sandmeier

The class of Aves is vastly diverse, with over 10,000 species in 27 different orders. The anatomy and physiology described within this chapter is based on that of parrots, raptors, passerines, pigeons and chickens. Various interesting variations seen in species of other orders are also described.

Musculoskeletal system

Avian bones can be summarized as lightweight but strong. Many bones are pneumatized. These include the skull, the vertebrae, the pelvis, the sternum and ribs, the thoracic girdle, the humerus and sometimes the femur. Charadriformes (waders) appear to be the only avian order with total absence of long-bone pneumatization (Cubo and Casinos, 2000). Trabeculae within this pneumatized cavity give strength. Bone pneumatization is achieved by projections of the air sacs.

Medullary bone is an inorganic structure, mainly comprising crystalline calcium phosphate, within the medulla of long bones. The formation of this medullary bone in females during the reproductive phase is controlled by oestrogens and androgens. For egg shell production, medullary bone can be mobilized in large amounts and within short periods (see 'Avian calcium metabolism').

Bone growth takes place by ossification of the cartilaginous epiphysis rather than the epiphyseal growth plate.

Figure 2.1 details the key differences between bird and cat and dog musculoskeletal systems, and their clinical significance.

Skull

The skull (Figure 2.2) comprises lightweight pneumatized bone. Unlike in mammals, the upper jaw (the premaxilla and nasal bones) is connected to the skull by a craniofacial elastic zone allowing individual movement of the upper jaw relative to the skull. In psittacine birds this craniofacial zone is not just a flexible hinge but a true joint. The mandible does not articulate directly with the skull but over the quadrate bone. This complex articulation of upper and lower jaw allows birds to use their beaks as a multifunctional tool adapted to each species' behaviour and feeding habits.

Bird	Dog and cat	Clinical relevance
Pneumatized bones	Bones not pneumatized	Birds are much lighter than similarly sized mammals; open fractures can cause infection of the respiratory system
Bone mineral content high	Bone mineral content lower	Avian fractures are often more complicated than those in mammals
Bone growth by ossification of epiphysis	Bone growth by ossification of epiphyseal plate	Instead of growth plates, immature avian bones have radiolucent ends on radiographs
Upper and lower jaw articulate to each other and skull	Only articulation between mandible and skull	Complex use of the beak as a multifunction tool; luxation of the upper jaw can occur
11–24 cervical vertebrae	7 cervical vertebrae	Birds have a very flexible neck, head can be rotated over 180 degrees vastly increasing field of vision; beak is a versatile tool
Thoracic as well as lumbar vertebrae and sacrum fused to notarium and synsacrum	Individual vertebrae	Avian vertebral fractures and subluxations are always located between the notarium and synsacrum
Coracoid is largest bone of the thoracic girdle	No coracoid bone	Assess for coracoid fractures on radiographs of birds with a drooping wing and no fractures of the wing bones

2.1 Musculoskeletal system of birds *versus* dogs and cats.

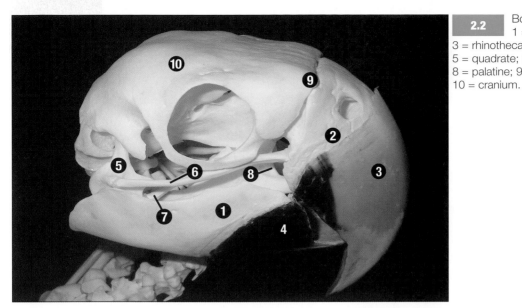

2.2 Bones of the skull (macaw).
1 = mandibular; 2 = maxilla;
3 = rhinotheca; 4 = gnathotheca;
5 = quadrate; 6 = jugal; 7 = pterygoid;
8 = palatine; 9 = craniofacial joint;
10 = cranium.

Vertebral column, ribs, sternum, thoracic girdle and pelvis

In contrast to mammals, which have seven cervical vertebrae, avian species have between 11 and 24 cervical vertebrae, resulting in a very flexible neck, head and beak. The vertebrae of the trunk are mostly fused to form a stable bony structure enabling flight. The majority of the thoracic vertebrae form the notarium. The caudal thoracic and lumbar vertebrae are fused together with the sacrum to form the synsacrum. The most caudal five or six coccygeal vertebrae are fused together to form the pygostyle, which supports the tail feathers (Figure 2.3).

The very stable avian thorax is formed by the fused thoracic vertebrae (notarium), the ribs and the sternum. The ribs are additionally reinforced by the uncinate processes, connecting the ribs to each other (Figure 2.4). The carina of the sternum is the origin of the main flight muscles.

The thoracic girdle consists of the paired scapulae, the fused clavicles (furcula) and the coracoid bones (which are not present in mammalian species). The coracoids act like a brace, prohibiting compression of the thorax during wing movement and keeping the wing and shoulder at a stable distance to the sternum (Figure 2.4).

The avian pelvis does not fuse to a complete pelvic girdle; the ischium and pubis do not fuse with the contralateral side, which allows birds to lay eggs. The pelvis, however, fuses to the synsacrum in order to stabilize the trunk for flight (see Figure 2.3). The ventral aspect of the ilium and synsacrum form the renal fossae protecting the kidneys, nerves and blood vessels.

Wings and flight muscles

The bones of the wings are the humerus, the radius and ulna (with the ulna being the structurally more important and stable bone), two carpal bones (the ulnar carpal bone and the radial carpal bone), the carpometacarpus (which is fused out of the distal carpal bones and the reduced metacarpal bones to a single two-strutted bone) and the three digits: the alula (corresponding to the human thumb) and the major and

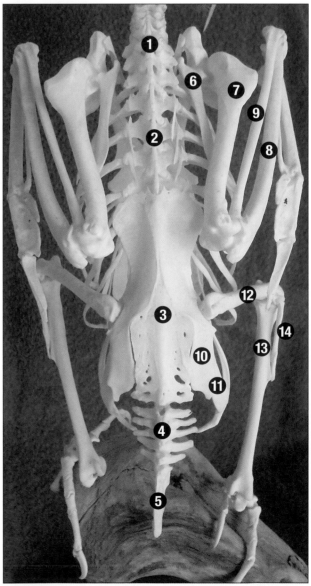

2.3 Dorsal view of the bones of the trunk and extremities (macaw). 1 = cervical vertebrae; 2 = notarium; 3 = synsacrum; 4 = tail vertebrae; 5 = pygostyle; 6 = scapula; 7 = humerus; 8 = ulna; 9 = radius; 10 = ilium; 11 = pubis; 12 = femur; 13 = tibiotarsus; 14 = fibula.

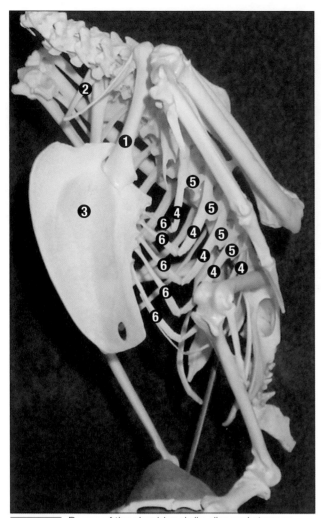

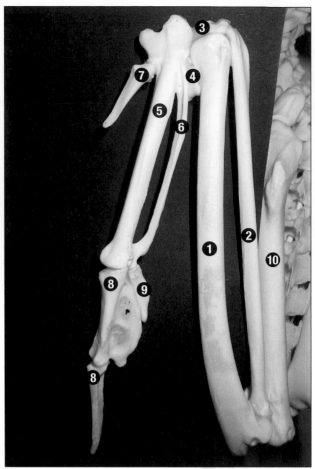

2.4 Bones of the shoulder girdle, ribs and sternum (macaw). 1 = coracoid; 2 = clavicle; 3 = sternum; 4 = vertebral ribs; 5 = uncinate process; 6 = sternal ribs.

2.5 Bones of the wing (macaw). 1 = ulna; 2 = radius; 3 = radial carpal bone; 4 = ulnar carpal bone; 5 = major metacarpal bone; 6 = minor metacarpal bone; 7 = alular digit (phalanx I); 8 = major digit (phalanx II); 9 = minor digit (phalanx III); 10 = humerus.

minor digits (corresponding to the second and third mammalian digits) (Figure 2.5). When extended, the elbow and carpal joints lock and the wing becomes very stable, moving only at the shoulder joint, whereas when flexed it remains mobile. The shafts of the secondary flight feathers are anchored into the dorso-caudal aspect of the ulna, and the primary flight feathers into the carpometacarpus.

The main wing muscles are on the carina of the sternum and wing movement is achieved by contractions of the pectoral muscle system. The superficial pectoral muscle is the strongest muscle that achieves the down stroke of the wing during flight. This muscle represents 15–20% of the total bodyweight. The contraction of the supracoracoid muscle, which passes through the triosseal foramen (formed by the articular surface of the three thoracic girdle bones), rotates the humerus, allowing elevation of the wing (Figure 2.6).

Legs and leg muscles

The bones of the legs are the femur, the tibiotarsus (the tibia fused with the proximal tarsal bones), the fibula (only the remnant proximal portion), the tarsometatarsus (the single metatarsal bone fused with the distal tarsal bone) and the phalanges of the four digits (Figure 2.7). The length of the tarsometatarsus and of the digits, as well as the alignment of the digits, depends

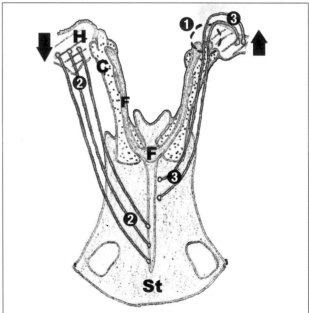

2.6 Schematic drawing displaying insertion and action of the flight muscles (modified after Nickel et al., 1977). The pectoral muscles (2) achieve downward movement of the wing, whereas the supracoracoid muscles (3) achieve lifting of the wing due to diversion of fibres via the triosseous foramen (1). C = coracoid; F = furcula (fused clavicles); H = humerus; St = sternum, with prominent carina. (Reproduced from the *BSAVA Manual of Raptors, Pigeons and Passerine Birds*, courtesy of RM Hirschberg)

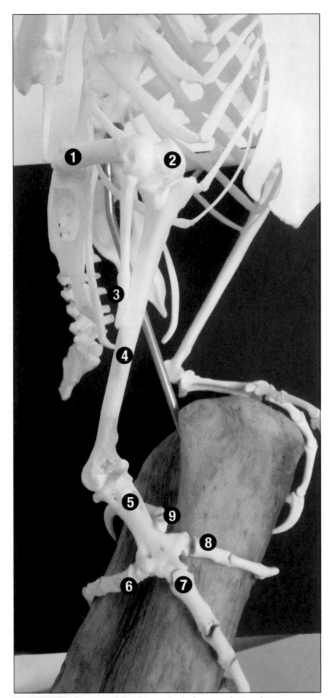

| | 2.7 | Bones of the lower limb (macaw). 1 = femur; 2 = stifle; 3 = fibula; 4 = tibiotarsus I; 5 = tarsometatarsus; 6 = phalanx II; 7 = phalanx III; 8 = phalanx IV; 9 = phalanx I. |

on the locomotion, stance and feeding habits of the bird species. Most avian species have an anisodactyl position with the first digit facing caudally and digits II, III and IV facing cranially. Some species, including psittacine birds, are zygodactyl, with digit IV also facing caudally and therefore have two caudal and two cranial digits. In other species, such as the ostrich, only digits III and IV remain.

The main leg muscles are located close to the body over the femur and tibiotarsus and, therefore, have long tendons down to the insertion points on the toes. A locking mechanism of the flexor tendons allows birds to sit with flexed toes around a branch with minimal muscle activity (Harcourt-Brown, 2000).

Cardiovascular system

Figure 2.8 details key differences between bird and cat and dog cardiovascular systems, and their clinical significance.

Heart

In comparison to mammals the avian heart is relatively larger and beats faster. In many species, the heart is 1–2.5% of the total bodyweight (compared with 0.4–0.7% in mammals); the heart rate of hummingbirds can be over 800 beats/minute. The arterial blood pressure is also higher than mammals; for example, 180/140 mmHg in the chicken (Smith et al., 2000).

As in mammals, the heart has four chambers. The heart valves are similar to those of mammals with exception of the right atrioventricular valve, which is only a muscular flap.

Bird	Dog and cat	Clinical relevance
Right jugular vein much larger than left	Both jugular veins similar sized	Jugular venepuncture on the right side (Note: not used in pigeons as jugular is hard to visualize, due to large capillary plexus)
Higher heart rate	Lower heart rate	Use of pulse oximetry difficult due to maximal heart rate capability of pulse oximeter
Nucleated red blood cells	Red blood cells without nucleus	Automated haematology systems cannot be used for avian blood samples
Heterophils	Neutrophils	More difficult to differentiate avian heterophils than mammalian neutrophils from eosinophils and basophils
No lymph nodes	Lymph nodes	Lymph nodes cannot be palpated

| | 2.8 | Cardiovascular system of birds versus dogs and cats. |

Blood vessels

The vascular system is similar to that of mammals; however, there are many species variations.

A jugular anastomosis at the head–neck border allows blood to be shunted from the small left jugular vein to the much larger right jugular vein.

See 'Urinary system' for information on the renal portal system.

Blood cells

For information on blood cells, see Chapter 12.

Lymphatic system

The central lymphatic organs of birds are the bone marrow, the thymus and the cloacal bursa.

The thymus is located along the length of the neck, but, as in mammals, it involutes with the onset of puberty. The thymus is the source of T-lymphocytes.

The cloacal bursa or bursa of Fabricius is a dorsal diverticulum of the proctodeal region of the cloaca (see Figure 2.13). Like the thymus, it also involutes during puberty. The cloacal bursa is the source of B-lymphocytes.

Peripheral lymphatic tissue is located within the spleen and the walls of the respiratory and gastro-intestinal tracts. This tissue aggregates to mucosal lymph nodules such as the caecal tonsils or Peyer's patches within the small intestine. Macroscopic lymph nodes are generally not developed in birds but can, for example, be observed in waterfowl as two paired lymph nodes near the thyroid glands and the gonads.

The spleen is located along the dorsomedial aspect of the proventriculus. In many species (e.g. passerines) it is an elongated comma-shaped organ, whereas in others such as psittacine birds or chickens it is round. As in mammals, it possesses red and white pulp. The function of the spleen includes production of lymphocytes and phagocytosis of erythrocytes, but the spleen does not function as a blood storage organ as it does in mammals.

Lymphatic ducts return extravascular fluid to the vessels and drain into the caval veins.

Body cavity

Due to the lack of a diaphragm the avian coelomic cavity is not divided into a thoracic and an abdominal cavity.

The coelomic cavity is divided into the air sacs (see 'Respiratory system'), the pericardial cavity, the intestinal cavity, as well as two dorsal and two ventral hepatoperitoneal cavities separated by the falciform and hepatic ligaments. The intestinal cavity contains the gastrointestinal tract from the stomach to the rectum, the gonads and the spleen. The kidneys and reproductive tract are located extraperitoneally (Figure 2.9).

The septa dividing these cavities are non-muscular and very thin and, unless there is ascites, are not recognized on radiographs or during post-mortem examination.

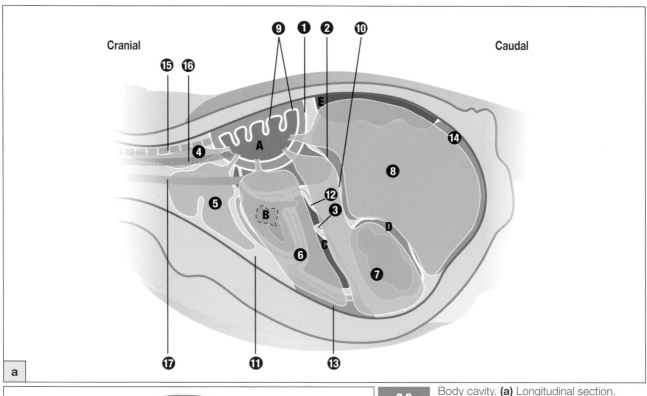

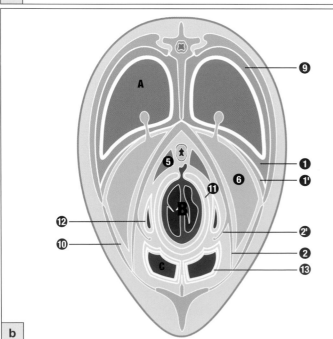

2.9 Body cavity. **(a)** Longitudinal section. **(b)** Sagittal section. 1 = horizontal septum; 1' = costoseptales muscle; 2 = oblique septum; 2' = hepatic ligament; 3 = posthepatic septum; 4 = cervical air sac; 5 = clavicular air sac; 6 = cranial thoracic air sac; 7 = caudal thoracic air sac; 8 = abdominal air sac; 9 = pulmonary cavity; 10 = subpulmonary cavity; 11 = pericardial cavity; 12 = dorsal liver peritoneal cavity; 13 = ventral liver peritoneal cavity; 14 = abdominal peritoneal cavity; A = lung; B = heart; C = liver; D = ventriculus; E = kidney.

Digestive system

The anatomy of the avian digestive system varies according to feeding habits and diet.

- Granivorous birds, such as chickens, pigeons, parrots and many passerines that eat a lot of hard vegetable fibres and seeds, have a short strong beak, a large crop with many mucous glands, a well developed ventriculus, longer intestines and often distinct caeca.
- Frugivorous birds that eat easily digested nutrients often have a rudimentary crop, a less distinct ventriculus, a short intestine and only rudimentary caeca.
- Birds of prey and other meat- and fish-eating species have a strong, often curved and pointed beak, a rudimentary ventriculus but a well developed proventriculus, a short intestine, a well developed pancreas and only rudimentary caeca.

- Insectivorous birds, such as many passerines, have a fine, longer beak, a rudimentary ventriculus but a well developed proventriculus, a short intestine and only rudimentary caeca.

Figure 2.10 details key differences between bird and dog and cat digestive systems and their clinical relevance.

Beak

The beak or 'rhamphotheca' is a horny skin structure of keratinized epidermis covering the upper and lower jaws. The size and shape of the beak is a good indicator of the diet eaten by a particular species (Figure 2.11). Seed-eaters have a strong wedge-shaped beak. Fruit-eaters and insect-eaters have a delicate pointed beak. The beak of ducks and geese is wide and flat, with horny lamella along the edge, allowing them to filter the water for food. Carnivorous birds have a strong pointed curved beak.

Bird	Dog and cat	Clinical relevance
Shape and size of beak indicate feeding habits	Shape and size of teeth indicate feeding habits	Choose diet of hospitalized birds according to beak shape
Oesophagus runs down right side of neck	Oesophagus runs down left side of neck	Tube feed anorectic birds from the left commissure of the beak
Crop for food storage (in most commonly seen species except small passerines such as canaries and finches)	No crop	Anorectic birds can be tube fed large volumes that then continuously move from the crop down into the gastrointestinal tract
Two stomachs with grit in ventriculus (in granivorous birds)	Single glandular stomach	On radiographs grit in the ventriculus is easily recognized, allowing orientation within the coelomic cavity Small amounts of grit must be added to diet
Cloaca collects faeces, urine and uric acid and voids all three parts together	Urine and faeces voided through separate body openings	Difficult for owners to differentiate between diarrhoea and polyuria Urine contaminated by faecal material; interpretation of urinalysis difficult
Haemoglobin metabolized to biliverdin in liver	Haemoglobin metabolized to bilirubin in liver	Birds with liver disease can be recognized through green colouring of urates (biliverdinuria)
Simple two-lobed liver	Multiple-lobed liver	Heart and liver form a typical hourglass shape on ventrodorsal radiographs

2.10 Digestive system of birds *versus* dogs and cats.

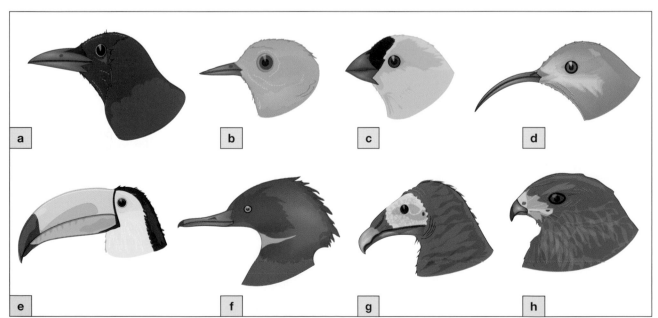

2.11 The size and shape of the beak is a good indicator of the diet eaten. **(a)** Omnivore. **(b)** Insectivore. **(c)** Granivore. **(d)** Nectivore. **(e)** Frugivore. **(f)** Piscivore. **(g)** Carrion eater. **(h)** Carnivore.

Oropharyngeal cavity

The oropharyngeal cavity is open to the nasal cavity through the choanal slit. During inspiration this slit is closed by the tongue. Caudal to the choana, the infundibulum is visible, which is the opening of the Eustachian tubes. The number of salivary glands in the oropharynx depends on the diet of the species and is higher in seed-eaters than fish- and meat-eaters.

Tongue

The size, form and function of the tongue varies according to feeding and living habits. In many birds it is used to move food within the beak; in others, such as hummingbirds and woodpeckers, it is used to collect food and can be obtruded. Nectar-eating species, such as lories and honeyeaters, have a specialized brush-tipped tongue. In psittacine birds the tongue also has a tactile function. In comparison to mammalian species, the avian tongue does not have many tastebuds.

Oesophagus and crop

The oesophagus runs down the right side of the neck adjacent to the trachea. The diameter and number of longitudinal folds is greater than in mammals, especially in species that eat large portions of food, for example, birds of prey and fish-eaters.

The crop is a dilatation of the oesophagus situated just proximal to the entrance to the pectoral cavity and directly under the skin (Figure 2.12a). The crop is generally larger in granivorous and carnivorous birds; in many insectivorous birds no distinct crop can be observed. The crop serves as a storage chamber allowing a continuous supply of nutrition to the gastrointestinal tract, including during resting periods. Although food in the crop is pre-digested by saturation of food with saliva and gastric fluids by retrograde oesophageal movement, there is no actual production of digestive fluid or enzymes by the mucosa of the crop wall.

Pigeons have the unique ability of producing crop milk. Under the influence of prolactin, the epithelial cells of the crop wall are desquamated producing a milk-like secretion that is fed to the nestlings by both male and female parents. Pigeon milk differs in composition to mammalian milk and consists of 9–13% protein, 9–11% fat, 0.9–1.5% carbohydrate, 0.8–1.1% ash and an energy content of 23.4–28.5 kJ/g (Denbow, 2000).

Stomach

The avian stomach is divided into a proventriculus and a ventriculus or gizzard (see Figure 2.12). The proventriculus is a glandular stomach producing digestive enzymes, similar to the stomach in dogs and cats. In seed-eating species, such as psittacine birds, chickens and pigeons, the ventriculus is extremely muscular and the mucosal surface is covered by a koilin layer (cuticle). Together with the grit within the ventriculus this achieves a grinding of seeds. In piscivores and carnivores the ventriculus has only a thin muscular layer and no cuticle.

Food in the stomach is propelled between the proventriculus and ventriculus in a series of cycles combining the mechanical and digestive functions of the stomach. In raptors, indigestible parts such as skin and bones are formed into a pellet within the ventriculus and then regurgitated.

Intestines

In general the avian intestine is shorter than that of mammals. Similar to the contrast between herbivorous and carnivorous mammals, the intestine of seed-eating birds is longer than that of fish- or meat-eating birds.

The duodenum is loop-shaped, surrounds the pancreas, and receives the opening of the bile and pancreatic ducts. The jejunum and ileum are arranged in a series of coils and allow digestion under the influence of bile and pancreatic enzymes (see Figure 2.12).

The colorectum is very short and opens into the coprodeum of the cloaca. Resorption of water from urine and faeces in the colorectum and cloaca is important for species living in arid climate regions.

Birds have paired caeca. In many species such as psittacine birds, passerines, pigeons and raptors, the caeca are vestigial, whereas in others such as chickens, waterfowl and ratites the caeca are very voluminous and contain lymphatic tissue. In the latter species cellulose is digested by the bacteria within the caeca. Content of the caeca is voided separately as a dark brown glutinous mass.

Pancreas

The pancreas is located within the duodenal loop (see Figure 2.12a). It features a dorsal and a ventral lobe as well as a small splenic lobe, which contains most of the endocrine tissue. The exocrine pancreas produces the same digestive hormones as in mammals (amylases, lipases and proteases). The endocrine pancreas also produces insulin, glucagon and somatostatin. Current evidence indicates that in avian species glucagon is the dominant pancreatic hormone, whereas in mammals it is insulin (Hazelwood, 2000).

Liver

The liver has a large right lobe and a small left lobe (see Figure 2.12b). The bile duct from each lobe drains into the duodenum. The right bile duct contains a gall bladder; however, this is missing in many species such as psittacine birds, pigeons and some passerines.

Due to the lack of biliverdin reductase, the end product of haemoglobin metabolism within the liver in avian species is biliverdin and not bilirubin. An icteric bird will therefore develop biliverdinuria, which can be recognized by green colouring of the urates.

Cloaca

The cloaca consists of three compartments and collects the excretions of the digestive tract, the urinary tract and the genital tract (Figure 2.13).

The proximal coprodeum is an extension of the colorectum and is not distinctly delineated. There is, however, a distinct fold between the coprodeum and the urodeum. During defecation the copro-urodeal fold is everted to the cloacal lips protecting the ureteral and reproductive openings from faecal contamination.

The urodeum contains the openings of the urinary and reproductive tracts. The ureters open dorsally and the spermatic ducts ventrolaterally into the urodeum. In females the oviduct opens ventrolaterally on the left side into the urodeum. The urodeum is separated from the proctodeum by the uro-proctodeal fold.

The proctodeum is the most distal short section of the cloaca between the uro-proctodeal fold and the vent. In juvenile birds it contains the dorsal opening into the cloacal bursa (see 'Lymphatic system'). Although most avian species have no phallus, some, such as ratites and waterfowl, do have an erectile phallus.

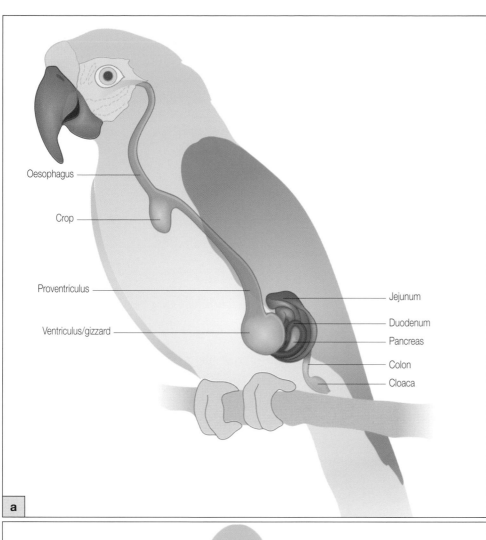

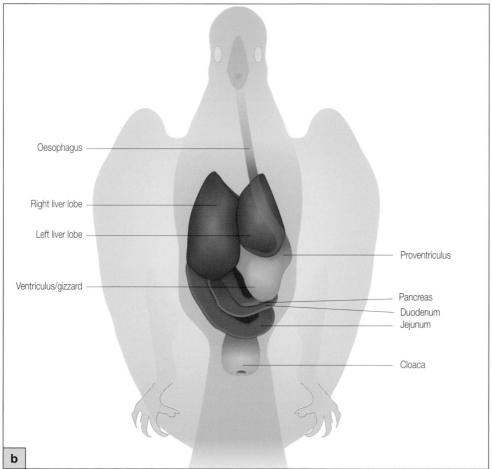

2.12 **(a)** Lateral view of the psittacine digestive system (liver not shown in this view). (Redrawn after Ritchie *et al*., 1994) **(b)** Ventral view of the psittacine digestive system and liver. (Redrawn after Ritchie *et al*., 1994)

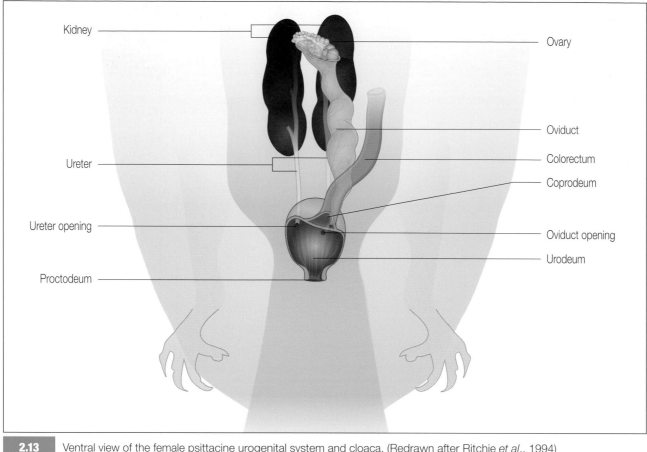

2.13   Ventral view of the female psittacine urogenital system and cloaca. (Redrawn after Ritchie *et al.*, 1994)

Respiratory system

Upper respiratory tract

The upper respiratory tract consists of the nares, the nasal cavity and the infraorbital sinus. The main function of the upper respiratory tract is to filter, warm and moisten the inhaled air.

Figure 2.14 details key differences between bird and dog and cat respiratory systems and their clinical relevance.

Nares

In most avian species the nares are situated at the base of the beak in a dorsal or lateral position. Wide species variations exist; in Kiwis, for example, they are located at the rostral point of the beak. In psittacine species the operculum, a horny structure, covers the opening into the nasal cavity.

Nasal cavity

The nasal cavity consists of three nasal conchae. The rostral concha is covered by cutaneous mucosa, the middle concha has a mucociliary epithelium, and the caudal concha is covered by olfactory epithelium. The base of the nasal cavity is not covered by the palatine, as in mammals, but is open through the choanal slit to the oral cavity.

Infraorbital sinus

The infraorbital sinus is situated within the upper jaw, rostroventrally to the eye. Large parts of the sinus are covered by soft tissue only. The infraorbital sinus has multiple cavities within the upper jaw, lower jaw and head, forming an air-filled cushion around the eye and helping to keep the weight of the head to a minimum (Figure 2.15).

Lower respiratory tract

The lower respiratory tract consists of the larynx, trachea, syrinx, bronchi, air sacs and lungs.

Larynx

In avian species the larynx is a simple slit between the two arytenoid cartilages, without any vocal cords. The syrinx at the proximal end of the trachea is responsible for sound production. The most important function of the larynx is to separate food and air during swallowing and breathing.

Trachea

Unlike in mammals, the avian trachea is stabilized by complete and closed cartilaginous rings. The trachea follows the oesophagus down the neck and ends at the bifurcation, where the syrinx is situated. In some species, such as swans and cranes, the trachea is especially long and folded into loops between the skin and the pectoral muscles, allowing them to make especially loud, resonant noises (Fitch, 1999). In penguins, the bifurcation is in the upper area of the neck without a visible syrinx and continues down the neck as a double tube.

The increased aerodynamic resistance of the longer avian trachea is compensated for by a wider trachea; however, this increases the dead space.

Bird	Dog and cat	Clinical relevance
Choanal slit opens into oral cavity/pharynx	No palatine cleft	Allows easy endoscopic evaluation and sampling of the nasal cavity through the choana
Infraorbital sinus consists of multiple cavities	Simple nasal and frontal sinuses	Avian species are more susceptible to sinusitis and more difficult to treat
Infraorbital sinus covered by soft tissue only	Nasal and frontal sinuses surrounded by bony structure	Sinusitis visible as infraorbital swelling Sinus can be opened and flushed through skin, no trephination necessary
Closed cartilaginous tracheal rings	Non-fused, C-shaped tracheal rings	Use non-cuffed endotracheal tubes for intubation in avian species
Longer, wider trachea	Shorter, narrower trachea	More dead space (anaesthesia) Increased susceptibility to respiratory disease
No vocal cords in larynx Sound produced by tympanic membranes in syrinx	Sound produced by vocal cords in larynx No syrinx at tracheal bifurcation	Birds with *Aspergillus* granulomas in the syrinx are often hoarse
Air capillaries No alveoli	Alveoli	More efficient gaseous exchange Less respiratory reserve as birds cannot vary lung volume but only respiratory rate
Air sac system	Simple in/out breathing system	Longer duration of residual air within the respiratory system, making avian species much more susceptible to respiratory infections, especially aspergillosis Allows easy endoscopic evaluation of the coelomic cavity without necessity of insufflation Placement of an air sac breathing tube is possible
No diaphragm Breathing through movement of rib cage, neck and wings	Breathing through contraction of diaphragm	Respiration impaired by placing the bird in a towel during clinical examination Respiration impaired by dorsal recumbency during anaesthesia Caged birds not allowed to fly have difficulty exchanging complete lung and air sac volume, leading to residual air in respiratory system and increased susceptibility to diseases of the respiratory system
Pneumatized bones	No connection between bones and respiratory system	Open fractures can cause infection within the respiratory system

2.14   Respiratory system of birds *versus* dogs and cats.

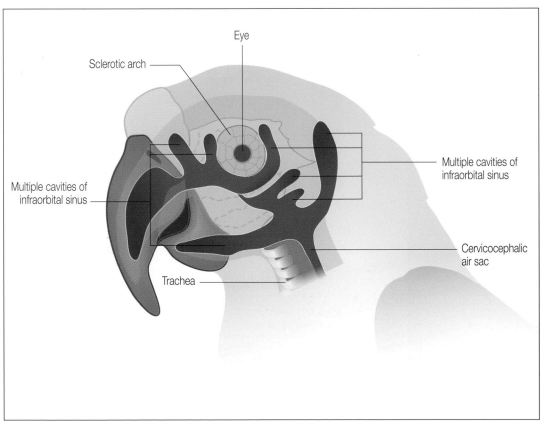

2.15

Psittacine infraorbital sinus. (Redrawn after Ritchie *et al.*, 1994)

Eye

Sclerotic arch

Multiple cavities of infraorbital sinus

Multiple cavities of infraorbital sinus

Cervicocephalic air sac

Trachea

Syrinx

The syrinx, situated at the bifurcation of the trachea, is responsible for sound production (Figure 2.16). The complexity of the syrinx anatomy differs considerably between various avian orders and species.

The tympanum is formed by modified tracheal cartilages at the proximal end of the trachea. The space between the last tracheal and first bronchial cartilage is spanned by the lateral and medial tympaniform membranes. The tension of these membranes is regulated by the syringeal muscles, allowing different tones to be formed. Whereas some passerine species have five or more pairs of syringeal muscles, other species, such as pigeons, have only one pair.

Whereas humans sing using a continuous expiration, passerines sing and tweet using very fast oscillating mini-expirations, in a frequency of up to 25 per second. Some passerine species are capable of oscillating the left and right membranes individually, allowing them to produce two tones at the same time.

Bronchi and lungs

The trachea branches at the syrinx into the two primary bronchi that enter the left and right lungs. The primary bronchi traverse the lungs and open at the caudal end of the lung into the abdominal air sac. Within the lungs numerous secondary bronchi arise from the primary bronchus and then further branch into parabronchi, which finally branch into air capillaries, where the gaseous exchange takes place. The parabronchi continue through the lung and back into the primary bronchus, where the air then empties into the air sacs. The lungs are situated within the dorsal aspect of the rib cage, closely connected to the thoracic wall. The volume and shape of the lung remains constant and does not change during inspiration and expiration.

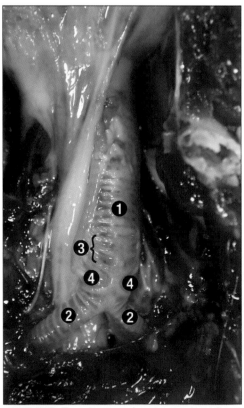

2.16 The pigeon syrinx. 1 = trachea; 2 = primary bronchus; 3 = tympanum; 4 = tympaniform membrane.

Air sacs

Air sacs are divided into caudal air sacs (abdominal air sac and caudal thoracic air sac) and cranial air sacs (cranial thoracic air sac, clavicular air sac and cervico-cephalic air sac). Whereas all air sacs originally develop as pairs, in most species the clavicular and cervico-cephalic paired air sacs fuse with the contralateral side. The cranial and caudal thoracic air sacs and the abdominal air sacs remain paired in adult birds. In most avian species air sacs form diverticula into pneumatized bones such as the humerus, sternum, vertebrae, femur and pelvis (Figure 2.17; see also Figure 2.9).

Movement of air through the respiratory system

The unique anatomy of the avian respiratory system allows gas exchange despite the missing diaphragm and the fact that lung shape and volume stay constant throughout the respiratory cycle (Figure 2.18).

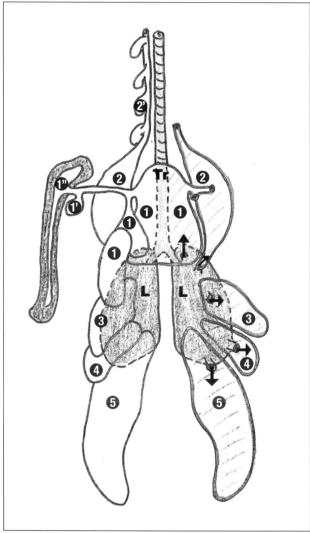

2.17 System of air sacs (modified after King and McLelland, 1984). The right side displays opening of the major bronchi supplying the respective air sacs. The colours indicate functional grouping into caudal (blue) and cranial (green) compartments. 1 = unpaired clavicular sac with axillary diverticulum (1') and the recess pneumatizing the humeral bone (1"); 2 = cervical air sac with vertebral recesses (2') pneumatizing the cervical vertebrae; 3 = cranial thoracic air sac; 4 = caudal thoracic air sac; 5 = abdominal air sac; L = lungs; Tr = trachea. (Reproduced from the *BSAVA Manual of Raptors, Pigeons and Passerine Birds*, courtesy of RM Hirschberg)

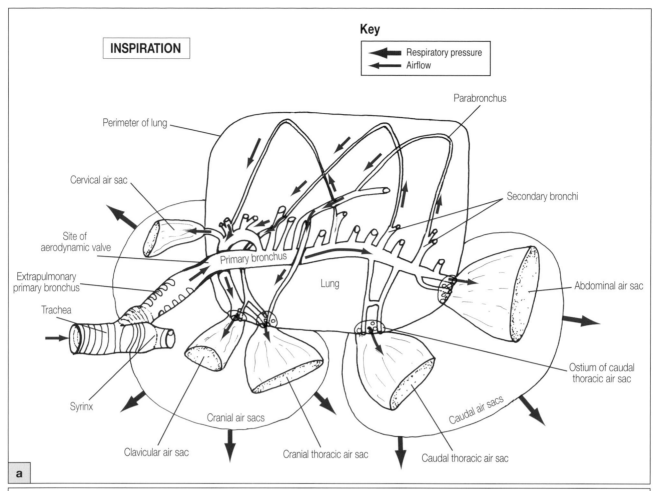

INSPIRATION

Key

⬅ Respiratory pressure
← Airflow

Parabronchus

Perimeter of lung

Cervical air sac

Secondary bronchi

Site of aerodynamic valve

Primary bronchus

Extrapulmonary primary bronchus

Lung

Abdominal air sac

Trachea

Ostium of caudal thoracic air sac

Syrinx

Cranial air sacs

Caudal air sacs

Clavicular air sac

Cranial thoracic air sac

Caudal thoracic air sac

a

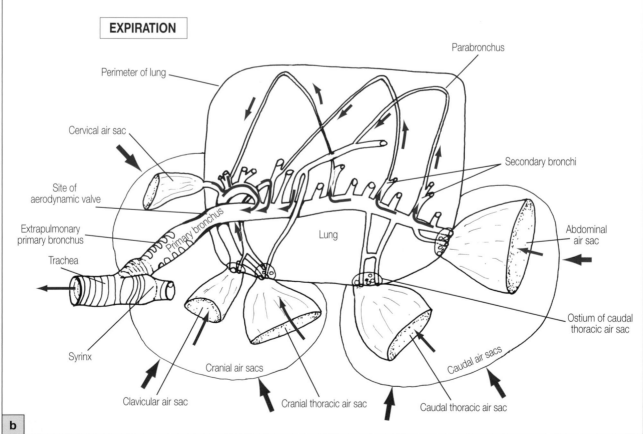

EXPIRATION

Parabronchus

Perimeter of lung

Cervical air sac

Secondary bronchi

Site of aerodynamic valve

Primary bronchus

Extrapulmonary primary bronchus

Lung

Abdominal air sac

Trachea

Ostium of caudal thoracic air sac

Syrinx

Cranial air sacs

Caudal air sacs

Clavicular air sac

Cranial thoracic air sac

Caudal thoracic air sac

b

2.18 Movement of air through the lung of a bird. **(a)** Inspiratory movements increase air sac volumes and **(b)** expiratory movements decrease them. The volume and shape of the lung remains the same. Because of the arrangement of the parabronchi and the possible presence of an aerodynamic valve, the air is moved unidirectionally through the parabronchi and therefore through the area of gaseous exchange. (© Nigel Harcourt-Brown)

During inspiration, respiratory movements of the body wall, as well as neck and wing movement, increase air sac volume, pulling fresh air through the bronchi and parabronchi into the caudal air sacs. At the same time, exhausted air moves from the lung into the cranial air sacs.

During expiration, the air from the caudal air sacs is bellowed back into the bronchi of the lung and the air in the cranial air sacs moves back into the primary bronchus and is exhaled.

This unique system with unilateral air movement through the bronchi and parabronchi allows a very effective gaseous exchange both during inspiration and expiration, but at the same time entails that inhaled air stays in the respiratory system over two breath cycles.

Gaseous exchange

Gaseous exchange takes place within the air capillaries and not in alveoli as in mammals. Air capillaries are smaller than mammalian alveoli and the blood–gas barrier is thinner than in mammals. This plus the fact that there are no blind-ending alveoli leading to dead space and residual air volume all improve the effectiveness of gaseous exchange in comparison to mammals.

Urinary system

Figure 2.19 details key differences between bird and dog and cat urinary systems, and their clinical significance.

Kidney

In comparison to mammals, the kidneys of birds are large and divided into a cranial, middle and caudal lobe. They are situated dorsally within the renal fossa formed by the synsacrum and iliac bone (Figure 2.20).

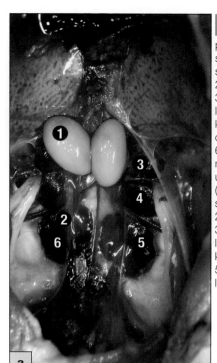

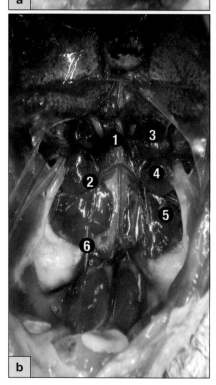

2.20 **(a)** The male pigeon urogenital system (breeding season). 1 = testes; 2 = ductus deferens; 3 = cranial kidney lobe; 4 = middle kidney lobe; 5 = caudal kidney lobe; 6 = ureter. **(b)** The male pigeon urogenital system (out of breeding season). 1 = testes; 2 = ductus deferens; 3 = cranial kidney lobe; 4 = middle kidney lobe; 5 = caudal kidney lobe; 6 = ureter.

The functional unit of the kidney is the nephron. Avian kidneys contain mammalian as well as reptilian nephrons. The mammalian nephrons are located within the medulla, have a well developed glomerulus and contain a loop of Henle, thus allowing the concentration of salts. The reptilian nephrons are located within the cortex and have a less developed glomerulus and no loop of Henle (Figure 2.21).

Uricotelism

Unlike mammals, but just as in reptiles, birds are urico-telic. The end product of nitrogen metabolism is uric acid. Uric acid is formed in the liver and excreted via the kidney. Although uric acid is also produced by glomerular filtration, the vast majority results from tubular

Bird	Dog and cat	Clinical relevance
Uric acid is the end product of nitrogen metabolism (uricotelism)	Urea is the end product of nitrogen metabolism	Birds excrete not only urine but also white pasty uric acid Birds are more prone to developing gout
Cloaca collects faeces, urine and uric acid and voids all three parts together	Urine and faeces voided through separate body openings	Difficult for owners to differentiate between diarrhoea and polyuria Urine contaminated by faecal material; interpretation of urinalysis difficult
The lumbosacral plexus passes between the cranial and middle kidney lobes and the pelvic bones	No association between kidney and lumbosacral plexus	Kidney swelling, especially neoplasia and other coelomic masses, can cause compression of the lumbosacral plexus and unilateral paresis
Renal portal system	No renal portal system	Medication injected into hind limbs may cause renal toxicity or be excreted without achieving required levels in the blood
Marine species have a salt-secreting supraorbital gland	No supraorbital gland	Marine avian species can drink seawater

2.19 Urinary system of birds *versus* dogs and cats.

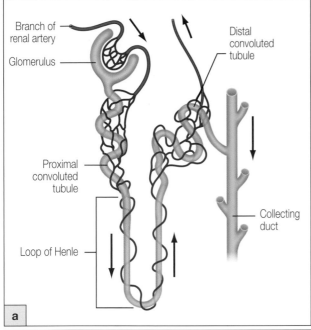

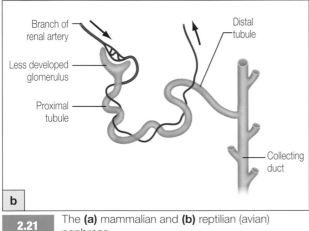

The **(a)** mammalian and **(b)** reptilian (avian) nephrons.

secretion and is therefore largely independent of urine flow rate. This water-saving mechanism allows waste excretion without loss of water.

Lower urinary system

Urine leaves the kidneys through the ureters, which flow into the urodeum of the cloaca (see Figure 2.13). Birds, therefore, have no bladder or urethra. Through retroperistaltic movement urine can be moved into the colorectum, allowing further water and salt reabsorption. Furthermore, marine and various other avian species have a supraorbital gland that excretes enough salt as a hypertonic fluid that these species can drink seawater. The supraorbital gland is a crescent-shaped organ that lies along the frontal bone above the orbit. Each salt gland is formed of a medial and lateral segment, each of these draining into a separate duct, which empty into the nasal cavity (Marples, 1932).

Renal portal system

The renal portal system collects venous blood from the hind legs and caudal parts of the body, which drains into the peritubular capillary system via the renal portal vein. About two-thirds of the blood entering the kidney comes from the renal portal vein and only approximately one-third from the renal artery. Renal valves

within the renal portal system allow direction of this renal blood either away from or through the kidney, therefore regulating waste product removal. This valve system is regulated by the autonomic nervous system (Figure 2.22).

Cloaca

For more information see 'Digestive system'.

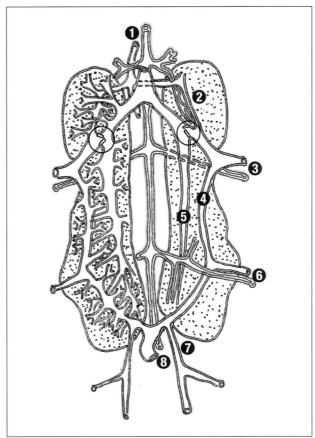

Schematic drawing showing the vascular system of the kidney (arteries are shown in red and veins in black) (modified after Baumel, 1993). The encircled areas show the localization of the renal valve that enables redirection of venous return. 1 = descending aorta and cranial vena cava; 2 = cranial portal vein; 3 = external iliac artery and vein; 4 = caudal portal vein; 5 = caudal renal vein; 6 = ischiadic artery and vein; 7 = internal iliac vein; 8 = median sacral artery and caudal mesenteric vein. (Reproduced from the *BSAVA Manual of Raptors, Pigeons and Passerine Birds*, courtesy of RM Hirschberg)

Reproductive system

Figure 2.23 details key differences between bird and dog and cat reproductive systems and their clinical significance.

Male

Unlike in mammals, the avian testes remain at their site of origin, analogous to the ovary at the cranial end of the kidney directly adjacent to the adrenal gland (see Figure 2.20). The size and vascularity of the testes vary greatly during the reproductive cycle.

Sperm produced within the testes is collected into the epididymis and emptied into the ductus deferens, which ends in the urodeum of the cloaca. Avian species have no accessory genital glands.

Bird	Dog and cat	Clinical relevance
Oviduct develops unilaterally on the left side only	Paired ovary and oviduct	Surgical endoscopic sexing is performed from the left side
Mucosal folds of the vagina can store viable sperm for several weeks	No storage of sperm within the vagina	Fertilization of follicles is possible several weeks after copulation
Mesovary attaching ovary to body wall is short and well vascularized	Mesovary easy to mobilize and ligate	Surgical ovariectomy is difficult in avian species
Testicles remain in the coelomic cavity cranially to the kidney	Testicles descend into scrotum	Castration is an intracoelomic procedure making it much more difficult than in dogs and cats

2.23 Reproductive system of birds *versus* dogs and cats.

The opening of the spermatic duct into the urodeum is called the cloacal promontory. In neonatal birds and during reproductive phases this external projection can be identified by the practised eye and used for sex determination in some species. During copulation, the cloacal lips of the male and female bird are pressed together. In some species, such as ostriches and other ratites, ducks and geese, a large erectile phallus allows the emptying of semen into the female cloaca.

Female
In most female birds only the left of the paired embryonic Müllerian ducts is fully and functionally developed, although in some individuals rudimentary ovaries and oviducts can be observed on the right side. Adult Kiwis consistently have paired ovaries and in some raptor species, especially Peregrine Falcons, this is also commonly seen (Kinsky, 1971).

The left ovary lies adjacent to the cranial pole of the kidney and the adrenal gland. It is attached by a short and well vascularized mesovarian ligament to the body wall. In immature birds and during non-reproductive phases the ovary surface has only small follicles, which then increase in size during reproduction.

The oviduct (Figure 2.24), which greatly increases in size and vascularity during egg production, contains five distinct parts.

- The follicle that ovulates from the ovary is encaptured by the **infundibulum**. Within the infundibulum the chalazae and first layers of albumen are produced. During this short period of time the egg cell is fertilized by sperm. Egg transport through the oviduct is primarily achieved by contractions that move the egg towards the cloaca (Johnson, 2000).
- Within the largest portion of the oviduct, the **magnum**, the rest of the albumen (egg white) is produced.
- The egg then passes into the **isthmus**, which is clearly distinguishable from the magnum by its thick circular muscle layer, where the shell membranes are produced.
- From the isthmus the egg passes into the actual **uterus or shell gland** where the calcified egg shell

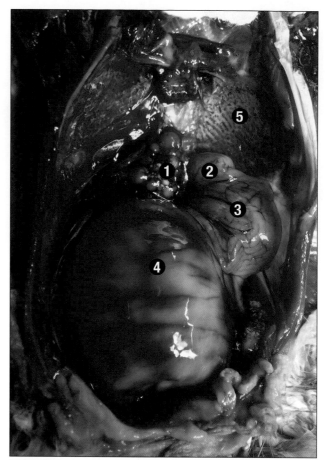

2.24 The active female pigeon reproductive system. 1 = ovary; 2 = infundibulum; 3 = magnum and isthmus; 4 = uterus (shell gland); 5 = lung.

is produced. The developing egg spends roughly 80% of its time in this shell gland.
- The final and most distal part of the oviduct is the **vagina**. This muscular section expels the egg through the cloaca as it is laid. The mucosal folds of the vagina store sperm that remains viable for several weeks.

Cloaca
For more information see 'Digestive system'.

Integument
Figure 2.25 details key differences between bird and dog and cat integuments and their clinical significance.

Function
The main functions of avian skin and feathers include protection, thermoregulation and allowing flight, as well as camouflage and decoration.

Skin layers
The outermost layer of the skin, the epidermis, is thinner than in mammals. Feathers are a complex structure of the epidermis. The dermis, the connective tissue layer, contains the feather follicles, the smooth muscles that move the feathers as well as nerves and blood vessels. The subcutis contains fatty tissue, often as circumscribed fat bodies, which functions as insulation and an energy source in migrating birds.

Bird	Dog and cat	Clinical relevance
Epidermis thinner	Epidermis thicker	Be aware of tearing skin when plucking feathers for surgery
Circumscribed fatty tissue in subcutis	Diffuse fatty tissue in subcutis	In fat birds (e.g. Budgerigars) formation of localized lipomas over breast or abdomen
Cere: waxy epidermal membrane between beak and nares	No cere	Blue, smooth cere in male Budgerigars Brown, rough cere in female and immature Budgerigars
Psittacids have strong sharp beaks	Teeth and lips	In psittacids, good fixation of head and beak is necessary during clinical examination
Raptors have strong sharp dirty claws	Sharp claws	In raptors, good fixation of feet and claws is necessary during clinical examination
Powder down feathers common in psittacids, especially cockatoos	No feathers	Fine white dust cover bird and surroundings, especially in feather pluckers; can cause nasal/respiratory irritation in some birds
Red feather colour produced by dietary uptake of carotenoids	No feathers	Flamingos and other species lose their colour if not fed carotenoid pigments
Down feathers important for insulation and thermoregulation	No feathers	Be aware of hypothermia caused by applying too much alcohol to small birds
Sheath of newly formed feathers is preened away	No feathers	Retained sheaths if bird is not preening (ataxia, pain in legs/feet, collared birds)
New feathers are formed by cell division within the feather follicle	No feathers	Broken/cut feathers remain in place until next moult Plucked feathers regrow immediately
Newly formed feathers contain blood vessels	No feathers	Heavy bleeding from damaged new feathers is possible; bleeding feathers must be plucked

2.25   Integument of birds *versus* dogs and cats.

Skin glands

Avian skin does not contain sweat or sebaceous glands. Specific keratinocytes within the skin form a thin oily layer protecting the skin from dehydration and microbes. Thermoregulation takes place over the respiratory system and via the feet. The uropygial gland at the dorsal base of the tail produces a sebaceous oil that birds distribute across their feathers and which acts as a conditioner. The large volume of finely distributed air within the interlocking hooks and barbules of the feathers, however, is the principal factor in the water-repellency of plumage (Fabricius, 1956). The uropygial gland is present in most species and it is relatively large in aquatic species. It is absent in other species, including the Ostrich, Emu, Cassowary, Bustard, Frogmouth, many pigeons, many woodpeckers, as well as in Hyacinth Macaws and all Amazon species (King and McLelland, 1984).

Special skin structures

The skin over the tarsometatarsus and toes is scaly. The scales are a cornified epidermal structure. In male chickens and other Galliformes, spurs are formed on the medial aspect of the scaly leg.

Ducks and geese have toe webs between their second and third, and third and fourth, toes, allowing them to use their feet as fins to propel themselves forward within the water.

The avian claw is a keratinized epidermal structure covering the tip of the most distal phalanx. The structure of the claw corresponds to the species-specific lifestyle; for example, claws may be used for grasping, digging, climbing or defence. Some groups, such as birds of prey, have a rudimentary claw on the alular digit of the wing. Toe pads are modified skin structures on the palmar aspects of the toes, cushioning ground contact.

The beak or 'rhamphotheca' (which consists of the rhinotheca covering the maxillary bone and the gnathotheca covering the mandibular bone; see Figure 2.2) is a horny skin structure of keratinized epidermis covering the upper and lower jaws. For more detail on the shape and function of the beak, see 'Digestive system'. The cere is a modified epidermal waxy membrane between the beak and the nares, seen, for example, in raptors and psittacine birds.

The oestrogen- and prolactin-regulated brood patch loses all feathers and becomes highly vascularized and oedematous during egg laying and breeding. The dense innervation of the brood patch and thermoreceptors located here are important for controlling incubation.

Feathers

Feathers are complicated epidermal structures unique to birds. They are formed in a feather follicle and are arranged in feather tracts (pterylae) that are separated by areas with no feather follicles (apteria) (Figure 2.26). Each feather consists of the shaft or rachis, the barbs, which branch off the shaft and then branch off again to the barbules. The barbicules interconnect barbules from one barb to the next, stabilizing the vane of the feather (Figure 2.27).

Contour feathers cover the body and wings, giving them their typical structure (Figure 2.28). They are characterized by a distinct shaft and the feather vane. Contour feathers include:

- Cover feathers on the body covering the down feathers
- Flight feathers on the wings (remiges)
- Steering feathers of the tail (retrices)
- Ornamental feathers in some species.

Flight feathers are divided into (normally 10) primaries, which are attached to the carpometacarpus (feathers 1–6) and major digit (feathers 7–10) and secondaries (in varying numbers from six in hummingbirds to 38 in albatrosses), which are anchored into the ulna.

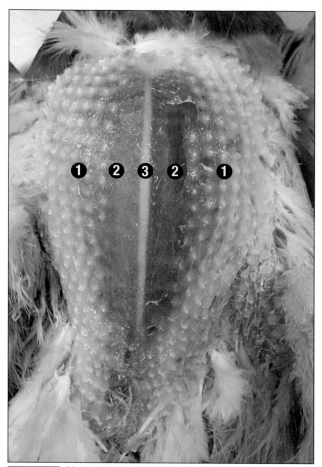

2.26 Ventral view of a plucked pigeon breast. 1 = feather tracts (pterylae); 2 = areas with no feather follicles (apteria); 3 = carina of the sternum.

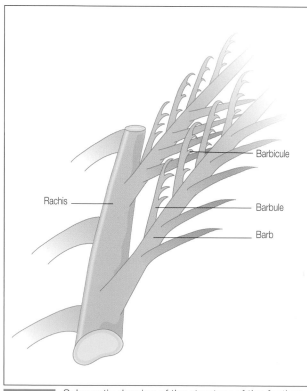

2.27 Schematic drawing of the structure of the feather vane of contour feathers.

Rachis — Barbicule — Barbule — Barb

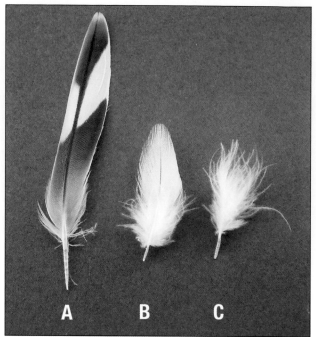

2.28 Feather types (Budgerigar). A = contour feather; B = semiplume feather; C = down feather.

The shafts of these flight feathers are covered by various layers of shorter cover feathers.

- Down feathers have a short shaft and long soft barbs (Figure 2.28). They are found under the contour feathers and help insulate the body.
- Semiplumes combine the structures of contour feathers and down feathers, with a soft downy base and a harder contour-type top.
- Powder down feathers are continuously growing white down feathers. The barbs at the tip dissolve forming a fine white dust that coats the bird. These are common in orders such as pigeons and psittacine birds.
- Filoplumes are associated with the contour feathers, but are not obviously seen until a bird is plucked. Filoplumes consist of a long thin shaft with only a few short barbs. They are presumed to have a sensory function in conjunction with the Herbst corpuscles assessing movement of the contour feathers during flight.
- Bristle feathers are short strong protective feathers mainly found around the eyes, nares and beak.

Moulting

Moulting is a necessary process to allow the replacement of neonatal feathers by juvenile and then later adult feathers, to replace damaged and worn out feathers, and to allow the formation of display plumage during courtship. Many birds will moult once a year, others twice a year, between courtship plumage and off-season plumage. Other birds, such as vultures, will only moult every 2–4 years. Normally a set moulting pattern is followed, for example, by losing the same flight feather on each wing at one time. Most birds will moult one pair of flight feathers at a time, allowing them to continuously be able to fly. Others, such as ducks, moult all at one time, and therefore cannot fly during this time. Moulting is regulated by a light-dependent endogenous rhythm and is dependent amongst other things on thyroid hormone and oestrogens (McNabb, 2000).

New feathers are formed by cell division within the feather follicle pushing the newly formed feather out of the follicle. The sheath of the newly formed feather is then preened away, allowing the vane to unfold. The vascular and nervous tissue within the newly formed feather gradually retracts, leaving the dead horny structure of the fully grown feather.

Feather colour

Feather colour is important for characterizing juveniles and adults, males and females, breeding status, courtship and display as well as for camouflage. Different mechanisms that form feather colours include:

- Carotenoid pigments form reds and yellows, such as in flamingos. These rely on dietary uptake and transfer to feather cells. These colours typically lighten if no dietary uptake is possible
- Melanocytes within the skin produce brown, black and yellow colours
- Turacoverdin and turacin are unique copper uroporphyrin pigments responsible for the bright green and red coloration of turacos. Unlike reds and greens in other species they are not derived from carotenoids (Gill, 2006)
- White and blue are structural colours. These are formed by absorption and reflection of light within the feathers. Iridescent colours are formed by refraction of light on melanin lamellae within the feathers.

Nervous system

Meninges

As in mammals, birds have three meninges: pia mater, arachnoid and dura mater. Cerebrospinal fluid is located within the subarachnoid space.

Brain and spinal cord

Relative to body size, the avian brain is not as large as in mammals but is larger than in reptiles. It is lissencephalic with virtually no convolutions and the cerebral cortex is very poorly developed. The optic lobe is massive whereas the olfactory centre is rather underdeveloped. As in mammals, the cerebellum is responsible for the coordination of movements. In many species, specific function-related characteristics of the brain can be observed. For example, the corresponding areas within the brain are well developed in food-storing passerines and also in homing pigeons.

The spinal cord is structurally similar to that in mammals. There is no cauda equina. The glycogen body is situated within the lumbosacral swelling of the spinal cord and consists of glia cells that contain a large amount of glycogen. The function of the glycogen body is not known; it may, however, be a sense organ for equilibrium.

Cranial and spinal nerves

Avian cranial nerves correspond to those found in mammals. The optic nerve (CN II) is especially large and more than half the diameter of the spinal cord.

The cervicothoracic swelling of the spinal cord represents the origin of the brachial plexus, which is formed by the ventral branches of three to five spinal nerves and innervates the wings. The lumbosacral swelling represents the origin of the lumbar, ischiatic and pudendal plexuses. These nerve roots lie between the pelvic bone and the kidneys.

Autonomic nervous system

Consisting of the sympathetic and parasympathetic systems, the autonomic nervous system is similar to that in mammals.

Senses

Olfaction

Many birds, such as passerines, have relatively poorly developed smelling capacities. Other species, however, such as albatrosses and petrels as well as vultures, react very sensitively to odour cues.

Gustation

In comparison to mammals, birds have few tastebuds. The greatest numbers are on the caudal surface of the tongue and the pharyngeal floor.

Many avian species respond to sweet tastes, especially psittacine species and nectar-feeders. Birds without nasal salt glands refuse concentrations of salt that are hypertonic to their body fluids. Birds with salt glands, such as gulls and penguins, will drink saltwater, but prefer pure water over saline solution.

Responses to sour and bitter are puzzling and no consistent taste behaviour can be correlated (Mason and Clark, 2000). In summary, birds probably do not share human taste experiences.

Hearing

Birds do not have an external ear. Owls, however, have a facial disc that reflects and amplifies sound. In addition, in some owl species, the left and right ears differ in height and direction of their openings, allowing detection of sound direction and elevation above ground. In diving birds the ear canal is reduced and protected by specialized feathers.

The tympanic cavity of the middle ear contains a single auditory ossicle and the inner ear consists of a cochlear organ and a vestibular organ.

The eye and vision

Vision is the most important sense in birds and the avian eye is very large. The weight of the two eyes exceeds that of the brain.

The majority of birds, being prey species, have a narrow head with the eyes located laterally, giving them a large field of total vision but only a small field of stereovision. Predatory species such as owls have broad heads and frontally located eyes, giving them a large field of stereovision but a limited total field of vision. The very flexible neck still allows owls good vision in all directions without having to change their body position.

The eye is protected by the upper and lower eyelids as well as the dorsolaterally located transparent third eyelid (nictitating membrane). The lacrimal gland is associated with the third eyelid, which spreads the tears over the cornea. The tears are then drained by the lacrimal duct in the nasal angle of the eye. The third eyelid is closed to protect the eye, for example, during diving under water or during the stoop in falcons.

The eyeball is held by a ring of bony scleral ossicles that circularly attach to the cornea. The ciliary body that holds the lens contains striated muscle that gives birds conscious control over iris and pupil size.

> Birds have striated muscles in the ciliary body of the eye, whereas dogs and cats have only smooth muscle. Birds are therefore able to consciously control the size of their pupil, which can make assessment of pupil size difficult, and mydriatic eye drops do not cause mydriasis in the avian eye

The cornea, which is thinner than in mammals, covers the small anterior chamber. The posterior chamber is larger than in mammals and differs in shape in various species. Diurnal birds have a disc-like flat or globular posterior chamber. These shapes allow the retina to have a broad visual acuity rather than the single region of acute vision found in mammals. Night-active owls have a tube-shaped posterior chamber. Accommodation is controlled by the posterior or anterior sclerocorneal muscles, which push the ciliary muscles towards the lens, increasing its curvature.

The avian retina is comparatively thick and avascular. The large number of cones, each of which has its own ganglion, allow excellent visual acuity. Night-active birds have more rods, which are grouped together to a ganglion, allowing very small amounts of light to trigger an impulse. The area centralis (representing a zone of increased optical resolution) contains the central fovea retinae, with a maximal optical resolution. The fovea retinae is small and round in seed-eating birds, allowing the bird to focus on a single object. Owls and raptors have an additional fovea temporalis allowing binocular, stereoscopic vision. The pecten is a thin pleated vascular and pigmented structure within the vitreous chamber. Its main function appears to be the supply of nutrients to the otherwise avascular retina and posterior segments of the eye (Figure 2.29).

Endocrine system

The avian endocrine system can basically be compared to that of mammals.

Pituitary gland

The pituitary gland is closely connected to the hypothalamus at the base of the brain.

The adenohypophysis produces the gonadotropins luteinizing hormone (LH) and follicle-stimulating hormone (FSH), thyroid-stimulating hormone (TSH), adrenocorticotropic hormone (ACTH), growth hormone (GH) and prolactin. Prolactin stimulates the production of crop milk in pigeons and doves, and is involved in incubation behaviour and broodiness.

The neurohypophysis produces arginine vasotocin (AVT) and oxytocin or mesotocin (8-isoleucine oxytocin). AVT correlates to antidiuretic hormone (ADH) in mammals and is the major antidiuretic hormone in birds. The avian uterus contracts in response to AVT, but much less so to mesotocin. Ovipositioning is therefore mainly controlled by AVT.

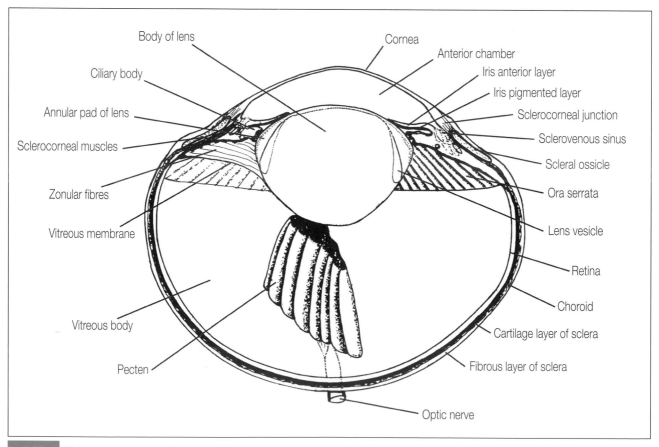

2.29 Schematic drawing of the structures of the eye. (© Nigel Harcourt-Brown)

Pineal gland

The pineal gland is located at the dorsal surface of the brain between the cerebellum and the two hemispheres of the telencephalon. Melatonin, the hormone produced in the pineal gland, inhibits all endocrine glands, especially the gonads, and therefore influences reproduction. Melatonin also controls the circadian rhythm.

Thyroid gland

The avian thyroid glands are paired oval glands located ventrolaterally to the trachea near the junction of the subclavian and carotid artery and are closely associated with the parathyroid and ultimobranchial glands.

Similarly to mammals, iodide is actively transported into the thyroid gland, where thyroglobulins are iodinated to triiodothyronine (T3) and thyroxine (T4). Whereas plasma concentrations of T3 are similar to those in mammals, the plasma concentrations of T4 are much lower.

> Birds have lower plasma T4 levels than dogs and cats, and therefore not all measuring techniques used in these species are suitable for measuring T4 in avian blood samples

Thyroid hormones influence the body metabolism, i.e. basic metabolic rate, heat production, and heart and respiration rates. They also regulate and promote growth and are important in processes such as hatching, moulting and reproduction.

> The high metabolic rate of birds means that fasting of small species prior to anaesthesia is contraindicated

Calcium metabolism

Due to egg shell production, calcium metabolism is especially important in birds. An egg-laying bird can mobilize calcium from the bone and intestine within minutes, whereas in mammals this can take over 24 hours. For the production of an egg a hen requires 10% of its total body calcium reserves. Parathyroid hormone, vitamin D_3 and calcitonin regulate this system (Figure 2.30) (Stanford, 2006).

Parathyroid hormone

The number of parathyroid glands in birds varies between two and four. They are situated directly caudal to the thyroid glands. Parathyroid hormone increases the blood calcium level by increasing osteoclast activity, increasing the reabsorption of calcium in the kidneys and increasing the absorption of calcium within the intestines. The oviduct uptake of calcium from the plasma is also regulated by parathyroid hormone.

Vitamin D

Provitamin D_3 is converted to vitamin D_3 under the influence of ultraviolet light in the skin. Vitamin D_3 is then metabolized in the liver and kidneys respectively to the active metabolite $1,25\text{-}(OH)_2D_3$. This active metabolite increases blood calcium levels mainly by regulating calcium absorption across the intestinal wall. Vitamin D_3 additionally regulates the uptake of calcium from the plasma pool into the oviduct.

Calcitonin

The ultimobranchial glands are located in close proximity to the parathyroid and thyroids glands. They produce calcitonin, which decreases the blood calcium level mainly by inhibiting the mobilization of calcium from the bones.

Prostaglandin and oestrogen

Prostaglandins facilitate bone resorption and therefore increase blood calcium levels. Oestrogens have a hypercalcaemic effect by promoting the formation of vitellogenins in the liver, which are calcium-binding lipoproteins that are incorporated into the egg yolk (Dacke, 2000).

> Common calcium-related pathologies in birds:
> - Osteodystrophy in growing birds (metabolic bone disease)
> - Hypocalcaemic seizures (especially in Grey Parrots)
> - Egg binding

Adrenal glands

The adrenal glands are located within the triangle between the cranial lobe of the kidney and the lateral

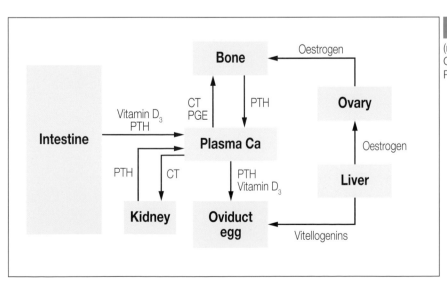

2.30 Summary of calcium (Ca) metabolism in the bird (modified after Causey Whittow, 2000). CT = calcitonin; PGE = prostaglandin E; PTH = parathyroid hormone.

aspect of the gonads. As in mammals they produce corticosteroids and aldosterone. Corticosteroids are regulated by ACTH. The regulation of aldosterone through the renin–angiotensin system is similar to mammals. Corticosterone is essential for survival in times of stress, whereas aldosterone regulates electrolyte metabolism.

References and further reading

Baumel JJ (1993) *Handbook of Avian Anatomy: Nomina Anatomica Avium.* Nuttall Ornithological Club, Harvard University, Massachusetts

Causey Whittow G (2000) *Sturkie's Avian Physiology, 5th edn*. Academic Press, New York

Cubo J and Casinos A (2000) Incidence and mechanical significance of pneumatization in the long bones of birds. *Zoological Journal of the Linnean Society*, **130(4)**, 449–510

Fabricius E (1956) What makes plumage waterproof? *Zoologisk Revy* **18**, 71–83

Dacke G (2000) The parathyroids, calcitonin and vitamin D. In: *Sturkie's Avian Physiology, 5th edn*, ed. G Causey Whittow, pp 473–488. Academic Press, New York

Denbow DM (2000) Gastrointestinal anatomy and physiology. In: *Sturkie's Avian Physiology, 5th edn*, ed. G Causey Whittow, pp 299–325. Academic Press, New York

Fitch WT (1999) Acoustic exaggeration of size in birds via tracheal elongation: comparative and theoretical analyses. *Journal of Zoology* **248**, 31–48

Gill FB (2006) *Ornithology, 3rd edn*, p 97. W. H. Freeman, New York

Harcourt-Brown N (2000) *Birds of Prey: Anatomy, Radiology and Clinical Conditions of the Pelvic Limb*. Zoological Education Network, Palm Beach

Harcourt-Brown N (2002) Avian anatomy and physiology. In: *BSAVA Manual of Exotic Pets: A Foundation Manual, 4th edn*, ed. A Meredith and S Redrobe, pp. 138–148, BSAVA Publications, Gloucester

Hazelwood RL (2000) Pancreas. In: *Sturkie's Avian Physiology, 5th edn*, ed. G Causey Whittow, pp 539–556. Academic Press, New York

Hirschberg RM (2008) Anatomy and physiology. In: *BSAVA Manual of Raptors, Pigeons and Passerine Birds*, ed. J Chitty and M Lierz, pp 25–41. BSAVA Publications, Gloucester

Hummel G (2000) *Anatomie und Physiologie der Vögel*. Verlag Eugen Ulmer, Suttgart

Johnson AL (2000) Reproduction in the female. In: *Sturkie's Avian Physiology*, 5th edn, ed. G Causey Whittow, pp 569–596. Academic Press, New York

King AS and McLelland J (1975) *Outlines of Avian Anatomy*. Ballière Tindall, London

King AS and McLelland J (1984) Birds: *Their Structure and Function, 2nd edn*. Ballière Tindall, Philadelphia

Kinsky FC (1971) The consistent presence of paired ovaries in the Kiwi (*Apteryx*) with some discussion of this condition in other birds. *Journal of Ornithology* **112**, 334–336

Marples BJ (1932) Structure and development of the nasal glands of birds. *Proceedings of the Zoological Society of London*, pp. 829–844

Mason JR and Clark L (2000) The chemical senses in birds. In: *Sturkie's Avian Physiology*, ed. G Causey Whittow, pp 43–46. Academic Press, New York

McNabb FMA (2000) Thyroids. In: *Sturkie's Avian Physiology, 5th edn*, G Causey Whittow, pp. 461–471. Academic Press, New York

Nickel R, Schummer A and Seifferle S (1977) *Anatomy of the Domestic Bird*. Verlag Paul Parey, Berlin

Ritchie BW, Harrison GJ and Harrison LR (1994) *Avian Medicine: Principles and Application*. Zoological Education Network, Palm Beach

Sealing LE (1994) Anatomy of the Umbrella Cockatoo, lateral and ventrodorsal views in a clear overlay system. In: *Avian Medicine: Principles and Application*, ed. BW Ritchie, GJ Harrison and LR Harrison, pp 1352. Wingers Publishing, Lake Worth

Smith FM, West NH and Jones DR (2000) The Cardiovascular System. In: *Sturkie's Avian Physiology*, ed. G Causey Whittow, pp 141–231. Academic Press, New York

Stanford M (2006) Calcium metabolism. In: *Clinical Avian Medicine, Volume 1*, ed. GJ Harrison and TL Lightfoot, pp 141–152. Spix Publishing, Palm Beach

Husbandry

Alan Jones

Bird keeping has a very long history. From prehistoric times, once hunter-gatherer humans realized that many birds and their eggs were a good source of food, they began to confine groups of species such as early poultry, waterfowl and pigeons to provide a readily available supply. These birds bred in captivity, providing eggs for immediate consumption and offspring for longer-term replenishment of stock.

In time, other species became associated with humans for other purposes: raptors for hunting; decorative birds for display and prestige; songbirds and mimics for their entertainment value. From the time ancient civilizations started to record their lives on stone tablets, papyrus parchment or pottery, birds have featured heavily in these records.

The keeping of birds is as old as civilized man, and in recent generations understanding of the welfare, husbandry and nutritional needs of birds has advanced significantly. This has led to considerable legislation concerning which species may be kept in captivity; dimensions and construction of enclosures or cages; as well as transport, breeding and slaughter. However, there remains considerable controversy regarding the ethics of confining many types of bird.

Accommodation

Some species, such as temperature-sensitive small passerines or tropical parrots, should only ever be housed within a building, providing shelter from the elements and additional heating when required. Others are better kept outdoors, for reasons of size, practicality or the need for fresh air and sunlight. Most collections of raptors on public display have outdoor quarters, as do larger parrot species and hardy passerines. Such facilities should still provide shelter from driving cold wind and rain, hard frosts or fierce midday sun. Figure 3.1 details the advantages and disadvantages associated with keeping captive birds outdoors *versus* indoors.

Few raptor species are housed fully indoors. Occasionally 'pet' individuals or juveniles that are being hand-reared may be kept in this way. Otherwise, most are kept in outdoor flights, or a combination of shelter with an attached flight or weathering. Hardy passerine

Accommodation	Advantages	Disadvantages
Indoor	■ Reduced risk of theft ■ Reduced risk of predators and vermin ■ Less noise disturbance to neighbours ■ More keeper–bird interactions	■ Lack of natural sunlight ■ Artificial extension of day length ■ Warm dry atmosphere ■ Household hazards
Outdoor	■ Fresh air ■ Sunlight ■ Natural rainfall ■ Exercise ■ Stimulating environment ■ Healthier plumage	■ Extreme weather conditions, e.g. frost ■ Increased risk of theft ■ Predators ■ Disease transmission from wild birds ■ Increased risk of parasites ■ Noise disturbance

3.1 Advantages and disadvantages of keeping captive birds in indoor/outdoor accommodation.

species can live year-round in aviaries, usually with an enclosed and heated shed section. More delicate species require a secure internal environment, protected from the elements. The same applies to collections of breeding parakeets: most are kept in outdoor aviaries, with a combined brick or wooden 'house' linked to an open flight. Some are maintained in purpose-built bird-rooms, or converted garages or outbuildings. Collections of breeding parrots may be kept in similar outdoor aviaries, or inside more substantial buildings, especially when their monetary value is high or when noise annoyance to neighbours is likely to be a concern.

Outdoor

Construction

If an outdoor aviary is to be used as year-round accommodation for birds, then security and weather-proofing are particularly important (Figure 3.2). In temperate climates, birds require protection from frost, rain and snow; in warmer climes they may require protection from tropical storms or flooding. Alternatively, flights may be used simply for daily exercise and fresh air or just for 'fair-weather' living. Either way, the ideal arrangement is a 'three-thirds' setup (Figure 3.3): one-third of the length of the aviary is secure,

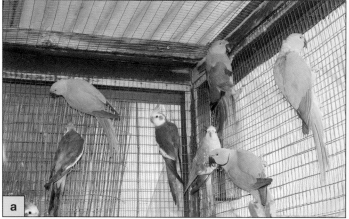
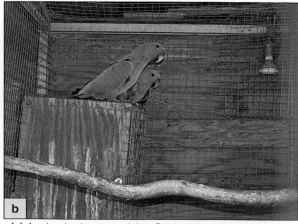

3.2 Outdoor aviaries must provide protection from the elements. **(a)** A mixed aviary containing Cockatiels and Indian Ringnecked Parakeets. The aviary is double-wired, with mesh attached to the inside and outside of the timber frame, reducing the risk of predator attack. The roof is covered with corrugated Perspex®, while the outer mesh is covered with clear plastic sheeting to provide some protection against wind and driving rain in inclement weather. There is also some reed screening at the back, providing additional seclusion. **(b)** Two male Eclectus Parrots sitting on top of a nest box in a metal-framed aviary clad with mesh and timber. There is a ceramic heat lamp in the corner of the aviary to provide heat when needed. This has been shielded from beak attack by a frame of wire mesh.

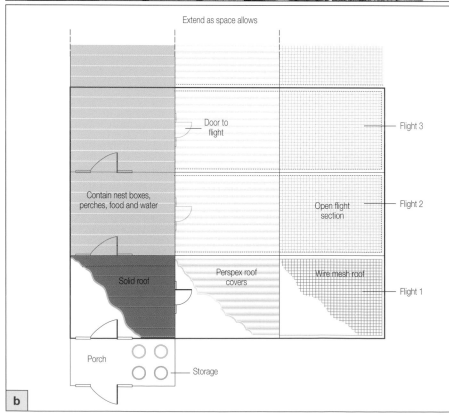

3.3 The three-thirds aviary setup. **(a)** A wooden-framed garden aviary for small parakeets, showing a door to a rear service corridor; a row of flights, each with a nest box and feeding dishes under the felt roof; an open section of flight with a perch to allow the birds access to sun and rain; a sloping floor of paving slabs for ease of cleaning and large shallow water dishes for bathing. The whole unit is incorporated into the garden as an attractive feature. Note that this aviary is not double-wired, thus leaving the birds vulnerable to predator attack. **(b)** Plan of an example three-thirds aviary setup. (continues) ▶

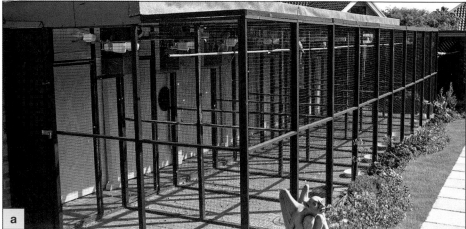

Extend as space allows

Door to flight

Flight 3

Contain nest boxes, perches, food and water

Open flight section

Flight 2

Solid roof

Perspex roof covers

Wire mesh roof

Flight 1

Porch

Storage

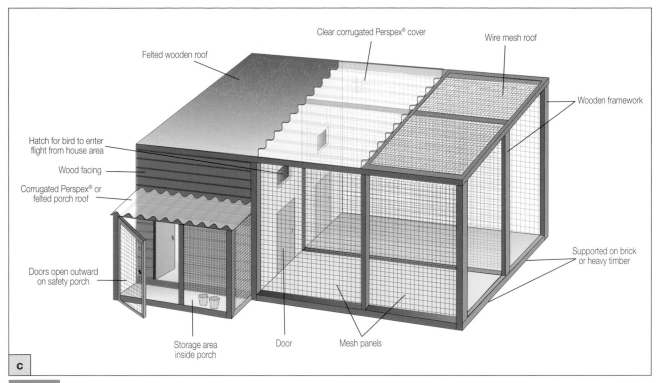

Felted wooden roof

Clear corrugated Perspex® cover

Wire mesh roof

Wooden framework

Hatch for bird to enter
flight from house area

Wood facing

Corrugated Perspex® or
felted porch roof

Doors open outward
on safety porch

Storage area
inside porch

Door

Mesh panels

Supported on brick
or heavy timber

c

3.3 (continued) The three-thirds aviary setup. **(c)** Diagram of an example three-thirds aviary setup.

sheltered housing; one-third is a wired flight that is covered with a roof; while the final third is a wired flight open to the elements.

The sheltered section of the flight gives the birds protection from the elements, security and a place to roost, feed and breed. The birds may be shut in this section by closing the access to the outside flight in order to reduce the noise nuisance to neighbours, to carry out cleaning or maintenance in the flight, or to facilitate capture, handling and treatment.

While in the outside flight, the occupants can shelter under the roofed area from hot sun or heavy rain or snow, but may choose to stay in the open area in fine weather or light showers.

The position of the aviary is important. If in a domestic garden, visibility from the house will allow better visual enjoyment, as well as improving security. Closed circuit television (CCTV) or an alarm system should be a major consideration. Screening from neighbours with a high hedge or fence is sensible, and the use of shrubbery bearing thorns will further deter intruders. Such screening will also provide protection against prevailing winds and rain. Space should be allowed for potential expansion.

Aviary construction should be appropriate to the species of bird. Most raptor and passerine aviaries are constructed of wood or combined wood and brick (Figure 3.4), and the same may be used for the smaller, less destructive parrot species. More destructive parrots, large macaws and large cockatoos may require completely brick-built, metal-framed aviaries or timber faced with metal sheets (Figures 3.5ab). The timber used should be treated with bird-safe preservative (Figure 3.5c).

Panels of aviary wire mesh attached to the framework prevent the birds from escaping. These are available in various gauges of wire thickness and wire spacing, and the keeper should choose a size and strength appropriate to the bird housed (Figure 3.6). The lower the gauge number, the thicker the wire used. Figure 3.7 gives a guide to the recommended sizes for various parrot species.

The quality of wire used is important. Using cheaper brands of galvanized wire, or housing large-beaked parrots in inappropriately small-gauge wire enclosures, introduces the potential for zinc poisoning. Stainless steel is the recommended – but most expensive – option. The risk of zinc poisoning may be reduced (but not eliminated) by washing down new panels of galvanized wire with a weak solution of vinegar and water, and then allowing the mesh to 'weather' in sun and rain, before allowing birds access. However, birds may still nibble at tags of the galvanized layer or the wire itself.

Birds of prey are often accommodated behind simple chain-link mesh or even nylon netting for smaller species (Figure 3.8). If such flights are accessible to visitors (e.g. in public collections), then a barrier will be required in front of the aviary to prevent direct bird–human contact. Adjacent aviaries should be double-wired – that is, there should be two sheets of wire mesh dividing each compartment, with a 5–7.5 cm gap between them. This will prevent birds attacking each other's feet while climbing the wire, which can be a particular problem during the breeding season. Some birds are better not seeing neighbours at all, in which case the flights should be divided with metal sheets or board fixed between the wire mesh.

The exposed fronts or ends of the aviaries should also be double-wired to prevent predator attack. Instances of passerines, parakeets and even birds as large as Grey and Amazon parrots being grasped through the wire by hawks, owls, foxes, cats or rats are common. Such cases may result in traumatic

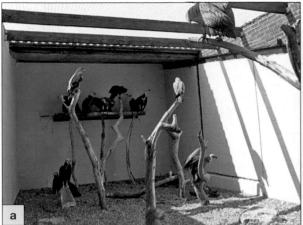

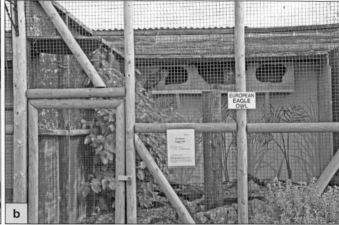

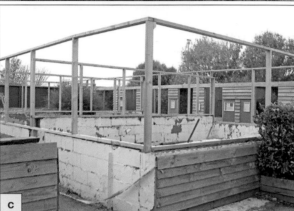

3.4 Raptor centre aviaries. **(a)** The wall of this eagle and vulture flight is painted blockwork; perching is provided by rocks, a wooden platform, and tree branches; the flooring is shingle; and the roof and front of the flight comprise simple wire mesh. Part of the roof is solid to provide some shelter above the wooden platform. This is a temporary holding area – this number of birds in an aviary this size would be considered overcrowded for permanent occupation. **(b)** An owl aviary comprising a simple wooden framework, with plastic-coated wire mesh; gravel floor with rocks and plants; and a roof part-covered at the back above the roosting boxes. A painted rear wall, and solid wood dividers between the flights, prevent interference with neighbouring birds.
(c) Renovation of old raptor aviaries. The existing blockwork walls are being clad with timber on the outside, while a wooden frame to support the wire mesh is built on top of the walls. Completed flights with labelling for visitor information are visible in the background.

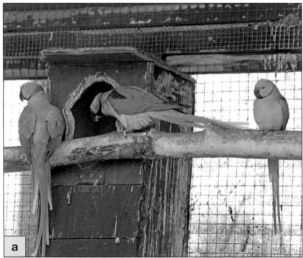

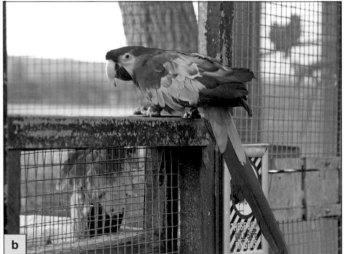

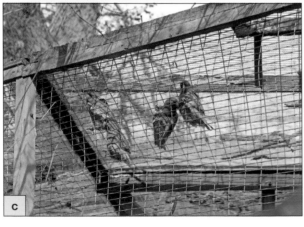

3.5 Choice of outdoor aviary materials is an important consideration. **(a)** Alexandrine Parakeets and a Ringnecked Parakeet showing the destruction these birds can do to timber. This flight is double-wired using the simpler (and cheaper) technique of a nylon mesh on the outside of the flight. **(b)** Scarlet Macaws in a timber-framed aviary, with metal facing on some wood to protect it from chewing and weathering. Note the swivel feeders to the right, allowing access to the food and water bowls from outside the aviary. **(c)** Tail-less Patagonian Conures in a wood and wire aviary that is in need of repair and renovation. There is no double-wiring or weather protection, and the timber is rotting and chewed.

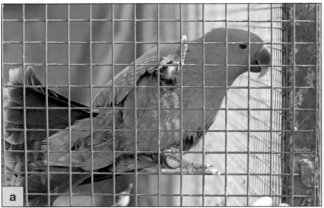 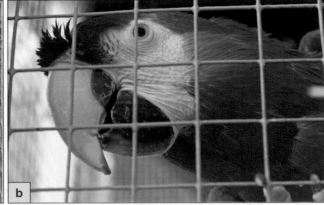

3.6 Choice of wire mesh gauge size should be made considering the species to be kept. **(a)** Male Eclectus Parrot in an all-metal aviary. **(b)** Scarlet Macaw clinging to metal weldmesh.

Wire gauge size (G)	Species
16	Small parakeets, Budgerigars and Cockatiels, most conures, lovebirds, rosellas
14	Larger parakeets, including ringnecks, pionus parrots, Amazon parrots, Grey Parrots, dwarf macaws, *Poicephalus* spp.
12	Larger macaws, most cockatoos
10	Hyacinth Macaws, Moluccan Cockatoos

3.7 Recommended wire gauge sizes for various species.

amputation (Figure 3.9a) or fatal haemorrhage. In this case, the outer layer of mesh does not need to be as substantial as the inner, since the birds' beaks will have no contact with it. A finer-gauge mesh, or even nylon netting, will suffice (Figure 3.9b).

For parrots, if resources allow and multiple birds are kept, it is a good idea to have a large communal flight (Figure 3.10). This will allow the birds to exercise and flock together, encouraging natural behaviour, including

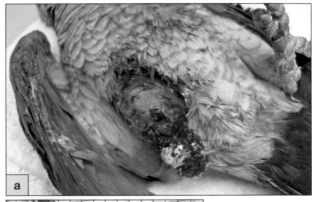

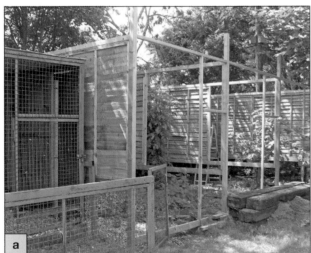

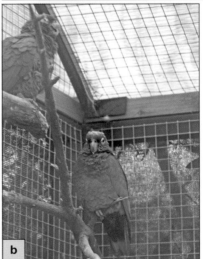

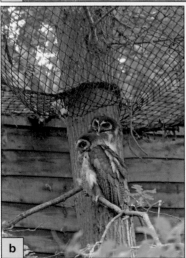

3.8 Materials for raptor aviaries. **(a)** The older aviaries on the left are of painted metal construction, with a gravel base; the newer timber constructions are supported on railway sleepers, and use fence panels as flight dividers. **(b)** A pair of Brown Wood Owls in a planted aviary. Simple soft netting is quite sufficient to keep these birds contained, as they do not chew wire unlike parrots.

3.9 Double-wiring of outdoor aviaries is recommended. **(a)** African Grey Parrot with traumatic amputation of its right leg following a predator attack (probably a fox) as it was clinging to the single layer of wire mesh around its aviary. **(b)** Maximilian Pionus in a timber-framed aviary, with metal roof supports, and natural wood branches for perching. External protection is provided in this case by simple nylon mesh, while the internal layer is standard weldmesh.

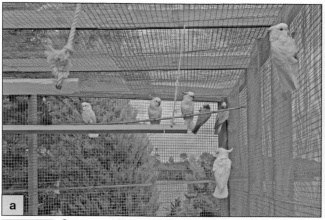
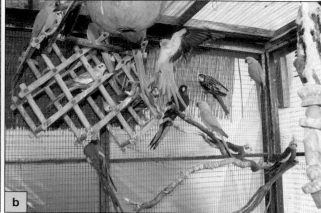

3.10   Communal flights. **(a)** A mixed group of cockatoos in a timber-framed exercise flight, with a variety of perches and double-wiring. **(b)** A variety of parakeets and Cockatiels in a timber-framed, double-wired aviary.

mutual preening. Young birds that have been bred or just recently acquired can grow together and learn social skills, and older birds may choose their own mates before being isolated in breeding aviaries.

A safety porch (Figure 3.11) is an essential feature of an aviary. It is too easy for a bird to fly out past the keeper if there is only one access door to the flight. This is especially true of swift-flying small passerines and aggressive parrots and raptors – particularly in the breeding season. Low-level doors that necessitate the owner crouching down to enter the aviary will reduce the risk, since birds are less likely to fly down so low to escape, but will not altogether negate it.

A bank of aviaries may have an access corridor along the back, allowing individual approach to each flight from within the corridor (Figure 3.12). The main door should be closed securely upon entering, and then any bird that escapes from its flight will be contained within the corridor. This system also makes

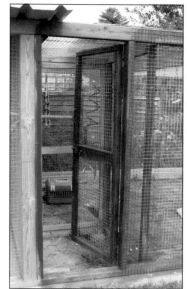

3.11   Access porch to the exercise flight, allowing closure of one door before the other is opened, to prevent birds escaping. An outward-opening door would have been preferable for ease of operation.

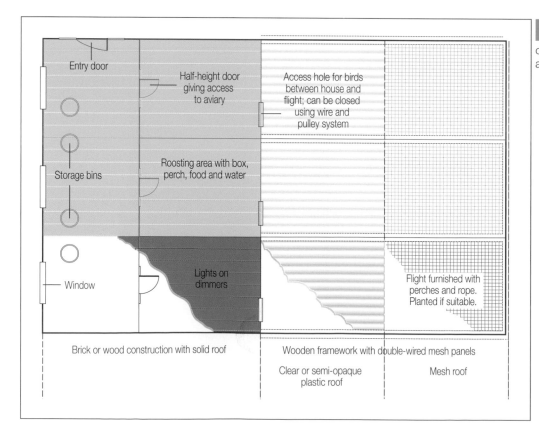

3.12   Plan of a bank of outdoor aviaries, featuring an access corridor.

Entry door

Half-height door giving access to aviary

Access hole for birds between house and flight; can be closed using wire and pulley system

Storage bins

Roosting area with box, perch, food and water

Window

Lights on dimmers

Flight furnished with perches and rope. Planted if suitable.

Brick or wood construction with solid roof

Wooden framework with double-wired mesh panels

Clear or semi-opaque plastic roof

Mesh roof

access for changing food and water and to clean each flight far easier than the alternative arrangement of having a single safety porch on the end of the bank of aviaries, with each flight then entered in turn from its predecessor. This latter set-up is more awkward (e.g. necessitates carrying multiple pieces of equipment through each flight) and poses a greater risk of disease transfer, as well as involving more disturbance to the birds.

Flooring

Bird keepers have a range of choices for flooring their aviaries. Bare earth or turf will allow natural foraging or digging activity for parrot species such as the Galah and other cockatoos and grass parakeets. However, intestinal parasites may be acquired or perpetuated in this way, as well as some infectious diseases. Birds kept in this manner should receive prophylactic worming treatments three to four times a year, or be subject to regular faecal screening for parasite eggs. Earth floors will also allow vermin such as rats to dig their way into the flight and injure or kill its occupants, unless the foundations are dug out and wire mesh is buried under the replaced soil.

Paving slabs (see Figure 3.3a) or concrete will prevent animals burrowing in and also make cleaning out easier – the surface may simply be swept over and hosed down. Solid floors should be laid on a slight slope to allow drainage of excess water.

Shingle (Figure 3.13a) is an excellent alternative: laid over a weed-suppressing membrane, it may be raked over and hosed down, making cleaning quick and easy. This is generally the substrate of choice for raptor aviaries. Some keepers use chipped bark; this has the same easy maintenance as shingle, but is notorious for harbouring potentially pathogenic fungal spores, especially when wet. Neither of these materials will prevent the ingress of rats, unless wire mesh is laid underneath the substrate.

Suspended flights are another alternative, although usually only for parrots (Figure 3.13b). Suspended flights allow waste food and droppings to pass through on to the ground underneath, where the birds cannot reach them, making hygiene and disease control very easy. However, access to retrieve a bird if required is difficult, as is the replacement of perches or other cage ornaments, especially if the flights are large. A trapdoor of mesh in the floor of the flight will enable the keeper to stand head and shoulders in the flight, which should not be so large as to prevent reaching all corners of the flight with a net, otherwise the bird will be uncatchable. Suspended flights are not suitable for birds that are natural ground foragers. It should also be noted that the wooden supports of suspended aviaries may still allow ingress of vermin; smooth metal legs or inverted cones may be required to prevent such invasion.

Perches and planting

The flight should be equipped with perches providing landing places for the birds to reach food, water and the entrance to the sheltered shed area, whilst still allowing the birds to fly the length of the flight without hindrance. Perches may be fixed rigidly to the wire mesh or the aviary framework, or they may be suspended on chains or ropes from the roof. Rope suspended as a loop makes a perfectly adequate perch (Figure 3.14a); however, the swallowing of fibres, which can lead to intestinal obstruction, is a potential hazard. Mobile perches provide more stimulation and exercise, and more closely mimic the living tree branches that birds would use in the wild. Large raptors often prefer a wooden platform (Figure 3.14b) or tree trunk.

In general, most types of wood are safe for birds of prey and passerines, which do not chew at their environment. However, non-toxic wood must be used for perches (and aviary framework) for inquisitive and destructive parrot species. Hazel, birch, chestnut, sycamore, maple, eucalyptus (Figure 3.15a), and any untreated fruit tree branches are all suitable. Willow, mallow, elder and buddleia are also suitable and, because they regenerate swiftly after cutting, are more environmentally sustainable. Branches should be scrubbed clean (e.g. of bird droppings, lichen and moss), disinfected and cut to size to fit the flight (Jones, 2011).

Actively toxic plants such as yew, laburnum and lilac should not be used. Care should also be taken with

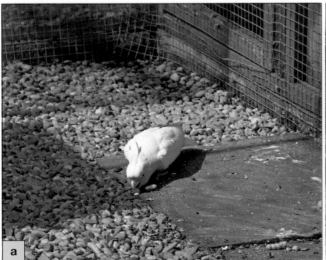
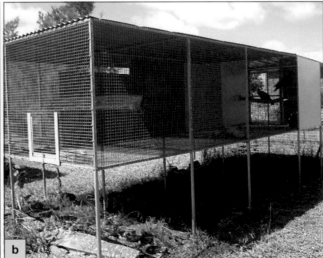

3.13 Flooring options for outdoor aviaries. **(a)** A Major Mitchell's Cockatoo foraging on the floor of its aviary. The substrate is a combination of gravel and paving slabs. Ground-feeding birds are at greater risk of intestinal parasites than are those that feed in trees and shrubs. **(b)** Suspended flights prevent the build-up of waste food and droppings, but make access to the birds difficult. (b, courtesy of RJ Doneley)

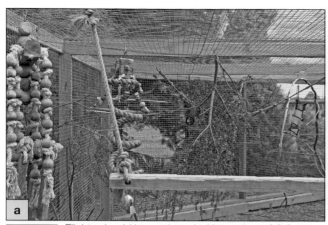
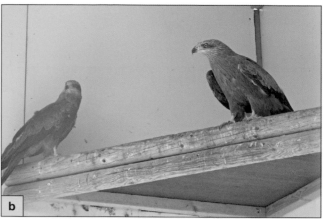

3.14 Flights should be equipped with perches. **(a)** Communal exercise flight, with a variety of perches and hanging toys. **(b)** Black Kites using a corner shelf in their flight. The walls are covered with melamine-faced board, for seclusion and ease of cleaning.

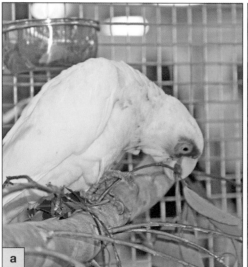
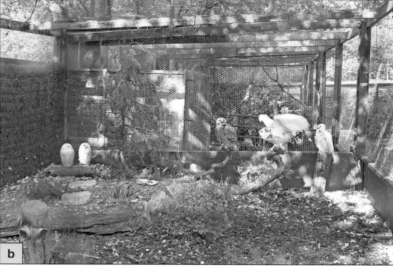

3.15 Planting of aviaries. **(a)** Long-billed Corella enjoying a perch made of a fresh eucalyptus branch. **(b)** A family of Snowy Owls in a semi-planted aviary of wood and simple wire mesh construction. The rear wall is covered with a reed screen, and the aviary floor is a combination of chipped bark and shingle. Note: that chipped bark is a potential source of *Aspergillus* spp., and could be a problem if used with species susceptible to aspergillosis, such as Gyrfalcons or Grey Parrots.

oak and beech because of the tannins in their bark, and pine trees because of their high resin content. Sawn pine off-cuts (where the bark has been removed) from a timber merchant are safe as long as they have not been treated with a chemical preservative.

Larger raptors rarely require much in the way of planting in their aviaries, but owls and small falcons will often benefit from some evergreen planting (Figure 3.15b). When breeding, freshly cut twigs or brushwood should be offered for nest building. Large owls generally lay their eggs in a simple scrape in the ground (Figure 3.16).

Planting of aviaries for parrots is contentious. Most parrots will rapidly destroy anything that is growing within the flight; however, some planting will not only improve the aesthetic appearance of the flight, but will also give the birds physical stimulation. Rapidly growing and regenerating trees or shrubs such as willow, elder, mallow or buddleia may survive the onslaught. Alternatively, shrubs may be planted outside the wire so that the birds can eat only the branches that grow through, and are not able to destroy the whole plant. Rapidly growing non-toxic climbing plants such as *Polygonum* spp. may be used in the same way. Trees

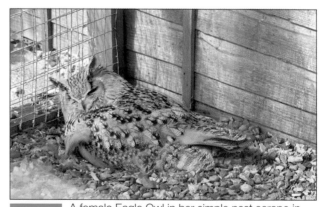

3.16 A female Eagle Owl in her simple nest scrape in shingle in the corner of her flight.

and shrubs provide shade, shelter and stimulation for birds; however, they may also provide an opportunity for ticks to reach the birds (see below). An alternative option is to plant tubs or pots, and move these in rotation in and out of the flights, giving them time to recover and regenerate on the outside. Old branches, tree trunks, barrels and boxes will also keep parrots occupied for hours.

Maintenance

Daily maintenance tasks should include an inspection of the birds. The aviary should be checked for signs of damage by its occupants, vermin or the weather. Food and water need to be replaced daily (or more frequently in hot weather) and bowls washed and disinfected. All birds must always have fresh water available, and this is usually supplied to raptors in broad, shallow bowls (Figure 3.17). This requirement should be emphasized to raptor keepers.

Weekly tasks include checking for signs of vermin; raking over or hosing down the floor of the aviary; and cleaning and replacement or repair of perches. Unlike their wild counterparts, captive birds perch on the same branches day after day, resulting in an accumulation of waste food and droppings that are not exposed to heavy rainfall and microbe-killing ultraviolet light.

Annual maintenance may include the replacement or repair of nest boxes; treating woodwork with bird-safe preservative; replacing worn locks, hinges or window fasteners; pruning any overgrown plants; renewing shingle or bark on the floor; and checking the integrity of roofing materials.

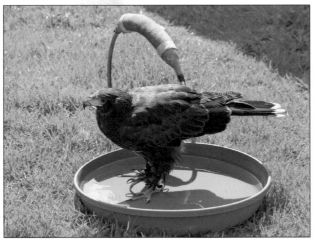

3.17 Harris' Hawk in front of its bow perch, standing in a shallow tray of water, used for drinking and bathing.

Indoor

Most pet parrots, parakeets and passerines are housed indoors with their keepers. This enables the keeper to watch and/or interact with their bird for a greater part of the day. Keeping birds indoors has associated advantages and disadvantages (see Figure 3.1); indoor birds are protected from the elements, predators and the risk of theft is reduced, in addition to the benefit that the bird and its behaviour can be observed at close range (Jones, 2011).

Cages

Birds that are going to spend most of their lives indoors should be provided with as large an area as can be afforded and accommodated in the house. In some cases bird keepers set aside a whole room for their birds (Figure 3.18a), or an 'indoor aviary' is built into an alcove. Most will be kept in cages for at least a portion of the day (Figure 3.18b). The selection of cage type follows many of the criteria involved with building aviaries. It should be appropriate in size, strength and wire gauge for the species of bird and the number of occupants. It should also be manoeuvrable and easily dismantled for cleaning and maintenance. Cages on wheels or castors are therefore easier to manage than those with plain legs (Figure 3.18c). The bird can then be moved from room to room with its owners or out into the garden or conservatory for a change of scenery. Simple but strong construction, with ease of access to the bird, perches and bowls, is paramount. There is a plethora of styles and shapes on the market. Ornate and fancy curlicues such as those favoured in the Victorian era look attractive, but their design creates danger points where birds may get their toes or other extremities trapped. Having selected a type of cage appropriate to the bird(s), the final choice will depend on how it fits in the home and the owner's personal preference of colour and material. The choice of bird and consideration of its needs should be the primary criteria for the choice of cage (Jones, 2011).

The bird's home cage is its primary dwelling where it may be left safe and secure while the owners are out,

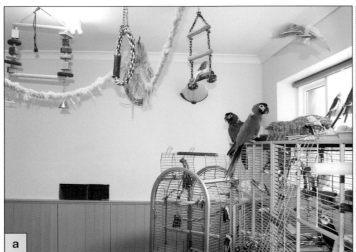
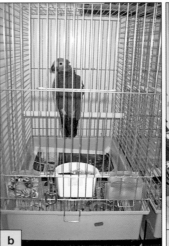
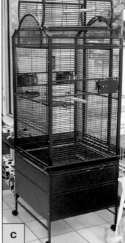

3.18 Examples of indoor housing and cages. **(a)** Room given over to housing a collection of birds, including Cockatiels, Budgerigars and Yellow-naped Macaws. This allows the birds considerable freedom and ample opportunity to exercise, but must be weighed against the potential difficulties of maintaining hygiene standards and controlling the spread of infectious diseases. **(b)** Young African Grey Parrot in a simple cage in a pet store. This size of cage would clearly not be sufficient for long-term housing of such a bird. **(c)** Powder-coated metal indoor cage, incorporating an opening top to allow some freedom and play; swivel feeders to enable access to bowls from outside the cage; 'skirts' to catch discarded food; useful drawer storage at the base; and castors on the legs to facilitate movement.

but a second, smaller cage may be used as a spare while the home cage is cleaned, as a 'night cage' for sleeping or as a garden cage (Figure 3.19a). A useful adjunct would be a play-stand or foraging tree, on which the bird can spend time playing, exercising and puzzle-solving, under supervision (Figure 3.19b). Finally, it may also be worth considering a travel carrier, to make transporting the bird to the veterinary clinic or holiday boarding easier (Figure 3.19c).

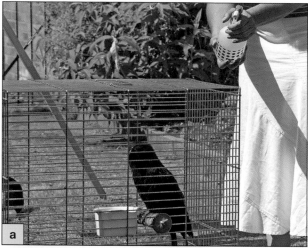

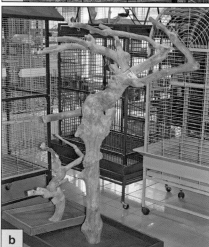

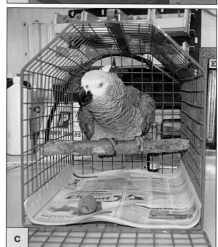

3.19 (a) Female Eclectus Parrot enjoying being sprayed with warm water out in the fresh air of the garden, but safely secured in a transport cage. (b) Large and small play-stands made from hard Java wood mounted on a wooden tray, in front of a variety of indoor cages. (c) African Grey Parrot at a veterinary clinic in a small plastic-coated wire pet carrier with a simple wooden perch.

Maintenance

Pet indoor birds are restricted to a comparatively small area, and keepers have a duty of care to their birds to prevent the build-up of waste food and excretions in order to minimize the risk of infection.

The cage or play-stand base may be lined with cat litter, dried corn waste, compressed paper granules, wood, bark chippings or sawdust. However, birds with free access to the substrate frequently scatter these materials around the room. Chipped bark is also a common source of disease-causing fungal spores, especially when damp, so is best avoided. The simplest option is to cover the base with several layers of old newspaper sheets (Figure 3.20). The top page may be removed each day, taking with it the discarded debris and droppings, and leaving the next clean sheet. Lories or lorikeets, which have liquid droppings, will require the removal of several sheets of paper, or the use of a more absorbent material. Some cages have a grid floor above the base tray, which allows waste food and droppings to pass through (Figure 3.20a), preventing the bird reaching discarded food and thus reducing the risk of potential contamination. This is a good idea in principle, but wasteful of food: most parrots will sort through their food bowls, searching for favourite items and evicting the rest, but will return to the discarded items later in the day. There is also the potential danger of feet or wings getting caught in the grid, especially if the bird panics for some reason.

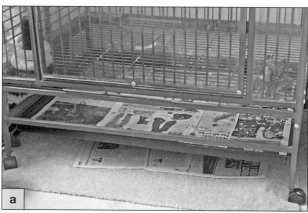

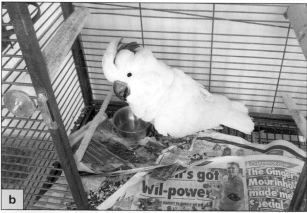

3.20 (a) Indoor metal cage on castors, with a lower tray covered with newspaper that is removable for cleaning. Above this is a metal grid, which allows waste food and droppings to fall through to the paper below, but also slides out for ease of cleaning. (b) Moluccan Cockatoo guarding his 'nest area' and shiny food bowl 'chick' on the newspaper-lined floor of his cage. Note how the lower wooden perch has been chewed to matchwood, and the rear bars of the cage have been bent and removed by this bird's powerful beak.

Once a week, the whole cage, tray and perches should be dismantled, washed thoroughly with soapy water, rinsed, dried and replaced. Plastic, wood or metal toys should be treated in the same way, cardboard is simply thrown away, while rope toys may be washed and dried (Jones, 2011).

Food and water bowls

These should be cleaned thoroughly every day. Many parrots will drop their food in their drinking water, and inappropriately placed perches result in contamination of bowls with droppings (Figure 3.21a). Fruits and vegetables deteriorate rapidly in warm weather, and accumulated waste food and droppings will rapidly form a rich culture medium for pathogenic bacteria and fungi. All birds must always have fresh water available.

The need for daily cleaning and replenishing of food and water bowls has led to a variety of designs intended to make access easy. The simple plastic D-cup (Figure 3.21b) hooks over horizontal bars or wires. Their removal necessitates opening the cage or aviary, and they are also easily removed by playful parrots. The plastic may split, crack, or become scratched and will be difficult to sterilize properly.

Stainless steel coop cups (Figures 3.21cd) are similarly suspended, but are more robust and generally easier to keep clean. The holding brackets may be wired to the cage to make them more difficult for the birds to remove. Some cages have a gap designed to receive a hard plastic cup (Figure 3.21e) that is then secured in place using a clip on the outside of the cage (the same comments about sterilization and cleaning apply as with the D-cup).

The final choice, especially useful in larger cages or aviaries, is a rotating mechanism whereby access to the bowls is achieved by rotating the holder from outside the cage (Figure 3.21f). Bowls may be removed, cleaned, replenished and replaced, and are usually locked in position, before rotating the holding mechanism back inside the cage.

Husbandry-related disease

Only a minority of avian disease conditions are caused by infectious agents. By far the biggest factors causing birds to become sick or die are poor diet (discussed in Chapter 6) and bad husbandry.

Outdoor birds

Feather condition

It is generally true that outdoor birds have much better quality plumage than indoor birds. There is typically more sheen to the feathers, with brighter, more vivid colours. This is a reflection of the general health benefits of more exercise, fresh air, soaking with rainwater and exposure to sunlight. The ultraviolet wavelengths in sunlight are essential for the synthesis of vitamin D in the skin and the preen gland (where present). Birds kept indoors have the same requirement, and if kept permanently inside will eventually suffer 'sunlight deficiency'. In parrot species, feather destructive disorders are a major problem in avian veterinary practice, but are less commonly encountered in parrots that are kept outside in aviaries compared with indoor birds. However, moving an indoor pet bird to an outdoor aviary because it plucks is not an accepted line of treatment.

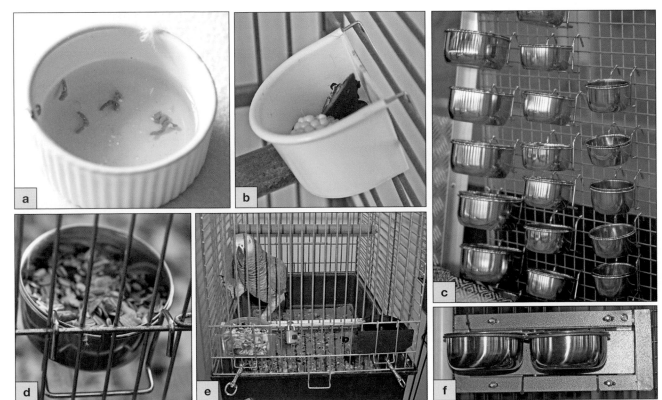

3.21 Food and water bowl options. **(a)** Water bowl contaminated with bird droppings because it was situated on the cage floor under a perch. **(b)** Simple plastic 'D-cup' containing pomegranate and sweetcorn clipped over the wire of a cage. **(c)** Stainless steel 'coop cups' in various sizes for holding food and water. **(d)** Stainless steel 'coop cup' containing parrot mix, clipped simply over the horizontal bars of a cage. **(e)** African Grey Parrot in a holding cage in a pet store; the plastic food and water dishes are held in their designed openings with spring clips, with additional security provided by dog clips. **(f)** 'Swivel feeder' mounted mailbox-style on the side of a cage. It rotates around its vertical central spindle, allowing access to the bowls from outside the cage or aviary.

External parasites

Outdoor birds are more likely to acquire external para-sites from wild bird species than are protected indoor varieties. Further detail on parasitology is given in Chapter 19, but organisms encountered include feather lice, mites and ticks. The latter are a particular problem in areas where hedgehogs, sheep and rabbits are present, and where vegetation is allowed to grow close to or overhang the aviary. Control of this problem depends on the prevention of birds from interacting with carriers (e.g. using an outer mesh or nylon net) and removal of overgrown vegetation from around the flight.

Internal parasites

These include protozoa and coccidia, although they tend to be less of a problem in parrots than in passer-ines and raptors. *Trichomonas* sp. causes canker in pigeons or frounce in birds of prey and is also com-monly found in Budgerigars, resulting in chronic vomit-ing and weight loss, similar to macrorhabdosis. For more information see Chapter 19. Roundworms are very common, especially in ground-feeding birds such as grass parakeets and some cockatoos. They may be passed in the droppings, and are 2–3 cm long, taper-ing at both ends.

Bacteria, viruses and fungi

Housing birds outdoors will allow the spread of infec-tious agents from wild birds and rodents. Common viral infections include avian poxvirus in raptors (from wild birds of prey and pigeons) and paramyxovirus in small parakeets (from pigeons and doves), and possibly avian bornavirus in larger parrots. Avian chlamydiosis (psitta-cosis) may be acquired from pigeons or ducks, while rodents may spread *Mycobacterium* spp., *Yersinia* spp. and other bacteria including *Salmonella* spp. and *Escherichia coli*. Fungal infections may be associated with chipped bark bedding or generally damp, unhy-gienic conditions; *Candida* spp. may be acquired from spoiled fruits and vegetables.

Injury

Attack by predators such as wild birds of prey, foxes, cats, stoats or rats may result in injury, hence double-wiring of aviaries is recommend. Snakes or predatory lizards may be a problem in some countries. Severe storms and strong winds can result in flooding or destruction of flights from falling branches or trees, injuring the inhabitants or enabling their escape. Care should be taken to shield electrical appliances or cables to reduce the risk of electrocution (Figure 3.22).

Poisoning

The ingestion of poisonous plants or fungi growing in or close to the aviary may result in poisoning; this is espe-cially common in inquisitive species such as parrots and parakeets. Zinc poisoning from galvanized wire has already been mentioned above. Smoke from plastic or rubber being burned on nearby bonfires will rapidly affect birds' respiratory systems, while insecticides or weed killers sprayed too close to the aviaries are also dangerous to avian species.

Indoor birds

The majority of diseases affecting indoor captive birds are related to husbandry and diet. Parrots particularly, are potentially long-lived, and long-term

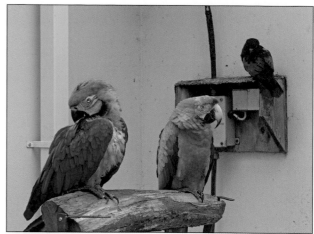

3.22 Macaws free-living outside at a public bird garden in the UK. The exposed electrical junction box is a potential hazard.

imbalances or deficiencies in their diet will manifest as fatty liver and kidney disease, obesity, poor feather condition, gout, hypocalcaemia and hypovitaminosis A, chronic recurrent secondary infections, and over-growth of beaks and claws. These conditions are cov-ered in more detail in Chapter 6.

Feather condition

Most human homes have a warm, dry atmosphere, but most parrots come from areas of high natural rainfall, and an arid atmosphere is damaging to their plumage. All passerine species bathe regularly in ponds, streams or puddles, or in rain showers. It is therefore important not to site the bird's cage too close to a radiator or other heat source. Humidifiers should be used and birds should be sprayed or bathed with clean warm water three to four times a week to keep the plumage in good condition (Figure 3.23a). In the summer months, this frequency may be increased to daily, or even several times a day. In addition, birds will benefit from having some time in a cage outdoors or in an outside flight (see Figure 3.19a).

Many of the feather problems seen in parrots are the result of prolonged dry-heat damage and insuffi-cient moisture on their plumage. Parrots will attempt to bathe in their water bowls – this is an indication that the bird is desperate for a bath. They will particularly indulge in this behaviour when there are loud noises/vibrations present (e.g. the vacuum cleaner or high-volume music). This is thought to be an instinctive reac-tion; in the wild, parrots are accustomed to tropical rainstorms and the associated noise of thunder, plus rain drumming on foliage. At these times, parrots will expect to get wet, and will spread their wings and hang upside down. Amazons especially will behave in this way when sprayed (Jones, 2011).

Bacteria, viruses and fungi

Infectious diseases tend to spread more rapidly when birds are housed indoors, because of the confined communal air space. Enteric and respiratory bacteria and viruses, and *Chlamydia psittaci*, spread rapidly in a housed collection. Single pet birds are less likely to suffer from infectious disease, unless they are mixed with other birds at times of holiday boarding or at bird shows, or they are acquired carrying an infectious agent with a long incubation period (e.g. psittacine

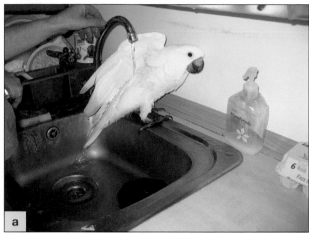

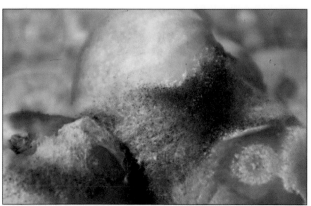

3.23 **(a)** Umbrella Cockatoo bathing under a tap. Regular bathing is essential for the healthy maintenance of birds' plumage. **(b)** This Sulphur-crested Cockatoo shows mild signs of feather destructive disorder, with contour feathers self-removed from the chest and abdomen. The damage that can be done if allowed unsupervised freedom is also shown.

beak and feather disease (PBFD, circovirus) or proventricular dilatation disease (PDD, avian bornavirus)).

Fungal diseases, such as aspergillosis (Figure 3.24), are common in confined indoor environments, especially where there is damp or heavy condensation, or birds are weakened by poor diet, irritation of the respiratory system by inhaled fumes, or underlying infections. Candidiasis is commonly encountered in fledgling birds being hand-reared, and may result from poor hygiene, dietary deficiency, overuse of antibiotics, a weakened immune system or, in the case of parrot chicks, feeding a formula when it is too hot.

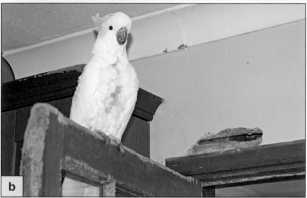

3.24 *Aspergillus* mould growing on peaches. Each of the black pinpoints arising from the grey hyphae is a conidium containing hundreds of minute fungal spores, which if inhaled may lead to serious aspergillosis in birds.

Foot problems

Simple smooth dowelling perches will lead to foot problems, exacerbated by arthritis and an unbalanced diet. Perches should be available in a variety of textures and diameters, and should include natural wood with bark on.

Circadian rhythm

Housed birds are usually subjected to an artificial extension of their day. Most parrots come from tropical or subtropical latitudes, and as such are adapted to an approximately 12-hour cycle of night and day. In a busy household, with family members rising early for school or work, but not retiring to bed until late at night, the bird may be exposed year-round to an unnaturally long day. This can cause stress and is a potential factor in the common problem of feather destructive disorder and other irritable behaviours.

This disruption to the bird's circadian rhythm may be compensated for in part by quiet periods during the day, when all humans are out of the house. In fact, this may even approximate the natural diurnal pattern of the wild parrot, which is active and feeding at dawn and dusk, but quiet and resting during the heat of the day. The bird's cage may also be covered in the evening to allow it to sleep before its owners do, although if left in the same room, most birds will not fully relax. It is therefore worth considering putting the bird in a night cage in a quiet room. However, most working owners will want to spend these few hours in the evening having contact with their pet.

Household hazards

There are many potential dangers for a bird in the average household. Parrots are inquisitive, and notorious chewers, and will investigate telephone cables and power leads (Figure 3.25). They will eat the leaves of houseplants, so poisonous varieties should not be kept anywhere near birds. Building plaster, paintwork and metal objects are all possible sources of danger. Quality curtains may have lead sewn in their lower hems to weigh them down, and curious birds may pick out this metal and swallow it.

Other pets in the household may at best be a nuisance to the indoor bird, but at worst they could seriously injure or kill it. However, the majority of dogs and cats will learn a healthy respect for birds once they have experienced the power of a large parrot beak or the talons of a raptor.

Perhaps the most serious of household hazards relates to toxic fumes. Birds have a highly efficient respiratory system in order to absorb the extra oxygen needed to power flight muscles (see Chapter 2), but any gas will be rapidly absorbed – not just oxygen. Therefore any noxious material in the air of the home will affect birds. Cigarette smoke, scented candles, incense burners, open fires, aerosol sprays – all will cause irritation to birds' lungs and air sacs, and chronic exposure can result in permanent damage. Affected birds will experience episodes of dyspnoea and may be predisposed to serious secondary infections such as aspergillosis.

The mostly deadly of toxic fumes are those associated with cooking. Overheated cooking oil releases a blue smoke that will rapidly cause a bird to gasp and choke, so caution must be exercised when using deep fat fryers and heating woks. Domestic irons, self-cleaning ovens that work at high temperatures, new

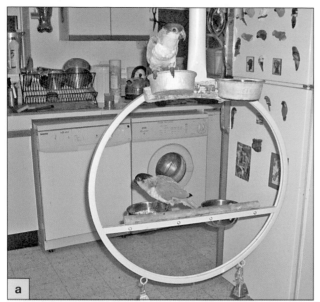

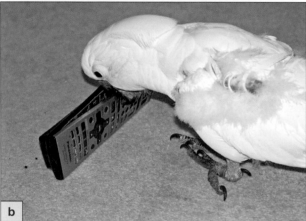

3.25 **(a)** Black-headed Caiques on a play-stand in a domestic kitchen. Such a room is full of potential dangers to birds (see text). **(b)** Umbrella Cockatoo destroying a TV remote control. The metal and plastic, as well as the batteries, in this instrument are a serious risk to birds.

grill pans and Teflon®-coated saucepans will all, if over-heated or allowed to burn dry, release toxic fumes that may make humans cough and their eyes run, but will kill a parrot in minutes. Birds that were hitherto healthy will suddenly start to gasp and cough, then collapse on the floor with wings spread, and die very quickly. Post-mortem examination in these cases reveals a distinctive bright cherry-red colour to the lungs, as the lung tissue is invaded with red blood cells.

The home can be a dangerous place for birds, so it is incumbent upon all bird keepers to take good care of their charges, and for veterinary personnel to be aware of such risk factors and to advise proactively.

Ethical considerations

Consideration must be given to the species kept, and possible interactions between them. Maintaining pred-ator species like raptors adjacent to prey species like passerines would be stressful for all concerned. Many parrots and parakeets flock in larger social groups for most of the year, but during the breeding season they split away in breeding pairs. Some species will become fiercely territorial of their chosen nest site, while others are happy to nest communally.

There is also no doubt that certain species are better kept in larger aviaries rather than small cages. Active flying and climbing birds like parrots and para-keets require space to move around and behave as naturally as possible. Small passerines fly continually from the nest or roost to feed and drink, and require the protection and seclusion of vegetation. Hence, they are better maintained (more 'naturally') in a planted aviary rather than a bare, limiting cage (Figure 3.26). For show and exhibition, show cages are acceptable (and many are tastefully decorated with plants and natural wood), but these are only ever intended as temporary accommodation for the few hours of the exhibition, and the birds should be returned to their more spacious aviaries as soon as possible.

The keeping of birds in captivity is an ancient prac-tice, but it is controversial. The idea of confining birds is anathema to many people. This section considers reasons why birds are kept in captivity and the ethical considerations of which keepers should be aware.

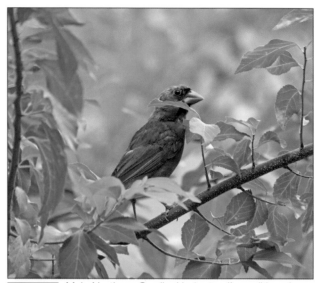

3.26 Male Northern Cardinal in 'natural' conditions in a planted aviary.

Falconry

As dogs and horses became domesticated to aid in the hunting of living prey, somewhere along the way humans also started using birds of prey. These raptors were tethered and used for controlled hunting of smaller birds to provide a meal for the humans, in return for which the birds were protected and given food. Thus began the development of falconry, a prac-tice that continues worldwide, although the keeping of birds of prey has widened beyond hunting to include conservation and education, breeding and hobby fly-ing. In a similar way, birds such as cormorants are used to catch fish for human consumption in Asia.

Modern falconry is widely popular in Europe, Asia and North America. Its status as a sport of the noble classes in mediaeval times is to a large extent retained in the Middle East, while in the Western world it is far less so. Many of the terms used in falconry reflect its ancient origins and there is still much tradition and folk-lore attached to the hobby; items such as jesses, hoods and bow perches all still feature in modern fal-conry (Figure 3.27).

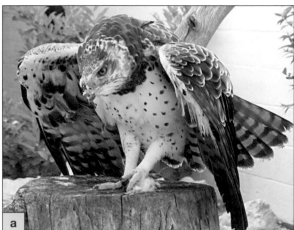
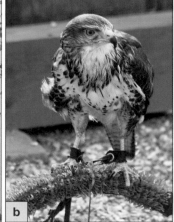
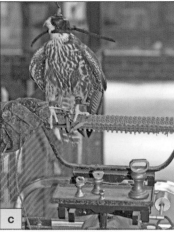

3.27 Many falconry terms reflect its ancient origins, such as 'tiercel' for a male falcon (a third smaller than females) and 'mews' for housing (from the French *muer*, to shed feathers). **(a)** Captive Martial Eagle 'mantling' its prey (shielding the prey with its wings). **(b)** Red-tailed Hawk tethered to a bow perch, which is in turn covered with artificial grass. Note the leather jesses, threaded through anklets on each leg, and attached to a tether. **(c)** Falcon on a perch mounted on weighing scales. Note the leather anklets and jesses, attached to a leash, which is in turn held by the falconer's leather glove (which gave rise to the phrase 'wrapped around his little finger', meaning to be under his control). The weights used are old-fashioned brass imperial measures, still used by most falconers, rather than using modern metric and digital scales. The bird wears a leather hood to keep it calm.

With regard to raptors, there is a fundamental debate about the ethics of using one animal to pursue and kill another. Raptors used for hunting are kept 'keen' by reducing food intake so that they remain hungry and therefore desire to hunt (Scott, 2008). At rest, many raptors are kept tethered to a perch (Figure 3.27b), another source of contention. In nature, such birds spend a minimum of time flying (e.g. to find food, a mate or a nesting site), since flight is such an energy-intensive process. For the rest of the day the birds perch in safety, preening and resting. Thus, a tethered bird is probably no less active than it would be in nature, but a high degree of care is required of the falconer to cater for its needs and protect against injury.

Showing

Many small parakeets, including Budgerigars, and passerine species (particularly canaries and finches), are involved in shows and exhibitions. There are numerous clubs and societies dedicated to this aspect of bird keeping, and considerable value can be attached to successful birds that win prize money. Such birds will be maintained in home aviaries or bird-rooms, as described above, but require transport carriers (see Chapter 9) for journeys over often long distances, as well as display cages for the exhibition (Figure 3.28). The latter are generally well maintained, furnished and displayed, but the conditions during transport are less well monitored. Birds may be confined for several days while being transported to the show, put on display for judging and exhibition for up to 3 days, followed by transport home again. Attention must be paid to their welfare during these periods, with ample food and water supplied. Extra vitamin supplements and/or probiotics are commonly used by owners to boost the birds during this time. However, it is debatable whether such action has any value provided the birds are fed and consume a properly balanced diet. Equally, birds that receive a diet that is seriously deficient or unbalanced in macronutrients are unlikely to be assisted significantly by the addition of a supplement in the drinking water.

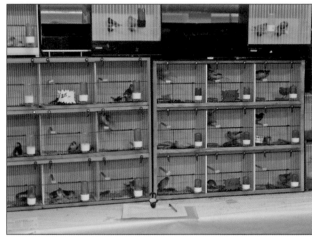

3.28 A selection of Zebra Finches and canaries in exhibition cages, awaiting judging at a bird show.

Pets

In the Western world, concern about the ethics of keeping birds such as parrots in cages as pets has led to a range of legislation governing cage sizes (see 'Regulations in bird keeping'). Minimum requirements are that a bird should be free to extend its wings completely in all directions – height, length and breadth – in the cage; however, it is unlikely that this minimum standard can offer enough enrichment for active birds (Figure 3.29a). Indoor pet parrots should have the largest cage area available to them, or an open 'play area' with time out of confinement (Figure 3.29b).

Wing clipping of indoor pet parrots is a contentious issue. It is discussed in more detail in Chapter 15, but a summary of the advantages and disadvantages is given in Figure 3.30.

Conservation and education

There is no doubt that many captive birds, provided their husbandry and diet are managed properly, will live longer and produce more young than their wild counterparts, as they are protected from predation and removed

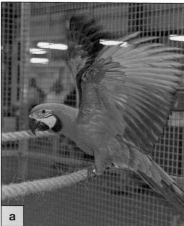

3.29 **(a)** Juvenile Blue and Gold Macaw on a rope perch in a display aviary, spreading its wings to show its magnificent colouring. These birds have a wingspan of around 120 cm. **(b)** Three young Amazon parrots on a Java wood play-stand, with a Galah on its cage, in a 'baby bird room' at a pet store. Customers may view the birds through the glass windows to the left, but are not allowed direct access to the birds unless genuinely interested, and only then with a staff member. This helps to reduce the risk of escape, customer injury and the spread of infection to the birds.

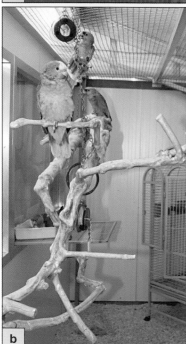

Advantages

- Bird is allowed to roam outside its cage without risk of it flying away
- Less damage to home
- Reduces risk of injury to the bird
- Taming is easier
- Temporary
- Useful for controlling mate aggression (clip cock bird to allow hen to escape)

Disadvantages

- Bird is unable to exercise fully
- Falling off items carries risk of crash landing and injury
- Birds are often more nervous
- Greater risk of feather destructive disorder
- Requires some level of expertise to clip correctly

3.30 Advantages and disadvantages of wing clipping of indoor parrots. Note that Jones (2011) recommends that young birds should be allowed to develop flying and landing expertise, and full pectoral musculature, before being clipped.

from competition for nest sites and food. This has a bearing in conservation projects for the maintenance and breeding of endangered species whose numbers in the natural environment are threatened. Conservation efforts have brought species such as the Scarlet, Blue-throated and Lear's Macaws back from the brink of

extinction in selected areas, and enabled repopulation back to the wild, where suitable 'safe' areas exist.

An extension of this aspect of bird keeping is educational. Thousands of people are given the opportunity to see birds of prey, fascinating songbirds and entertaining parrots that they would otherwise never see in nature, through visiting public collections and zoos (Figure 3.31a). Educational visits by students, seminars and meetings, and flying displays (Figure 3.31b) held at such centres all serve to bring to the attention of a wider public the biology, lifestyles, behaviour and plight in the wild of these fascinating creatures (Figure 3.31c).

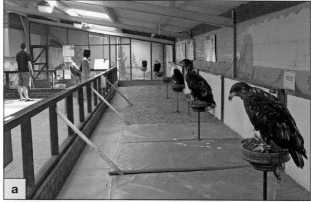

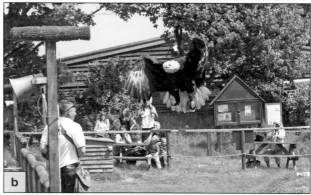

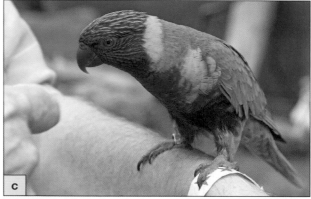

3.31 **(a)** Display of vultures and eagles in a raptor centre. Note the barriers to prevent public access to the birds; floor coverings of mixed concrete, shingle and washable plastic-coated pads; the block perches to which the birds are tethered; and the informative signage. **(b)** American Bald Eagle flying to an artificial grass-covered T-perch during a flying display at a raptor centre. The falconer wears a shoulder bag containing food items with which to reward the bird. Such centres provide excellent opportunities for people to get close to and observe these birds and their behaviour. **(c)** Rainbow Lorikeet in a walk-through aviary. These birds are accustomed to human contact, probably through hand-rearing, and allow the public to get close-up. Note the stainless steel identity ring (band) on the bird's right leg.

Breeding

Many species kept by humans have changed significantly over the centuries. Poultry provide a prime example, with a wide variety of breeds and sizes now developed from the original jungle fowl. Pigeons and doves, ducks and geese have been similarly developed. Ornamental and hobby types have also been affected, especially those that mature early and breed quickly, such as the Budgerigar and Zebra Finch. The native wild Budgerigar is a small green bird, but generations of selective breeding for exhibition have changed this popular parakeet into a much larger bird, occurring in a wide variety of colours (Figure 3.32a). The Zebra and Gouldian Finches also now have a range of colour varieties.

The trend continues with many captive parakeets and passerine species. Rare naturally occurring colour mutations such as albinism or lutino varieties are mated back to parents or siblings to perpetuate these recessive colours. In their natural environment, such individuals usually do not survive very long because they are easily spotted by predators, or are ostracized by their own kind and thus unable to breed. However, in captivity these varieties are highly prized, and command higher prices than their 'normal' counterparts (until the colour variant becomes widespread) (Figure 3.32b). Modifications to feather size and quality have also been developed, in Budgerigars and poultry particularly.

However, achievement of these modifications is often the result of inbreeding to hasten the perpetuation of the chosen genes. Inbreeding also concentrates less favourable characteristics, so such selective breeding comes with attendant reduction in immunity and health. Inbred individuals are genetically not as robust.

There are instances where the original nominate species are now rare. The Splendid Parakeet is now endangered in the wild, yet many thousands of mutation colours and varieties exist within aviculture, to the point where species enthusiasts find it difficult to find a 'normal' Splendid (Figure 3.32c). Even individuals that have apparently normal colouring carry mutation genes, and will not breed true.

However, this extent of modification has not extended to the species of birds that have been associated with man for centuries – birds of prey. Although some species are hybridized (Peregrine Falcons with Saker or Lanner Falcons, for example), and there are natural colour morphs found amongst Gyrfalcons, the development of colour or plumage mutations has not been excessively developed by the falconry fraternity.

Regulations in bird keeping

At the time of writing, there are several Acts and Orders within the UK appertaining to the keeping of birds in captivity. These include the Wildlife and Countryside Act 1981, the Pet Animals Act, the Animal Welfare Act, the Zoo Licensing Act, and the Performing Animals Act; as well as the Diseases of Poultry Order, the Zoonoses Order, and the Psittacosis or Ornithosis Order, among others (Scott, 2008). The Balai Directive controls the movement and quarantine of birds within member states of the European Union (EU). Other countries will have their own equivalent legislation, with full current details available online.

Of greater importance internationally is the Convention on International Trade in Endangered Species (of wild fauna and flora), usually abbreviated to CITES (Scott, 2008). The Convention was drafted as a result of a resolution adopted in 1963 at a meeting of members of the International Union for Conservation of Nature (IUCN). The text of the Convention was finally agreed at a meeting of representatives of 80 countries in Washington, DC, USA, on 3 March 1973, and on 1 July 1975 CITES entered into force (www.cites.org). Hence, it is alternatively known as the Washington Convention.

CITES is an international agreement to which States (countries) adhere voluntarily. States that have agreed to be bound by the Convention (CITES members) are known as Parties. Although CITES is legally binding on the Parties – in other words they have to implement the Convention – it does not take the place of national laws.

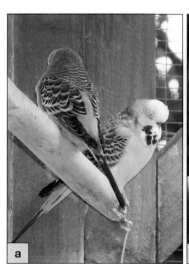
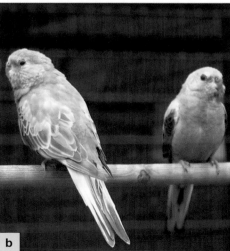
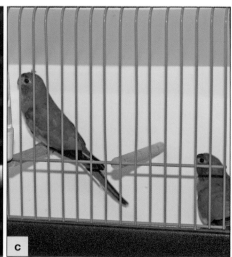

3.32 **(a)** A grey and a sky-blue Budgerigar – two of the many colour mutations of this familiar parakeet. **(b)** Two Rosa Bourke's Parakeets, a pale pink variation of the nominate race, which have darker wings and head, and a pale blue rump. This species is highly popular in captivity and is a gentle, easily managed bird. **(c)** Blue mutations of the Splendid Parakeet in a show (exhibition) cage. The nominate race of this species has a blue head, neck and wing flashes, but with a green back and tail, yellow abdomen and scarlet chest.

CITES provides a framework to be respected by each Party, which has to adopt its own domestic legislation to ensure that CITES is implemented at the national level. This Convention was established, as its name suggests, to protect endangered species of plants and animals by controlling trade and trafficking. This significantly affects many species of birds that are currently kept in captivity.

There is a considerable range of species control levels (Appendices) set by the Convention, and species may be moved from one Appendix to another as their status in the wild changes. To confuse the issue further, there is a further categorization into Annexes A, B, C and D (at least within the EU).

Many endangered parrot species are listed in Annex A, including several cockatoos, Amazon parrots, macaws and parakeets. These birds may not be traded within the European Community without official CITES and, in the UK, Defra (the Department for Environment, Food and Rural Affairs) paperwork. Such birds must be identified by a closed leg ring (band) and/or an unalterable microchip meeting ISO standards.

All European species of raptor are included in Annex A and, as well as the above trading restrictions, CITES requires under the terms of Article 10 that anyone breeding, exchanging or displaying for commercial gain any species (including cadavers or hybrids, and body parts such as feathers) must have a 'specimen-specific' licence (Scott, 2008). This is colloquially known by raptor keepers as an 'Article 10 licence', and is issued in the UK by Defra.

Some of this legislation is vague and equivocal. For example, in large areas of Western Europe and the Americas, small parrots such as Indian Ringnecks and Monk (Quaker) Parakeets that have escaped from captivity have established successful feral colonies. So successful has their breeding in the wild become that in places they are rapidly becoming pest species (Figure 3.34). At the time of writing in the UK, the official Defra

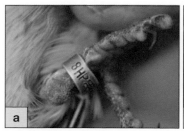
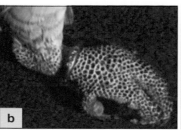
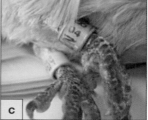
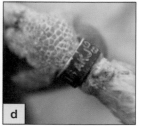

3.33 **(a)** Coloured aluminium leg band showing breeder's code. **(b)** Stainless steel leg band with veterinary code. **(c)** Leg bands may show the year of hatching of the bird. **(d)** If the leg band fitted is too small for the bird's fully grown size this may lead to compression of the circulatory system and, ultimately, loss of the foot.

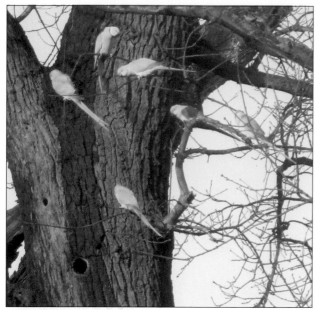

3.34 Feral Ringnecked Parakeets around a nest hole in an oak tree in a Buckinghamshire park, UK.

position is that 'Ringnecked Parakeets are non-native invasive species, and that Schedule 9 of the Wildlife and Countryside Act offers some level of protection. Thus it is illegal to take these birds from the wild to maintain them in captivity, neither is it legal to release such birds into the wild.' Yet, equally, there is no official requirement for legally captive Ringnecked Parakeets (that have been bred and maintained for many generations) to be permanently identified with a closed ring (band) or microchip.

In summary, it may be said that legislation covering the keeping, movement and trade of most birds is varied and complex, and those working in the field of avian medicine are advised to check current lists and rules on the relevant websites.

Ethical conclusions

Whatever an individual's feelings may be on the ethics of keeping birds in captivity, there is no doubt that many millions of birds will continue to be confined in close association with humans. Those that are raised for food are probably most closely supervised, although some would argue that welfare regulations do not go far enough. It is up to veterinary professionals to ensure that their patients are maintained in as desirable, humane and healthy a condition as is possible. This includes advising owners on the suitability or otherwise of housing and management, and bringing to their attention any omissions of care, or even illegalities, in their husbandry.

References and further reading

Jones AK (2011) *Keeping Parrots – Understanding Their Care and Breeding.* The Crowood Press, Ramsbury

Scott PW (2008) Legal, zoonotic and ethical considerations. In: *BSAVA Manual of Raptors, Pigeons and Passerine Birds*, ed. J Chitty and M Lierz, pp. 377–383. BSAVA Publications, Gloucester

Reproduction

Bob Doneley

Reproductive problems, including medical, physiological and behavioural, are a common occurrence in avian practice. Veterinary surgeons (veterinarians) are frequently presented with birds with egg binding, yolk peritonitis, gonadal neoplasia, excessive egg laying, and aggression. Less frequently, veterinary surgeons are called upon to investigate fertility and production problems in breeding facilities.

All of these problems require the clinician to have a sound knowledge of avian reproduction including anatomy, physiology, breeding behaviours and chick rearing. This chapter seeks to provide a foundation of knowledge in these areas to provide the clinician with the necessary tools to work-up and diagnose reproductive problems, and then to treat them. (The anatomy of the reproductive tract is discussed in Chapter 2; Treating a sick baby bird is discussed in Chapter 31.)

Sexing birds

Sex determination
The sex of birds is determined genetically by the inheritance of a combination of non-homologous sex chromosomes, Z and W. Unlike mammals, the male bird is homogametous with two identical sex chromosomes (ZZ) while females are heterogametous (ZW) (Figure 4.1). The W chromosome carries little genetic material and it appears that, in nearly all birds, sex is determined by the Z chromosome (Z dosage) rather than the presence/absence of the W chromosome; two Z chromosomes make a male, while only one makes a female (Smith, 2010).

Sex identification
Although aviculturists have a vested interest in knowing the sex of their birds, pet owners may query the necessity (and expense) of knowing. However, many health and behavioural problems are linked to the sex of the bird (e.g. egg binding and nest-site aggression), making knowledge of the bird's sex an important clinical tool.

To the human eye many birds are sexually monomorphic (e.g. many South American and African parrots, many raptors and Columbiformes; see Appendix 2). Some are initially monomorphic, later becoming dimorphic (e.g. many Asiatic parakeet cocks develop a

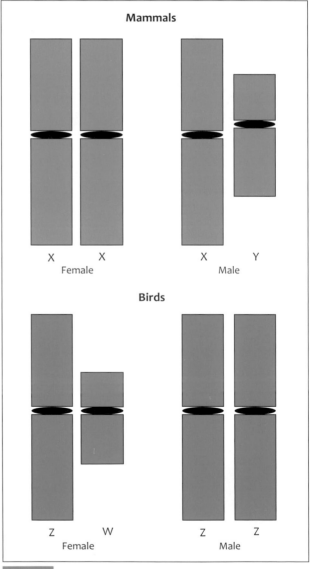

4.1 Sex chromosomes in mammals and birds.

black neck ring at 2–3 years of age (Figure 4.2a); there are size differences between different sexes of some mature raptors). Other species, such as the Eclectus Parrot (Figure 4.2b), are obviously dimorphic from the time of fledging. The ability of birds to see in the

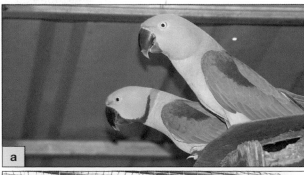

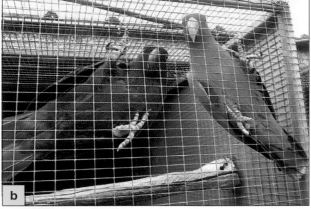

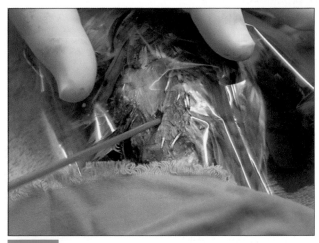

Endoscopic (surgical) sex determination.

4.2 **(a)** Delayed sexual dimorphism is seen in this pair of Alexandrine Parakeets (left, male; right, female). **(b)** Sexual dimorphism is illustrated in this pair of Eclectus Parrots (hen on the left).

ultraviolet (UV) spectrum of light is believed to make sex identification more feasible; dimorphism may be apparent in plumage coloration not visible to the human eye (Note: this ability is not conferred to humans simply by the use of a UV light such as a Wood's lamp.)

There are several techniques employed by avian veterinary surgeons and aviculturists to identify the sex of monomorphic birds.

DNA sexing

DNA sexing uses polymerase chain reaction (PCR) to identify genes that are associated with the Z and W chromosomes. It is important that the laboratory doing the testing knows what species is being tested, as there are species-specific differences in these genes. This test uses blood or feather pulp or epithelial cells from freshly plucked feathers as the source of DNA. Some laboratories offer testing from the remnants of inner shell membranes inside hatched egg shells, but this source is subject to contamination from the parents and siblings. Some of the laboratories performing DNA testing often claim 99.9% accuracy, but anecdotal reports from aviculturists suggest the accuracy from some laboratories may be lower.

Surgical sexing

Surgical sexing is the endoscopic inspection of the gonads performed under anaesthesia (Figure 4.3). This technique allows identification of the gonads, evaluation of the bird's maturity and examination of other internal organs. In experienced hands this technique has an accuracy of approximately 98%, but risks exist – there is a mortality rate of less than 0.2% for even experienced surgeons. Errors in identification using this technique usually occur in very young, small, or very obese birds (author, personal observation).

'Wait and see'

'Wait and see' is relevant for those species that develop dimorphism later in life. The age at which these differences develop varies between species. Cockatiels (with the exception of some colour mutations) develop dimorphism after the first juvenile moult, usually at 6 months of age. Asiatic parakeets, on the other hand, do not show dimorphism until they are 18–24 months old (see Figure 4.2a).

Other techniques

Other techniques, used by field researchers, include analysing faecal steroid levels or karyotyping from feather pulp or blood samples. These techniques are not readily available to clinicians.

There are aviculturists and others who maintain that techniques such as palpating the width between the pubic bones or holding a wedding ring or needle on a thread over the bird (to see which way it swings) are valid sexing techniques. There is no evidence to support these beliefs.

Reproductive characteristics

Avian species differ substantially in their reproductive characteristics, including physiology and timings such as incubation, rearing and development. Figure 4.4 details reproductive characteristics for selected species of birds kept in captivity.

Physiology

Most birds are seasonal breeders, with substantial variation between species in their reproductive strategies. There is variation in the environmental cues used to trigger reproduction, the developmental stage of the chick at hatch, and the extent of parental care. There are both endogenous and exogenous mechanisms controlling breeding seasons.

Endogenous factors are poorly understood, but are reflected in the fact that many captive birds held in constant environmental conditions still show seasonality, as do migratory birds (going through a wide range of environmental changes) and tropical birds (with little variation in photoperiod). It is possible that other environmental factors, such as humidity or food availability, may play a more important role than photoperiod in these birds.

Species	Clutch size	Incubation period (days)	Fledging age (days)	Weaning age (days)	Sexual maturity
Psittaciformes					
Macaws					
Blue and Gold Macaw	2–4	24–25	90–100	90–110	5–7 years
Green-winged Macaw	2–3	27	100	110–140	3–5 years
Hyacinth Macaw	2	28	100	180–270	5–7 years
Military Macaw	2	26	90	110–120	2–3 years
Red-shouldered Macaw	2–4	24	55	70–85	2–3 years
Scarlet Macaw	2–4	24–25	105	90–110	5–7 years
Amazon parrots					
Blue-fronted Amazon	3–4	28	55–65	90–120	4–6 years
Double Yellow-headed Amazon	2–3	26	65–77	90–120	4–6 years
Yellow-fronted Amazon	2–3	26	65–77	90–120	4–6 years
Yellow-naped Amazon	2–3	26	65–77	90–120	4–6 years
Cockatoos					
Galah	3–4	23–25	42–49	85–95	2–3 years
Gang-gang Cockatoo	2–3	25–30	50–60	75–100	3–4 years
Greater Sulphur-crested Cockatoo	2–3	25–28	63–90	120–150	3–4 years
Little Corella	2–4	26	49–56	110–120	3–4 years
Long-billed Corella	2–3	26	49	85–95	3–4 years
Moluccan Cockatoo	2	28	90–100	100–120	3–5 years
Palm Cockatoo	1	30–35	100–110	142–152	7–8 years
Red-tailed Black Cockatoo	1–2	28	75–95	180–220	4–5 years
Umbrella Cockatoo	2	28	84	95–105	5–6 years
Conures					
Green-cheeked Conure	4–6	22–24	50	55–75	9–18 months
Sun Conure	3–4	24–25	49–55	55–75	2–4 years
Cockatiels, Budgerigars and lovebirds					
Budgerigar	4–8	18	30	30–40	6–9 months
Cockatiel	4–7	18–21	35	40–50	8–12 months
Lovebirds (*Agapornis* spp.)	7–8	22–23	35–40	45–55	6–12 months
Lories and lorikeets					
Chattering Lory	2	26	70–80	85–100	2–3 years
Rainbow Lorikeet	2–3	23–25	55–60	60–70	1–2 years
Red Lory	2	24	70–80	85–100	2–3 years
Other psittacine groups					
African Grey Parrot	2–3	28	75–85	100–120	4–6 years
Alexandrine Parakeet	2–4	24	50	85–100	2–3 years
Caiques (*Pionites* spp.)	2–4	25–28	70	95–105	2–3 years
Eclectus Parrot	2–3	28–30	72–80	80–90	3 years
Indian Ringnecked Parakeet	4–6	23–34	50	70–90	2 years
Jardine's Parrot	3–4	23–25	42–49	95–105	3–4 years
Meyer's Parrot	3–5	24–25	60–65	70–90	2 years
Monk Parakeet	5–7	23–24	40–50	50–60	1 year
Neophema spp.	4–6	18–19	28–35	50	1 year
Princess Parrot	4–6	20	35	50–55	1–2 years
Psephotus spp.	4–6	19	28–35	40–50	1 year
Regent Parrot	4–6	20	35	50	2 years

4.4   Reproductive characteristics of selected bird species. (continues)   ▶

Species	Clutch size	Incubation period (days)	Fledging age (days)	Weaning age (days)	Sexual maturity
Other psittacine groups continued					
Rosellas (*Platycercus* spp.)	4–5	20	35	50	2–3 years
Senegal Parrot	3–5	24–25	60–70	70–90	2–3 years
Timneh African Grey Parrot	2–3	27–28	75–85	95–105	3–5 years
Passeriformes					
Domestic Canary	4–5	14	18	20–25	10 months
Mynahs	2–3	13–17	25–28	60	2–3 years
Raptors					
Hawks					
Cooper's Hawk	4–5	32–36	27–34	60	2 years
Harris' Hawk	3–5	32–34	35–45	60–90	1 year
Northern Goshawk	3–5	32–34	35–45	70	1–3 years
Red-tailed Hawk	1–5	30	42–46	70	2–3 years
Falcons					
Gyrfalcon	3–5	32–33	49–55	90–120	2–3 years
Lanner Falcon	3–5	31–33	40	90–120	2–3 years
Peregrine Falcon	3–5	31–33	42–46	90–120	2–3 years
Saker Falcon	3–5	31–33	45–50	65–85	2–3 years
Eagles					
Golden Eagle	2	43–45	63–70	100	4 years
Owls					
Barn Owl	4–7	29–34	50–70	70–100	1 year
Eurasian Eagle Owl	1–6	31–36	120–160	170	1–3 years

4.4 (continued) Reproductive characteristics of selected bird species.

Exogenous factors are better understood. They can be either *ultimate factors* that select for individuals that will breed when there are optimum conditions for offspring survival (e.g. food availability) or *proximate factors* that vary from year to year. These proximate factors are further broken down into:

- Initial predictive factors that initiate gonadal development in anticipation of breeding (e.g. photoperiod)
- Essential supplementary factors that supplement the initial predictive factors and initiate final stages of gonadal development. These include: social cues (e.g. breeding plumage, mate availability, courtship behaviour (Figure 4.5a)); territorial behaviour; climate (e.g. rainfall); and nutrition (in particular, an increase in fat and sugars in the diet (Figure 4.5b))
- Synchronizing and integrating factors that regulate the sequence of breeding behaviour, such as social interaction between a pair (Figure 4.5c)
- Modifying factors that can disrupt the breeding cycle, for example, loss of a mate or disturbance of the nest site (Figure 4.5d).

All of these factors have hormonal modulators. The input of these modulators into the hypothalamus has an effect on the release of gonadotropin-releasing hormone (GnRH), which in turn stimulates the pituitary gland to release follicle-stimulating hormone (FSH) and luteinizing hormone (LH). In the hen, FSH supports ovarian and oviductal growth, gametogenesis and steroidogenesis, while LH also supports steroidogenesis. This steroidogenesis results in the release of oestrogen, which has effects on follicular and oviductal growth, calcium metabolism and vitellogenesis. Some secondary female behaviours are also influenced by oestrogen, such as courtship and nesting. In males, FSH initiates growth of the seminiferous tubules and results in increased spermatogenesis, while LH promotes development of the testosterone-producing cells of Leydig. This in turn gives rise to secondary male characteristics such as plumage changes, nesting activity, courtship behaviour and territorial behaviour.

Progesterone is produced by granulosa cells in the large follicles as they develop, under the influence of LH. This in turn causes a surge in LH production from the pituitary just before ovulation. This surge of LH stimulates the production of prostaglandin PGF2a from ovarian follicles, causing the follicular stigma to rupture, allowing ovulation. Progesterone inhibits further ovulation and induces behavioural and physical changes associated with incubation and brood care.

Prostaglandins PGF2a and PGE (1 and 2) are released by the F1 and post-ovulatory follicles. PGE2 and PGF2a bind at specific sites in the shell gland and vagina; PGF2a binds preferentially at the shell gland, allowing PGE2 to potentiate its effects and to facilitate relaxation of the vagina during oviposition. Therefore, PGE (1 and 2) allows relaxation of the utero-vaginal sphincter, while PGF2a stimulates shell gland contractions. Uterine contractility stimulates arginine vasotocin (AVT) release from the pituitary, which stimulates further contractility and release of uterine prostaglandins.

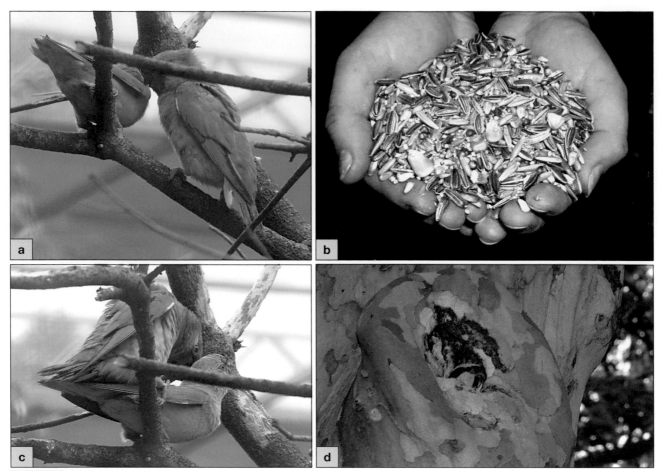

4.5 **(a)** This pair of Little Lorikeets are engaged in courtship feeding. **(b)** The typical seed diet fed to many birds is an essential supplementary factor driving reproductive behaviour. **(c)** This pair of Little Lorikeets have synchronized their proximate factors to result in mating. **(d)** Disturbance of this Musk Lorikeet's nest site (e.g. by a predator) is likely to disrupt breeding behaviour, resulting in abandonment of the nest site or loss of interest in breeding.

Eggs are laid until a clutch is formed: indeterminate layers continue to lay if eggs are removed, while determinate layers will lay only a set number of eggs. Incubation is performed either by the hen only (25% of species), by both sexes (54% of species), by the males only (6% of species) or by mixed strategies. Plasma prolactin levels are elevated in both sexes during incubation, which then has an inhibitory feedback on GnRH release.

Incubation

Incubation of eggs in captivity can be done either naturally under the parent (natural or foster) in the nest or artificially in an incubator (Figure 4.6). Artificial incubation is rarely as efficient or as effective as natural incubation, but it may be utilized for a variety of reasons.

- To allow increased production, particularly in rare or valuable species; removing an egg shortly after it has been laid often induces an indeterminate layer to lay a replacement.
- Poor parenting by some birds means that eggs and/ or chicks can be lost in the nest.
- Traditionally, it was thought that hand-rearing birds made them bond closer to people; therefore, artificial incubation was (and still is) widely practised to provide 'bonded' chicks for the pet market.
- In some cases artificial incubation is used as a means of disease control. Pathogens that are not

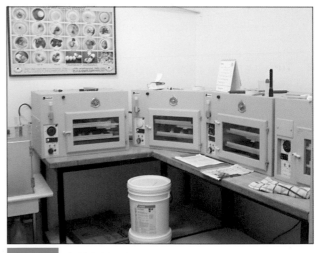

4.6 Artificial incubation of parrot eggs.

vertically transmitted through the egg, but can be horizontally transmitted, can be reduced or eliminated by artificial incubation.

The incubation period varies between species, but is generally between 14 and 28 days, with smaller species hatching earlier (see Figure 4.4). Incubation can be divided into three trimesters, each approximately one-third of the incubation period. The first trimester is a period of rapid cellular division and differentiation, with the development of blood vessels and embryonic membranes, followed by the central nervous system and other organs. During the second trimester these organs further develop and grow. The final trimester is characterized by the completion of organ growth, the chick positioning ready for hatching, the withdrawal of the yolk sac and, finally, the hatching process – internal pipping, external pipping and then hatching. The embryo is most vulnerable to disturbances during the first and third trimesters and these are the peak times for embryonic death.

A successful incubation, whether natural or artificial, is dependent on a number of factors.

- **The temperature at which the egg is incubated.** There are slight variations between species, but the average temperature is in the range of 34–37°C. Too cold, and the chick is slow to develop and may hatch late. Too warm, and the chick develops too rapidly and may hatch early, before final organ development and fluid loss is complete. Either situation leads to late embryonic death or weak chicks that fail to thrive and usually die.
- **The amount of water lost from the egg during incubation.** As the chick grows, water held in the yolk and albumen is lost through the shell, at a rate dependent on the thickness and porosity of the shell and the relatively humidity of the air around the egg. Too much water loss (greater than 17% weight loss) during incubation frequently results in dehydrated chicks ('sticky chicks') that have difficulty hatching and frequently die within the first day or two. Too little water loss (less than 10% weight loss) results in oedematous chicks ('wet chicks') that also have difficulty hatching and frequently die.
- **Gas exchange during incubation.** Gas exchange (respiration) also occurs across the egg shell and is limited by the shell thickness and porosity, as well as by the provision of fresh air around the egg and the humidity level in the incubator.
- **Turning of the egg during incubation.** This was originally thought be important in stopping the chick 'sticking' to one part of the egg. It is now known that turning encourages healthy blood vessel development in the embryonic membranes and stops nutrients from settling in one part of the egg. However, excessive turning and jarring of the egg during the incubation may disrupt the chick's growth.
- **Cleanliness of the egg, nest and incubator.** Dirty eggs, nests and incubators can result in bacterial and fungal agents crossing the egg shell and causing infections that will usually kill the embryo. Eggs should be cleaned with a dry brush before setting in the incubator, and the incubator cleaned and sterilized between broods. The selection of disinfectant and hygiene regime may be determined by the pathogens known or suspected to be present (e.g. enveloped viruses *versus* non-enveloped viruses; bacteria *versus* fungi).

Hatching usually occurs over 1–2 days, in three stages. Firstly, the chick positions its beak against the air cell within the egg and rubs the internal shell membrane until it ruptures, allowing the chick to move its head into the air cell space and begin breathing air.

This process is known as the 'drawing down' of the air cell and then internal pipping. As carbon dioxide (CO_2) builds up in the air cell, the chick is stimulated to use its 'egg tooth', a keratin tip on the rhinotheca, to break through the egg shell (external pipping). The amount and pattern of breakthrough varies between species, but the result is that the chick is now able to breathe room air. After a short period of time (usually minutes) to regain its strength after the exertions of pipping, the chick crawls out of the shell, completing the hatching process (Figure 4.7).

When artificially incubating eggs, the egg about to hatch is frequently moved to a hatcher, where the temperature is slightly less, the humidity slightly higher, and there is no turning of the egg.

In a well run incubation setup, 85–90% of fertile eggs should hatch without difficulty (author, personal observations).

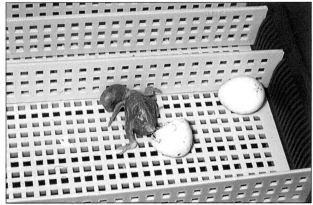

4.7 A newly hatched Cockatiel chick in an incubator tray.

Chick rearing

Most pet bird species and raptors hatch **altricial chicks** (near-naked, blind, deaf and totally dependent); some species (such as ratites and poultry) hatch **precocial chicks** (fully feathered, eyes and ears open and much less dependent). The rearing of altricial chicks, whether by the bird parents or by human keepers, is an intensive process.

Development of the altricial chick

The relative growth rate of all chicks follows a similar pattern, with an initial period of rapid growth that peaks at weaning, then drops down to a plateau at the adult weight. Growth rate charts are available in avicultural literature for many different species and are useful tools in assessing a chick's development.

In the wild and in the aviary, chicks are reared in nesting hollows, characterized by their dark, often cramped, conditions. This close confinement keeps the chicks relatively immobile and reduces the amount of stress placed on developing long bones. In some captive rearing nurseries, chicks are kept in large, brightly lit enclosures; the excessive movement this encourages may contribute to bowing and rotation of the long bones, particularly the tibiotarsus and femur.

Depending on the species, some chicks are hatched naked, or with wispy down feathers, whereas others are covered in fluffy down feathers. A second wave of down feather growth begins at 1–3 weeks of age, although this can occur later in some species. Pin feathers begin to emerge at 2–3 weeks of age. The body contour feathers emerge over the shoulders first; the pattern of emergence after that varies between species, although usually the body contour feathers emerge at the same time as or shortly before the secondary flight feathers on the wings. Primaries may begin to develop before secondary feathers, but usually mature after them. Final feather maturity is usually not complete before the bird has weaned.

The eyes begin to open at 10–28 days, and then take several days to open completely. Most Australian and African parrots hatch with their ears open. The ears of Eclectus Parrots and South American species should be open within 2–3 weeks of hatching.

Fledging – the age at which a chick is ready to leave the nest – varies between species. After leaving the nest the chick learns a range of behaviours – socialization, flying, foraging and feeding, and predator avoidance – under the supervision of watchful parents. The chick is still fed by the parents, albeit with reduced frequency and amounts, until it is finally weaned and ready to move on (see Figure 4.4).

Hand-rearing

Wherever possible chicks should be left in the nest for the parents to rear, as humans cannot replicate the round-the-clock feeding and socialization that natural rearing provides. However, aviculturists may choose to hand-rear chicks (Figure 4.8) for many of the same reasons they choose to incubate eggs: to increase production; to take over from dead or poor parents; to produce pet birds; or to reduce the exposure of chicks to disease in the aviary. The basic considerations when developing a hand-rearing operation are detailed below.

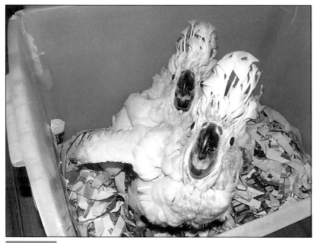

| 4.8 | Hand-reared Moluccan Cockatoo chicks. |

When to start: Unless eggs are artificially incubated, when hand-rearing has to start from hatching, it is often best to allow the parents to do the initial 'hard work' and rear the chick to 2–3 weeks of age. Many aviculturists take chicks from the nest at this age and take over all feeding. A growing movement in aviculture advocates taking the chicks only for a few hours each day, feeding them and socializing with humans before returning them to the nest. This system allows the bird to gain social interaction experience with humans while learning and retaining bird behaviours.

What to feed: There are many commercial hand-rearing formulae available to aviculturists today and these should be utilized. Homemade recipes, usually using milk powders and other ingredients not normally consumed by birds, rarely achieve a balanced diet. A good-quality commercial diet, fed according to the manufacturer's directions, removes much of the guesswork from chick rearing. The food should be fed at approximately 41°C (avian body temperature), but never heated using a microwave (this can produce small 'hot spots' in the formula capable of burning the crop mucosa). Only enough food should be prepared for one feed at a time; it does not keep well even when refrigerated, with bacterial and yeast overgrowth a common occurrence.

How to feed: A variety of tools can be used to feed chicks, including syringes, spoons and feeding tubes (crop needles). The tool used is usually determined by the skill and experience of the person doing the rearing. A good feeding response should be elicited from the chick before feeding with a syringe or spoon. All implements should be cleaned and disinfected between feedings. When using a tube, care must be taken to avoid iatrogenic trauma to the crop wall when a feeding chick is vigorously bobbing its head. Care must also be taken to ensure that the tube is securely attached to the syringe, to avoid it dislodging and being swallowed by the chick.

How often and how much to feed: The frequency of feeding is dependent on the species and age of the chick; newly hatched chicks may require feeding every 1–2 hours around the clock, while chicks at 3–6 weeks of age are fed every 4–6 hours. Chicks older than fledging age are usually fed every 8–12 hours, reducing to once daily at weaning age (see 'Weaning'). The amount fed at each feed is usually calculated at 10% of the chick's bodyweight (Australian species, especially cockatoos, are usually fed 8–10% of their weight, while macaws are fed at 12% of their weight). In a healthy chick, the crop should empty nearly completely between 4 and 6 hours after feeding.

Weaning: The age at which a chick weans is species dependent, and avicultural literature should be consulted as a guide (see also Figure 4.4). The frequency of hand feeding and the amount of feed given is reduced at the same time as a variety of foods are offered (e.g. pellets, seed, vegetables and fruit) in a flat dish to encourage the chick to 'play' with the food, exploring and tasting it. As the chick is observed to be eating more solid food, the amount of hand-rearing formula is reduced further until it is eliminated completely. The evening feed is the last to be dropped from the feeding regime. This is a stressful time for both the chick and the keeper, and a growing trend is for some breeders to sell unweaned chicks to novices, claiming that finishing off the hand-rearing process will create a closer bond between the bird and the new keeper. This unethical practice should be strongly discouraged. Many new owners are novices at hand-rearing and certainly with weaning; the result is often stunted, malnourished chicks and tired, dispirited keepers who have lost the bond with their charge. Some birds, especially strong-feeding species like macaws, risk perforation of the oesophagus when fed by inexperienced persons.

Nursery management: Chicks should be kept in small, dark containers and not encouraged to exercise until they have reached fledging age. Species that usually have multiple chicks in a clutch should be reared in small groups to prevent the development of behavioural problems. The substrate in the container should be inert, non-toxic, absorbent, and not readily ingested. Paper towel or recycled paper cat litter is preferable to wood shavings or corn cob bedding. Active heating should be supplied, initially at 32°C for newly hatched chicks and then reduced by 1°C each week. Humidity can be provided by placing a bowl of wet cotton wool in the container, replacing it each day.

Strict hygiene must be practised, particularly in multi-bird nurseries. Chicks should not be moved from one container to another, and new chicks should not be mixed with older chicks. The practice of 'contract hand-rearing', where chicks from several different owners are mixed and reared together, invariably results in disaster (in the form of explosive outbreaks of infectious diseases) and should be discouraged.

As the chicks reach fledging and weaning age, it is important to provide some form of environmental enrichment to develop normal inquisitive and foraging behaviours appropriate to this age. Simply placing food in a dish, while convenient, does not encourage normal eating and foraging behaviours. Offering a wide range of different foods in a wide flat dish encourages the chick to explore and taste different foods.

Reproductive diseases

Male

Orchitis

Orchitis (Figure 4.9), caused by infection with bacteria (e.g. *Escherichia coli*, *Salmonella*, *Pasteurella* spp., *Chlamydia* or *Mycobacterium* spp.) or fungi, can be spread via a haematogenous route or through an ascending infection from the cloaca/phallus. There are usually no clinical signs unless the bird is septicaemic. The diagnosis can be made by aspiration cytology or endoscopic biopsy. Treatment with antimicrobial therapy as indicated by culture and sensitivity testing, or surgical orchidectomy, may be required.

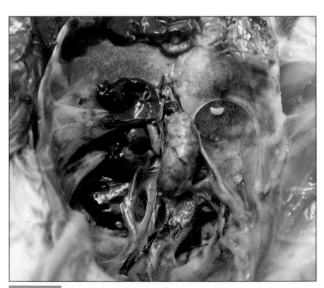

4.9   Orchitis due to salmonellosis in a domestic pigeon.

Neoplasia

Numerous species have been reported as having a variety of tumours. Sertoli cell tumours are the most common, but interstitial cell tumours, seminomas, teratomas, lymphosarcoma, leiomyosarcoma and carcinoma of the ductus deferens and epididymis have all been reported. Affected birds may demonstrate chronic weight loss, coelomic distension and sometimes unilateral paresis of a leg (due to sciatic nerve compression) (Figure 4.10). In Budgerigars, a change in the cere colour (from blue to brown) is sometimes seen, but it should be noted that this colour change is not pathognomonic for Sertoli cell neoplasia. Diagnosis can be made by endoscopic examination and biopsy; on endoscopic examination the testicle may appear cystic, and can be confused with an immature ovary. Treatment requires orchidectomy, and carries a good prognosis if no metastatic disease is present and the surgery is performed by an experienced surgeon.

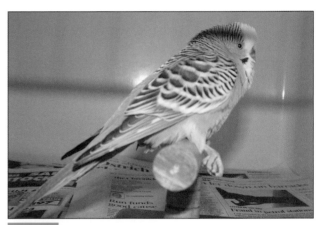

4.10   Paresis due to testicular neoplasia in a Budgerigar.

Cloacal prolapse

In male birds, especially cockatoos, cloacal prolapse has been associated with masturbatory behaviours. Surgical treatment requires ventoplasty (temporary or permanent) or cloacopexy. Prevention of recurrence requires behavioural intervention and possibly the use of hormonal manipulation (e.g. deslorelin implants) combined with dietary, social and environmental modification (see 'Chronic or excessive egg laying').

Female

Oophoritis

Oophoritis can arise from the haematogenous spread of a bacterial infection (e.g. *Salmonella* spp., *Mycobacterium* spp.), fungal infection or viral infection (e.g. herpesvirus), or spread from adjacent air sacculitis or peritonitis. It can also develop following the rupture of follicles and extrusion of yolk into the ovarian stroma. Infectious oophoritis is often part of a systemic illness, and many birds will present for generalized weakness. In milder cases there may be an infertility problem or increased embryonic deaths. Endoscopy may reveal abnormally coloured or shaped ovaries, which are often haemorrhagic and have abnormal follicles. In the case of infectious disease, antimicrobial therapy combined with drainage of the affected follicle(s), being careful not to contaminate the abdomen, may be successful. Partial or complete ovariectomy may be required for chronically infected and caseated follicles.

Ovarian cysts

Congenital and acquired (secondary to neoplasia or oophoritis) ovarian cysts are not uncommon (Figure 4.11). If the cysts are small, there may be no clinical signs, but large cysts may cause coelomic distension and dyspnoea (through compression of the air sacs). Ultrasonography or endoscopy can be used for diagnosis, or an exploratory coeliotomy can be performed. Aspiration, either blind or guided by ultrasonography or endoscopy, can be used to relieve immediate clinical signs. Ovariectomy (partial or complete) is difficult to achieve successfully because of the complex vascularity of the ovary. It should only be attempted by an experienced avian surgeon using good magnification (e.g. an operating microscope). Hormonal therapy, using deslorelin (4.7 mg implant), leuprolide acetate (100–750 µg/kg q14 days for three treatments) or human chorionic gonadotropin (500 IU/kg on days 1, 3, 7, 14 and 21), has been suggested to reduce or resolve ovarian cysts in birds and offers a non-invasive treatment option. This is, however, assuming that the cysts are primary in origin, and are not secondary to other disease processes (e.g. neoplasia, oophoritis) and are responsive to hormonal manipulation. In the author's experience, these conservative treatments are rarely effective.

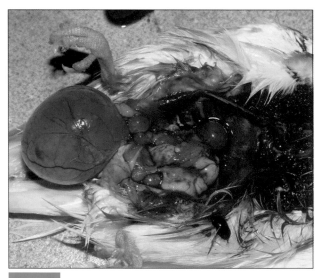

4.11 Ovarian cyst in a Budgerigar.

Ovarian neoplasia

Ovarian neoplasia (Figure 4.12), including granulosa cell tumours, ovarian carcinomas, dysgerminomas, arrhenoblastomas and teratomas, is less commonly seen. As with ovarian cysts, small tumours may not cause any clinical signs while large tumours may cause abdominal enlargement and dyspnoea. Granulosa cell tumours (and possibly other reproductive tract tumours) may be functional and cause increased plasma hormone levels. This can result in hormonally induced changes such as polyostotic hyperostosis (normally only seen in reproductively active hens). Ultrasonography and radiography may show gonadal enlargement, with endoscopic or surgical biopsy used to confirm the diagnosis. Treatment requires partial or complete ovariectomy, possibly combined with adjuvant chemotherapy and/or radiation therapy. The prognosis is guarded.

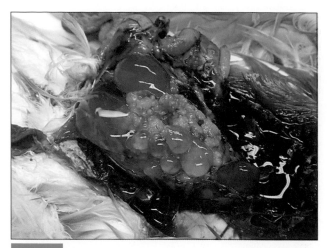

4.12 Ovarian neoplasia in a Sulphur-crested Cockatoo.

Salpingitis and metritis

Salpingitis (inflammation of the oviduct and mesosalpinx) and metritis (inflammation of the shell gland) are relatively common conditions in domestic birds (Figure 4.13). Predisposing factors include the age of the bird, obesity, excessive egg laying, egg binding and other reproductive disorders. Primary infections are rare, but secondary infection (either haematogenous or ascending infections) with bacteria such as *E. coli*, *Klebsiella* spp., and *Pseudomonas* spp. can occur. Clinical signs include weight loss, ruffled plumage, anorexia and lethargy. If the bird is still laying eggs, these eggs may be malformed (e.g. soft shells, stress lines, abnormal shape) or have streaking of blood on the shell. Physical examination of the bird may show a distended coelom, a flaccid vent and, occasionally, a cloacal discharge. In some birds the oviduct, distended with caseous pus, can be palpated. Radiography and ultrasonography may reveal retained eggs, an enlarged oviduct or the presence of coelomic fluid. Conservative treatment (reproductive rest, anti-inflammatory drugs and antibiotics) is usually unsuccessful. If there is material in the oviduct (e.g. caseous pus, eggs or fluid) the use of prostaglandins may be indicated. Using PGE2 (0.1 mg/kg per cloaca) to relax the uterovaginal sphincter and stimulate oviductal contractility may assist in this regard. Great caution must be exercised with this therapy, as chronic cases may have developed adhesions to the oviductal wall, and strong contractions may

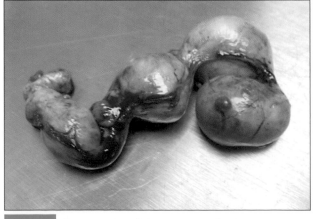

4.13 Pyometra in a Sulphur-crested Cockatoo.

lead to rupture of the oviduct. Definitive treatment usually requires a salpingohysterectomy. In all probability, a diagnosis of salpingitis or metritis indicates that the bird's reproductive life is almost certainly over. If the patient is a prized breeder, this must be communicated to the owner before commencing any treatment.

Yolk peritonitis

This is an inflammatory reaction to the presence of free yolk material in the coelomic cavity. It can be caused by retropulsion of yolk from the oviduct into the coelom (possibly associated with metritis/salpingitis, neoplasia, oviductal cystic hyperplasia or oviductal impaction, or with exuberant reverse peristalsis) or by failure of the infundibulum to 'capture' ovulating yolk (due to obesity, trauma or disease). It is usually seen in high-producing hens, especially Cockatiels, and is usually sterile. The inflammatory reaction may result in thick caseous adhesions or, more commonly, large volumes of fluid. Clinical signs are therefore related to the presence of this fluid and include dyspnoea, coelomic distension (Figure 4.14) and weakness. The bird usually stops laying, or may lay malformed eggs. If it becomes septic, signs are consistent with severe septicaemia. Secondary diseases may develop as a result of yolk peritonitis: neurological signs due to yolk emboli ('yolk stroke'; note that this is not pathognomonic for yolk peritonitis); pancreatic disease, including diabetes mellitus; hepatitis; nephritis; and splenitis. Ultrasonography confirms fluid distension of the coelom, rather than organomegaly. Caseous material (inspissated yolks) may be detected. Coeliocentesis reveals brown or yellow-pink fluid. Cytology demonstrates mesothelial cells, leucocytes and pink yolk globules. Short-term therapy (coelomic drainage, anti-inflammatory drugs, antibiotics, and hormonal manipulation to stop ovarian activity) may help initially, but most cases will require surgery to lavage the coelom and perform a salpingohysterectomy.

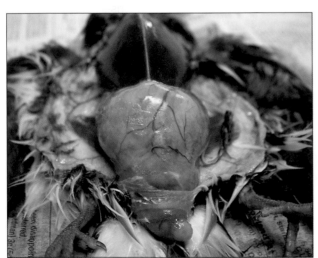

4.14   Coelomic distension associated with yolk peritonitis (post-mortem examination).

Egg binding

Egg binding (dystocia) (Figure 4.15a) is one of the most common reproductive problems seen in clinical practice. Very young and very old birds are more frequently affected, particularly overweight, unfit birds with a history of excessive egg production. Although commonly attributed to a calcium deficiency, other causes

include oversized or abnormally shaped eggs, oviductal muscle dysfunction or myositis, concurrent salpingitis or metritis (possibly with strictures), other concurrent illnesses (e.g. neoplasia), hypothermia, hypoglycaemia and environmental stress. Running a 'cage-side' test for ionized calcium and blood glucose (e.g. i-STAT®) may help to differentiate between metabolic and physical causes of egg binding.

In early-onset cases egg-bound birds are usually presented with excessive straining and an upright 'penguin-like' posture. As the condition worsens, the affected bird may become dyspnoeic, paretic in the legs and even collapse. Palpation usually reveals an egg, but soft-shelled eggs (Figure 4.15b) can be difficult to detect, requiring radiography or ultrasonography.

If the bird shows no, or only mild to moderate, signs of discomfort and distress, the time the last egg was laid should be confirmed – eggs are usually laid 23–26 hours apart, and the patient may not be ready to lay. The bird should be placed in a heated hospital cage with adequate humidity and given calcium gluconate by intramuscular injections (10 mg/kg q1h) as needed. Tube feeding highly digestible, high-sugar supplements should be considered to provide a rapid source of energy, with stress and handling minimized, and the bird kept in a dark, quiet environment.

If the bird fails to respond to this treatment, intracloacal PGE2 gel (0.1 mg/kg) will usually produce uterovaginal sphincter dilation and straining within 5–10 minutes. Oxytocin (3–5 IU/kg i.m.) may be given, but there is controversy over its efficacy (and safety) in birds. If necessary, the egg can be manually manipulated into the cloaca and delivered. If the bird is distressed, performing this procedure under anaesthesia may be advantageous. Caution must be taken not to push the egg dorsally, as it is possible to crush the kidneys against the spine.

If the bird is distressed or dyspnoeic, the clinician may have to consider ovocentesis and egg collapse as an emergency procedure. With the patient under anaesthesia, the egg is held against the skin or cloaca.

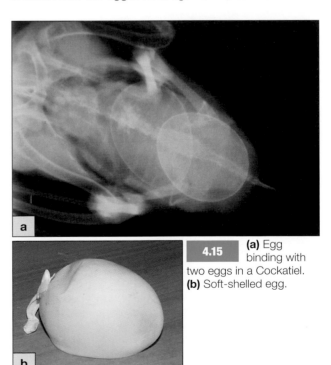

4.15   (a) Egg binding with two eggs in a Cockatiel. (b) Soft-shelled egg.

Wherever possible, the egg should be moved into the cloaca so it can be visualized, even if it cannot be passed. Care should be taken not to stretch or tear the cloacal and oviductal mucosa whilst manoeuvring the egg. A large-gauge needle should then be introduced into the egg either directly (preferably) or through the cloacal mucosa or coelomic wall and the contents aspirated, simultaneously collapsing the egg with digital pressure. (Note: percutaneous aspiration carries a higher risk of peritonitis and metritis.) The egg shell can then be removed or is usually passed within 48 hours of this procedure. If this procedure is used, the owner should be warned that metritis and further egg binding is probable. Coeliotomy and caesarean section may be necessary in some cases.

The earlier the bird is presented, the better the prognosis. Simple cases have an excellent prognosis, while cases that have reached the stage where the bird is collapsed, dyspnoeic and unable to use its legs properly have a more guarded prognosis.

Oviductal prolapse

Oviductal prolapse is an uncommon condition, and may follow both egg binding and salpingitis. On initial examination some cases can be confused with cloacal prolapse, but careful inspection (especially with an endoscope) reveals the characteristic mucosal folds of the oviduct (Figure 4.16). Very mild cases can be treated by reducing the prolapse (ensuring the oviduct has been completely reduced into its correct position, not just into the cloaca), performing a temporary ventoplasty, treatment with anti-inflammatory drugs and antibiotics, and managing the bird's reproductive activity (see 'Chronic or excessive egg laying'). More severe cases often require a coeliotomy to assess for internal haemorrhage (from torn vessels in the dorsal mesosalpinx) and may indicate salpingohysterectomy.

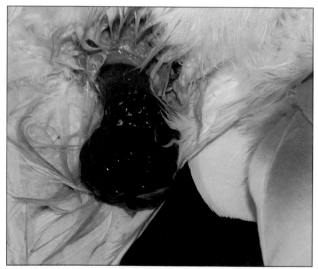

4.16   Oviduct prolapse in a Major Mitchell's Cockatoo. Note the characteristic mucosal folds of the oviduct.

Ectopic eggs

Ectopic eggs occur when an egg-bound bird ruptures its oviduct at the level of the shell gland, leaving a fully shelled egg loose in the coelom. These cases present clinically very similar to egg-bound birds, with the same aetiology and clinical signs, but the hen fails to pass the egg, regardless of the treatment given. Radiography reveals a normal-looking shelled egg, which may be in an abnormal position within the coelom. Treatment requires a coeliotomy to remove the egg and repair the oviduct. The prognosis is good, and some of these birds return to egg laying uneventfully, provided they are given several months to recuperate.

Retained eggs

Retained eggs differ from egg binding in the chronicity of the problem. In many cases the egg may be retained in the oviduct, but has collapsed, leaving only the shell. In other cases the egg may still be intact, but the bird is not straining to pass it. The egg is often located in the anterior coelom, and usually does not cause dyspnoea. These birds may present with coelomic distension, or may be asymptomatic. Diagnosis is usually made radiographically and treatment requires salpingohysterectomy.

Chronic or excessive egg laying

Chronic or excessive egg laying (Figure 4.17) is most commonly seen in Cockatiels, but any species can be affected. Left untreated, many of these birds deplete their calcium reserves and develop problems such as egg binding and pathological fractures. Many will develop salpingitis/metritis and subsequent yolk peritonitis. Chronic egg laying results from the interaction of a number of proximate factors inadvertently activated by the bird's husbandry. They include:

- Extended photoperiod; these birds are often housed indoors and do not have an appropriate diurnal rhythm
- Readily available food and water, especially high-fat and sweet foods (e.g. seeds and fruit)
- A potential mate. This may or may not be another bird; in many cases it is the owner who has allowed an 'unnatural' bond to develop between themselves and the bird. It is not just the sight of the 'mate' that is a potential trigger – even the sound of the 'mate' may be enough to initiate reproductive behaviour
- A secure nest site, which may be anywhere in the house or cage where the bird has established territoriality.

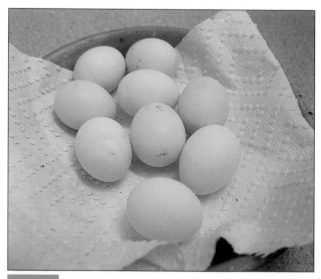

4.17   Chronic egg laying in a Cockatiel.

Treatment requires eliminating or neutralizing these proximate factors and can be broken down into three categories:

- Environmental modification
- Behavioural modification
- Nutritional modification.

Environmental modification:

- Re-establish normal diurnal rhythms. In some cases it may be necessary to drastically reduce daylight hours artificially (to 8 hours or less) until the egg-laying behaviour has stopped, and then bring the bird up to normal rhythms. Note that in species where day length has little effect on breeding (e.g. Budgerigars), changing day length will have little effect on reproductive behaviour.
- Remove nest sites (if possible). If the bird chooses an unconventional nest site (e.g. on the floor of the cage) rearranging the area may effectively remove its attractiveness as a nest site.
- Change the bird's environment; for example, add new or rearrange existing cage furniture or reposition the cage on an irregular basis. This induces a certain amount of environmental stress and reduces territoriality.

Behavioural modification:

- If appropriate (and possible), remove the companion bird. Note that care must be taken not to trigger other behavioural issues such as separation anxiety if the mate is removed.
- Establish a normal relationship between human and bird through the introduction of basic behavioural training and client education. The keeper must be taught what behaviours may sexually stimulate the bird (e.g. stroking the bird's back).
- Removing the eggs of an indeterminate layer, such as a Cockatiel, will only induce further egg laying. Leaving the eggs in the nest, or replacing them with artificial eggs, will often result in a hen laying a normal-sized clutch and then brooding the eggs. This shuts down (temporarily) the production of eggs. The eggs can be removed after 3–4 weeks or when the hen abandons the nest.

Nutritional modification:

- Reduce fat and sugar in the diet by converting to a commercial formulated diet and/or removal of fruit from the diet.
- Encourage foraging behaviour. Typically, wild birds spend 80% of their day foraging for food, leaving 20% of the day to groom, socialize and 'nap'. In captivity, this time allocation is nearly completely reversed, with birds only having to spend a small amount of time looking for food. By introducing foraging activities, there is less time for pair bonding and other reproductive activities.

Hormonal manipulation: If the above changes are not sufficient to stop or reduce egg laying, hormonal manipulation may be indicated. Note that hormonal therapy does not work in isolation. Unless the modifications in environment, behaviour and diet are instituted beforehand or concurrently, there will be minimal or no response to the use of hormones. Drugs that have been used include:

- Leuprolide acetate at 100–700 µg/kg every 2–4 weeks for three or four treatments, then as required
- HCG at 500–1000 IU/kg every 2–4 weeks. Antibodies to HCG develop quickly, limiting its efficacy. It has been suggested that dexamethasone be administered concurrently to suppress the production of these antibodies, but this risks generalized immunosuppression
- Medroxyprogesterone acetate at 5–25 mg/kg every 6 weeks. Side effects (e.g. diabetes mellitus, obesity, hepatopathies and sudden death) limit its use, and great care should be exercised. The author recommends that it is only used under the direction of a specialist avian veterinary surgeon
- Deslorelin implants (Figure 4.18), placed every 5–18 months, have been used by many veterinary surgeons, with mixed results
- Cabergoline at 10–20 µg/kg q24h for 1 week, then once weekly (or more frequently if required), has been reported to be effective (Chitty et al., 2009).

Surgery, in the form of a salpingohysterectomy, has been proposed as a means of controlling egg production. Unfortunately, it appears that, by itself, this does not stop reproductive behaviour and subsequent ovulation, which then results in yolk peritonitis. Surgery should therefore be reserved as a 'last resort' therapy only.

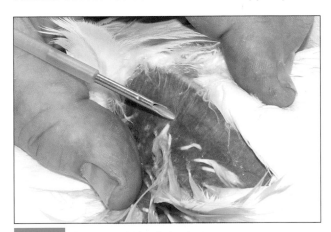

4.18 Placing a deslorelin implant.

Behavioural problems associated with reproduction

Behavioural problems associated with a bird's reproductive drive can include masturbation, excessive egg laying, territorial aggression, one-person bonding (with aggression exhibited towards other people), redirected aggression and attention-seeking behaviour. These behaviours can result in isolation of the bird from the household (and lead to other behavioural problems), surrender and rehoming of the bird, or euthanasia. An international survey conducted in 2009 suggested that 43% of parrots surrendered for rehoming were done so for behavioural problems including biting, aggression, noise and feather destructive disorder (Clubb, 2011). Some of these problems can be attributed to reproductive issues. Ford (2009) emphasized that 'the undesired behaviour is not the problem – it is a symptom of an incongruity between the bird and its environment, its management, or its owner's expectations.'

How does this situation develop? It must be emphasized that no single factor leads to reproductive behavioural problems; rather, it is the result of a complex interaction of the proximate factors discussed earlier. In some cases, the bird may be exhibiting normal behaviour, but this behaviour is inappropriate for its environment and the owner's lifestyle and expectations. Other cases develop when the behaviour is inadvertently reinforced by the owner. Understanding these problems requires a detailed examination of the bird's early social development and learning, its current relationship with its owner (and others in the household), its health, diet, husbandry and environmental cues.

Understanding these behaviours and how they develop

Avian behaviour can be categorized into two functional groups:

1. **Self-maintenance behaviours**, designed to accomplish a specific task to maintain the health of the individual. These include feeding, feather care (Figure 4.19a), locomotion and concealment.
2. **Social behaviours**, designed to communicate information to another individual. These behaviours include territoriality (Figure 4.19b), concern or fear, and courtship.

Some of these behaviours are believed to be innate or instinctive; others are learned. All are reinforced by the reaction the bird receives. Captive parrots, especially those hand-reared as pets, may not have the opportunity to learn normal social behaviours. Their instinctive behaviours – particularly as they reach maturity – may then bring them into conflict with their human 'flock'.

Problems seen in clinical practice can be attributable to one of two causes:

1. **Failure of the socialization process.** This is usually the result of an individual bird being hand-reared in isolation and not being taught basic social skills. Once weaned, the bird is often ignored as its novelty value wears off. This process often results in attention-demanding behaviour (e.g. begging calls, screaming, feather chewing), displacement behaviours such as biting, feather destructive disorder (Figure 4.20), phobias and sometimes even self-mutilating behaviour.
2. **Failure of the human 'flock'.** Failing to understand normal parrot behaviour, and expecting birds to 'fall into line' with human expectations. It was once said that there are no abnormal behaviours – just normal behaviours expressed inappropriately. Behaviours such as screaming morning and night, displaying territoriality and certain reproductive behaviours are examples of normal behaviour that are inappropriate in a companion bird scenario.

It is this second group that includes reproductive-based problems. Young captive birds need continued mentoring and behavioural moulding, and require guidance for the establishment of a normal bird–human flock relationship. This includes a range of normal social behaviours for flock interaction, with appropriate rules regarding conflict resolution, and appropriate self-maintenance and social behaviours.

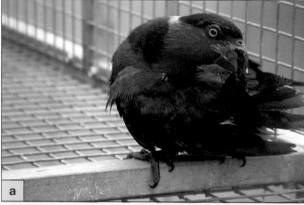

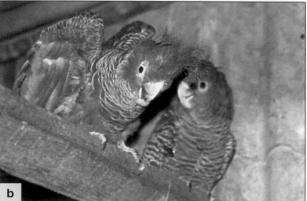

4.19   **(a)** Feather care is a self-maintenance behaviour. **(b)** Gang-gang Cockatoo displaying territorial behaviour – the direct eye contact and the outspread wings are a warning to intruders that an attack is imminent if the intruder does not withdraw. Whether this attack occurs will depend on the individual bird and circumstance.

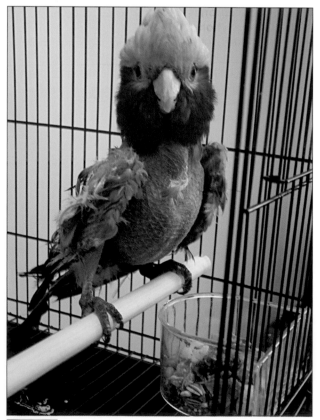

4.20   Feather-destructive Galah.

Failure to be taught – or learn – these behaviours means that many young birds are not prepared for a life in captivity, and may develop behavioural problems. In the absence of imposed rules, birds will develop their own 'rules', based on immediate gratification and revolving around perceived value; however, these rules may not be socially acceptable to their keepers. The bird becomes unable to socially interact with humans appropriately, and therefore a series of displacement or defensive behaviours develop (e.g. aggression and biting). As these antisocial behaviours develop, the bird may become even more isolated, and therefore be more vocal or aggressive in trying to re-establish contact with the 'flock'.

Modifying these behaviours

Unfortunately, these problems are often chronic by the time the bird is presented to a veterinary surgeon, and correspondingly difficult to overcome. They may also have been modified, by either negative or positive reinforcement, to an extent that the presenting problem may not resemble the original. Early recognition and treatment are much more likely to result in a successful outcome; prevention through education of bird keepers is the preferable approach. Incorporating behavioural training into annual wellness examinations is an important step in preventing problems, and should be practiced vigorously by all those involved in the well being of birds.

Reproductive-based behavioural problems are most commonly associated with one-person bonding. In order to overcome this it is essential to normalize social interactions between the bird, the person it is bonded to, and the rest of the household. This has to be done on two levels:

1. **The interactions between the bird and the person to whom the bird has bonded have to be modified.** Interactions such as picking up the bird, scratching its head and body and playing with it have to be stopped or reduced dramatically while the modification programme is being implemented. The bonded person can clean the cage and put in fresh food and water; however, the less interaction the better.

2. **Other members of the household need the opportunity to interact positively with the bird.** To avoid distracting the bird or triggering protective or territorial aggression, it is best if the bonded person is not around while this is being undertaken and, when 'out of cage' training is being performed, the bonded person should bring the bird to a place where it does not exhibit territorial behaviours. The bird should learn to interact with other people using a combination of positive reinforcement and incremental exposure. For example, the new person can drop a preferred food reward in the bird's food bowl and then walk away. If this is done often enough, eventually the bird will react positively to seeing the new person. This person can then try offering the reward to the bird through the cage bars. Eventually the reward can be offered for stepping up on the hand as well as other cooperative behaviours. Alternatively, working in a neutral territory, the other members of the household can cue the bird to perform simple behaviours the bird already knows how to do. This gives the bird an activity on which to focus, while at the same time receiving rewards from people other than the one person the bird has bonded to. This can help build a positive relationship with the rest of the household.

The goal with these two levels of modification is to limit the positive experiences with the bonded person and, at the same time, increase the positive experiences with the new person. However, it may never be possible for the new person to interact with the bird at the same level as the bonded person, and it is unlikely that positive interactions will occur while the bonded person is in the room (see also Chapter 5).

References and further reading

Chitty J, Raftery A and Lawrie A (2009) Use of cabergoline in companion parrots. *Proceedings of the Annual Conference of the Association of Avian Veterinarians Australasian Committee*, Adelaide, pp. 105–109
Clubb SL (2011) Parrot relinquishment in the US: why are birds losing their homes? *Proceedings of the Association of Avian Veterinarians: 32nd Annual Conference and Expo with the Association of Exotic Mammal Veterinarians*. AAV, Seattle, pp. 279–284
Ford SL (2009) Reproductive complications in companion parrots. *Proceedings of the Wild West Veterinary Conference*, Nevada
Smith CA (2010) Sex determination in birds: a review. *Emu* **110(4)**, 364–377

Behaviour

Deborah Monks

Many birds, particularly parrots and passerines, are social animals with a diverse range of communication tools. Vocalization and various body postures telegraph a rich variety of information to their conspecifics. Unfortunately, the subtleties of avian behaviour are often lost on many owners. The failure to interpret cues can lead to owners:

- Inadvertently rewarding inappropriate behaviour
- Misunderstanding subtle threat behaviours, leading to lunging and biting
- Failing to provide basic social and emotional needs for the bird, leading to screaming, feather destructive disorders and other maladaptive syndromes.

Despite these obstacles, many bird owners experience deep affection for their avian pets (Figure 5.1), and would greatly benefit from more focused guidance in this area.

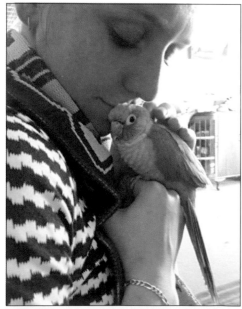

5.1 This owner has a deep regard for her Green-cheeked Conure, and is very happy for any behavioural advice she can get to improve the welfare of her pet. Although 'cuddling' can lead to inappropriate sexual behaviours, this owner has a robust training programme that offsets this potential issue. (© Deborah Monks)

In most developed countries, avian adoption and rescue centres are struggling to keep up with the number of birds given up to them. Behavioural problems are a primary cause of a large proportion of bird surrenders in many countries. While some birds are rehomed due to genuinely unavoidable changes in owner circumstances, many birds are surrendered because they did not meet their owner's expectations. Numerous owners take on birds without researching their physical and behavioural requirements. For instance, an owner taking on a falcon will need to exercise the bird regularly. If that is not done, various physical and psychological problems will arise. An owner taking on a parrot, needs to understand that these are messy creatures, with a predilection for destruction. Canaries and other songbirds vocalize regularly and quite loudly, and while many people find passerine song soothing, it causes considerable irritation to others. It is strongly advisable that novice bird owners do thorough research into the costs, physical needs, behavioural needs, and time involved in avian ownership. A significant number of 'problems' reported by owners are actually just normal avian behaviours.

However, some birds do have true behavioural pathologies, usually secondary to a long-term inability to fulfil normal avian social and environmental needs. Some of these pathologies are amenable to focused modification by experienced behaviourists. Some deficits, such as failure to play independently, can be taught. Other birds may be left with behavioural shortcomings, but can be integrated sufficiently for rehoming after appropriate intervention. Sadly, some birds are permanently behaviourally dysfunctional. These individuals may exhibit feather and skin destructive disorders. They may exhibit non-functional repetitive behaviours and/or be incapable of interacting normally with humans and/or other birds. Managing these behaviourally end-stage birds is problematic.

This chapter aims to give the veterinary surgeon (veterinarian) a brief guide to normal parrot behaviour and first-line problem-solving skills for behavioural issues. In the case of complex or escalating behavioural problems, referral to a qualified, experienced avian behaviourist or specialist practitioner must also be considered.

What is behaviour?

Behaviour is a term that is used in many different contexts. A single behaviour is the directed set of actions exhibited by an individual toward a specific outcome. This may be something like a parrot husking a seed or nut, or foraging within a tray looking for food. Single behaviours can be specifically described and analysed using the science of applied behaviour analysis.

Behaviour can also be used as a general descriptor of the bird. The problem with classifying a bird as either 'well behaved' or 'badly behaved' is that it tends to make the bird the focus of the behaviour (or behavioural problem) and remove owners from their part in the development of that behaviour (or behavioural problem). Classifying or anthropomorphizing the psychological state of a bird is not useful when trying to change its behaviour. It is very difficult to formulate a plan to change a 'grumpy', 'sweet', 'hormonal' or 'territorial' bird; it is far easier to formulate a plan for the owner to be able to change the food dishes without being bitten.

For the remainder of this chapter, the word 'behaviour' will be used to describe a single action or set of actions.

Applied behavioural analysis

It is crucial that veterinary surgeons use and understand correct behavioural terms. This section defines behavioural terms that are used to describe all actions.

The **antecedent** is what happens immediately *prior* to the behaviour. A deliberately applied antecedent is often called a **cue**. During training, the antecedent should be the cue that the trainer is using to elicit a particular behaviour. (Note: the owner's perception of the 'cue' may not mirror the bird's perception of the cue.)

Cues need to be simple, obvious and consistent. They may be visual (such as presenting the hand to the bird for stepping up, or using a hand signal for a particular trick) or auditory (using a whistle, a word or a particular sound). Each requested behaviour should have a unique and easily distinguishable cue; cues that are too similar lead to confusion.

Outside training, however, the antecedent can be any number of things, such as proximity of other individuals, the phone ringing and particular movements of other individuals or objects. In a complex situation, detecting what event is actually the antecedent often takes determined, repeated observation. It is, however, crucial that the precise antecedent is determined.

The **behaviour** is the action that is elicited from the bird after the antecedent. During training, this may be precise (such as raising a foot, stepping up or lifting wings). Outside of training, this can be much more complex and variable.

The **consequence** is the result of the behaviour. Externally applied consequences are described as reinforcement or punishment (Figure 5.2). Birds can have internal reinforcement of behaviour (for instance, flying may be internally reinforcing in the same way that some humans find exercise to be enjoyable). During training, consequences should be positive reinforcement of some type (e.g. verbal, food, toy, touch) that will 'seat' the behaviour in the bird's repertoire as a valuable action. Consequences can be described as either reinforcing or punishing, which can often cause confusion.

- **Reinforcement** is the application of an external consequence to a particular behaviour that is likely to *increase* that behaviour. Reinforcement can be positive or negative. Positive reinforcement is the addition of something valued by the bird, whereas negative reinforcement is the removal of something that the bird finds aversive.
- **Punishment** is the application of an external consequence designed to *decrease* a particular behaviour. Punishment can also be positive or negative. Positive punishment is often called correction, and is the addition of something aversive in response to undesired behaviour. Negative punishment occurs when a desired stimulus is removed from the bird after an undesired behaviour is displayed.

	Reinforcement	Punishment
Positive	Verbal praise Food treat Favoured toy	**STRONGLY NOT RECOMMENDED** Tapping beak (aggressively) Physical force
Negative	Removal of disliked object (such as towel, less favoured person)	Removal of favoured toy Removal of food treat Time out (removal of owner attention)

5.2 Examples of reinforcement and punishment in bird training.

> ### WARNING
>
> It is never recommended to use positive punishment when training a bird. While positive punishment may appear effective in the short term, the detrimental effect to the bird's trust of the owner will cause longer term complications in their relationship

Birds that have been trained using positive reinforcement will tend to offer *more* than the minimum behaviour required, and be much more complicit in the training process. The benefits to the owner–bird relationship are immense.

It is imperative that bird trainers realize that the application of consequence only works when the bird understands the causal relationship between the behaviour and the consequence. To do so, the consequence must be immediate, it must be consistent and it must be directly applicable to the action. For instance, to reward a bird for stepping up, having the trainer walk to the cupboard to get out a treat after the bird has stepped up will be ineffective in increasing the likelihood of future stepping up. The bird will not associate the two actions. The trainer needs to have food treats in the hand, ready to use, when the bird initially steps up. Trainers must *plan* the timing of requests, and the likely outcomes, and have positive reinforcers prepared. This will allow precise application of the reinforcer, at exactly the right time.

The reinforcement should also be conditional on the behaviour being performed within a short timeframe. For instance, asking a bird to step up, and then reinforcing stepping up behaviour after 10 minutes of waiting with the hand extended, will lead to a less immediate response to subsequent requests than removing the hand (and the opportunity for reinforcement) after 15 seconds of non-responsiveness. The same request may be made a short time later, but with the same defined 'window of opportunity' for response. This consistency of timing of reinforcement will reinforce a faster response to future requests. This mechanism can also be used to increase the speed of response to regularly provided behaviours. The trainer can ask for a specific action, but only positively reinforce the action within a certain timeframe. That timeframe can be changed as the bird begins to respond more rapidly.

Most bird trainers use food and toys as **primary positive reinforcers** (Figure 5.3). A primary reinforcer is something that has intrinsic value to the bird, so is immediately rewarding to receive. Some commonly used food reinforcers for parrots are listed below. Individual birds will have different preferences, and some birds will vary their preferences over time. Laying out a 'smorgasbord' of favourite foods in front of a parrot and seeing which foods are chosen first is a good way to determine those of value to the parrot. Choices of positive reinforcement for passerines vary more widely. Raptor training (e.g. demonstration flying) tends to be done using food reinforcers.

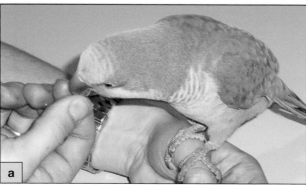
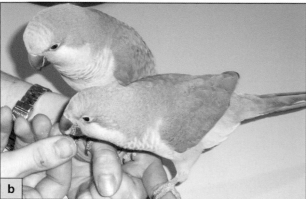

5.3 **(a)** This Monk Parakeet has successfully stepped up, and is being given a small piece of almond as a reward. **(b)** These two Monk Parakeets have been asked to sit quietly and calmly together on the owner's finger (this is a form of stationing). The owner is rewarding each of them, in turn, for continuing to sit appropriately. Please note that this level of physical proximity is not always desirable, and may precipitate biting and other traumas in certain birds. (© Deborah Monks)

Commonly used food reinforcers for parrots

- Slivered or flaked almonds, broken into pieces of 1–2 mm
- Dried fruit, broken into pieces of 1–2 mm
- Pureed fruit from a syringe (often useful for lorikeets as it is one of their favourite treats)
- Walnuts, crushed into small pieces
- Rice puffs

When using primary reinforcers for a training session, it is important to be able to dole out very small amounts at a time, so that the training session is not delayed waiting for the bird to finish eating or playing. As it can be difficult trying to administer food or toys at the precise moment that positive reinforcement needs to be given (that is, at the *exact* moment of the required/requested behaviour), many trainers will couple the primary reinforcer with sound (single words, such as 'good', or clickers are the most common). The sound acts as a secondary reinforcer, which does not have intrinsic value to the bird, but has become associated with a primary reinforcer over time, and has developed value to the bird. This process is called **bridging**. Bridging is useful because it precisely marks when a desired behaviour has been performed, allowing the trainer time to administer the primary reinforcer. Secondary reinforcers, if not continually paired with primary reinforcers, can lose their efficacy.

A reinforcer is applied *after* the behaviour has occurred. If a reinforcer is applied before the behaviour has occurred, then it becomes a **lure**, rather than a reinforcer. While luring is often used early in a training plan, to promote a behaviour that is not likely to occur naturally (see 'Basic training'), it should be phased out quickly. It is not recommended to use luring as a long-term strategy to elicit behaviour. Birds that are continuously lured tend to perform desired behaviours only when the lure is present.

Lastly, although implicit in any positive reinforcement training plan, it needs to be said that a bird should *always* have the option to 'decline' a specific behaviour. At best, forcing a bird that is not compliant to perform a specific behaviour is negative reinforcement. At worst, it becomes positive punishment. Either way, the negative consequences of such training will be to decrease long-term compliance and likely avoidance behaviour. Biting may result. A bird may generalize avoidance of that specific behaviour to other aspects of the bird–owner relationship.

While initially cumbersome, describing training in these constituent parts allows intervention to be precisely targeted. Describing problem behaviours in this way allows the focus to be on the changeable parts of the issue, rather than on the individual bird and its perceived 'personality'. It is worthy of note that human involvement is critical in terms of both the antecedent and the consequence and that these stages are available for human manipulation. The bird is only 'responsible' for the actual behaviour. The antecedent and the consequence are both changeable. Differing the antecedent and changing the consequence make massive differences to the actual behaviour performed. This, then, puts the onus of forming or changing bird behaviour firmly back on owners.

Basic training

Like many young animals, young hand-reared birds tend to find human attention intrinsically rewarding, and are very keen to be near to and interact with humans. Birds are therefore perceived as easy to train, as the reinforcement for appropriate behaviour occurs unintentionally. As these birds mature, and (hopefully) become more independent, simple human attention tends to lose efficacy as a primary reinforcer. Owners that have not instigated positive reward-based training programmes begin to notice that their birds are less accepting of human modulation of their behaviour. Often, nipping or biting behaviour begins, and may progress to actually drawing blood.

Prepared owners start training their new bird soon after acquisition. They will have a list of basic desirable behaviours for a pet bird. These should include stepping up; stepping down; staying on a station (perch) for a period of time; and allowing hand entry into the cage (or human entry into an aviary). These basic desirable behaviours are the equivalent of a dog being able to sit, lie down, heel and come, and are considered a minimum standard for an indoor companion bird. Outdoor birds (or indoor, untame, caged birds) may have a different set of behavioural criteria. However, it is still possible to train these birds to calmly accept certain interventions. For instance, a large raptor could be trained to station on a perch to allow safe human entry into the enclosure.

Initially, training can be as simple as adding cues and reinforcers to behaviour that the bird is already readily performing. The behaviour will thus be cemented into the bird's repertoire. Once a bird understands the training process – human request, bird acquiescence, and provision of reward – subsequent cued behaviours tend to be easier to train.

Continued reinforcement of behaviours already firmly in the bird's repertoire is a sort of 'maintenance' reinforcement. This should be applied to all desired behaviours performed by the bird. Maintenance training should ideally occur periodically and regularly throughout all owner–bird interactions. The owner does not need to set aside a special training session for this. Unfortunately, what normally happens is that established behaviours tend to become progressively less rewarded, leading to breaks in the bird's compliance. This can easily be rectified by returning to a high-frequency reinforcement schedule.

As well as maintenance training, it is advisable for owners to also complete 'novel training'. That is, training cued behaviours that are not already within the bird's repertoire. Novel training serves the combined benefits of: providing structured interaction for the owner and bird (good for new owners); keeping the relationship between bird and owner healthy (good for owners and birds); and giving the bird mental stimulation (good for birds).

There are two potential methods for instilling new cued behaviours. The first is to wait until the bird performs the behaviour unsolicited, and then to reinforce it. This works well to capture common behaviours, such as raising the wings or raising a foot. It is also successful for rewarding talking. However, it can take a long time for those behaviours to be performed at a time and in a manner that is amenable to immediate reinforcement. Careful and clever manipulation of the environment to increase the likelihood of the behaviour occurring can speed this process. For instance, if the bird tends to raise its wings in the shower, then the keeper can begin to reinforce that behaviour in the bathroom, using praise and a food or toy treat. The keeper would then seek to couple the behaviour with a verbal cue to allow the behaviour to be captured, all the while continuing primary reinforcement and praise. The behaviour would be requested (still in

the bathroom) and reinforcement would begin to shift from continuously to only immediately after being requested. Once the behaviour was performed consistently via cueing, the owner would begin generalizing the behaviour to other areas of the house or aviary, using a similar process. Generalization tends to occur more quickly than the initial training. Regularly trained birds tend to be less traumatized after negative interactions (such as forced restraint and non-compliant medication techniques).

The second method is for behaviours that are never performed unsolicited. For these behaviours, the owner can use approximations. Below is a training plan for waving goodbye with a foot, using approximations.

Training a parrot to wave goodbye with a foot (Figure 5.4)

1. Prepare to request 'step up', but stop just short as the bird lifts a foot.
2. Audible 'marker' (e.g. 'good' or a using a clicker) followed by food treat reinforcement for lifting the foot.
3. Once the action is performed reliably, start using a different cue to signal 'foot lift' rather than 'step up'.
4. Once the foot lift is being performed reliably to the new cue, start reinforcing for a higher lift of foot rather than standard.
5. Continue incrementally increasing the height of the foot hold, before reinforcement.
6. Once height is appropriate, begin reinforcing slight movement of foot when at that height, rather than foot held still.
7. Continue incrementally increasing the amount of foot shaking exhibited before reinforcement.
8. Once action is clearly a wave, begin only reinforcing the full wave, rather than any earlier approximating behaviour.

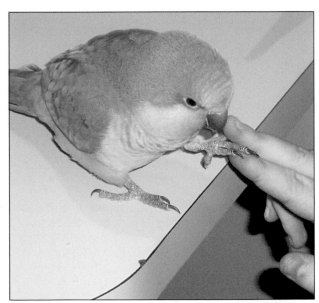

5.4　A Monk Parakeet starting to learn how to give a 'wave'. The owner has an approximation plan, allowing the bird to gradually move into the new behaviour. (© Deborah Monks)

The benefit of a written plan is that it gives owners a more realistic expectation of training progression. Should the training of a particular action become derailed, it also allows rational backtracking to a point at which the bird was performing well, and provides the pathway for continuing the training.

Novel training is extremely useful in acclimatizing the bird to medical handling. Basic medical training includes: consenting to being wrapped in a towel; consenting to foot and wing examination; holding wings elevated for examination of the underwing area; standing on scales for weighing; and taking medication from a syringe. Advanced medical training could include: consenting for venepuncture; consenting for aspiration of masses; and consenting for examination of the oral cavity, eyes and ears.

Many owners enjoy training their bird to do tricks. Although not required for husbandry or health care, trick-trained birds are usually highly willing to participate in human–bird interactions, and are often more behaviourally robust.

Birds, like people, have individual variation in their peak productive times. Many birds train best early in the morning; some do better training later in the day. Keepers should monitor their birds to assess times at which their pets are most likely to be responsive to a training session. Sometimes, removal of food from the cage a short while before a training session can increase the motivation of the bird to work for food rewards (this is the basis of training many raptors). Obviously, food should not be removed for long periods of time, as hypoglycaemia, weight loss and negative metabolic consequences can occur.

Training a parrot to be transported in a pet carrier

1. Place the carrier on a table.
2. Release the bird, and reward for approaching the carrier. **Do not** force the bird to approach.
3. If the bird does not wish to interact with the carrier, reward for simply looking in that general direction. As the bird becomes more comfortable, increase the requirement for reward to:
   a. Looking directly at the carrier
   b. Leaning toward the carrier
   c. Stepping toward the carrier
   d. Touching the carrier.
4. Place a favoured treat or toy just inside the cage ('luring'). Give auditory secondary reinforcement for taking this.
5. Continue the luring by placing the treat further and further into the carrier, until the bird is comfortable entering and standing in the carrier. If the carrier has openings through which treats can be given, then switch from luring to giving the reward through the openings.
6. Once the bird is calmly entering the cage, then begin slowly closing the carrier door. Monitor for any subtle signs of distress. If distress is seen, stop the movement of the cage door until the bird begins to relax, and then reward. Gradually, repeat the above, over repeated sessions, each time closing the carrier door more and more until it is fully shut.
7. Finally, take the carrier (with the bird within) for short 'trips' around the room, stopping to reinforce regularly.

Training a parrot to be held in a towel

1. Place the towel on a table.
2. Release the bird, and reward for approaching the towel. **Do not** force the bird to approach.
3. If the bird does not wish to interact with the towel, reward for simply looking in that general direction. As the bird becomes more comfortable, increase the requirement for reward to:
   a. Looking directly at the towel
   b. Leaning toward the towel
   c. Stepping toward the towel
   d. Touching the towel.
4. Suspend the towel securely between two positions (e.g. tall cans or chair backs), and reward the bird for walking underneath the towel. If the bird does not wish to do this, return to step 3, and continue through that, but using the suspended towel rather than the towel placed on a table.
5. Start to reward the bird for waiting underneath the towel for a short period of time rather than walking straight through.
6. Continue the approximation by drooping the towel lower and lower, continuing to reward the bird for walking underneath.
7. Once the bird is calmly walking underneath the towel, while the towel is touching the body, then remove the suspension devices (be they cans or chair backs) and use hands to suspend the towel. Continue rewarding for waiting calmly while the towel is touching the bird's back. Cease rewarding for exiting the towel.
8. Begin draping the towel over the bird, and rewarding for calm acceptance. Monitor for any subtle signs of distress. If distress is seen, immediately elevate the towel and reward the bird once it calms.
9. Once the bird is comfortable with draping the towel, then begin to apply very gentle lateral pressure, through the towel, to approximate the beginning of being held. Continue rewarding calm acceptance of this behaviour.
10. Start to gently lift the bird in the towel, and continue small approximations until the bird is completely held within the towel.
11. Increase the length of time for which the bird is held before administering reward.

If a bird refuses to perform a particular behaviour, then the owner should simply not use the positive reinforcer, and retreat for a moment. The bird can be invited to perform the behaviour again after a short break. If the bird refuses on more than two consecutive occasions, the owner should consider stopping the training on that particular behaviour. The bird may be tired, or not motivated at that particular point. It is a good idea to return to a simpler behaviour that the bird is more likely to perform, and then reward that behaviour instead. If refusal occurrs at multiple training sessions, the owner should consider some of the possibilities discussed in Figure 5.5. It is better to end a training session on a positive note, if at all possible.

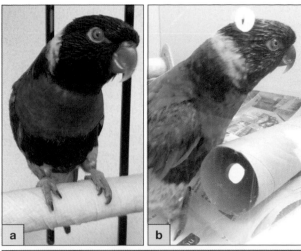

Problem	Potential causes	Solution
Bird not interested in positive reinforcer	Reinforcer no longer primary preference	Try alternative reinforcers (different foods, toys)
	Bird not sufficiently motivated for food reinforcer	Try different foods Try short periods of food removal prior to training session (avoid starvation and monitor bird's weight) Ensure reward not part of normal diet
Previously consistent behaviour no longer consistent	Inconsistent 'marking' of correct behaviour	Improve consistency of verbal secondary reinforcer as a marker exactly at the point of the behaviour
	Moving through approximations too fast	Retrace a few steps of the approximation plan and start again
	Insufficient reinforcement as 'maintenance' behaviour	Increase frequency of primary reinforcement
Loses interest in training session	Requested behaviour too complicated	Reassess approximation plan and retry smaller increments
	Session too long	Reduce length of session Consider increased frequency
	Poor concentration	Try varying time of day, place of training session (may be too many distractions); owner energy level may be poor

5.5 Potential causes of poor training outcomes.

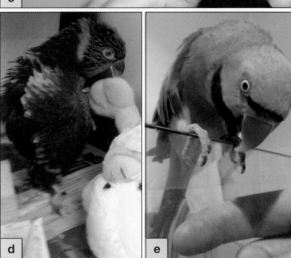

Avian body language

It is obvious that bird keepers need to have as great an understanding of avian body language as possible, relevant to the species for which they are responsible. An owner that can interpret behavioural signs can more accurately judge receptiveness to training, and when it is advisable to terminate a training session. They can differentiate when a bird is interested for more food from when it is uninterested in cooperation and would be best left alone (Figure 5.6).

There are a number of DVDs and internet resources available to assist novice owners, and there are some useful websites given at the end of this chapter. The importance of interpreting subtle body language cannot be overstated.

5.6 **(a)** Rainbow Lorikeets are commonly surrendered due to biting problems. In the wild, they are a pugnacious species, and this can be problematic in the human environment; these birds often express their displeasure with a situation. This bird is watching carefully, but is not displaying overt aggressive signs. **(b)** This Rainbow Lorikeet now has constricted pupils and tight feathering across the head, and should be approached with caution, as a bite may ensue. **(c)** This young Monk Parakeet is very comfortable training with its owner (in this case, learning to 'ladder'). The head and facial feathers are relaxed. **(d)** This Rainbow Lorikeet is playing with a soft toy. His posture is excited, and he is rubbing his head on it, as well as lifting his feet over it. This sort of play is quite sexual in nature, and this bird is quite likely to react negatively to humans trying to touch or remove this object. **(e)** This Moustached Parakeet, with tight feathering and constricted pupils, is clearly not interested in interacting at this moment. (© Deborah Monks)

As time progresses, most owners will learn that there are specific situations in which their bird is likely to be less responsive to human intervention. Figure 5.6d shows a Rainbow Lorikeet playing with a soft toy. The method of play is sexual, and the bird is quite excited. This bird should be approached with caution, and owners should be aware that it may react negatively to that particular toy being touched or removed. Examples of body language which should flag a cautious approach include:

- Sudden stillness
- Pinning of the pupils (abrupt miosis)
- Rapidly changing pupil size
- Fluffed head feathers with a stiff body posture
- Open beak with head held low and forward (Figure 5.6e)
- Using beak or foot to 'push' the hand away.

PRACTICAL TIP

It is often forgotten that behaviour occurs to fulfill a need. Therefore, simply removing the ability to perform a particular behaviour is not 'solving' the problem. The internal need fulfilled by that behaviour will remain. So, it is crucial that bird trainers ensure that there is a replacement behaviour offered for every 'undesirable' behaviour removed from the behavioural repertoire

Successful bird trainers will keenly observe their birds, and take steps to avoid or manipulate situations in which there is likely to be a poor outcome. For instance, they may avoid giving the bird a favoured sexual object, but replace it with a more food-oriented object (Figure 5.7). The potential biting has been avoided, but the bird's total interaction has not been reduced.

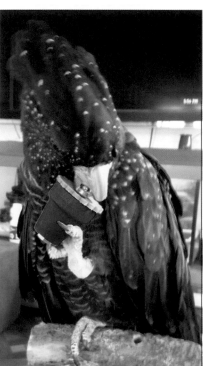

5.7

This Red-tailed Black Cockatoo is being kept positively occupied with a foraging toy. (© Deborah Monks)

Problem behaviours

Problem bird behaviours can be divided into two groups (Figure 5.8). Type 1 is normal avian behaviour that is perceived as problematic by humans. These behaviours are completely normal within the bird's behavioural repertoire, and although they may be modulated, are never likely to be extinguished; these behaviours are functionally appropriate for birds, whether or not they are perceived as appropriate by humans. In these cases, the veterinary surgeon needs to manage client expectations.

Behaviour group	Psittacines	Passerines	Raptors
Type 1 (species-appropriate behaviour, but deemed unacceptable by humans)	Vocalization Environmental destruction Some territory defence Specific wariness of new objects	Vocalization Specific wariness of new objects	Vocalization
Type 2 (species-inappropriate behaviour, pathological behaviour, stereotypes)	Feather destructive disorder Continued distress vocalization Biting Generalized aggression Generalized neophobia	Generalized neophobia	Feather destructive disorder

5.8 Typical 'problem' behaviours presented to veterinary practitioners.

Type 2 behaviours are either species-inappropriate behaviours, or appropriate behaviours that have now become pathological. An example would be a bird that has feather destructive disorder, as an extension of normal preening. These behaviours require behavioural intervention, as there is usually an underlying problem with the bird's adjustment to its environment that needs to be addressed.

As a general rule, parrots are loud, active, destructive pets. They most commonly live in groups (although that is not always the case) and communicate with loud vocalizations. They use their powerful beaks to explore and shape the world around them. They use their inquisitive minds to manipulate their environment, and interact with conspecifics. These factors contribute to the attractiveness of parrots, but are often part of their downfall as captive pets. (See Chapter 1 for some insight into different species' needs and behaviours.)

With the exception of Harris' Hawks, raptors are often more solitary individuals (except when breeding). As a gross generalization, more ecologically solitary individuals tend to have a lesser behavioural repertoire, not needing to interact as much with conspecifics. Raptors therefore tend to present less with Type 1 behavioural complaints.

For passerines, the rate of perceived behavioural problems also appears to be lower. Excess vocalization seems to be the most common issue.

This section covers some common avian behavioural 'problems'. The advice given in this section is general, and may need to be fine-tuned or adapted for each individual case. Each bird is an individual, and each situation is unique, so it is important to remember to custom design any behavioural intervention programme.

Vocalization

The 'dawn chorus' is a term that has permeated common usage, referring to the propensity of many avian species to greet the new day with vocalization. Parrots and passerines particularly embrace vocal communication at this time. This is not an unnatural behaviour, although it not uncommonly causes conflict for humans sharing the birds' environment. Birds often have periods of more intense vocalizing at other times during the day as well.

While it is not possible to eliminate this 'normal' behaviour, it can often be modulated. The following strategies can be employed:

- Minimize the opportunity for vocalization. Pre-empt times at which the bird is likely to make noise (for instance, when guests arrive) and distract the bird just prior to those times
- If the bird consistently begins vocalizing at a particular time, then offer distractions such as food, foraging treats and training exercises just prior to that time
- Do not reinforce the behaviour by shouting. (Note: be careful with separation anxiety as this is not likely to be extinguished by simply avoiding reinforcement. In fact, in many cases ignoring vocalization due to separation anxiety without providing an alternative route of behaviour expression will **worsen** the noise)
- Reinforce quieter vocalizations with (quiet) verbal responses or reinforce alternative vocalizations (for instance, substitution of whistling for screaming behaviour). In behavioural terminology, this is differential reinforcement of an alternative behaviour (also called counterconditioning).

Most birds are social creatures and like to stay in auditory contact with one another. Parrots will frequently call out to their owners when out of visual contact, so that they can track the owner's proximity throughout the day. Humans who wish to reduce the noise produced by a parrot can pre-emptively call, whistle or sing to their parrot when not in the bird's room. The bird can then track the owner's position within the house.

It is worth reiterating the social nature of birds. Buying a bird that has evolved to live in a social group and confining it to virtual solitary confinement is not only a recipe for excessive vocalization but is ethically concerning. The 'five freedoms' are a series of requirements, espoused by most animal welfare organizations, for the keeping of animals under human control. The fourth freedom enshrines the freedom to express (most) normal behaviour, and specifically mentions the 'company of the animal's own kind'. Many behavioural 'problems' could actually be circumvented with better attention to the normal behavioural needs of the individual and species. Owners are often concerned that their bird will not interact with them if it has conspecifics. While a bird housed with avian company is not reliant on human company, a well adjusted bird is able to maintain a relationship with humans and with birds.

If the owner has instituted these general strategies, and nothing has worked, then an Antecedent-Behaviour-Consequence (ABC) analysis should be undertaken (see 'Case examples').

Environmental destruction

Most birds will do some 'readjustment' of their environment. This can vary from the shuffling of sticks or newspaper, to the large-scale havoc wreaked by the beak of a large parrot on wooden furnishings. In the latter case, any and all internal house furnishings are at risk.

The destructiveness of parrots leads to significant problems – intoxication, electrocution, gastrointestinal and respiratory foreign bodies, and trauma are potential sequelae. The most common intoxication is heavy metal poisoning. Lead, zinc, copper and arsenic (in treated timbers) are commonly implicated. Foreign bodies can include synthetic (and some natural) fibres. Rope fibre obstruction is becoming increasingly common in smaller parrots. Trauma can include punctures, lacerations, limb fracture and dislocation, and even getting caught on cage furnishings.

The astute owner will absolutely ensure the safety of the bird's cage or aviary. Safety needs to be balanced with the provision of sufficient environmental enrichment to supply the bird's foraging and activity needs. If the bird is allowed out of the cage, then the area to which the bird has access needs to be safeguarded. Intrinsic safeguarding involves the removal of any dangerous items that the bird can access. If dangerous items remain, then the owner must exert diligent monitoring.

Common household dangers for birds

- Heavy metals:
  - Electrical cords
  - Leadlight
  - Solder
  - Curtain weights
  - Pewter
- Fibres:
  - Towels
  - Clothes
  - Ropes
- Caustic agents:
  - Bleach
  - Hydrochloric acid
  - Many other cleaners
- Other toxins:
  - Pot plant fertilizer
  - Insecticide
  - Insect baits

Birds can be distracted from less desirable destruction by offering more favoured items. For instance, the owner may save a preferred toy for out of cage time, which will distract the bird from chewing on computer cabling.

Within the cage, environmental enrichment is the provision of species-appropriate items to promote the bird interacting with its surroundings. Examples include providing browse, altering and providing more natural perches and providing non-toxic flowers.

Captive foraging is the act of harnessing a bird's natural propensity to search for food. It can be as simple as covering the food bowl with a piece of paper for the bird to remove, or as difficult as having to solve a complex puzzle for normal food (Figure 5.9). At all times, it is important to ensure that the bird can

5.9 Examples of foraging toys available for parrots. (© Deborah Monks)

access adequate caloric intake. Done successfully, captive foraging dramatically improves the quality of life of captive birds. Done poorly, it merely frustrates and starves them.

Resource aggression

Birds, like many animals, are instinctively programmed to protect resources. Darwinian evolution ingrains a need to preserve genetics (i.e. produce offspring), and this is incumbent on having sufficient food, a mate and private areas for reproduction. It is therefore a common complaint of owners that their birds are 'aggressive' around a particular resource. That resource could be the cage, a favourite toy or food. Whatever the item that triggers this behaviour, the outcome is often that a bird that is normally tractable becomes less so around that specific item.

It is often best to avoid the use of terms such as 'aggression' or 'territoriality' with bird owners. Although these phrases may accurately describe the behaviour, the emotional connotations surrounding them tend to distract from the objective scientific analysis required to put a solution into place.

Direct confrontation is not the solution for this sort of behavioural conflict. The outcome will almost invariably be an escalation of the antagonistic behaviour from the bird. For instance, a bird that was merely spreading its wings and lunging may progress to actual biting, or a bird may begin to bite hard enough to draw blood.

This is clearly a situation in which careful planning and pre-emptive manipulation of the situation can reap rewards. For instance, if the bird is biting when hands are put into the cage, then it may be possible to remove the bird from the cage on a stick (having previously trained this behaviour with positive reinforcement), and to station the bird on a stand with a time-consuming food treat or toy. The owner can then clean the cage unscathed.

Another example might be a bird that starts to bite when the owner attempts to remove a particular toy. One option may be to simply restrict access to the toy, but another (preferred) option would be to train the bird to move away from the toy for a large food reward. Motivation can be increased by short-term food restriction prior to playtime.

Inappropriate pair bonding

Occurring particularly (but not exclusively) in hand-reared birds and in birds kept without conspecific companionship, inappropriate pair bonding is a common problem in avian practice. This occurs when a bird fixates on a human as its 'mate', and can lead to a number of issues.

It is normal for a bonded bird pair to defend a territory as they prepare a nest, lay eggs and raise chicks. In the situation of an inappropriate pair bond, the bird often begins to defend the 'mate' against other members of the family, as well as becoming less comfortable with intrusions into the cage. This can result in injury to other family members. Sometimes displaced aggression will be seen, in which the bird will bite the favoured person, in an attempt to drive them away from the perceived threat. This often results in the bird having less interaction with humans, and coming out of the enclosure less frequently, which are poor welfare outcomes. In species in which wild pairs are together constantly, the formation of a bond with a human who is not continuously present can lead to distress, resulting in inappropriate behaviours (such as screaming and feather destructive disorder). Hens may begin to continuously lay eggs, which can lead to malnutrition, egg binding and other reproductive problems. Cock birds can start obsessively masturbating.

It is far better for the keeper to avoid forming a pair bond with the bird, by having ample social time that avoids behaviours that are sexually ambiguous for birds. Humans are, generally speaking, a tactile species, and enjoy having close contact with their avian pets. Unfortunately, these physical intimacies are often used in avian courtship and pair-bond maintenance. Avian couples also engage in mutual feeding, so owners should avoid feeding birds from their mouths (which has hygiene-related issues as well). Petting and stroking should be limited to above the shoulders, if at all. Owners should ignore all sexual behaviour of their birds, and only reward non-sexual interactions (such as tricks, stepping up or other trained behaviours).

If a pair bond has formed, then it is very important to break the bond humanely. Simply terminating interaction can be very stressful for the bird, so it is important to have replacement behaviours that will satisfy the bird's need for social interaction without reinforcing the sexual component. Environmental factors that promote sexual behaviour and breeding should be minimized. These include, but are not limited to: dark hiding places that mimic nest hollows; high-fat diets; long day lengths (for particular species); and, for some species, high rainfall (Figure 5.10; see also Chapter 4).

Sexual behaviour	Initial replacement	Intermediate replacement	Final replacement
Feeding from keeper's mouth	Feeding from keeper's hand	Feeding from table or food bowl, but with owner present	Feeding as a communal activity; food should be offered by the owner only as training reward Provide foraging opportunities separate to owner within cage
Cuddling and full-body stroking	Head scratching, with body contact between owner and bird	Head scratching only, without body contact	Head scratching, as a reward for training exercises
Time spent in dark 'nest hollow'	Remove access to darkened area Provide environmental enrichment to occupy bird (may initially resemble nesting material)	Continue to deprive bird of access to darkened area Change focus of environmental enrichment so that material used is not likely to be interpreted as nesting material	Focus on continuing environmental enrichment and starting to use foraging behaviour to occupy time that otherwise would have been spent nesting
Masturbating behaviour	Try to avoid getting the bird out at times when it is likely to masturbate Change cage position Rearrange cage furnishings Remove furnishings that are likely to trigger masturbation Reduce fat in the diet, or (more ideally) change to balanced pelleted diet	Ignore masturbating behaviour If occurring on owner, then remove bird Request an already trained behaviour, then reward with attention, food and/or toy once performed	Encourage flying to tire bird out physically Encourage bathing behaviour as an enjoyable, but not sexual, activity

5.10 Replacement behaviours for inappropriate pair bonding.

Conclusion

It is worth repeating that behavioural problems, whether perceived or actual, are very serious to the owners and require appropriate attention. The general practitioner should be prepared to refer cases that are escalating, or are beyond their abilities to assist. It is helpful to establish a relationship with a local avian veterinary specialist, or an experienced avian behaviourist.

Useful websites
Barbara Heidenreich
www.goodbirdinc.com
Susan Friedman
www.behaviorworks.org

Case example 1: Finches flying frantically when disturbed

Presentation

A client has a large indoor cage containing four finches. The aviary is positioned just inside the front door of the house. Increasingly, as humans approach the front door, the finches fly erratically around the cage and hit the cage sides. One finch has caught her leg on the wire, and one has damaged pin feathers. The behaviour seems to be increasing in severity.

History

Upon detailed anamnesis, it is discovered that the birds used to be positioned opposite the front door, which is glass. The cage was moved because the owner did not like the look of the messy birdcage immediately upon entering the house. Soon after moving the cage, friends of the family visited, with their four young children and Rottweiler. There was an incident as the friends were entering the house, and the cage was knocked to the floor. The owner is now trying to enter the house as quietly as possible. When the birds startle, the owner tries to leave the vicinity of the cage as fast as possible so that the birds do not get hurt.

The fact that the behaviour is worsening shows that there is likely a learned response to some of the behaviour, even if it began as instinctive fright which was an appropriate response to a dangerous situation.

Possible antecedent 1:
- Humans entering the house

Possible antecedent 2:
- Human appearing suddenly and unexpectedly next to the cage (after entering the house)

Behaviour:
- Birds fly around the cage and injure themselves

Consequence:
- Owner moves away from the cage (negative reinforcement; removal of unpleasant stimulus)

Recommendations

Examining the chain of events more closely, the owner could begin by modifying her actions to alter possible antecedent 2. For instance, she could reposition the cage so that the birds have a better view of the front door, but are further away from people entering directly through the door. The owner could vocalize as she is approaching, to warn the birds of her approach.

The owner should also change the consequence of the birds' frantic flying. Currently, the birds are 'rewarded' by removal of the human as they are flying and hurting themselves. If the birds take flight, an alternative consequence is to enter the house calmly, and stop just inside the front door. Standing quietly, with non-threatening body language, she could wait until the birds had settled before progressing any further into the house.

Once the severity of the flying behaviour is reduced, the owner could increase the distance that she moves into the house before standing quietly.

If the finches are accustomed to taking food from the owner directly, then that would be an ideal positive reinforcement to reward non-flying behaviour. If the birds are not used to taking food directly, then the solution to the problem depends solely on the removal of negative reinforcement.

Case example 2: Galah 'aggression' towards family members

Presentation

A client brings her Galah for a general health check. She mentions that the bird 'hates' her teenage son, and tries to bite him when he walks past the cage.

History

The cage is positioned in the hallway, between the bedrooms and kitchen. Further questioning reveals that the son points and yells at the bird when he passes by. When outside the cage, the bird tries to bite the son. This is a particular problem for the family because the owner is planning an overseas holiday in 6 months and the son is the only family member available to look after the bird while she is gone.

> **Antecedent:**
> - Proximity of son to bird's cage and pointing/yelling at bird by son
>
> **Behaviour:**
> - Bird tries to bite son through bars of cage
>
> **Consequence:**
> - Son moves away from cage (negative reinforcement)

Recommendations

The solution to this type of problem involves candid discussion with all family members about the desired outcome, the degree of effort that will be expended in the pursuit of the outcome, and also the possible consequences should nothing change. In the case of a large parrot, the behaviour modification plan must be predicated on avoidance of bites. In this particular case, the son actually did desire a closer relationship with the bird, and was keen to alter their interactions.

It can be seen, similarly to the first case study, that the consequence of the bird's behaviour is negative reinforcement (removal of a negative stimulus: the son's proximity to the cage), with the antecedent being application of the negative stimulus (proximity of the son to the cage and pointing/yelling behaviour). The son agreed to immediately cease the pointing/yelling behaviour. Repositioning the cage (to remove the other antecedent) was discussed, but was not possible. The family elected to look at ways to positively reinforce the presence of the son at the bird's cage.

A new stainless steel bowl was placed in the bird's cage, and was kept empty. Every time the son approached the cage, he dropped a small, hard, favoured food treat into the bowl, which resulted in a small 'pinging' noise. This treat was acting as a 'lure' (positive reinforcement before the behaviour), with the pinging noise acting as a marker for the presence of the lure. After only a few days, the bird began moving toward the food bowl when she saw the son moving past the cage. At this point, the timing of dropping the food into the bowl was changed to after the movement of the bird had commenced. This changed the pinging noise to a marker of desired behaviour, and the food treat from a lure to a positive reinforcer. The method of delivery kept the son safe from any biting while the relationship was being redefined.

Once the bird was reliably moving toward the food bowl and being positively reinforced for that movement, the timing of the treat was again changed to occur when the bird was progressively closer to the bowl (approximation). After 8 days, the bird was coming right up to the cage bars, and waiting for the delivery of the food treat into the food bowl. The son then offered the food treat directly to the bird (taking good care to protect his fingers in the event of a bite attempt). On the fourth attempt, the bird took the treat from the son directly. Over the next few weeks, the son worked regularly with the bird, and was able to look after the bird while his mother was away.

Case example 3: Bird–owner misunderstanding

Presentation

A client brings in her Moustached Parakeet for lameness. While examining the bird, the owner mentions that the lameness began after the bird had a fall from her hand. She had asked the bird to step up, but it grabbed her hand with its beak. When she pulled her hand away, the bird fell and bounced off a table. Soft tissue damage only is diagnosed and non-steroidal anti-inflammatory medication prescribed for 3 days. After the bird is put back into the cage, it tries to climb up on to the clinician's hand again. It reaches out with its beak to stabilize the move from the perch to the hand, and gently holds the finger as it moves its feet on to the back of the hand. The owner points and says that that is exactly the same behaviour the bird showed when it tried to bite her the day before.

History

Since that time, the client says that the bird is reluctant to step on her hand and is starting to bite harder. The last time it bit her, it drew a small amount of blood. She feels that the lunges are getting faster, and the bites harder, with each interaction.

Recommendations

This situation is a classic mismatch of bird and client perceptions. Looking at the applied behavioural analysis:

> **Antecedent:**
> - Owner offers hand for stepping up
>
> **Behaviour:**
> - Bird reaches out with beak and grasps hand
>
> **Consequence:**
> - Owner moves hand away and bird stumbles

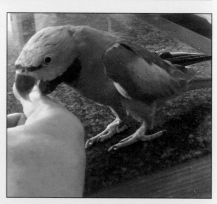

Once the ABC is examined, it can be seen that the offering of the hand has actually become an antecedent for the bird stumbling (and yesterday, falling and hurting itself), hence the bird is starting to grab the proffered hand more firmly. There are several solutions for this sort of problem. Often, a simple, fast remedy is to teach the bird to step up on to a ▶

Case example 3 *continued*

stable stick. That way, the owner and the bird can rapidly restore confidence in the process. Other times, once the situation is demonstrated, the owner is able to train themselves to provide a more stable hand for stepping up.

Note: it is wise to pay attention to the body language of each party before dispensing this sort of advice. Sometimes, the bird is actually exhibiting non-verbal cues that indicate impending biting, and it would be a mistake to counsel an owner to continue offering a hand in that situation. There are now some DVDs which provide inexperienced owners with some assistance in the interpretation of avian body language.

Case example 4: Galah reluctant to 'step up'

Presentation

The client presents with a 10-year-old Galah. The client has been in possession of this bird for 1 year. He says that initially the bird would step up, but then it became reluctant to do so.

History

The client knew that it was bad for birds to get away with being naughty, so he persisted with pushing on the bird's chest and unbalancing it to get it to step up. After a while, the bird began vocalizing and lunging when the owner would put his hand in the cage. The bird continued to need to be pushed on the chest in order to step up. Recently, the bird has begun biting the owner and drawing blood whenever the owner puts his hand in the cage. The owner has begun removing his hand when this occurs.

At this point in the behaviour, the ABC analysis is:

> **Antecedent:**
> - Owner puts hand in cage
>
> **Behaviour:**
> - Bird bites owner's hand
>
> **Consequence:**
> - Hand is removed from the cage

Recommendations

It is evident from this analysis that the biting behaviour is, in fact, being rewarded and is likely to continue. Historically, some ill-informed behaviourists would say that the solution is for the owner to hold his hand in the cage and 'prove' to the bird that biting is not successful. Unfortunately, many birds are able to cause such significant trauma that no normal human will be able to withstand the pain without moving their hand! In this particular scenario, a more sensible approach is to start to habituate the bird to viewing the human hand as positive. The 'positive bowl reinforcement' strategy from Case 2 should be employed to start to safely rebuild positive interactions. That could be combined with

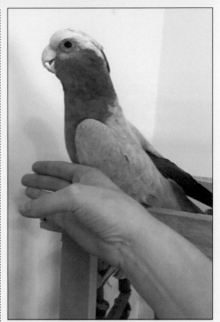

(Courtesy of Emma McMillan)

teaching the bird to step up on a wooden stick (with the option to comply or not – pushing the bird to step up by force will negate this option and the problem will quickly end up escalating again).

Nutrition

Brian Stockdale

It has been reported that malnutrition is responsible for up to 90% of pet bird disease, and is the most common cause of death in pet parrots (Harrison, 2011). Therefore, it follows that correcting malnutrition and nutritional disease will have a greater beneficial effect on the welfare, health and longevity of captive birds than any other veterinary discipline. To correct the problems that lead to avian nutritional disease the veterinary surgeon (veterinarian) needs an understanding of the issues that promote malnutrition. The following sections of this chapter are written from the perspective of a holistic approach to the principles of nutrition rather than a review of individual nutrients, although these are discussed where appropriate.

Overview of avian nutrition

Natural history

There are over 10,000 species of birds recognized worldwide (Del Hoyo et al., 1992), although the number commonly kept in captivity is confined to a few hundred species. Over time, birds have evolved gastrointestinal tract morphology and metabolic capabilities designed to exploit a wide range of habitats and the diversity of food that these provide.

Morphological convergence, due to similar nutritional and ecological pressures, means that many species of birds from unrelated families share common nutritional strategies; for example, New World hummingbirds (Trochilidae) and Old World sunbirds (Nectariniidae) have both evolved long beaks and tongues for efficient nectar extraction. For ease of general classification, birds can be placed into groups based on their preferred food substance (Figure 6.1).

Monophagy, reliance on one specific food item, is extremely rare in wild birds. A case could be made for the Lesser Flamingo, a filter feeder whose bill structure only allows passage of spirulina, a blue-green alga, but this bird will adapt to other diets once in captivity. Most species of birds are, within their designated category, more diverse in their eating habits.

The digestive anatomy of many species of birds is dynamic and plastic in its ability to move from one food source to another. This may be seasonal (e.g. a move from insectivory to frugivory in blackbirds during winter)

or age-dependent (e.g. many species of seed-eating British finches rear their young almost exclusively on invertebrates during their major growth period rather than seeds, which would not sustain the rapid growth rate required by these passerines).

It is the preferred food substances of wild birds that form the basis for captive diets, either by direct provision or comparable substitution; for example, the use of dead day-old chicks provides a suitable substitute for raptors that are mostly generalized faunivores, and commercially produced crickets and mealworms are used as a substitute for the wide range of invertebrates foraged by insectivores.

Whilst the nutrient composition of the variety of foods eaten by birds is extremely varied, ranging from the high sugar levels consumed by nectarivores to the high fat and protein levels in the diet of faunivores, the chemical composition of birds across the different orders is almost identical, especially where ash content is concerned. This suggests that, irrespective of the food source, the basic requirements for nutrients are very similar, and it is the methods by which species have evolved to procure these nutrients that differ. The behavioural, morphological, functional and biological adaptations that give a bird the capacity to consume, digest and metabolize the nutrients in its food are referred to as the bird's nutritional strategy (Figure 6.1). When considering captive diets this 'strategy' should not be overlooked, nor should the nutritional requirements placed on a bird by captivity.

Principles of avian nutrition

Basic nutritional requirements

Nutrients in the diet supply the energy to fuel metabolism and provide the precursors for the synthesis of structural and metabolic macromolecules. These nutrients are generally categorized as macronutrients (fats, proteins, carbohydrates and water), with dietary levels that can be measured in grams, and micronutrients (vitamins and minerals) that are required in micrograms.

Nutrient requirements are not static and a bird's physiological state is a major determinant of its dynamic needs. The demands of growth, breeding, incubation, moulting and thermoregulation increase nutritional needs above maintenance, and the pathological states

Nutritional strategy category	Species commonly kept in aviculture	Morphological adaptations	Diets most commonly provided in captivity	Notes
Faunivores: high-protein and high-fat diets, low carbohydrate. Generally adequate vitamin and mineral levels				
Insectivores: Arthropods, insects and other invertebrates (e.g. molluscs, annelids and crustaceans) Variable nutritional profile depending on species and life stage Good general amino acid and fat levels Poor calcium levels and calcium:phosphorus ratio High levels of indigestible material (e.g. chitin, shell)	Passerines: thrushes; blackbirds; robins; wagtails; redstarts; species of starling	■ Modifications of flight for 'hawking' ■ Beak is generally longer and thinner than that of granivores for probing ■ Ability to separate digestible soft tissue from relatively indigestible shells and exoskeleton ■ In general, insectivorous birds have smaller crops and larger proventriculi (for increased acid production)	■ Proprietary softbill pellets ■ Soaked dog, trout or ferret food ■ Commercially bred live food: mealworms, locusts, wax moth larvae, crickets, flies, earthworms ■ Hard-boiled eggs ■ Supplementary vitamins and minerals, some fruits	■ Most are opportunistic in their choice of prey item ■ Some birds are highly insectivorous during part of the year (facultative insectivores) ■ Most granivorous and frugivorous birds also feed their fast-growing young on invertebrates
Carnivores/piscivores: Mammals, birds, reptiles, amphibians and fish Relatively constant nutrient composition When consumed whole represents a complete nutritional package (even water)	Raptors: owls; falcons; hawks	■ Beak designed for capture and tearing flesh, allows separation of digestible from non-digestible food ■ Ability to egest pellets ■ Expandable oesophagus to swallow whole prey ■ Owls have large water-absorbing caeca ■ Acidic proventriculus pH	■ Variety of commercially bred small rodents and quail ■ Fish if appropriate ■ Dead day-old chicks are considered to be almost a complete diet for adult raptors ■ Avoid shot prey and roadkill smaller birds ■ Arthropods, pieces of day-old chicks, minced meat and protein pellets	■ Urate production is generally high relative to faecal matter compared with other types of birds, reflecting the high-protein nature and high digestibility of the food that reaches the small intestine
Florivores: foods of plant origin are more diverse in their chemical and nutritional composition than foods of animal origin, resulting in a wider range of digestive strategies across this category				
Nectarivores: Nectar is a dilute solution of various sugars and is the most nutrient-dilute food consumed by birds	Lories and lorikeets	■ Most birds have long beaks and tongues to aid nectar extraction from flowers ■ Lories have a 'brush' tip to their tongues to assist with nectar and pollen acquisition ■ Lories have small proventriculi and ventriculi and short bowels, making for poor protein digestion	■ Reconstituted proprietary nectar and pollen powders ■ Sweet fruits and small insects	■ No bird is completely nectarivorous, as nectar alone cannot meet the required amino acid needs (<15%) ■ Augmentation with soft-bodied arthropods and pollen is required ■ Pollen digestion is limited by rapid gut transit time ■ High daily urine output necessitates additional iron replacement from insects and direct mineral sources ■ Substitution of nectar with sugar-water is inadequate to sustain nectarivores. Protein/mineral enriched sugar-based powder foods reconstituted by adding water are commercially available for this purpose
Frugivores: Fruits vary widely in their nutrient content and can be divided into: nutrient-dilute, with a high water and sugar content and low protein and fat content (e.g. grapes, apples, citrus) characterized by a high energy to amino acid ratio; and nutrient-dense, with a low water content and high lipid and protein levels (e.g. ivy, holly and rowan berries, figs, dates) Sugar types vary between fruits. For birds such as thrushes and starlings that lack sucrose activity, these fruits can induce osmotic diarrhoea	Cedar Waxwings; touracos; fruit doves; toucans; barbets	■ Due to the availability and ease of procurement, few morphological adaptations are required by fruit eaters. Some have enlarged gapes and a dilatable oesophagus to facilitate ease of swallowing ■ Ventriculus musculature varies from poorly developed to reasonably well developed (and containing grit) in some species of fruit-eating doves and pigeons that use the mechanical action of their ventriculus as a mechanism for fruit removal from 'stoned' fruits. Gut length is short	■ Fresh and tinned fruits ■ Natural hedgerow fruits ■ Cooked/fresh vegetables, sweetcorn, peas Depending on the species and the degree of frugivory: ■ Pellets – often low iron (see 'Iron storage disease') ■ Mineral supplements	■ Frugivores eating nutrient-dilute foods have a high-intake/high-throughput strategy ■ Poor sugar digestion but relatively efficient amino acid digestion coupled with high-volume intake does, to some extent, offset the poor energy:amino acid balance of these fruits ■ Birds eating nutrient-rich fruits have a digestion rate and transit time more in keeping with that of insectivores ■ Almost all frugivores will augment their diet with invertebrates at some point to offset the inadequate protein levels of fruit

6.1 Nutritional strategies and corresponding adaptations of birds commonly kept in captivity. (continues)

Florivores: foods of plant origin are more diverse in their chemical and nutritional composition than foods of animal origin, resulting in a wider range of digestive strategies across this category continued

Nutritional strategy category	Species commonly kept in aviculture	Morphological adaptations	Diets most commonly provided in captivity	Notes
Granivores: ■ Many birds eat grains and other hard dry seeds and nuts as their primary dietary component for the majority of the year ■ For many temperate-living species, facultative granivory is commonplace when insects become scarce in winter ■ Seeds have the highest nutrient density of any part of the plant and are rich in starch and moderate to low in protein ■ Oil level varies with the type of seed ■ Seeds are usually low in calcium and have a moderate level of phosphorus; however, much of the phosporus, is a component of phytate, which is not efficiently digested by birds (see 'The seed *versus* pellet debate')	Canaries; finches; sparrows; pigeons; parrots	■ Seeds are protected by an outer coat which varies in its degree of hardness. Many birds dehull seeds prior to eating (e.g. finches and parrots), increasing their digestibility and nutritive quality; others consume the seeds whole (e.g. doves) ■ Beaks have evolved structural adaptations to deal with accessing the seeds (e.g. goldfinch's thin beak for removal of fluffy thistle seeds) and subsequently processing them (e.g. ridges and grooved palates to position seeds prior to cracking them, or producing large mechanical forces due to enlarged jaw muscles and a flexible cartilaginous hinge between the beak and cranium to absorb the shock of seed cracking) ■ Large crops for storage and softening of the seeds prior to digestion; very large and muscular ventriculus, particularly in pigeons ■ Relatively long small intestine and well developed pancreas	Small seed-eaters: ■ Canary seed, millet, rape seed, hemp, various smaller seeds Pigeons: ■ Legume seeds, dari Parrots: ■ Sunflower seeds, safflower, flaked maize, nuts – pine, almonds, walnuts, 'peanuts' ■ Vitamin and mineral supplements ■ Formulated diets	■ Representative species of about 20% of avian families eat seeds as an important part of their diet but only around 2% are obligatory granivores ■ Many species of granivores that swallow seeds whole also consume insoluble grit that lodges within the gizzard and assists with the mechanical action of grinding ■ Seeds from wild plants are generally harder to digest than from cultivated crops (this has some direct bearing on seed consumption and energy satiation in captive parrots)
Herbivores: ■ Plants are highly abundant but are high in fibre and generally low in nutrient value ■ Protein content can range from 5–35% dry matter, but the presence of the cellulose, lignin and often silica-impregnated cell walls makes digestion a problem	Ratites, geese and species of ducks and swans	■ Beaks often have serrated edges to permit harvesting ■ Large muscular ventriculus for grinding plant material – usually contains grit	■ Lucerne and alfalfa (fresh and pellets), fresh greens, vegetables and 'grazing'	■ Vegetative parts make up a significant proportion of the diet of only about 3% of birds ■ Some species of herbivores practice coprophagy ■ Low level of protein in plants means that the chicks of many avian herbivores are more faunivorous and granivorous than their parents

Omnivores

- One-third of all avian families consume a wide variety of plant and animal foods on any given day and can be considered omnivorous; they are nutritional generalists rather than the specialists mentioned in the preceding sections
- Meat-biased: corvids; Pekin robin; starlings (e.g. Common Starlings); laughing thrushes
- Fruit-biased: barbets; toucans; starlings (e.g. Hill Mynahs); tanagers
- Many birds placed in a respective category regularly consume quantities of food from another designated category
- Others are seasonally facultative in their approach to eating foods rather than eating all types of food over any individual period
- Ability of the gastrointestinal system to modulate its structure and function is an important response to shifting nutritional regimes
- Levels of major pancreatic digestive enzymes and some intestinal brush border enzymes change in proportion to the dietary content of their respective substrates
- Retention time also appears to be adjusted to diet composition

6.1 (continued) Nutritional strategies and corresponding adaptations of birds commonly kept in captivity.

of stress, disease and injury also modify nutritional requirements. For some nutrients the difference between basal levels and maintenance is large (e.g. energy), while for others (e.g. some amino acids, minerals and vitamins) it is minimal. The roles of individual nutrients within the body are well documented (MacDonald, 2006).

A bird's energy needs are considerably more variable than other nutrient requirements. Birds eat to meet these demands and as such consumption varies with activity, temperature and the energy concentration of the diet. If a bird decreases its intake because of lower needs, due to decreased energy expenditure or by eating more energy-dense foods, there is a need for a proportional percentage increase in other nutrients within the diet. This simple equation has a fundamental part to play in the pathogenesis of avian nutritional disease.

The importance of ultraviolet (UV) light should also be mentioned. Exposure to UVB light has the effect of activating vitamin D within the skin. Many caged parrots are never exposed to unfiltered sunshine and as such are unable to activate their own vitamin D. While exposure to natural sunshine would be best, this is not always practical and specific UVB light bird lamps should be used to ensure adequate exposure and help with calcium metabolism.

Principles of good nutrition

- Provide captive birds with a diet that will deliver adequate levels of both macronutrients (fats, carbohydrates and proteins) and the micronutrients (vitamins and minerals) appropriate to the species or individual
- Nutrients need to be supplied in a form that is appropriate to the species being fed; the bird needs to have the anatomical and digestive capabilities to be able to consume and utilize the food provided
- Food, whilst having an appropriate chemical nutritional profile, must also deliver these nutrients upon digestion

---

The seed *versus* pellet debate

The majority of pet parrot owners feed commercially constructed 'parrot mixes' to their birds containing a variable range of grains, seeds and nuts, most of which are foreign to the experience of their free-living relatives. The choice of seeds (usually based on size) varies from mix to mix, generally depending on the target species at which the food is aimed. These seed products are either grown specifically for bird food or are second-grade leftovers from the human food market. It is important to consider the following points:

- The effects of storage have a profound effect on the nutritional quality of the seeds
- Not all components of parrot mixes are consumed by all birds
- Of those components that are eaten, the majority provide inadequate levels of many of the essential nutrients required to maintain healthy cellular function.

The nutritional value of seeds varies considerably. Fresh 'milky' seeds have higher levels of protein and vitamins, but storage in this 'semi-ripe' form is impractical. The large majority of the dry seeds fed to both seed-eating passerines and parrots are considered to be deficient in many of the essential nutrients (Figure 6.2). Some seeds, particularly the 'oil seeds' such as sunflower, are initially well supplied with vitamin E, which acts as an antioxidant preventing the fats from becoming rancid, but prolonged and poor storage (resulting in damage to the shell permitting oxygen to enter) depletes these stores. When considering seeds as a food source one should bear in mind that seeds are not designed to be eaten (unlike fruits), and so it should not be surprising that seeds are not replete in vitamins (acquired by photosynthesis) and minerals (acquired from the soil via roots once the seeds germinate).

Commonly used seeds (as fed) are missing 32 essential nutritional ingredients from eight groups	
Vitamins	Vitamin A, choline, niacin, pantothenic acid, riboflavin (B$_2$), cyanocobalamine (B$_{12}$), biotin (H), vitamin D$_3$, vitamin E, vitamin K, folic acid
Minerals	Calcium, phosphorus (70% tied up as non-digestible phytates in plant products), sodium
Trace minerals	Selenium, iron, copper, zinc, manganese, tin, iodine, chromium, vanadium, bismuth, boron
Pigments	Chlorophyll, canthaxanthin
Essential amino acids	Lysine, methionine
Fibre	Mucopolysaccharides – soluble and insoluble
Vitamin precursors	Beta-carotenes converted to vitamin A in the liver
Fatty acids	Omega-3

6.2 Essential nutrients potentially found lacking in an all-seed diet.

Notwithstanding their type, size or source, it has been well established that seeds are a deficient source of essential nutrients, and whilst the nutrients available from each individual type of seed or nut vary, no seeds come close to fulfilling the dietary requirements of birds (Ullrey *et al.*, 1991). Even if a cultivated seed mix that would meet the nutrient requirements if completely consumed could be assembled, it would be difficult to prevent the preferential self-selection of favoured, but nutritionally unbalanced, foods by birds.

- **Protein:** much is made of the level of protein in a diet. The percentage levels needed for breeding, growth and moulting are often quoted (Murphy, 1996). Whilst dietary levels of protein are relevant, it is protein quality, based on the profile of the essential amino acids that it is made from, that is crucial. Ten of the 20 or so amino acids that make up proteins are described as essential in birds. The proteins found in seeds are deficient in a number of these essential amino acids: lysine (necessary for good growth) and the sulphur-containing amino acids methionine and cysteine (needed for feather growth) can be highlighted. This is one of the reasons why many seed-eating birds, for example, finches and sparrows, move away from seeds as a diet for rearing their young and feed a high percentage of insects and arthropods. The quality of seed is insufficient to promote quality growth.

- **Calcium, phosphorus and vitamin D:** for effective bone growth, reproduction and metabolic function, a bird's diet needs to contain around 0.1% calcium – seeds have around 0.03%. However, looking solely at the levels of calcium in a diet can be misleading. A diet containing a calcium:phosphorus ratio of around 2:1 is considered optimal. In broad terms for seeds the ratio is around 1:4 or worse (1:7 in sunflower seeds) and this, along with a lack of active vitamin D in the diet (or exposure to UVB light), is a big contributor to the calcium deficiencies observed in many pet parrots.
- **Vitamin A:** the group of chemicals collectively called vitamin A are not present in plants; they are exclusively an animal or synthetic product. Plant tissues contain carotenoids, the vitamin A precursors that are converted in the bird's body into vitamin A. In general, seeds are short of these vitamin A precursors and so are considered to be 'vitamin A deficient'. Vitamin A is responsible for a number of functions within the body. Two of its main roles are as part of the immune system and being responsible for the quality of epithelium.

Wild *versus* captive bird seed consumption

From observation of wild parrots it is known that seeds represent a high percentage of their dietary intake, for the majority of species. This can be misleading for keepers seeking to provide their birds with a 'natural' diet.

One thing that seeds do provide is a rich source of calories. This can be in the form of carbohydrate (e.g in corn and canary seed), fat (e.g. sunflower, hemp, rape and nuts) or protein (e.g. legumes). Birds, wild and captive, eat to satisfy an energy need, but the energy expenditure of wild and outdoor aviary birds is several times greater than that of captive indoor caged birds and their feeding habits are driven by a quest for this energy. In eating a larger volume of food to satisfy this higher energy need, wild and aviary birds accumulate, by virtue of greater intake, adequate levels of the essential micronutrients. Caged birds, eating to a lower energy requirement, fail to do so.

Wild parrots also have a much wider range of food types available and tend to eat semi-ripe seeds, not dried, which have a much higher level of nutrients. Their diet is also augmented with fruits and invertebrates, all of which provide them with a much richer nutrition than caged birds.

The requirement for macronutrients of wild and free-flying aviary birds should not be compared with that of captive indoor birds.

Induced monophagism

Why do certain parrots become fixated, almost to the exclusion of everything else, with eating only one or two type of seeds, the so-called 'sunflower seed junkie'?

Dietary habits in parrots are based on a number of factors:

- Food availability and ease of procurement
- Digestive capability of the bird
- Palatability
- Taste (although a parrot has relatively few taste buds, around 350 compared with around 9000 in humans, which are mainly situated towards the back of the throat rather than on the heavily cornified tongue)

- Shape and colour (have been quoted as important, and possibly are to the owner, but doubt has been cast over their significance)
- Learning
- Energy intake.

Learning is the most fundamental principle in formulating the eating habits of birds, influenced by owners and companion birds. Providing a wide range of food types at an early age promotes ready acceptance of new food types later; restricting birds, particularly at weaning, to a limited range of foods (e.g. seed only) effectively creates the principles for their dietary habits for the rest of their lives. In later life, the new foods are often not perceived as 'food', and are thus ignored in preference for the bird's accepted diet. Previous dietary experience has a considerable bearing on the eating habits of older captive parrots.

Energy intake is also a particularly significant factor in birds' eating habits (see 'Wild *versus* captive bird seed consumption'). Although captive birds expend less energy their eating habits are still driven by energy needs. Easy 'fixes' such as high-fat seeds and nuts provide a readily accessible source of energy and satiation is generally reached quite quickly. The line between hunger and appetite often becomes blurred. Whilst the energy expenditure of captive birds is much lower than that of wild birds, their need for trace elements for vital body functions is not. In fact, one might suggest that it is higher as stress requires a high level of nutrients.

As a consequence of lower intake of foods of generally lower (micro)nutritional quality, pet parrots can become micronutrient deficient. **Diets for captive birds should therefore be lower in energy to stimulate appetite and higher in trace elements to take into account the lower ingested levels and greater needs.**

Client education

Bird keepers must take some of the responsibility for the existence and persistence of avian malnutrition, and it is important for the veterinary clinician to educate their clients in appropriate nutrition practices.

- Nutritional misconceptions and inappropriate feeding regimes such as those mentioned in the sections above perpetuate the problem.
- Many owners may have acquired their feeding advice from pet shops that, in many cases, allow economics to dictate their sales of 'bird food' to the public.
- An anthropomorphic approach to their bird's eating habits, taking pleasure from their pets liking for and desire to eat large quantities of unsuitable foods because 'he enjoys them', often makes owners feel they are 'doing right' by their bird.

> **'Mother Nature knows best'**
>
> It is a commonly held belief, but sadly a misconception, that pet parrots will selectively eat foods that are rich in certain micronutrients as and when their bodies require them. With very few exceptions (e.g. increased calcium intake by certain species of birds prior to egg laying) the 'Mother Nature knows best' philosophy does not apply. Whilst pet parrots do selectively eat foods high in fats, they do not select for micronutrients

Correcting diets for captive parrots

Mineral and vitamin supplements

Many parrot owners supply mineral and vitamin supplements. For those feeding a seed-based diet this is done primarily in an attempt to correct the known nutritional shortfalls of the basic diet. Whilst correction is undoubtedly required, initially feeding a diet in the knowledge that it is deficient and then trying to correct the deficiencies seems (to the author at least), at best, counterintuitive.

Dietary correction should not (and cannot) be a top-up of presumed deficient nutrients. Clinicians are unable to distinguish individual nutrient deficiencies so owners cannot be expected to simply 'replace' them with supplements, which in themselves may only contain a limited range of nutrients. However, continuing to feed a seed-based diet without the use of additional supplements would be to promote even greater nutritional issues.

Regulating intake can be problematic. The misguided philosophy that 'if one is good, two is twice as good' must be discouraged, and yet sprinkling powder on to the soon-to-be-discarded seed husks to fall to the bottom of the food bowl also seems less than satisfactory. Fortification of nutrients through water is problematic as aqueous solutions of vitamins and minerals are very unstable, prone to spoilage and water consumption is very variable (Koutsos et al., 2001). In all cases, supplements must be used as per manufacturer guidelines, using only reputable brands. Ideally supplements should be used to supplement specific needs and always with the aim of balancing the micronutrients.

The use of supplements does not prevent deficiency diseases – and certainly has no effect on the excessive intake of fats. Many birds on mineral and vitamin supplements are still presented suffering from clinical nutritional disease. One specific example is hypocalcaemia: birds that are being given regular calcium and vitamin D supplementation are still presented exhibiting signs. This is one of the few deficiencies that can be confirmed with a blood sample (see 'Malnutrition and nutritional disease'). The risk of hypervitaminosis (A and D_3) is also well documented (Koutsos et al., 2001). Whilst treatment of malnutrition should include a holistic nutritional reappraisal and not a top-up of presumed deficiencies, vitamin and mineral supplementation (e.g. calcium, iodine, vitamins A, D and E), initially by injection or orally, should be considered in the initial stage of treatment. In certain conditions this will provide a rapid increase in the body's reserves and act as a temporary depot while dietary correction is being undertaken. It will often improve both appetite and metabolism during dietary conversion.

Alternative foods to seeds and nuts

If it is accepted, from nutritional analyses, that seeds and nuts are both deficient in many of the essential nutrients and in general oversupplied with fats, then providing alternative foods, within the digestive capabilities of the species, would seem like a sensible alternative.

Fruit, vegetables and table foods are fed in varying amounts to pet parrots. It is worth commenting that this discussion has been considering 'the parrot' as a generic species; however, it should be noted that different species of parrots (unlike different breeds of dogs) have evolved different nutritional strategies. For example, Amazon and Eclectus Parrots are more frugivorous and their diet should contain more fruit and vegetables than that of the more omnivorous Grey Parrots.

Formulated (pelleted) diets

Formulated diets play an integral role in feeding farm animals, poultry and domestic pets; there are not many cat and dog owners who do not feed a formulated diet (wet or dry) to their pets. The use of seed mixtures as food for captive parrots has a long-abandoned historical precedent in the poultry industry.

Due to the problems in achieving a balanced diet through feeding a mixture of foods, many nutritional experts consider formulated diets to be the best method of feeding our pets. Avian veterinary surgeons generally agree that the feeding of formulated diets represents the biggest advance in captive avian health and welfare seen over the last 30 years.

The principal aim of formulated diets is to provide a balanced level of essential nutrients in an acceptable and palatable form. The natural foods of the species are used as the general matrix and then, following analysis, supplements are added to attain the required levels for each essential nutrient relative to dietary intake. Energy levels are kept reasonably low to ensure that a high level of eating is encouraged and micronutrient intake levels are maintained.

The extrusion process used in the production of pellets enhances the digestibility of the ingredients, by breaking down many of the naturally occurring digestion inhibitors and reducing potentially harmful mycotoxin levels.

By taking this approach to feeding, an owner ensures not only that all the essential nutrients are provided within the diet (something the use of mineral and vitamin supplements fails to address), but also that their pet is unable to 'buffet feed' on selected seeds. Organic formulated diets are available and may further enhance the health benefit to captive birds.

Conversion from a seed to a formulated diet: Weaning a bird on to a formulated diet is often reported to be difficult. Whilst some birds convert readily, some do undoubtedly take longer than others to change their, often habituated, eating habits. However beneficial the change to a formulated diet may be, there is no place in a conversion programme for starving a bird into submission. Apart from the obvious welfare issue, rapid mobilization of body fats can result in potentially fatal liver collapse, especially in obese birds that may already be suffering from hepatic lipidosis. Breeding and aviary birds are generally easier to convert than the tame pet parrot. There are many reasons why birds do not immediately accept formulated diets and the owner should be reassured that failure to readily convert is not an indication that the foods are neither palatable nor nutritious. As mentioned above, dietary habits are learned, usually at an early age. A change in dietary behaviour requires re-education (often of the owner as well as the bird) and this can take a period of time. There are a number of ways in which conversion can be helped; one is to wean baby and young birds on to a formulated diet as soon as possible whilst their dietary tastes are still being fashioned. Other ideas are explored in Figure 6.3.

Monitoring of the volume and consistency of the bird's droppings during the conversion process will assist in establishing the amount of food being eaten. Regular weight checks should be undertaken during the conversion period (daily in small birds and twice weekly in larger birds) to ensure that there is no significant weight loss. A weight loss of >5% in small birds and >10% otherwise should not be exceeded in the first week of conversion (assuming the bird was not initially obese). If excessive weight loss occurs, the conversion process should be halted while the bird is stabilized.

1. **Reduce food availability.** For about 7–10 days prior to conversion, the owner should be instructed to limit the volume of 'normal' food that is provided to between 1 teaspoon (5 g for Budgerigars) and 2 tablespoons (50 g for macaws) at any one time (**not per day**). This prevents the bird from buffet feeding and encourages it to eat what is available. Food is only replenished when all of it has been eaten.
   - For medium and larger parrots, a small amount of vegetables and fruit should also be provided, even if the bird is not generally keen to eat them.
   - The use of a water-soluble mineral mix (including iodine) should be used to replace deficits and may help stimulate appetite. This can be discontinued once the bird is eating 80% of the formulated diet.
   - Water dish hygiene needs to be exemplary.

2. **Weaning the bird off its old diet.** Offer a small amount (see above) of the usual food in the morning and then remove the bowl from the cage either once the food has all been eaten or after about an hour. Place some of the formulated diet (less than would cover the bottom of the bowl) in the usual feeding bowl. This should be the only food that is available to the bird during the main part of the day. If the new food is eaten then additional formulated diet in small amounts can be given throughout the day. In the evening some fruit and vegetables should be offered, and a little more of the usual food. Over subsequent days the amount of seed offered in the morning and evening should be reduced until such time as only formulated diet is offered from the start of the day and the previous diet can be completely withdrawn.
   - Pet parrots are generally habituated to eating from the same place in the cage and the same bowl; they will tend to ignore or play with novel food placed elsewhere.
   - Limiting the amount of formulated diet provided to a few pieces at a time helps prevent the bird from removing the food from the bowl to uncover its normal food or generally wasting it.
   - By offering the bird its normal diet for limited periods during the day, the owner can be reassured that the bird will not starve during the conversion period. The quality formulated diet will be available during the majority of the time should the bird become hungry.

3. **Add fruit juice to the food.** Many birds can be encouraged to taste the food and will readily consume it if a small amount of fruit juice is added. Pieces can be moistened (but not soaked, or some of the essential nutrients may be lost) with the juice of the bird's preferred fruit or vegetables (e.g. some birds particularly like the taste of peppers) so that they have a flavour that they know and enjoy. Over time the amount of juice can be reduced until the food is served dry.

4. **Heat and/or spoon-feed food.** Heating the food slightly can stimulate the bird to accept it. This can be also be combined with adding fruit or vegetables (see tip 5). If the bird is hand-reared then it may still readily accept warm moist food from a spoon (the size of the pieces may initially need to be reduced). Spoon feeding initially small pieces can be progressed to larger pieces and then pieces in the bowl.
   - This method may work if the bird is familiar with hand feeding from a spoon, or may instinctively associate it with either a parent or potential mate. The younger the bird, the more likely it is to remember being fed and the more readily this will work.

5. **Mix the pieces with fruit or vegetables.** Some birds will take to eating formulated diets if they are mixed in with their normal seed, but this is generally not recommended. However, crumbling the formulated diet and mixing it with pieces of fruit and vegetables that the bird is known to eat and enjoy is an alternative, as the moist fruit and vegetables improve the palatability of the formulated diet.
   - The problems with providing a formulated diet mixed with the basic seed mix are self-explanatory. The bird will reject the 'foreign objects' in the food bowl in favour of its usual seeds. This (non) method of conversion is one of the issues that alienates owners from formulated diets ('The food is no good (wasted) as the bird would not eat it').

6. **Eat it yourself and/or feed the bird at mealtimes.** Many pet parrots are used to eating with their owners at mealtimes; this can be a good tool for encouraging conversion. The food should be placed on a plate and the owner instructed to move it around with a finger or a spoon and eat or pretend to eat it in front of the bird. Most formulated diets are a little bland for human tastes but are palatable, and many birds are encouraged to try the food if they see their owners eating it.

7. **Use a converted bird as a role model.** If there is already a converted bird in the household it can be housed near the bird in the process of being converted. If compatible, the birds can be placed in the same cage; the converted bird becomes a 'trainer bird'.

8. **Change the bird's environment.** For small psittacines, moving the bird into a novel environment (e.g. light box, a repurposed aquarium or even a new cage) can work. All the toys, perches and bowls should be removed and the formulated diet offered loose on the floor. Sprinkling food on a mirror or sheet of white paper placed on the bottom of the cage can work especially well for Budgerigars: a bird old enough to be socialized may eat to compete with the 'rival' in the mirror; white paper draws attention to the food.

9. **Manufacturer's tips.** Specific manufacturers will offer tips for conversion oriented towards their products. These can usually be found on their websites, and offer additional hints.

10. **Veterinary supervised conversion.** Some birds do not convert readily. The owner's emotional attachment to their pet may lead to 'lapses' in a conversion protocol; others fear that they are starving their bird into dietary submission to the detriment of its health. Veterinary supervised conversion within the veterinary clinic, where regular monitoring can be undertaken, may often be necessary and successful.

'Failure' to convert. The biggest stumbling blocks to efficient conversion are the owners either giving in to 'parrot pressure' early in the conversion process or not persisting for long enough. Allowing a parrot to dictate its eating habits is the surest way of establishing malnutrition. If conversion steps do not work the first time (a period of at least 10–12 weeks should be attempted) then the owner can revert to feeding familiar foods for a short period of time (whilst instigating tip 1) and then try again. The effort is worth the long-term health benefits for the bird.

6.3   Converting birds from a seed diet to a pellet-based diet.

Feeding strategies of commonly kept birds

Psittacine birds

Psittaciformes represent a range of nutritional strategies (Figure 6.4), and research into the particular requirements of the species being kept is necessary to make informed decisions when devising a captive diet.

Fruit and vegetables (with some seeds and nuts) should constitute 20–40% by volume of a captive frugivorous parrot's diet, and 10–15% for more granivorous/omnivorous species. Commercially available formulated (pelleted) diets, as discussed earlier, are recommended as the primary nutrition source.

Nutritional strategy	Examples
Florivores	Blue and Gold Macaw Military Macaw
Nectarivores	Lories and lorikeets
Frugivores	Green-winged Macaw Orange-winged Amazon *Pionus* spp. Eclectus Parrot
Granivores	Budgerigar Cockatiel Hyacinth Macaw Rosellas Black-headed Caique Lovebirds Galah
Omnivores	Eastern Rosella Sulphur-crested Cockatoo African Grey Parrot

6.4 Nutritional strategies of commonly kept psittacine birds.

The group of parrots commonly called lories and lorikeets are more specialist feeders. They feed on the nectar of various blossoms and soft fruits, preferably berries. They have specially adapted tongues with a 'brush-like' fringe that helps with the removal of pollen and nectar from plants (and gives rise to the genus name of *Trichoglossus*, literally translating as hair-tongue). In captivity, commercially formulated nectar substitutes are generally fed. These are fortified with proteins. Additional pollen is also provided. Feeding formulated diets is also recommended, softened with honey water or similar, to offset the low protein and mineral content of the rest of their diet.

Fruit alone should not be seen as a complete diet for parrots and other psittacine birds. In general, cultivated fruit, because it is designed for the human palate, tends to be high in sugars but low in minerals and vitamins. Wild fruits and berries are better sources of micronutrients and contain higher levels of phytonutrients. These are complex products with diverse metabolic actions, some of which are considered to offer an 'added extra' to the food. Their value in a diet is as yet unproven.

Vegetables are generally higher in minerals than both fruit and seeds, and dark-coloured vegetables such as peppers, carrots, spinach and broccoli provide good levels of carotenoids. Mineral content is wholly dependent on the levels of minerals available to the plant from the soil in which it is grown, and as such is highly variable.

Some types of table foods do no harm to pet parrots, including limited amounts of rice, pasta, potato, bread and well cooked chicken, and will provide carbohydrate and protein to the diet but little more. Some human food items should be avoided, such as those that have been cooked in fats or contain high levels of fat (e.g. chips and crisps), as these have the potential not only to do harm but to create undesirable eating patterns. The main issue with feeding table foods is that, whilst most will do no harm, the energy levels of the birds are being met with foods that do not contain adequate levels of micronutrients. In general, feeding table food is more likely to exacerbate problems than correct them.

Formulated diets, foraging and environmental enrichment

Wild parrots spend a high percentage of their day foraging for food. Many species have recognized 'meal-times' interspersed with varying degrees of social interaction. In comparison, in captivity the provision of food, irrespective of its form, available in a bowl throughout the day, frees up large periods of time for the captive parrot to fill. It is this 'free time' that is often cited as the cause of 'boredom'-related behavioural issues (see Chapter 5).

Criticism is levelled at formulated diets for contributing to this potential problem by reducing the time taken to eat the pellets and for their 'boring' uniformity. Feeding *per se* should not be a substitute for environmental enrichment and owners should be encouraged to devise foraging toys in which food can be hidden to provide stimulation to the bird. The provision of edible branches (e.g. fruit, willow, hazel and alder) can also be used as a nutritional source of environmental enrichment.

Passerines

The order Passeriformes includes over half of the known species of birds. They range in weight from no more than 4–5 g to those weighing around 1.5 kg. This large range of species also features a wide range of dietary habits. Within aviculture, the majority of species kept can be divided into two groups; those nominally designated as seed-eaters and those referred to as softbills (see Figure 6.1).

Seed-eating passerines

The type of seeds fed to seed-eating birds is in general governed by two criteria: species preferences (based mainly on their ability to manipulate, crack and hull the seed); and commercial availability and cost. The nature of the seeds fed, in terms of nutrition, also falls into two basic categories: those seeds providing maintenance levels of energy and protein (which are fed throughout the year); and 'minority' seeds (fed at certain times to enhance nutrition during breeding and moulting).

The basic maintenance seed mixture for most foreign finches comprises varieties of millet seeds (for non-native finches) and canary seed (for canaries), which is a type of grass (Figure 6.5). These are grown in large quantities specifically for the bird market and so are relatively cheap.

Many of the 'minority' seeds are oil-based (e.g. rape, sunflower, hemp and linseed), which, if fed at high levels throughout the year, would result in obesity and potentially organ disease. Many other types of seed are available (at least 50 types are listed on feed sites), but can be quite expensive; the seeds from teasel are enjoyed by all British finches and canaries but the cost is around 12–15 times the price of millet or canary seed, reflecting the fact that teasel is a biennial plant, and the specialist harvesting techniques required to obtain it.

Many seeds are sold as species-specific mixtures, incorporating seeds based on the preferences of the birds in question. A canary mix will generally comprise 60–70% canary seed, with red and black rape, linseed, hemp and occasionally other smaller seeds. Some mixes may also contain 'egg-biscuit' (this resembles small pieces of hard yellow dog biscuit) but this, whilst nutritionally sound, is often not eaten in preference to

Species	Basic seeds	Additional seeds	Notes
Canary	Canary seed	Rape, hemp, linseed, soaked seed mix	Often all sold as a 'mixed canary seed'
Non-native finches: Zebra Finch, Bengalese, waxbills, Gouldian, mannikins, Australian finches	Millet: red, Japanese, white, pannicum; canary seed	Grass, small seeds such as maw, niger	The basic seeds are often sold as 'foreign finch mix'
British finches: Bullfinch, Greenfinch	Canary seed, buckwheat, hemp, linseed, niger, small stripped sunflower, groats, safflower, black rape, Japanese millet, wheat, 'wild seeds'		
Crossbills, grosbeaks, cardinals, Hawfinch	Variety of middle to larger-sized seeds: pine nuts, small sunflower, hemp, safflower, canary, buckwheat, peeled oats		
Java sparrows	Millet: red, Japanese, white, pannicum; canary seed, paddy rice, peeled oats		
Smaller finches: Siskin, Linnet, redpolls, Goldfinch	Smaller seeds: canary, niger, grass, teasel, perilla, lettuce, 'wild seeds'	Hemp, linseed	'Wild seed' mixes often contain small amounts of native plant seeds such as thistle, charlock and wild carrot

6.5   Seed mixes for passerines.

the seeds. These mixes can result in health issues as the bird will generally pick out the oil-rich seeds first.

Dedicated fanciers often make up their own mixtures, which may include seeds such as clover, lettuce, maw, chia, quinoa and perilla. Many of the mixtures are made from rapidly germinating seeds and these are specifically used as 'soaked seed'. The seeds are soaked and germinated to try to replicate a more natural seed supply during breeding. Soaking softens the seeds and stimulates chemical changes reducing digestion inhibitors and breaking down proteins and carbohydrates, all of which improve their digestibility when fed to chicks.

Supplementary feeding for seed-eating passerines: Many species of seed-eating passerines require additional protein when breeding. This is often supplied as live food (see 'Softbills') or as 'egg food'. This is a commercially available dry egg-based biscuit crumb, which is reconstituted with water to make a moist crumble. The additional protein (and vitamins and minerals) comes primarily from the egg.

Many seed-eaters will also consume appreciable amounts of green food. Salad herbs, weeds such as dandelion (including the roots, which are said to stimulate breeding) and chickweed (*Stellaria media*), peas and grated carrot are regularly fed to canaries and British finches. These green foods provide a reasonable level of vitamins and minerals, balancing (to some degree) those missing from the seeds. This is further enhanced by the provision of ripe seeding grasses and weeds when available and mineral and vitamin supplements.

Whilst seed-eating passerines hull their seeds (unlike Columbiformes and granivores), they still require a strong functional ventriculus to assist food breakdown.

Non-soluble grit should be provided to assist with this task. Soluble grit, generally in the form of crushed oyster shells, is also provided to assist with the need for increased calcium levels during breeding and moulting.

Nutritional disease in small seed-eaters is not often described. This may be due to underreporting or an acceptance, by their owners, that these small birds have a short life expectancy. However, poor moult and feather colour, poor reproductive performance (including egg binding) and some dermal conditions may all have an underlying nutritional component. One commonly encountered nutritional condition seen in pet cage-bound canaries (as opposed to fanciers' canaries) is obesity due to overconsumption of oil seeds. A similar issue is seen with pet Zebra Finches fed *ad libitum* millet sprays. Pet birds of this type should be kept on a more austere diet to offset the lack of exercise. 'Head twirling' or 'star gazing' has been attributed to lack of B vitamins and supplementation has been reported to bring about a resolution, although specific cases cannot be confirmed and other causes (e.g. viral disease, brain abscesses and husbandry issues) provide alternative aetiologies.

Softbills

The term 'softbill' is a blanket term to cover a range of birds (usually non-seed-eaters), whose diets generally consist of fruit and soft-bodied invertebrates; not all of these birds are passerines. The nutritional strategy of these species varies, with some being more frugivorous and others more insectivorous or – in the case of corvids – more omnivorous (see Figure 6.1).

Most softbills will eat a range of commercial fruits and soft hedgerow berries when in season. Fruits, whilst rich in sugars, are generally lacking in protein and minerals. Most captive softbills are also fed a commercial insectivorous diet. This generally consists of either small pellets or a dry 'pate' mix which includes dried invertebrates (e.g. brine shrimp). Many bird keepers make up their own food with soaked dog/cat/ferret food or trout/koi pellets forming the basis. While these provide a good level of animal protein and vitamins, the level of iron could be a potential issue, as many softbills (especially members of the starling family) are prone to iron storage disease (see 'Iron storage disease).

'Live food' will generally be provided to the majority of softbills. Commercially available mealworms, wax moth larvae, crickets and locusts are the most common. These are generally disease-free; however, worms, either commercial or 'home grown' from compost heaps, may contain gapeworm. Thrushes seem particularly susceptible to this parasite. For the larger softbills and omnivores, 'pinkies' and other small rodents and pieces of dead day-old chicks are also provided.

Nutritional disease is encountered more frequently in softbills than in seed-eaters due to the general lack of nutrients in commercial fruit and the poor calcium levels in most live food (and very low calcium:phosphorus ratio). Calcium supplementation is required, and this is generally provided by using a mineral mix on the food or by dusting the live food with a high-calcium powder. Softbills tend not to drink much as they get most of their water from their food, therefore water-soluble supplementation (and medication) is not recommended.

As already mentioned, many softbill species are prone to iron storage disease (haemochromatosis).

Paediatric osteodystrophy is also a common finding, particularly in hole-nesting softbills such as starlings, as they are less exposed to UV light. Gut impaction from the head parts of mealworms is reported (many body parts of invertebrates are high in relatively indigestible chitin) and some breeders will remove this when feeding birds with small young – many parent softbills can be observed removing extraneous chitin-rich body parts such as legs and wing cases prior to feeding to their young; others systematically chew the prey back and forth in their beaks to soften it up prior to feeding.

The resolution of apparent blindness and neurological problems associated with a nest of thrushes fed exclusively on live food, following the administration of a vitamin B complex, has been anecdotally reported; live food is generally deficient in vitamin B_{12} and thiamine, as well as other vitamins and minerals (Finke, 2002).

As with oil-based seeds, overindulgence on fat-rich mealworms will result in obesity and fatty liver disease.

Raptors

Raptor, derived from the Latin *rapiō* (to seize or take by force), is a general term for species of birds from the orders Strigiformes (owls), Falconiformes (falcons) and Accipitriformes (including hawks and eagles). Many are kept as individual pets, as professional falconer's birds, or as part of zoological or educational collections. Although there are some species that are very specific in their prey choice (e.g. the Snail Kite feeds almost exclusively on apple snails), the nature of the diets of most raptors is broadly similar, consisting of meat in some form or other, and most can be considered as opportunistic feeders. The captive raptor diet tends to therefore be simplified and standardized for most species and comprises mainly dead day-old chicks. These are generally obtained frozen as 'waste' from commercial hatcheries. Alternative birds, such as quail, and dead rodents and rabbits are also provided. These prey species do have a much higher cost, so in general tend to be used sparingly as a 'nutritional balancer' for a predominantly chick diet. Fish-eating and large carrion-eating raptors such as vultures are rarely encountered in general practice.

It is possible to make a comparison between the diets of captive parrots and those of captive raptors in that a compromise has been reached between a diet based on 'natural foods' (whatever these may be, as ornithological knowledge is far from complete on this subject) and the foods readily available. Where the two differ is that captive raptor diets tend to reflect more closely the types of food eaten as a group of birds than do those commonly fed to parrots (see Figure 6.4).

This does not mean that the diets of raptors are without nutritional issues, and many of these are similar to those of parrots. Poor feather quality, integument disease and musculoskeletal system problems (e.g. metabolic bone disease), brought on by the poor calcium:phosphorus ratio of day-old chicks and other foods, are all encountered. The practice of underfeeding to reduce bodyweight and increase hunting instinct is still encountered in falconry. This can lead to hypoglycaemia when the bird is worked hard. Conversely, overfeeding will lead to obesity, predisposing to cardiovascular and liver disease.

Toxicities (e.g. lead shot) and disease (e.g. trichomonosis from pigeons) can be a problem if wild caught animals or roadkill is fed.

Whilst a generic day-old chick diet may be suitable for most captive raptors, Merlins are more insectivorous and should therefore be fed a diet lower in fat or risk hepatic lipidosis (Forbes and Flint, 2000).

Malnutrition and nutritional disease

If good nutrition is the 'provision, through the intake of food, of appropriate levels of essential nutrients necessary to maintain healthy cellular function', then malnutrition is a failure to provide these appropriate levels, predisposing to suboptimal cellular function. Suboptimal cellular function leads to organ and system dysfunction and subsequent disease.

Malnutrition is experienced by all classes of birds, wild as well as captive. Along with predation, malnutrition is responsible for the largest number of wild bird fatalities. In general, the nutritional issue facing wild birds is that of finding adequate food and fulfilling gross energy needs. Climatic conditions, seasonal availability, territorial disputes, individual disease and anthropogenic activity all have a part to play in the availability of food supplies. Rarely is lack of specific nutrients an identifiable issue in wild birds. However, in captivity, whilst food bowl protection and inter- and intraspecies aggression may prevent feeding in certain situations, particularly amongst softbills (e.g. despite their size, hummingbirds are highly territorial and protective of their nectar supplies even in captivity), malnutrition by way of starvation should never be a problem, although clinicians may encounter cases of hypoglycaemia in working raptors where their weight has been 'dropped' too low by the falconer to encourage 'keenness'. Specific nutrient deficiency and excess, however, is common.

Nutritional diseases are a range of conditions arising from lack of optimal cellular function. Depending on which tissues are affected and to what degree, nutritional disease can manifest with a wide range of clinical pictures.

Disease may be clinically overt, presenting as:

- **Acute:** a clinical emergency (e.g. hypocalcaemic fits)
- **Chronic:** taking many years for the clinical signs to manifest themselves (e.g. hepatic lipidosis (fatty liver disease))
- **Acute manifestations of chronic disease**: such as sudden-onset feather destructive disorder.

Or subclinical:

- **Unperceived:** immunologically compromised or subclinical, where disease is present but undetected, predisposing to other secondary conditions (e.g. infected sinusitis). The bird may survive, but not thrive.

When discussing nutritional diseases with an owner, the veterinary surgeon should not lose track of the fact that malnutrition is the single biggest disease suffered by pet parrots and is preventable. The issue should not be whether an owner elects to change their bird's eating habits, but how quickly they can, if the health of their bird is to be improved or protected. Whilst this is not the forum in which to discuss the ethical aspect of feeding an all-seed diet to a parrot, given the weight of information directly implicating this type of diet with nutritional disease (see 'The seed *versus* pellet debate'), it would seem safe to suggest that this manner of husbandry borders on infringing one of the 'five freedoms': freedom from disease. Malnutrition is one of the most clinically relevant health issues of captive birds.

> When discussing malnutrition with owners it is important to clarify some simple definitions:
>
> - **Nutrition** is not another word for feeding
> - **Feeding** is what is put in the feeding bowl and should not be confused with diet
> - **Diet** is what the bird actually eats from the foods that are fed
> - Nutrition comes from the assimilation of the nutrients from the foods that the bird actually eats. Food selection and quality obviously have a strong bearing on nutrient levels, as does nutrient interaction and the bird's general health. Malnutrition can be a downward spiral

Diagnosis of malnutrition

The way in which the body stores and processes nutrients means that there are few simple diagnostic procedures that can be used to identify malnutrition. As with many conditions, the clinician's best diagnostic tools are observation, clinical examination and history taking. Simply knowing what the feathers of a healthy parrot should look like and that the presented bird lives on sunflower seeds are informative guides to diagnosis. There are, however, a few additional tests that can be done to assess the extent to which malnutrition has progressed, aid prognosis and provide diagnostic 'proof' to owners.

Biochemistry

Some specific nutrients can be tested for (e.g. bile acids, cholesterol, uric acid, ionized calcium) but, while abnormal levels are significant and strong pointers towards non-effective nutrition, they are essentially used as additional confirmation of what an avian clinician has already diagnosed from the physical examination and observation of the bird in front of them.

The volume of blood required and cost of testing for vitamins makes specific tests of this nature impractical in most circumstances.

PRACTICAL TIP

When assessing calcium concentration, it is important to measure the levels of ionized calcium, which is the portion that is immediately available to the bird. Total calcium levels can be influenced by blood protein levels and the hormonal status of female birds

Radiography

Similarly, whilst radiography will often clarify the extent or severity of certain nutritionally related conditions, such as metabolic bone disease or an enlarged liver, more often they are used to confirm what the clinician already suspects from their clinical examination.

Faecal Gram stain

A lack of gut flora is a general indication of poor intestinal homeostasis (note: parrots have a natural healthy gut flora, healthy seed-eating passerine birds do not). There are many conditions that will lead to a disruption of gut flora: toxicities including heavy metals; bacterial and viral diseases; high levels of stress; and general organopathies. Excessive dietary fat and lack of micronutrients both have an adverse effect on the viability of gut flora (Harrison, 2011) and, either as a primary problem (if no other aetiological cause can be found) or as part of the resolution of a primary condition, dietary change with or without the use of probiotics should be instituted to re-establish healthy gut flora.

Management of malnutrition

Nutrition is not a static process; it is dynamic and influenced by not only life stage and lifestyle, but by a range of interrelated metabolic processes occurring within a bird's body. Similarly, malnutrition is dynamic both with clinical expression and over time.

Prevention

Prevention is centred around the provision of a suitable diet from pre-egg (maternal under-funding of the egg can have subsequent lifelong issues for the chick) and throughout all life stages including metabolically demanding periods such as moulting and reproduction. A 'complete' diet should be used from as early as possible in the life of the bird because to play 'nutritional catch-up' is, in a lot of cases, not possible. The effects of juvenile metabolic bone disease, for example, will not be corrected by a change to a nutritionally complete diet; even minimal deficiencies or excesses have a cumulative effect on the bird's body that can result in unresolvable conditions (e.g. iron storage disease and hepatic lipidosis).

Treatment

Treatment of malnutrition may involve a 'short sharp fix' of injectable or oral nutrients but inevitably will involve a complete reassessment of both diet and feeding protocols.

'Cure'

Many conditions can be greatly improved. Some may even be 'cured' in that the observed effects of the deficiency are no longer present (e.g. hypocalcaemic fits), but nutritional disease can be subtle, insidious and permanent, and to suggest that the effects of malnutrition will be cured by treatment would be, for many conditions, optimistic.

Definition of a nutritionally complete diet

There are no definitive levels determined for the nutrient requirements of pet parrots and most other captive bird species (with the exception of poultry). When attempting to assess nutritional needs in order to construct a satisfactory diet for an individual bird it is necessary, therefore, to use data from a range of sources, considering:

- General nutritional knowledge as to what levels of nutrients sustain health
- Levels of nutrients that sustain optimal growth and health in young birds of the species under question
- Information researched directly from psittacine species

- Prudent extrapolation from other species (e.g. poultry)
- Pre-existing nutritionally related disease and its resolution.

Diets are then designed to ensure that minimal levels of all nutrients are met, based on the above guidelines and the digestibility and availability of the food source.

Nutritional and dietary correction
Overcoming the problem of malnutrition requires more than simply correcting macro- and micronutrient levels. Dietary correction is also much more than just a nutritional appraisal and overhaul; it generally involves a holistic approach to husbandry as well, and often a change of mindset by the keeper. When presented with a case of nutritional disease, it is important for the veterinary surgeon to:

- Make the owner aware of the existence of malnutrition in their bird, and the importance of their role in treating it
- Highlight the clinical signs and serious knock-on effects of dietary deficiencies/excesses
- Discuss the shortfalls in the bird's current diet and dietary regime and suggest alternative dietary approaches
- Offer a realistic prognosis: observable improvement will take time, and will require long-term (potentially lifelong) treatment, and does not equal cure.

Clinical signs of nutritional disease
When identifying the effects and underlying pathogenesis of avian malnutrition, it should be emphasized that nutritional disease is:

- Multifactorial in its cause (very rarely isolated to a deficiency of one or two specific nutrients)
- Multisystemic in its effects
- Multipresentational in its signs.

Integument
The skin and feathers are perhaps the easiest areas in which to recognize cellular dysfunction; cell turnover is high, therefore the consequences are more readily observable (Figure 6.6). The production of the wide range of keratin proteins is complex and heavily dependent on vitamin A for accurate biosynthesis, therefore low dietary levels of vitamin A (or the carotenoid precursors) and a lack of appropriate essential amino acids lead to poor protein construction, resulting in poor feather and epithelium quality. The integument is susceptible to a wide range of conditions often resulting in a similar clinical appearance. A full clinical investigation should be carried out to assess the possible causes (see Chapter 30).

Metabolic diseases
Metabolic disease has multiple aetiologies: bacterial, toxic and viral, as well as nutritional (Figure 6.8).

Clinical sign	Comments
Dry flaky skin (itch)	Poor quality epithelium leading to excessive desquamation; lack of skin oils (holocrine nature of avian epithelium); preen gland dysfunction
Bleeding blood feathers	Poor quality keratin formation of feathers leading to ease of fracture (often exacerbated by an inappropriate wing clip)
Stress bars (Figure 6.7a)	Poor protein supply to feather follicle during feather growth. Either primary nutritional or secondary due to raised corticosterone levels (Stockdale, 2011)
Overgrown/flaky beak Overgrown/misshapen claws	Poor keratinization of beak or claws; effects of poor protein deposition (liver disease); disruption to germinal layer
Failure to shed shafts	Poor keratin production of sheaths; poor follicle blood supply
Slow to moult (Figure 6.7b) Poor feather durability (melanin shows through) (Figure 6.7c)	Nutrient needs not met for both general metabolism and nutrient-intense new feather production (Murphy, 1996) Slow to moult results in retention of feathers for longer – resultant effect is greater wear and tear, particularly surface abrasion with resultant exposure of black melanin base pigmentation showing through
Abnormal feather colour (Figure 6.7d)	Direct failure to manufacture pigments due to follicular disease in psittacines or lack of carotenoids in passerines results in abnormal feather pigmentation (Stockdale, 2013)
Preen gland dysfunction/abscessation/impaction	Secretory dysfunction due to cellular abnormalities within the gland. Accumulation of cellular debris blocks ducts
Change in feather lustre	In parrots, the colour green is produced by the effect of light passing through feathers in which both yellow and blue pigments have been deposited. Both feather quality (the keratin nanostructure of feather barbs and barbules) and the effects of light on the feather oils play an important role in its production. Lack of preen gland (and skin) oils alters the optical affect, reducing or removing the 'sheen' from the feathers (Stockdale, 2013)
Lack of skin elasticity (especially the propatagium and tail)	Poor quality production of elastin reduces the capacity for skin to stretch and results in fissures. These result in pain and can lead to feather plucking and self-mutilation
Feather plucking and self-mutilation	Whilst feather destructive disorder is invariably multifactorial, any accessible skin lesions will invariably lead to progressive self-inflicted trauma. Although general malnutrition plays an important role in the pathogenesis of feather plucking, hypocalcaemia and hypovitaminosis A have been strongly linked as primary catalysts
Ulcerative pododermatitis ('bumblefoot')	Whilst this condition is multifactorial, poor quality pedal epithelium has been implicated
Secondary bacterial and fungal infections	Lack of antimicrobial action of preen gland and body oils (Shawkey et al., 2003)

6.6   Clinical signs of malnutrition affecting the integument and feathers.

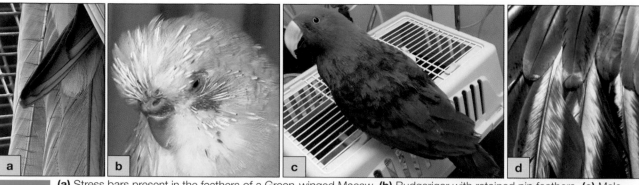

6.7 **(a)** Stress bars present in the feathers of a Green-winged Macaw. **(b)** Budgerigar with retained pin feathers. **(c)** Male Eclectus Parrot with melanin pigmentation. **(d)** Blue and Gold Macaw with abnormal feather coloration.

Metabolic disorders related to malnutrition		Clinical signs and comments
Obesity		Obesity is readily apparent. High levels of fat intake caused by inappropriate nutrition and feeding behaviour, and exacerbated by a lack of exercise, are obvious causes of this problem. Fat can be visualized as yellow deposits under the thin skin of birds, but also occurs around and within internal organs. An inability to visualize the dark pectoral muscles often implies a fat layer. All birds are susceptible; Amazon parrots, Galahs, Cockatiels and Budgerigars are particularly predisposed
	Atherosclerosis	Accumulation of cholesterol, often with secondary calcification in blood vessels, can occasionally be visualized radiographically
	Cardiomyopathy	Often resulting from obesity, but also as a primary condition due to vitamin E deficiency. May result in ascites
	Pancreatitis	Production of 'popcorn' faeces
	Diabetes	Polydipsia/polyuria in birds can have many causes, one being diabetes, which is not uncommon in Cockatiels. Diagnosis necessitates the measurement of fructosamine
	Xanthomas (Figure 6.9a), lipomas (Figure 6.9b) and fibrolipomas (Figure 6.9c)	Accumulation of cholesterol clefts within a range of tissues gives rise to the yellow nature of xanthomas. There is some species predilection for lipomas, with Budgerigars, Cockatiels, some Amazon species and Galahs particularly prone
	Hypothyroidism	Primary hypothyroidism due to a lack of iodine was a common condition up until the 1960s when iodine blocks became available. Secondary hypothyroidism is now more common; this is a lack of normal thyroid function following metaplastic change within the thyrocytes and lowered thyroxine output. Increasing dietary levels of vitamin A may resolve the problem; off-licence treatment with thyroxine-type drugs is not recommended as avian thyroid levels are hard to monitor and overdosage can occur
	Fatty liver disease	Almost every enzyme/metabolic function of the body
	Hernias (Figure 6.9d)	Obesity, increase in liver size and abdominal thinning all predispose to abdominal hernias
Iron storage disease (haemochromatosis)		Iron is an essential mineral, but its excessive accumulation gives rise to disease. The main organ of accumulation is the liver, where the primary presenting signs are a palpable enlargement of the liver (posterior to the sternum) and ascites. Certain groups of birds are particularly prone to iron storage disease, including mynahs, toucans, birds of paradise and frugivorous starlings. The aetiology of this condition is multifactorial, but the environmental ecology of the bird's eating habits (low dietary iron intake) seems to predispose to accumulation rather than excretion. A diet low in iron (<80 ppm) is recommended. See 'Iron storage disease' and the *BSAVA Manual of Raptors, Pigeons and Passerine Birds*
Hypocalcaemia		Calcium is required for healthy bones and egg shells, as well as being needed for the smooth working of the muscles and nervous system. Low circulating blood calcium will result in acute seizures, which, if untreated, can be fatal. A combination of low calcium intake (e.g. a seed-based diet) coupled with inadequate levels of active vitamin D and/or non-exposure to unfiltered sunlight will predispose to hypocalcaemia. Marginal ionized calcium levels are often detected in feather plucking birds. Grey Parrots are relatively frequently presented with this condition, probably a reflection of their predisposition to monophagy and that they are naturally equatorial tree-top dwellers and therefore rely on UV light for vitamin D synthesis to aid calcium metabolism; they are more clinically sensitive to low (or marginal) blood calcium levels
Gout (Figure 6.9e)		Birds are uricotelic; uric acid is the principal product of nitrogen metabolism. High dietary protein levels have been postulated as being responsible for the production of both articular and visceral gout by 'overloading' both the liver and kidneys, but there is no published evidence (Koutsos *et al.*, 2001). The dietary implications of gout production focus more on renal cellular dysfunction and the production of cellular liths within the tubules disrupting uric acid filtration (Ritchie *et al.*, 1994). The exact aetiology of gout in birds is unresolved
Hypervitaminosis toxicity (vitamin competition)		The excessive supplementation of vitamins, especially vitamins A and D_3, can lead to toxicity problems. Both these vitamins can be synthesized by the body using precursor carotenoids and inactive vitamin D_2, respectively. Both have a negative feedback system attached to their production, whereas exogenous dietary levels are absorbed without restraint. Fat-soluble vitamins (A, D, E, K, carotenoids) all compete for the same absorption sites within the gut wall. In diets overly abundant with one or two fat-soluble vitamins, competitive displacement occurs and a deficiency of the others may be induced (Koutsos, 2001; MacDonald, 2006). Hypervitaminosis is reported to resemble hypovitaminosis in clinical signs; dietary history and histopathology should assist in distinguishing between the two conditions

6.8   Metabolic disorders with a possible nutritional aetiology.

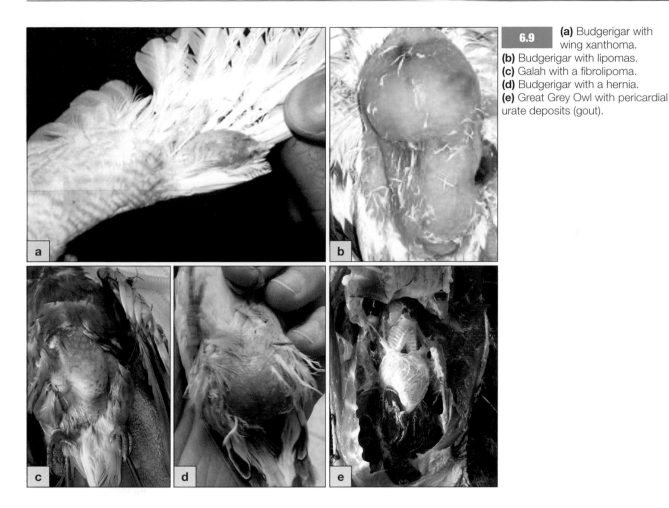

6.9 **(a)** Budgerigar with wing xanthoma.
(b) Budgerigar with lipomas.
(c) Galah with a fibrolipoma.
(d) Budgerigar with a hernia.
(e) Great Grey Owl with pericardial urate deposits (gout).

Iron storage disease: Iron storage disease (haemochromatosis) is a common finding in frugivorous birds kept in captivity. It can be a primary or secondary disease, causing iron deposition within tissues. Although the condition can affect a wide variety of species, not just frugivores, the most common groups of birds to suffer from iron storage disease are:

- Toucans, toucanettes and aracari (Ramphastidae)
- Mynahs, birds of paradise, species of starlings (Sturnidae)
- Turacos (Musophagidae)
- Some parrots (Psittaciformes).

In general, frugivorous, insectivorous and omnivorous birds tend to accumulate more iron in their liver and, thus, are more prone to the disease than carnivorous, piscivorous and granivorous birds.

The most common presenting clinical sign in these birds is respiratory disease brought on by the accumulation of abdominal fluid, attributable to liver cirrhosis and associated circulatory problems. The abdominal contour of affected birds is often convex rather than concave or flat and the presence of fluid will generally be appreciated on palpation. The enlarged, swollen distal edge of the liver can also sometimes be felt extending beyond the edge of the sternum. Care should always be taken when handling any bird with suspected ascites, as tipping the bird on its back, for example, can result in sudden death due to 'drowning'. Sudden death is also a common sign of iron storage disease and an initial presumptive diagnosis may be made at gross post-mortem examination in advanced cases by cutting through a piece of affected liver and observing it to be fibrotic and 'gritty' in texture due to the accumulation of iron deposits.

Although the exact pathogenesis of iron storage disease has not been elucidated, the following contributory factors are considered important:

- Absolute and relative (to species) dietary iron level is the greatest contributory factor
- Genetics: species-specific physiological adaptations to natural low iron availability in the diet/habitat (canopy birds with little direct mineral intake and water contaminated with rotting leaves resulting in high tannin levels)
- Iron bioavailability:
  - Other dietary components (tannins, phytic acid, fibres, ascorbic acid, organic acids, minerals) affect iron bioavailability
  - Stress and immunological reactions may induce iron accumulation in the liver
  - The variation in dietary iron absorption is due more to differences in the bioavailability, than to a variation in iron content.

Even if diagnosed in sufficient time, treatment and corrective dietary changes are often too late to affect the ultimately fatal conclusion to the condition. One treatment that has been suggested is regular phlebotomy, which involves removing up to 10% of blood volume (about 1% of bodyweight) on a bi-weekly to monthly basis, the rationale being that blood regeneration will draw on iron deposits to create new haemoglobin. Both the practicalities and success rate of this regime are debatable. Control of the problem is dependent on preventive dietary and husbandry measures.

- **Restriction of total dietary iron** is the most obvious measure: empirically based data suggest a maximum iron level of 100 ppm; <50 ppm, with 25 as ideal, is recommended but hard to achieve.
- When formulating diets for frugivorous birds, **raw materials with low iron levels** should be selected. Eggs are a good source of low-iron protein, as is poultry meat rather than red meat. Legumes and nuts in general have low iron content, as do pears, tomatoes, grapefruit, apples, tangerines, plums, oranges, apricots and papaya.
- **Ferrous (Fe^{2+}) haem iron *versus* ferric (Fe^{3+}) non-haem iron**. Haem iron, present in haemoglobin and myoglobin, is more readily absorbed and absorption *is not* influenced to any great extent by dietary modification. Non-haem iron found in fruit and vegetables is less well absorbed, but absorption is influenced both positively and negatively by other dietary factors.
  - Iron-chelating agents in the food, such as tannins (provide dilute tea as drinking water or 'spent' green-tea leaves mixed in with food) and plant phytates reduce the bioavailability of non-haem iron by forming insoluble complexes.
  - Ascorbic acid, organic acids or a low dietary pH *enhance* iron absorption by reducing Fe^{3+} to the more readily absorbed Fe^{2+}. Ascorbic acid in particular is a strong promoter of iron absorption and has a counteracting effect on phytate and polyphenols, therefore, it is recommended that fruits and vegetables high in vitamin C (such as peppers, citrus fruits, dark green vegetables such as broccoli and strawberries) are not fed at the same time as other (potentially) iron-rich foods.
  - Where practical, avoid feeding ferrous-rich meat products.
- If appropriate, **special mineral premixes without iron-containing** supplements should be used.
- **Formulated diets for frugivorous birds should be low iron.**
- **Feed foods high in iron blockers**, such as tea (even in water), beans and sorghum (high phytates).

Respiratory system

Pet parrots are commonly presented with sneezing, chronic nasal discharge, sinusitis, respiratory noise and, occasionally, more severe respiratory distress (Figure 6.10). The lining of the nares and sinuses is designed to inhibit the inhalation of foreign particles and to act as an active barrier to microorganisms. To function properly the cellular lining must have the ability to secrete mucus and generate normal healthy epithelium. Malnutrition has a profound effect on the lining of the sinuses and its ability to function effectively. Often designated as a vitamin A deficiency due to the role of this vitamin in cell division, there is a progressive change in the nature of the cellular lining of the sinuses from mucus-producing ciliated columnar epithelial cells to dry, metaplastic cells. These cells die and flake off within the sinuses and nares, initially causing inflammation, and then accumulating as swellings.

Primary agents affecting the respiratory system can be bacterial, viral, fungal, toxic, allergic and parasitic. All these possible aetiologies need investigation prior to arriving at a nutritional cause. Secondary bacterial infections are also common, especially in the upper respiratory system.

Reproductive system

Adequate nutrition is required for a hen to breed successfully and to produce healthy offspring. Egg production is a nutritionally demanding process.

- **Parrots form eggs from the nutrition that they receive at the time of laying**. A diet specifically designed for egg laying in parrots should not be necessary if a female bird is being provided with a good plane of quality nutrition that has optimized body condition (particularly the capacity to form intramedullary bone).

Respiratory disorders related to malnutrition	Clinical signs and comments
Upper respiratory tract (URT) infections, (rhinitis, nasal discharge)	Poor quality epithelium lining the nares, mouth, sinuses and oral cavity gives rise to loss of localized and structural defence mechanisms allowing colonization of the denatured tissue with opportunistic bacteria. This problem is commonly encountered in Amazon parrots, resulting in sneezing, rhinitis and nasal discharge. The problem will often resolve with antibiotic medication but return as the underlying cause has not been addressed. When assessing conditions of the URT, therefore, whatever the cause it is essential that the integrity of the mucosal epithelium is also addressed. Poor nutrition (normally vitamin A deficiency) will exacerbate the condition and may be the underlying cause of the initial problem. Whilst treatment with antibiotics may effect short-term remission in bacterial sinusitis, for example, treating the nutritional deficiencies either by dietary correction and short-term vitamin A injections or supplements is an essential part of long-term therapy
Sinus 'abscesses' (Figure 6.11a)	Where there is continued desquamation of the lining cells these will often accumulate, mix with nasal secretions and form sinus 'abscesses'. These are seen as discrete hard swellings around the eyes. Removal is usually simply achieved by incision over the swelling and squeezing/curetting the material out
Rhinoliths (Figure 6.11b) and destruction of the nares	Where desquamated cells have easy access to the nares, accumulations will often form, giving rise to rhinoliths. Removal is by curettage; however, the nasal tissue is often inflamed and, because it may bleed, some veterinary surgeons recommend leaving rhinoliths in place whilst local treatment is carried out. The presence of rhinoliths causes the destruction of local nasal tissue resulting in enlarged nares that rarely resolve. Large nasal openings are occasionally encountered during a general examination, often accompanied by grooves in the keratin of the upper beak extending from the nares, and can be considered the result of chronic nasal discharge or previous rhinoliths
Oral 'abscesses' (Figure 6.11c)	The oral cavity is subject to the same epithelial changes as seen in the skin and sinuses. Salivary glands become metaplastic and 'abscess' formation, resulting in the accumulation of inspissated material, occurs

6.10   Respiratory disorders with a possible nutritional aetiology.

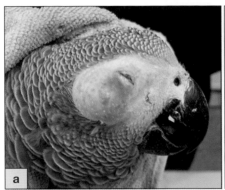
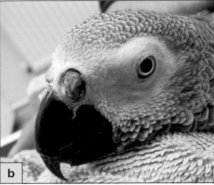
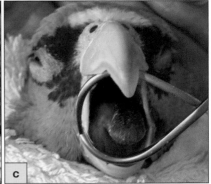

6.11 (a) Sinus abscess in an African Grey Parrot. (b) African Grey Parrot with a rhinolith. (c) Mitred Conure with a lingual abscess.

- **Malnourished hens will use a boost in nutrients to replenish their own reserves.**
  Nutrients will not specifically be used to breed, and any eggs produced may not be funded with as high a level of nutrients as would be optimal for good embryo development and hatchability. Eggs laid will be progressively poorer in quality, and calcification of the shell may also suffer, with the potential for thin shells and dystocia (see Chapter 4).

For male birds to produce good levels of quality sperm (high count and viability), and to protect the sperm from peroxidation, they have to have good levels of essential vitamins and antioxidants.

The majority of the issues encountered during reproduction can be directly attributed to husbandry and nutrition (Figure 6.12). Differential diagnoses include infectious disease and ovarian or testicular disease or neoplasia.

Reproductive disorders related to malnutrition	Clinical signs and comments
Egg binding (Figure 6.13)	Dystocia, failure of oviposition or 'egg binding' has a number of contributory factors in its aetiology (see Chapter 4). Oviduct inertia due to hypocalcaemia is the most commonly quoted nutritionally related cause. Undoubtedly, low circulating blood calcium levels have an important role to play in the condition. However, many eggs that fail to be laid successfully can be viewed per cloaca having effectively traversed the length of the oviduct before becoming stuck. Failure of the cloaca to stretch to allow successful oviposition can be due to lack of hormonal preparation, but also in malnourished birds to a lack of tissue elasticity of the pericloacal tissue prohibiting full dilatation, and a nutritional overhaul should be put in place in these cases rather than solely a top-up of calcium (see text)
	<table><tr><td>■ Egg peritonitis ■ Cloacal prolapse ■ Prolapsed oviduct</td><td>All of these potentially fatal conditions can arise from episodes of egg binding</td></tr></table>
Infertility	■ Lack of libido ■ Low sperm count and viability. Sperm production requires high levels of dietary antioxidants to ensure good protection against peroxidation of the fat-rich cells ■ Failure to ovulate ■ Failure to incubate; multiple nesting attempts. Both overprovision as well as underprovision of food can have an adverse effect on breeding patterns. A gross lack of or an inappropriate diet will often result in nest desertion during incubation or rearing as the investment in personal nutritional sacrifice cannot be sustained. Overprovision of (energy-rich) diets will often stimulate multiple nesting attempts with egg production but a failure to incubate. This is often seen in small finches such as Zebras and Bengalese
Poor parenting	Inappropriate diet can lead to a failure to provision the chicks adequately. An initial poor diet or inappropriate food selection can lead to, for example, metabolic bone disease or crop/ventriculus impaction
Inappropriate sexual activity	Breeding in birds is controlled by both intrinsic and extrinsic factors. Food, both availability and quality, is a strong extrinsic factor in a large number of bird species, parrots and the majority of passerine birds in particular. Too high a caloric intake (coupled with a strong bird–human relationship) will often trigger misdirected sexual activity. This can have a number of potentially unwelcomed sequelae
	<table><tr><td>■ Bonding ■ Aggression/ screaming</td><td>These are often misplaced manifestations of normal breeding behaviours – mate and nest protection, for example. Mate separation can also lead to feather plucking due to 'frustration' (see Chapter 5)</td></tr><tr><td>■ Feather destructive disorder</td><td>Part of the complex matrix that is 'feather plucking'. Physiological malfunctions during reproductive episodes are potential aberrations of misplaced mate preening or nest lining</td></tr><tr><td>■ Masturbation (leading to cloacal abrasions) or cloacal prolapse; regurgitation</td><td>Male birds (whether they are owner bonded or not) will occasionally indulge in misplaced sexual activity</td></tr><tr><td>■ Chronic egg laying</td><td>Predisposing to egg binding (see above), hypocalcaemia, osteoporosis (potential fractures – layer fatigue)</td></tr></table>

6.12 Reproductive disorders with a possible nutritional aetiology.

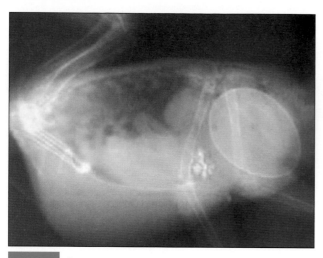

6.13   Radiograph of egg-bound African Grey Parrot.

Paediatric birds: Inappropriate nutrition during hand-rearing or parent-rearing can equally predispose to a variety of problems during growth (Figure 6.14).

Of equal importance is the effect that suboptimal nutrition has on the baby bird's immune system, depressing it and potentially predisposing the chick to a wide range of infections (see also Chapter 31).

Behaviour

Behavioural problems in captive birds are common (see Chapter 5). Many are a direct consequence of captivity and husbandry, some may be medical (e.g. viral or heavy metal toxicity), and some are a direct consequence of poor nutrition (e.g. marginal hypocalcaemia).

A lack of essential nutrients means that normal organ functions are not carried out. Where this influences the production of enzymes, hormones and other biochemicals that regulate normal metabolic activities within the brain, or result in the production of or non-breakdown of toxins and metabolites that have an adverse effect on normal function, atypical and often undesirable behaviours may arise. These can manifest in many ways, from subtle changes the owner could mistake as normal behaviour for their bird to more discernible changes such as self-mutilation, screaming or aggression (Figure 6.16).

Paediatric disorders related to malnutrition		Clinical signs and comments
Failure to grow ('stunting')		Quality and quantity of the food provided can affect the growth rate of neonates
Slow crop emptying		May be primary or secondary to *Candida* infection. Nutritional causes include inappropriate types and size of food, poor quality food (e.g. badly stored), dehydrated food (i.e. poorly prepared)
Skeletal	Metabolic bone disease (osteodystrophy; Figure 6.15a)	Metabolic bone disease (MBD) may be a direct consequence of incorrect feeding. A diet that is inadequately provisioned with calcium, vitamin D or has an imbalanced calcium:phosphorus ratio will result in varying levels of MBD. MBD is often encountered in hand-reared parrots where homemade mixes have been used instead of a nutritionally balanced commercially available mix. Where birds have been parent-reared, selective feeding of one or two specific food items by the parents can also lead to MBD, most commonly with seed-based diets. Commercially produced live food is generally low in calcium and has a poor calcium:phosphorus ratio, so many insectivore breeders dust the live food with a calcium preparation or pre-feed the insects with a high calcium diet (gut loading). MBD is commonly seen in parrots, raptors and pigeons/doves
	Splay leg and tibiotarsal rotation	The aetiologies of both conditions involve husbandry and diet. Poor underfoot nesting substrate combined with a diet deficient in calcium/vitamin D and too high in protein may predispose to femoral head rotation and cause a similar problem to rotation of the tibia in long-legged precocial birds. If diagnosed early, splay leg can be treated using soft material and padding to reposition the malalignment. Once calcification is advanced, correction is problematic. Seen in ratites
	Angel wing (airplane wing, slipped wing, crooked wing and drooped wing)	This syndrome manifests in young birds, where the carpal joint twists outwards with the wing feathers pointing laterally, instead of lying against the body. A high-calorie, high-protein diet and/or a diet low in vitamin D, vitamin E, calcium and manganese predisposes to the condition, but the exact aetiology is not known. Rapid feather growth would seem to cause a mechanical strain on the underdeveloped wing muscles, causing rotation around the carpal joint. Clinical signs include stripped remiges or remiges protruding from the wings at odd angles. In extreme cases, the stripped feathers may resemble sickly blue straws. In adult birds, the disease is incurable and affected birds are rendered effectively or totally flightless. In young birds, wrapping the wing and binding it against the bird's flank, together with feeding it a more appropriate diet, may reverse the damage. Angel wing is primarily seen in ducks and swans, but has also been reported in Goshawks and psittacine birds including Budgerigars, macaws and conures
Inappropriate food intake	Obstruction	Feeding foods that need to be cast to young raptors not yet able to egest pellets can result in obstruction, as can feeding oversized foods
Dead in shell (Figure 6.15b)		A chick is only as good as the egg from which it has hatched. An egg produced by a nutritionally replete hen is normally a rich source of amino acids, essential fatty acids, energy and all the vitamins, minerals and antioxidants required for development of a healthy embryo. An egg produced by a nutritionally deficient hen is not ideal for embryo development. This is particularly true of the funding of antioxidants (vitamin A, carotenoids, vitamin E, selenium and vitamin C); at the time of pipping, the chick moves from anaerobic to aerobic metabolism and free radical production increases. Early embryonic death, dead in shell, malformation or problems with subsequent growth and development, and neonatal infections due to poor immune status, can all be consequences of a poor female diet (Stockdale, 2005)

6.14   Paediatric disorders with a possible nutritional aetiology.

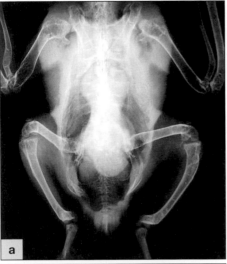

(a) Radiograph of a chick with metabolic bone disease. **(b)** 'Dead in shell'.

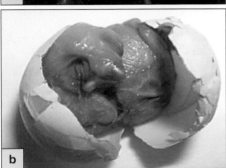

- Aggression/restlessness
- Feather chewing/barbering
- Self-mutilation
- Pica
  - Grit impaction
  - Foreign body ingestion
  - Heavy metal poisoning
- Poor parenting
  - Egg/brood desertion
  - Feather plucking (Figure 6.17)
  - Chick mutilation

6.16 Behavioural disorders with a possible nutritional aetiology.

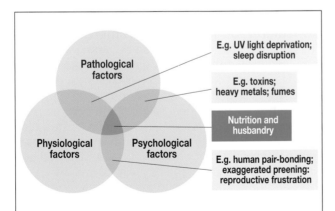

6.17 Model of feather plucking. The proportional size of the circles varies with the type of species under examination. For Grey Parrots, for example, the pathological and psychological factors are generally of more importance than the physiological factors. For Cockatiels the physiological factors tend to predominate, and for Amazons the pathological factors are most important. The one common denominator to all these causes can be nutrition. UV = ultraviolet.

The immune system

The most subtle but arguably one of the most significant consequences of malnutrition is suppression of the immune system. The immune system protects the body against attack from potentially pathogenic organisms (viruses, bacteria, fungi and parasites) and toxins, both internally and externally. Failure of the immune system predisposes the body to disease. The immune system comprises a wide range of cells, biological structures and processes that require essential nutrients to maintain their function. Whilst a lot of the structures and chemical responses that constitute the immune system are complex, others are not. For example, poor quality cells lining the sinuses affords reduced protection and allows colonization by opportunistic pathogens.

One of the major lines of defence within the body is provided by white blood cells. There are a range of conditions that will result in a reduction of white blood cells (leucopaenia) and stress haemograms, including viral conditions (circovirus) and toxicities. Birds that are presenting clinical expression of malnutrition almost invariably (in the experience of the author) also have a low white blood cell count when tested. Where blood samples have shown leucopaenia in apparently 'normal' birds where no cause can be identified, it may suggest that diet is involved (see also 'Faecal Gram stain').

References and further reading

Brue RN (1994) Nutrition. In: *Avian Medicine: Principles and Application*, ed. BW Ritchie, GJ Harrison and LR Harrison, pp. 63–78. Wingers Publishing, Lake Worth

Chitty J and Lierz M (2008) *BSAVA Manual of Raptors, Pigeons and Passerine Birds*. BSAVA Publications, Gloucester

Del Hoyo J, Elliott A and Sargatal J (1992) *Handbook of the Birds of the World – Volume 1*. Lynx Edicions, Barcelona

Finke MD (2002) Complete nutrient composition of commercially raised invertebrates used as food for insectivores. *Zoo Biology* **21(3)**, 269–285

Forbes NA and Flint CG (2000) *Raptor Nutrition*. Honeybrook Farm Animal Foods, Evesham

Harrison GJ (2011) 43 years of progress in pet bird nutrition. Available online at: http://avianmedicine.net/content/uploads/2013/03/43years.pdf. [Adapted from: Harrison GJ (1998) Twenty years of progress in pet bird nutrition. *Journal of Avian Veterinary Medicine and Surgery* **212(8)**, 1226–1230]

Karasov WH (1994) Digestive adaptations of the avian omnivore. In: *Nutrition in a Sustainable Environment*, ed. W Wahlqvist *et al.*, pp. 494–497. Smith-Gordon, Huntingdon

Klasing KC (1998) *Comparative Avian Nutrition*. CAB International, Wallingford

Koutsos EA, Matson KD and Klasing KC (2001) Nutrition of birds in the order Psittaciformes: a review. *Journal of Avian Medicine and Surgery* **15(4)**, 257–275

MacDonald D (2006) Nutrition and dietary supplementation. In: *Clinical Avian Medicine*, ed. GJ Harrison and TL Lightfoot, pp. 86–107. Spix Publishing, Palm Beach

Murphy ME (1996) Nutrition and metabolism. In: *Avian Energetics and Nutritional Ecology*, ed. C Carey, pp. 31–60. Springer Publishing Company, New York

Ritchie BW, Harrison GJ and Harrison LR (1994) *Avian Medicine: Principles and Application*. Wingers Publishing, Lake Worth

Shawkey MD, Pillai SR and Hill GE (2003) Chemical warfare? Effects of uropygial gland on feather-degrading bacteria. *Journal of Avian Biology* **34(4)**, 345–349

Stockdale BC (2005) Funding the optimal egg. In: *Proceedings of the 8th European Association of Avian Veterinarians Conference*. 23 April–1 May 2005, Arles

Stockdale BC (2011) Stress line: gaps in our feather knowledge. In: *Proceedings of the 11th European Association of Avian Veterinarians Conference*. 26–30 April 2011, Madrid

Stockdale BC (2013) The colour of flight – a veterinary perspective. In: *Proceedings of the 12th European Association of Avian Veterinarians Conference*. 20–26 April 2013, Wiesbaden

Ullrey DE, Allen ME and Bear DJ (1991) Nutrition of caged birds: formulated diets versus seed mixtures for psittacines. *Journal of Nutrition* **121(11 Suppl)**, S193–S205

Zsivanovits P, Monks DJ and Forbes NA (2006) Bilateral valgus deformity of the distal wings (angel wing) in a Northern Goshawk (*Accipiter gentilis*). *Journal of Avian Medicine and Surgery* **20(1)**, 21–26

The bird-friendly practice

Aidan Raftery

A bird-friendly practice must provide good clinical medicine and be properly equipped to satisfy its clients' expectations. For a veterinary surgeon (veterinarian) to expand their remit to include avian medicine requires the average small animal clinician to acquire a large amount of extra knowledge before they are able to provide the same level of primary care that they provide for dogs and cats. It is essential, if accepting birds as clinical cases, to have a basic knowledge of avian anatomy, physiology, husbandry and medicine, as well as being familiar with conditions that affect the species that will be seen.

The practice

There are certain basic essentials required for avian medicine that would not be usual in a small animal practice that does not treat exotic pets. The full range of specialized equipment needed is dependent on the level of avian medicine that will be delivered and the range of avian species that will be accepted.

Waiting room requirements

The waiting room should be designed to prevent escape and minimize stress for avian patients. Ideally, it should have a relatively low ceiling (less than 2.5 m). Ornamental coving is not recommended as it provides perching areas for escaped birds, enabling them to elude capture. Ceiling- and wall-mounted lights and cameras may also provide areas beyond capture and, therefore, should be recessed. A long-handled net is useful for capturing escaped birds. Windows should be fixed closed and the glass must be 'made visible' to the birds (e.g. using posters) to prevent collision injuries. Doors should be fitted with automatic closers that are set to close slowly. Temperature and ventilation should be controlled by an air-conditioning unit so there is no temptation to jam the door open in hot weather. Protective grilles should be in position over any air inlets and outlets.

Clients should be advised to arrive with their birds in transport boxes or carriers to prevent potential accidents (Figure 7.1). Refer to Chapter 9 for information on the safe transport of different species.

Owners with birds from the same taxonomic orders should be seated in opposite corners of the waiting

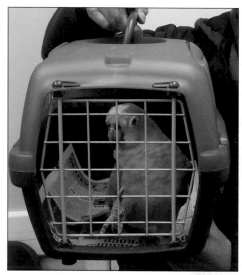

7.1 Birds should be transported to the clinic in a suitable carrier.

room as many avian pathogens are airborne. For example, all clients with Galliformes species in the waiting room should be kept as far apart as possible, as should clients with species in the order Psittaciformes.

Consulting room/area requirements

The consulting room should also be arranged to minimize escapes and make it easy to recapture any escapees: there should be no high potential perching points; the tops of cabinets should be boxed in to eliminate high ledges. The ideal height of the avian consulting room is approximately 2.5 m. High ledges also allow the accumulation of dust that may harbour infectious pathogens. Using a room with no (or blacked out) windows is a big advantage as it will be dark when the lights are turned off, allowing for much easier capture of escapees and, where necessary, facilitating the capture of some birds within their carrier. If the room cannot be darkened then a net may be needed for the recapture of escapees (see Chapter 9).

All the necessary equipment needed for an avian examination should be readily available in the consulting room. Availability of accurate weighing scales is essential (Figure 7.2). Scales capable of weighing up to 2 kg in 1 g increments are needed for most birds. Birds weighing <100 g require scales that weigh in 0.1 g increments.

BSAVA Manual of Avian Practice: A Foundation Manual. Edited by John Chitty and Deborah Monks. ©BSAVA 2018

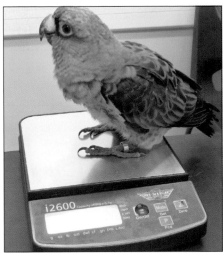

7.2 Weighing a bird in the consulting room. Use of a small rubber mat placed over the scales would provide a non-slip surface making it easier for the bird. Less tractable birds will need to be weighed in a container, using the tare function on the scales.

A separate clean towel or tea towel should be available for capture and restraint of each patient (Figure 7.3). For birds <130 g, disposable paper towels can be used instead. Clean towels should be stored either in the consulting room cupboard or outside the consulting room.

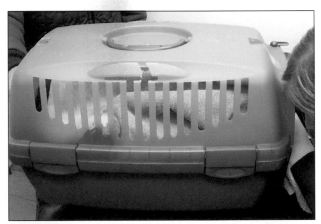

7.3 Capture from within the transport box using a towel. Note any holes that could catch the feet or wings.

Consulting room equipment

- Gram scales
- Weighing boxes
- Towels for restraint
- Avian oral specula (a selection of sizes)
- Light source (e.g. otoscope, pen torch, Finoff Transilluminator)
- Ophthalmoscope (indirect ophthalmoscopy is most useful in avian medicine)
- Magnification (e.g. head loops or magnifying examination lamp)
- Cotton buds
- Examination gloves
- Cotton wool
- Topical antiseptic preparation (e.g. chlorhexidine or povidone–iodine preparations)
- Sink with hot and cold water ▶

Avian-specific disposables

- Sterilized cotton tips (small packs of these are very good for atraumatic tissue manipulation during surgery, and also good for removing haemorrhage and putting pressure on bleeding vessels deep in the coelomic cavity)
- 29 G needles
- 0.5 ml syringes
- Soft crop feeding tubes (a range of sizes)

Hospitalization area requirements

The hospitalization area for avian patients should be separate from the dog and cat hospitalization area; it is very stressful for many birds to be within the sight and sound of dogs and cats. Likewise, predatory bird species such as hawks and falcons should be kept away from potential prey species. Birds require a higher environmental temperature when hospitalized, which can be more easily achieved by heating the room. Hospitalization cages for birds should be easily transportable so birds can be moved into different air spaces if necessary. The cages must be easy to clean and disinfect, and any perches used must be made of a non-porous easily disinfected material.

There are differing opinions as to whether the view of one bird to another should be blocked to reduce stress. Birds in full view of one another will often visually display to each other and behave differently from when they have the visual security of not being observed. It is useful to have a webcam so that hospitalized birds can be observed remotely, as their behaviour changes when they know they are being viewed. On the positive side, hospitalized birds will often vocalize to each other, and the sight of another bird eating may stimulate foraging and/or feeding behaviour.

Hospital cages should be available for which the oxygen concentration can be increased, internal temperature controlled and nebulizers connected, if required (Figure 7.4). There should be a range of sizes appropriate for the range of species accepted as patients (see Chapter 11).

A range of appropriate normal foods should always be available in the practice, including food for carnivores, omnivores, frugivores, insectivores and granivores. Hand-rearing formulas can be stored frozen in small dated bags to defrost when needed, and it is equally important to have a range of foods suitable for nutritional support in severely compromised patients (see Chapters 6 and 11).

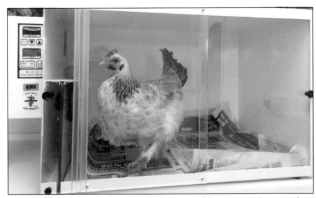

7.4 Critical care hospital cage with temperature and humidity control.

Hospitalization area equipment and supplies

- Appropriate cages
- Perches that can be easily disinfected
- Oxygen enrichment
- Nebulization
- Nutritional support foods
- Gavage tubes and feeding needles in a range of sizes (Figure 7.5)
- Intraosseous catheters, particularly useful in birds <400 g (use 20–22 G for birds >400 g). Hypodermic needles can be modified for use as intraosseous catheters with a trocar made from orthopaedic wire)
- Fluid warmers (Figure 7.6)

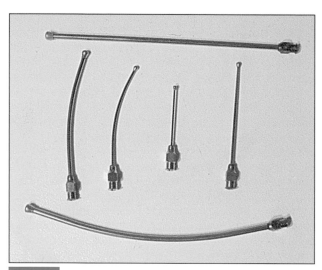

7.5   A selection of smaller gavage feeding tubes.

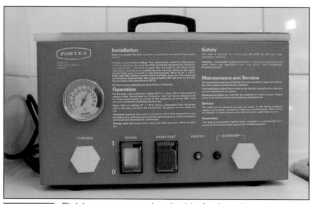

7.6   Fluid warmers are invaluable for keeping parenteral fluids at body temperature.

Surgical requirements

Most avian patients are significantly smaller than the dogs and cats more commonly presented as surgical patients. Thus, considerably more skill and manual dexterity are required; the effects of haemorrhage and tissue trauma are much greater in avian surgery. The instruments required are of normal length, but the tips have small delicate points. Use of microsurgical instruments is preferred for the safe manipulation of the more fragile avian tissues. Microsurgical instruments are rounded and counterbalanced to allow a rolling action by the fingers, giving finer control while manipulating delicate tissue.

Having some form of magnification is significantly beneficial in avian surgery, especially for the smaller species. Tissue manipulation will be far more dexterous under magnification than with the naked eye. Even small amounts of haemorrhage are significant in birds, and magnification allows the source to be more readily identified and ligated.

Radiosurgery, although not essential, is a very useful addition. The monopolar electrode is mainly used for cutting through skin and other tissues. It must, however, be correctly adjusted to avoid collateral damage. The bipolar handpiece is invaluable for controlling haemorrhage deep in body cavities. Monopolar electrosurgery is not recommended due to the risk of burns from the ground plate in smaller patients.

Surgical equipment

- A good set of retractors (e.g. Lone Star®) will increase access to tissues and thus facilitate more gentle tissue handling, which will result in an improved outcome
- Heated operating table or heated pad
- Anaesthetic monitoring equipment
  - Doppler flat probe to measure blood pressure
  - Capnography
  - Temperature probe
- Anaesthetic circuits with minimal dead space
- Avian size appropriate endotracheal tubes, non-cuffed
- Anaesthetic induction masks in a range of suitable sizes
- Avian ventilator
- Orthopaedic equipment for tiny bones
- Small suture materials
- Translucent surgical drapes
- Surgical magnification (surgical loupes or an operating microscope)

Diagnostics

Radiography capability

Radiology is more useful in birds than in mammals and is therefore a more common diagnostic technique in birds. Clinicians will need training to be able to interpret the radiographs unless the plan is to refer these cases. The majority of avian patients will be 50–500 g in bodyweight, therefore high-definition radiographs are essential (see Chapter 18 and 'Training and continuing professional development').

Endoscopy capability

To handle respiratory emergencies, the clinician will need to be able to perform at least a tracheoscopy and preferably also a coelioscopy. These are often required for an early diagnosis and appropriate treatment, which is more likely to result in a successful outcome (see Lierz, 2008, for more detailed information).

Laboratory requirements

Most veterinary practices that treat birds are able to at least run a basic avian biochemistry screen, test packed cell volume (PCV) and to interpret haematology smears. It is especially important in emergency cases to have this information early, when the results will provide important information for treatment and the next diagnostic steps. Disease in avian species progresses at a much faster rate than in dogs and cats (see Chapter 12).

Laboratory equipment

- Microhaematocrit tubes
- Small volume heparin and EDTA blood collection tubes
- Minimum biochemistry database capability: electrolytes, glucose, ionized calcium, uric acid, aspartate aminotransferase (AST) and creatine kinase
- Plain blood collection tubes
- Microswabs (plain and with transport media)
- Microscope slides and coverslips
- Good quality microscope
- Cytology stains

Additional equipment required for treating avian patients

- Selection of ring removers for different sizes of rings and different ring materials
- Rings for identification after surgical sexing in a selection of different sizes
- Beak repair materials
- Net for capture of escapees
- Dremel for beak and nail reshaping (see Chapter 15)
- Supplies for making and applying tail guards (see Chapter 11)

Practice personnel

Reception team

Receptionists in veterinary practices accepting avian cases should be trained in avian telephone triage (see Chapter 8). A list of clinical signs that require attention as soon as possible (emergencies) is provided below, together with presenting clinical signs that should be seen within 12 hours (urgent cases). This list must not be regarded as definitive and receptionists should seek a second opinion from the veterinary surgeon if there is any doubt. Birds tend to hide signs of illness so, by the time signs are recognized, the bird will often be severely ill and in need of urgent attention. If there is any doubt, an emergency appointment should be scheduled. A list of species competencies of the veterinary surgeons in the practice and a list of any presentations that should be redirected to more specialized colleagues should also be available. Receptionists should refer to their practice policy and Chapter 8 regarding the provision of first aid advice if required; they should consult the veterinary surgeon about what advice can be given for a particular case.

If a bird has already been treated at another practice, the receptionist should aim to have the previous medical records available by the time of the scheduled consultation.

It is important for receptionists to be able to identify the species seen in the practice. Any additional husbandry knowledge they have is also helpful for interacting with the clients, although they should refrain from offering definitive advice. This should be left to the veterinary surgeon during the consultation (see Chapter 8 for further information).

Receptionists are often called upon to give estimates for treatment. They should be aware of the pricing structure and be able to give some idea of cost for common procedures. They should also be aware of the procedures undertaken in the practice, although they do not need to be able to discuss them.

Telephone triage for birds

Emergency (see as soon as possible):

- Injury from a predator
- Profuse blood loss
- Acute respiratory distress
- Unable to stand
- Acute enlargement or swelling of any body part

Urgent (see within 12 hours):

- Decrease in food intake
- Change in attitude, personality or behaviour
- Fluffed-up posture
- Decreased vocalization
- Change in breathing or abnormal respiratory sounds
- Vomiting or regurgitation
- Discharge from eyes, nostrils or mouth
- Decrease or increase in water consumption
- Change in number and appearance of droppings

Nursing team

Veterinary nurses should have basic husbandry knowledge of the variety of species that will be seen, including awareness of normal diets and familiarity with foods used for nutritional support.

Handling expertise is essential (Figure 7.7a), as well as the ability to perform basic clinical techniques such as intramuscular injections and gavage feeding (Figure 7.7b) (see Chapter 11). Familiarity with the normal behaviour of different species will allow for species-specific nursing and critical care.

There are continuing education courses available in avian medicine and there are also some very good avian reference textbooks written for the nursing team. The *BSAVA Manual of Exotic Pet and Wildlife Nursing*, in conjunction with chapters in the textbooks listed in 'References and further reading', will provide most of the information required.

Client expectations

Clients will expect the staff of the veterinary practice to be familiar with the species they accept as patients and to be able to give an estimate of the potential cost, although staff should make the client aware that the latter is not always possible until after the consultation. They also expect the practice to be suitably equipped and able to deal with any potential complication that might arise during a procedure.

Clients may have been getting contradictory information from sources such as the internet and books; they will expect to be able to discuss these topics and obtain more evidence-based information from practice personnel.

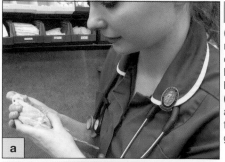

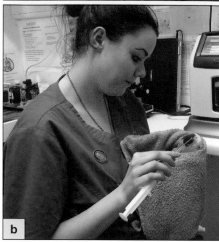

7.7

(a) A veterinary nurse demonstrating her avian handling skills. **(b)** Nurse administering fluids by crop gavage.

Clients will also expect their practice to provide out-of-hours emergency cover. Veterinary practices in the UK are required by the Royal College of Veterinary Surgeons to provide 24-hour availability in all their specialties, or they should, by prior arrangement, direct clients to an alternative source of appropriate assistance. If a dedicated emergency clinic is used for out-of-hours cover, the emergency clinic staff should have at least some basic training in avian emergencies and be able to call in more expert help when required.

When a client brings in their new bird for a health check, this is an ideal opportunity to discuss diet, husbandry, environment, training and appropriate handling. For young birds, behavioural problems that manifest in adulthood can be avoided with the correct advice. This initial visit will take much longer than a normal consultation period so an extended appointment should be booked.

Clients will often arrive with a list of their own questions to ask about everything from potential disease risks to queries about normal behaviour in different species. They may also expect to discuss controversial management techniques, such as the trimming of flight feathers, and the clinician should be able to do so without bias (clients often find it difficult to source objective factual information on these topics).

Clients will expect the nursing and reception team to be able to identify the species treated in the practice and to have basic husbandry knowledge. They should not expect them to have in-depth knowledge or to be able to discuss the advantages and disadvantages of the different husbandry methods. Staff will also be expected to be familiar with commonly used hobbyist terms, for example falconry terms (Figure 7.8) (see Appendix 5). Nurses and reception staff should avoid discussing avian medical matters, referring these questions back to the veterinary surgeon.

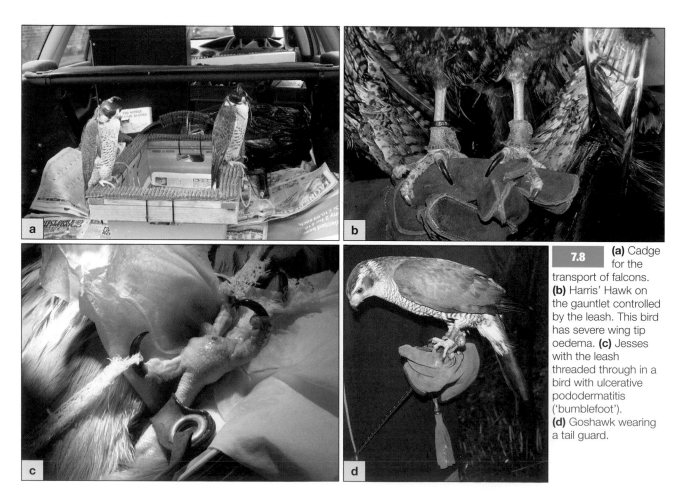

7.8 **(a)** Cadge for the transport of falcons. **(b)** Harris' Hawk on the gauntlet controlled by the leash. This bird has severe wing tip oedema. **(c)** Jesses with the leash threaded through in a bird with ulcerative pododermatitis ('bumblefoot'). **(d)** Goshawk wearing a tail guard.

Training and continuing professional development

Veterinary surgeons preparing to offer avian medicine at a primary care level should follow a structured course of learning, preferably including working alongside an experienced colleague prepared to act as a mentor and supervise progressive training. In the absence of a mentor, home study complemented by continuing education courses is an alternative start.

In addition to the information contained in this Manual, there are a number of core texts that avian practitioners utilize for anatomy and physiology information (e.g. King and McLelland, 1984; Whittow, 2000; O'Malley, 2005).

Diet is a key area of misunderstanding; there is a lot of conflicting information on the internet and it is important to be able to provide evidence-based advice to clients, particularly when a bird's current diet is causing harm to its health. There are many different feeding practices for a given species and the avian clinician must be familiar with a wide range and have the background knowledge to be able to evaluate unusual diets to ascertain if they are nutritionally complete. Diets can also provide environmental enrichment and, in many species, need to promote normal wear of the beak and gut function. (See Chapters 6 and 11 for more information on normal nutrition and critical care nutritional support.)

Behaviour is another complex area, with many published texts about parrot behaviour for veterinary surgeons (e.g. Luescher, 2006) and owners (e.g. Moustaki, 2005). It is recommended that veterinary surgeons read information published for owners as well as the standard veterinary texts, to get a good overview of the information available. Chick behaviour, particularly around weaning, is an important area of focus as inappropriate management at this stage will have implications for behaviour throughout life. Evidence-based information on raptor and passerine behaviour is more difficult to find, and books written for owners may be the best source, although caution should be exercised when evaluating this information.

Discussion with clients about husbandry and the environment in which the bird is kept should be a part of every consultation. There are many good resources (e.g. Heidenreich, 1997); see Chapter 3 and the *BSAVA Manual of Raptors, Pigeons and Passerine Birds* and the *BSAVA Manual of Psittacine Birds* for more information. Veterinary surgeons should also be familiar with the types of cages and aviaries, perches, toys and other cage equipment available.

In the examination room, clinicians should be able to competently and confidently capture and handle birds, in order to minimize stress, avoid damage to the bird and facilitate clinical examination, sample collection and safe administration of medication and/or nutritional support (Figure 7.9) (see Chapters 9 and 10).

Continuing professional development and training must also include avian anaesthesia (see Chapter 16), radiology (see Chapter 18) (Samour and Naldo, 2006), medicine (key texts include Altman *et al.*, 1997; Fudge, 2000; Harrison and Lightfoot, 2006; Tully *et al.*, 2009) and surgery (Figure 7.10) (see Chapter 17) (Orosz *et al.*, 1992). Post-mortem examination requires a good understanding of all the topics mentioned above and is very useful as a learning aid (see Chapter 14) (Schmidt *et al.*, 2003; Campbell and Ellis, 2007).

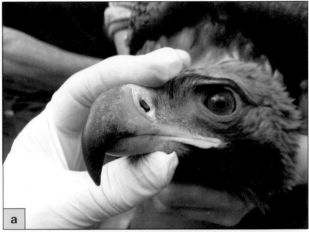

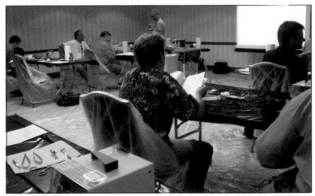

7.9 **(a)** Clinical examination of a large and potentially dangerous bird, such as this Golden Eagle, requires expert handlers. **(b)** Restraint of a Peregrine Falcon.

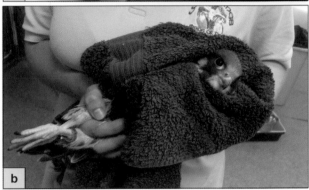

7.10 Microsurgery wet lab at an Association of Avian Veterinarians conference.

Referrals

Avian medicine is a well developed branch of veterinary medicine and most conditions have tried and tested treatment protocols. In most cases there is an answer, and if the veterinary surgeon is unfamiliar with the condition then referring the case to an experienced colleague will be an opportunity to learn as well as it being the best decision for the bird.

The Royal College of Veterinary Surgeons Code of Professional Conduct states that 'Veterinary surgeons should recognise when a case or a treatment option is outside their area of competence'. This is when cases should be either redirected or referred.

A redirection is when the bird has not been seen at the practice but treatment is recommended elsewhere. The reception team should be aware of the limitations of their veterinary team: what species and presentations are outside their area of competence. It is better for the bird and the owner if these cases are identified early and redirected rather than delaying treatment by scheduling a consultation and then having to refer the bird.

A referral is when a clinical case under investigation is sent to a veterinary surgeon with more expertise and/or the facilities to continue its diagnosis and/or treatment, and may occur before or after diagnosis (Figure 7.11). An early referral before the client asks about a second opinion is preferable.

Veterinary surgeons referring a case should promptly provide the referral veterinary surgeon with the full case history, including copies of any laboratory tests and diagnostic images.

Economics

The standard models of economics created from small animal practice do not apply to bird-exclusive situations. A significant percentage of consultations will be annual health checks and grooming procedures; however, this does not nearly amount to the level of revenue from routine vaccinations in small animal practice. Consultations are longer than normal due to the need to collect and discuss a much more detailed history. The number of cases seen is lower, so the cost of equipment and training has to be shared between a smaller number of cases. These are the main reasons why a different pricing structure is necessary for avian consultations compared with small animal practice. As a consequence clients need to be attracted from a much wider geographical area per full-time avian veterinary surgeon compared with the geographical area needed to sustain a full-time dog and cat veterinary surgeon.

References and further reading

Altman RB, Clubb SL, Dorrestein GM and Quesenberry K (1997) *Avian Medicine and Surgery*. WB Saunders, Philadelphia

Campbell TW and Ellis CK (2007) *Avian and Exotic Animal Hematology and Cytology, 3rd edn*. Blackwell Publishing, Ames

Chitty J and Lierz M (2008) *BSAVA Manual of Raptors, Pigeons and Passerine Birds*. BSAVA Publications, Gloucester

Fudge AM (2000) *Laboratory Medicine: Avian and Exotic Pets*. WB Saunders, Philadelphia

Harcourt-Brown N and Chitty J (eds) (2005) *BSAVA Manual of Psittacine Birds, 2nd edn*. BSAVA Publications, Gloucester

Harrison GJ and Lightfoot TL (2006) *Clinical Avian Medicine*. Spix Publishing Inc., Palm Beach

Heidenreich M (1997) *Birds of Prey: Medicine and Management*. Blackwell Science, Oxford

King AS and McLelland J (1984) *Birds: Their Structure and Function, 2nd edn*. Baillière Tindall, London

Krautwald-Junghanns ME, Pees M, Reese S and Tully T (2010) *Diagnostic Imaging of Exotic Pets: Birds, Small Mammals, Reptiles*. Schlütersche, Hannover

Lierz M (2008) Endoscopy, biopsy and endosurgery. In: *BSAVA Manual of Raptors, Pigeons and Passerine Birds*, ed. J Chitty and M Lierz, pp. 128–142. BSAVA Publications, Gloucester

Luescher A (2006) *Manual of Parrot Behavior*. Wiley-Blackwell, Ames

Moustaki N (2005) *Parrots For Dummies*. John Wiley & Sons, Oxford

O'Malley B (2005) *Clinical Anatomy and Physiology of Exotic Species: Structure and Function of Mammals, Birds, Reptiles and Amphibians*. Elsevier Saunders, Edinburgh

Orosz SE, Ensley PK and Haynes CJ (1992) *Avian Surgical Anatomy*. WB Saunders, Philadelphia

Samour JH and Naldo JL (2006) *Anatomical and Clinical Radiology of Birds of Prey: Including Interactive Advanced Anatomical Imaging*. WB Saunders, Philadelphia

Schmidt RE, Reavill DR and Phalen DN (2003) *Pathology of Pet and Aviary Birds*. Blackwell Publishing, Ames

Silverman S and Tell LA (2009) *Radiology of Birds: An Atlas of Normal Anatomy and Positioning*. WB Saunders, Philadelphia

Tully T, Dorrestein G and Jones A (2009) *Handbook of Avian Medicine*. WB Saunders, Philadelphia

Varga M, Lumbis R and Gott L (2012) *BSAVA Manual of Exotic Pet and Wildlife Nursing*. BSAVA Publications, Gloucester

Whittow GC (2000) Sturkie's *Avian Physiology, 5th edn*. Academic Press, San Diego

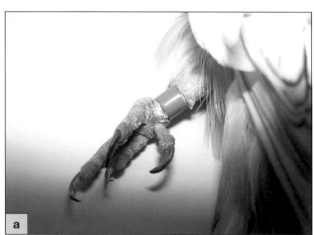

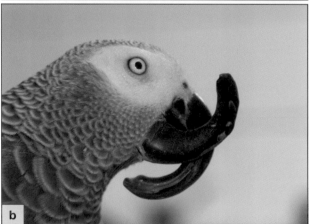

7.11 Referral may be required if the clinician is inexperienced or a case is complicated. **(a)** Ring removal can be extremely difficult even with plastic rings as in this case. **(b)** Correction of this beak deformity will require in-depth knowledge of the normal anatomy.

Reception guide for the general practice

Alistair Lawrie

Birds of any species are adept at disguising signs of illness. It is not in the best interests for survival of a wild bird if it exhibits signs of malaise or injury as predators will recognize weakness and target the sick or injured bird as an easier kill. As a result, a commonly held belief is that sick birds are 70% dead when noticed by their owners and 90% dead by the time they are presented to the veterinary surgeon (veterinarian). This means that there is a greater urgency for the veterinary practitioner to see birds suspected to be unwell compared with other cases. The majority of birds that are showing signs of illness require emergency, or at least same day, attention.

Reception staff guidelines for avian patients

It is absolutely essential that all staff, and especially those carrying out reception duties, have a basic knowledge of bird problems and that they have absolutely no doubt about what constitutes an avian emergency. Their 'telephone triage' and basic advice may be the difference between a successful outcome and a dead bird.

Reception staff must not only have the confidence and ability to take decisions about the relative urgency of cases but also must be able to offer basic first aid advice to the owner of the patient. In some cases this may be life-saving advice that will keep the patient alive until it can be examined. Reception staff should also be able to advise the veterinary staff of the nature of the emergency that is going to arrive in order that preparations can be made (e.g. incubators may be heated; a warmed and humidified oxygen supply prepared).

One of the complicating factors of bird emergencies is the fact that not only are there so many different species that differ in their biological needs, but also that there is an enormous variation in size (and therefore metabolic rates), anatomy and physiology within the different bird families. For example, a few days of not eating may not be particularly worrying if the patient is an eagle, whereas one might be dealing with a potentially fatal case if the patient were a Merlin. Similarly, one might contrast a macaw with a parrotlet or a Common Hill Mynah with a St Helena Waxbill (Figure 8.1). Small birds have a much higher metabolic

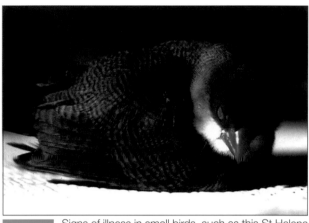

8.1 Signs of illness in small birds, such as this St Helena Waxbill, should be treated as an emergency.

rate and a greater surface area to body mass ratio, and thus cannot afford to be anorectic for very long. They can also become hypothermic more easily. Differing approaches to giving advice and to supportive care are required, depending upon the species in question.

The level of expertise of the bird's owner should also be gauged as this may be important in the triage of the case. Expert bird keepers (e.g. raptor keepers and professional keepers/breeders of psittacine species) may be more likely to have a better avicultural knowledge than someone keeping a pet finch or Budgerigar – but this should not be taken for granted.Having access to internet sources may mean that a bird's owner may seem well informed, but they may have come to an erroneous conclusion about their bird's condition.

General signs of illness, such as the bird being described as 'fluffed up', anorexic or not perching, always warrant investigation, especially in a small bird. The art of triage is to be able to recognize how ill a patient is and then to prioritize the acutely unwell from the chronically sick, as well as recognizing which cases are emergencies, urgent or more routine (Figures 8.2 and 8.3). At this stage there is not an attempt to make a diagnosis and, as many sick birds will show similar signs, this is generally not plausible over the telephone.

What constitutes an emergency?

All signs of illness that a client may report are concerning, but sitting on the bottom of the cage, bleeding, prolonged anorexia, respiratory distress, vomiting, convulsions or obvious trauma are all cases that need to be seen urgently

- What appears to be the problem?
- How ill does the bird appear to be?
- Are there any obvious signs of illness (e.g. prolapse, fracture, diarrhoea)?
- When was it last seen to be acting normally?
- Is it sitting on its perch or on the floor?
- Caged or aviary bird?
- Is it still eating?
- Is it vocalizing?
- Has any first aid been administered?
- Is the bird under the care of another veterinary surgeon and, if so, is it a referral or a second-opinion case?

8.2 Questions that a receptionist should ask of a client calling about their sick bird.

Urgent clinical signs that require first aid and emergency veterinary attention

- Abandoned chicks/nestlings
- Acute respiratory distress (tachypnoea or dyspnoea/mouth breathing)
- Air sac rupture
- Burns to skin
- Cloacal prolapse
- Collapse/shock (including egg binding and exhaustion)
- Crop burns/fistulae
- Crop stasis and 'sour crop'
- Contamination of feathers with oil (e.g. frying pan oil/waste oil)
- Convulsions
- Dehydration
- Diarrhoea
- Eye injuries/infections/discharges
- Fractured wings/limbs/toes (open or closed)
- Haemorrhage (from wound or blood in droppings)
- Hypothermia/frost bite/wing tip oedema
- Poisoning (inhalational or heavy metal ingestion)
- Trauma/concussion from attack
- Vomiting

Non-urgent clinical signs that can be investigated in a routine appointment

- Chronic diarrhoea/polyuria without weight loss
- Feather plucking/feather conditions unless involving skin damage/self-mutilation
- Reproductive failure
- Investigation of body masses
- Weight loss but not emaciated

8.3 Urgent *versus* non-urgent clinical signs.

Bird-keeping terminology

One confusing aspect of aviculture for the non-expert is the variety of terms that are used for describing birds' bodily functions, their husbandry and bird-keeping equipment. This is particularly true of falconry where many medieval terms are still used. An understanding of these terms is necessary, not least to uphold the credibility of the whole practice. Figure 8.4 lists the most commonly used terminology in relation to passerine and psittacine birds. See Appendix 5 for falconry terminology.

Term	Definition
Closed rings	Slid on to the tarsometatarsus of chicks within a few days of hatching, these are a means of identification. As bird grows they cannot be removed without cutting; birds with closed rings are generally bred in captivity
Cuttlefish bones	Cuttlefish bones are placed in the cages of small birds so that they have access to a calcium source
Droppings	Material voided from the cloaca (i.e. faeces, urates and urine). Vary in consistency depending upon the bird's species and diet and whether there is diarrhoea or polyuria
Egg food	This is a mixture of hard-boiled egg yolk and biscuit crumbs that is moistened and fed to passerines before and during the breeding period. May also be used as an adjunct during hand-rearing
Feather plucking/picking	Some birds 'pluck' their feathers and pull them completely out of the follicles, which is different to those that 'pick' at their feathers and disrupt the integrity of the feathers so that they appear fluffy or downy. Picking is usually a chronic condition but sudden onset of feather plucking or feather loss warrants relatively urgent attention
Fluffed up	Describes any bird that is unwell and is ruffling its feathers so that they trap more air in an effort to reduce heat loss from the body
Going light	Losing weight; non-specific and has many causes
Loose droppings	'Wet' droppings can have many causes, but severe diarrhoea in a small bird is a serious situation. Cases of polyuria may not need such urgent investigation
On the floor	Healthy birds do not normally sleep or spend time on the floor of the cage being fluffed up. This is a sign of unwellness or lameness. Some birds, of course, do not habitually perch (e.g. quail and other ground dwellers)
Lost its voice	Vocalization is the first activity to stop when a bird becomes unwell and it is generally a positive sign when a recovering bird starts to speak or vocalize again. Changes in the 'normal' voice of the bird are also a significant sign of airway disease
Training cage	These are small cages of a standard size for getting birds accustomed to being exhibited for competition purposes
Head under wing	Any bird that is sleeping a lot, especially when it would normally be alert, is ill
Split rings (leg bands)	These can be fitted at any time in the bird's life by closing a 'C'-shaped ring around the leg with pliers
Soft	A small bird that is 'soft' is one that is sitting with slightly ruffled feathers and showing subtle signs of illness without being overtly ill. It will generally still be eating and moving about but fluffs its feathers out when at rest and looks slightly sleepy
Vitamin/mineral/ nutritional supplements	Examples include: Zolcal D®, Collo-Cal® D, Avipro®, Daily Essentials, ACE-High, Vetark® Critical Care, Poly-Aid, Emeraid® Critical Care Formula

8.4 Terms and phrases commonly used by keepers of passerine and psittacine birds.

Clinical signs

Character of droppings

For more general information about droppings, see Appendix 4.

- **Absent/scanty:** scanty droppings are indicative of reduced appetite, whereas the complete absence of droppings is very concerning and may be a sign of either intestinal blockage or anorexia. Note that birds may still produce urates without any faecal component to the droppings. Quite specific questions need to be asked.

- **Diarrhoea:** this is a serious condition in a small bird and can rapidly lead to dehydration and death.
- **Polyuria:** excessive drinking and excreting more urine than normal needs investigation but generally would not be an emergency situation unless the bird is very unwell or others in the group are dying.
- **Colour of urates:** the normal colour of urates is white. Variation in the colour is important and the presence of green or red urates warrants urgent investigation. Golden yellow urates can sometimes be seen after the administration of vitamins.

Vomiting/regurgitation

Vomiting and regurgitation should always be regarded as serious signs, with the exception of courtship regurgitation by male birds.

- **Sticky/malodorous:** if the bird is vomiting very mucousy or 'smelly' fluids it is in need of urgent attention since dehydration can quickly ensue. In a raptor this may be due to 'sour crop'; in other birds it could signify gastrointestinal stasis (e.g. proventricular dilatation disease). In the smaller bird, vomiting may be evidenced by the patient having 'sticky' feathers on the crown of its head as it throws its head about and attempts to clear its oral cavity of the vomited material (Figure 8.5).
- **Regurgitating seed by an otherwise well bird:** some male birds (e.g. Budgerigars) will regurgitate seeds when they are in breeding condition and may 'feed' their mirrors in the absence of a mate. These birds are always in good condition and are not ill. The seeds can be adhered together in small 'tubes' but are never malodorous.
- **Vomiting fluids:** there are many causes ranging from heavy metal poisoning to acute hepatic disease or intestinal obstruction. Patients with these signs require urgent stabilization and thorough investigation.
- **Retching:** attempting to vomit can be caused by many conditions, ranging from crop infections and ingested foreign bodies to problems lower down the gastrointestinal tract (e.g. *Macrorhabdus ornithogaster* infection, formerly known as megabacteriosis). The urgency of these cases will depend upon whether the bird is still able to eat and whether it is exhibiting signs of being really ill.

Paediatric problems

With the popularity of hand-rearing birds, especially parrots, there has been an associated increase in the paediatric problems that need to be dealt with. Some conditions may be congenital, but more are developmental or a result of improper hand-rearing. Developmental problems (e.g. limb and beak deformities) do need to be attended to when they are first observed and the bird is still growing, but they are not 'emergencies' requiring immediate attention or first aid. Simple advice may be given so that the condition can be prevented from getting worse until the bird is seen.

- **Splayed legs:** these need to be examined reasonably promptly but are not emergency cases. The birds can be placed in a deep padded cup until they are seen (Figure 8.6).
- **Wryneck:** this condition needs to be attended to and the neck supported, but it is an urgent case rather than an emergency (Figure 8.7). A simple neck support made from a section of foam pipe insulation would be sensible first aid advice, always given with the proviso that it does not interfere with breathing or crop emptying.

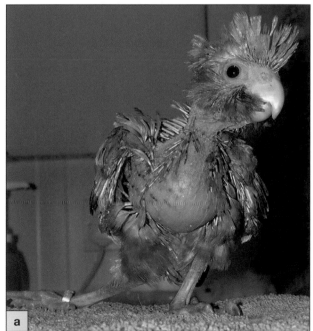

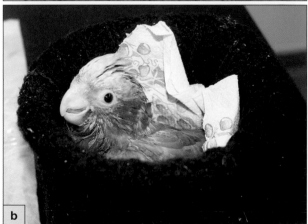

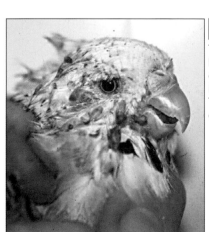

8.5 This Budgerigar's head is covered in crop contents, indicating vomiting. This is an urgent case.

8.6 **(a)** Galah chick with leg splay, which is not an emergency. This chick also has nasal accretion of food, which needs to be cleared but is not urgent. **(b)** Placing the chick in a deep nest prevents further leg deviation.

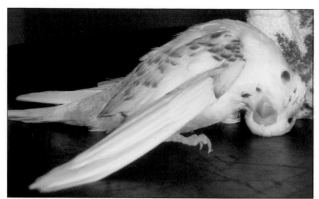

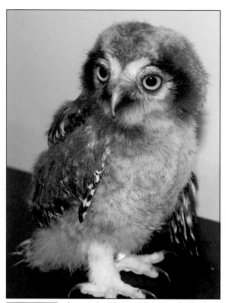

8.7	Wryneck (torticollis) in a Budgerigar should be seen urgently.

- **Angel wing:** this is another developmental problem of the young bird that is rapidly growing wing feathers (Figure 8.8). Supporting the wing, increasing calcium and reducing protein content of the diet may be advised until professional help and assessment are available. It is not an emergency situation so long as the wings are supported, but it needs to be corrected quite quickly before there is permanent deviation of the developing carpal area. The urgency will also depend upon how long the owner has been aware of the condition. If very recently noticed then next-day attention would be sensible. However, in cases of established angel wing there may be no easy cure.
- **No feeding reflexes:** lack of feeding reflexes indicates a very sick baby bird and necessitates immediate first aid if possible, for example, tube feeding and increasing the environmental temperature, and emergency veterinary attention.
- **Delayed crop emptying:** this may be as a result of low temperature of the chick (or the brooder), feeding hand-rearing formula that is too cool, or due to disease or infection (e.g. candidiasis). First aid advice is to increase the temperature of the brooder, provide more liquid feeds (Figure 8.9) or fluids and to gently massage the crop contents. If there is no rapid improvement then examination is required.
- **Dehydration/hypothermia:** dehydration may be suspected if one is able to cause prolonged 'tenting' of the skin by gently pinching it between the fingers. In the case of hypothermia, the chick will feel cold to the touch and is likely to be extremely quiet. Increasing the temperature and giving extra oral fluids may suffice but these small birds must also get an energy source. Most newly hatched birds will initially derive their nutrition by reabsorption of their yolk sacs. Advice would always be to examine these birds if there is no rapid improvement (within an hour or two).
- **Sudden death amongst nestlings:** from a triage point of view, the important advice to be given in these cases is that post-mortem examination of the dead individuals is imperative in order that a definitive diagnosis may be made. This is urgent and would be classed as an emergency.
- **Inability to move:** if the condition is orthopaedic and the bird is alert and feeding then it is not an emergency, but as with all paediatric conditions it needs to be attended to relatively quickly.

8.8	An owl chick with metabolic bone disease and 'angel wing' is an urgent case. The sooner this case is seen, the easier it will be to treat.

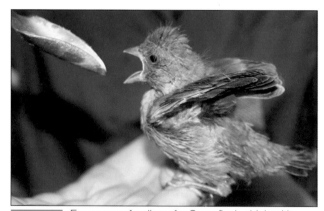

8.9	Emergency feeding of a Greenfinch chick with a beak-shaped spoon.

- **Swollen toes:** Macaw, Eclectus and Grey Parrot chicks may be observed by the owners to have swollen toes. Not uncommonly this will also occur in young and adult passerines where nesting fibres have caused a constriction around the digit or foot with a compromised blood supply to the extremities being the result. In the case of passerines, if fibres are visible, then the owner should be advised to remove the constriction or bring the bird in for examination. Psittacine birds with constrictions generally require immediate attention because minor surgery may need to be performed on the toes in an attempt to re-establish the circulation by incising the tight bands that form around the digits. Owners should be advised to keep the toes moist until they can be examined by applying emollient cream.
- **Beak deformities/deviations:** these cases are non-urgent, but are in the 'need to be seen soon' category so that they can be assessed and corrected. Older (mature) birds with these problems are definitely not urgent cases (Figure 8.10).
- **Crop burns/fistulae:** hand-rearing formula that has been fed at too high a temperature to the chick may result in thermal necrosis of the lining of the crop and skin with a resultant fistula. All cases will

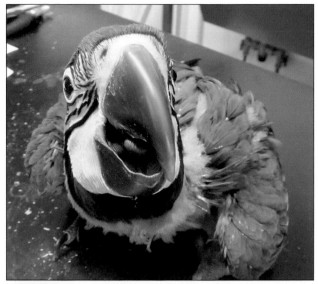

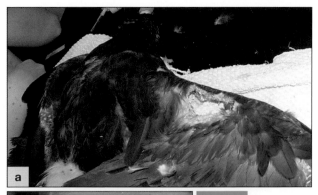

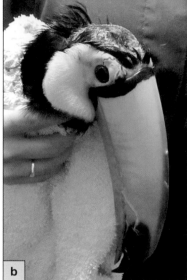

8.10 The deviation in this Blue and Gold Macaw's beak is not an emergency.

8.11 (a) Propatagial membrane laceration in this Harris' Hawk should be examined by a veterinary surgeon urgently. (b) A Toco Toucan with a head laceration such as this is also an urgent case.

need to be seen and the fistula repaired. They are all in the urgent category of needing attention and, to a certain extent, the size of the fistula, fluid and food loss, age and health of the chicks as well as the time since the problem was noticed can all change the speed with which the chick requires attention.

Traumatic injuries

- **Lacerations:** the majority of lacerations of any significant size will need to be examined and repaired (Figure 8.11). The severity and position of the laceration and whether there is associated haemorrhage will determine whether it is an emergency or just urgent. Some lacerations that look fairly dramatic (e.g. propatagial web lacerations) will need suturing but would not be classed as life-threatening emergencies.

- **Haemorrhage:** significant haemorrhage is always potentially life-threatening and appropriate advice needs to be given even before arranging for an emergency admission. This may range from simple pressure pads or bandaging, to tourniquet application. Simple, but often problematic, haemorrhages that concern owners greatly are those from beaks and nails. Significant amounts of blood can be lost and it can be difficult to arrest the bleeding.

- **Loss of nail or talon 'sheath':** these will not necessarily be emergencies, but owners will need appropriate advice regarding first aid and management of the injury (e.g. keeping clean and moist) until an appointment can be arranged within 24 hours.

- **Inability to use leg:** if there is any suggestion that the limb may be fractured then an urgent appointment is indicated, together with appropriate advice on support of the limb and carriage to the practice (Figures 8.12 and 8.13).

- **Severely drooped wing:** one wing that is hanging down may be the result of trauma (e.g. fracture) or acute joint disease (e.g. septic arthritis). These are urgent cases (Figure 8.14). Both wings drooping down in a sick-looking bird may indicate general malaise.

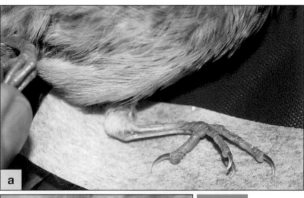

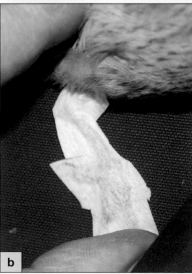

8.12 (a) Splinting of a Canary's leg using microporous tape. (b) Completed splint with second piece of tape applied and trimmed.

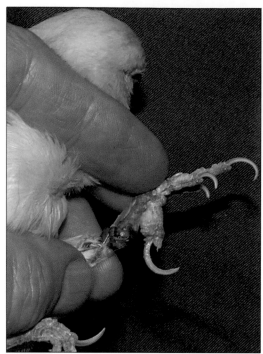

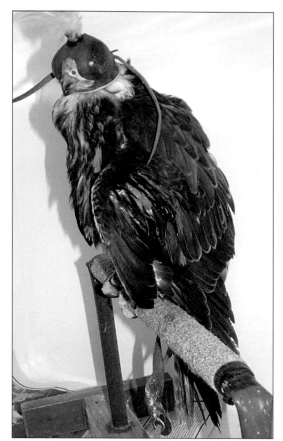

- **Wing tip oedema:** a particularly concerning sign in a raptor would be slight drooping of the wing(s) with fluid-filled swellings around the carpal joint area (Figure 8.15). These fluid-filled vesicles may or may not be leaking and the wing usually feels cold. This is likely to be wing tip oedema and definitely warrants emergency action and early diagnosis by a veterinary surgeon. Immediate steps must be taken by the owner to try to improve the circulation to the distal extremities of the wing even prior to examination.
- **Electrical or thermal burns:** these two events are emergency situations.

8.13 Domestic Canary with a vascular occlusion and injury caused by a too tight leg ring; this case is urgent.

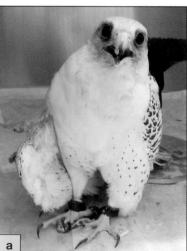

8.14 **(a)** This Gyrfalcon has a fractured wing in urgent need of support. **(b)** Harris' Hawk with tibiotarsus fracture adequately supported.

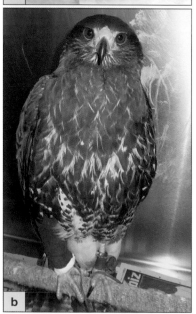

a

b

8.15 Signs of wing tip oedema, as displayed in this young Peregrine hybrid, should be investigated as an emergency.

Convulsions

These are always serious cases and merit immediate attention. Owners need to transport the bird quietly, safely and in a darkened container to the veterinary clinic. In certain instances (e.g. a raptor that is suddenly convulsing whilst it is being worked at low bodyweight and possibly in adverse weather conditions) immediate administration of a glucose solution may be indicated before further transportation – assuming that it can be administered safely without risk of the bird regurgitating and then inhaling the fluid.

Acute respiratory distress

This is always an emergency situation and these patients need to be seen quickly, but at the same time distress must be minimized. The extra stress of handling or catching the bird can sometimes result in a bird that was just managing to survive being over-stimulated, leading to rapid deterioration and death.

These risks should be clearly explained to the bird's owners and steps taken to minimize the distress whilst at the same time encouraging them to get attention for the bird. This may involve administering oxygen and/or inserting an air sac tube depending upon the clinical signs. Birds in this situation should be transported in containers that maximize the passage of fresh air and their breathing must not be restricted (e.g. by wrapping them in towels).

Basic first aid advice for owners

'First aid' is the initial response and treatment of a patient in a situation where there is acute illness or injury. It has three distinct components:

- Preservation of life
- Prevention of any further harm occurring to the patient by minimizing tissue damage or removing the patient from the source of harm whether physical or toxic (e.g. inhaled fumes)
- Promotion of recovery by taking whatever supportive action is needed.

The first point of contact between the owner and the practice is usually a telephone call and, given that the owner may be stressed and is probably not an expert in avian medicine, determining the patient's health status can be challenging. Using the owner's initial description, the reception staff will need to deduce what course of action needs to be taken. Questioning (see Figure 8.2) and history taking are vital. Advice can then be divided into the following categories:

- Emergency cases with first aid advice given that will help to preserve life until arrival at the practice for examination
- Non-life-threatening cases that need to be seen as soon as possible (e.g. leg or wing fracture) (Figure 8.16). Advice may need to be given to minimize further injury during transport
- Chronic problems that may only need advice about supportive care until a routine appointment can be arranged
- Cases which can be managed at home with appropriate advice.

Much of the advice given will be general advice that relates to the majority of cases where a bird is ill or in shock, namely the provision of warmth (26.7–29.4°C), fluids and a quiet dimly lit environment that is as stress-free as possible.

Abandoned chicks and nestlings

Advice depends upon the species of bird. In all species if a bird has lost the 'gape' or begging for food reflex then urgent attention is needed because it will be weak, hypoglycaemic and possibly dehydrated. If the bird is otherwise 'healthy' (i.e. bright and looking for food), then simple feeding will suffice: hand-rearing formula, baby food or egg food for psittacine birds and passerines; and small pieces of day-old chick for raptors.

It is essential that chicks are put on to a recognized balanced diet as soon as possible, ensuring adequate calcium intake. Chicks that are less lively can be given a critical care formula. If no proprietary critical care

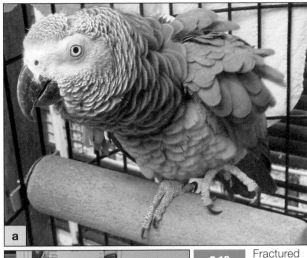

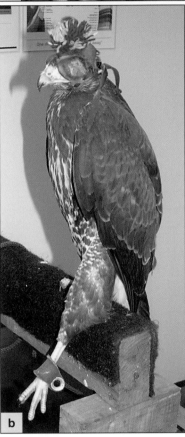

8.16 Fractured legs, as in this **(a)** African Grey Parrot and **(b)** Harris' Hawk, are urgent cases that need to be seen as soon as possible.

formula is available then honey or glucose diluted with warm water can be given until they can be examined by a veterinary surgeon.

Warmth is essential and chicks must be kept at a suitable temperature (approximately 38°C). Hypothermia and/or feeding food that is too concentrated or too cool will result in crop stasis. If absolutely no food is available then small amounts of boiled water (allowed to cool to an appropriate temperature; see Chapter 4) should be administered by syringe or dropper or, for very small birds, drops off the end of a small paintbrush, until they can be given professional attention. In general terms, they should not be fed again until the crop is virtually empty. Note that it is quite normal for parrot chicks to 'crash out' after being fed and for their heads to hang down. If they are strong and healthy then they will exhibit a violent 'pumping' action of the head when they are being fed (see Chapter 31).

Air sac rupture

This can be quite a concerning problem when the owner is presented with a 'blown up' or inflated bird. The cause will need some investigation but, unless there is associated respiratory distress, it is not a desperate emergency. If there is respiratory distress, a prominent and more transparent area of distended air sac may be punctured/incised with a sterile needle. This will allow escape of the trapped air and time to transport the bird to a clinic for further treatment. If left without treatment the air sac will usually re-inflate and become distended again (see Chapter 22).

Bite trauma

Bites from cats, dogs or other animals will generally require antibiotic cover and analgesics/anti-inflammatory drugs. Homecare first aid is limited to copious flushing of wounds with warm saline and povidone–iodine solution, arresting any haemorrhage, and then covering the area with a sterile dressing.

Bleeding/haemorrhage

Advice given depends upon the origin of the haemorrhage. The most important thing is that bleeding is arrested as soon as possible. Initially, the bird should be gently restrained in a soft towel and the cause of the haemorrhage identified.

- **Nails or beak tip bleed:** if there is haemorrhage from the nails or beak tip then pressure and/or a styptic (e.g. silver nitrate, ferric chloride, potassium permanganate) should be applied. If a styptic is not available then cornflour or talcum powder can be applied to promote clotting. If the haemorrhage cannot be controlled then the site of the bleeding may need to be cauterized with heat; the bird should be brought to the surgery as an emergency as this is a veterinary procedure.
- **Feather bleed:** the skin around the base of the feather should be firmly gripped and the bleeding feather pulled sharply out of its follicle using haemostats or tweezers. The wing must be held firmly as there is a deep and strong attachment of the feather to the periosteum. Gentle pressure can then be applied to the follicle and the haemorrhage is usually easily resolved (note: this is not suitable for primary/secondary feathers in raptors since feather follicle damage may ensue, resulting in non-regrowth of feathers).
- **Tongue bleed:** generally the best advice is for urgent veterinary examination since owner-administered first aid is difficult and lacerations may need suturing. Asphyxiation is possible from excessive bleeding into the oropharyngeal area in small birds. Owners should be advised to incline the bird's head forward and try to keep the mouth clear of blood clots.
- **Soft tissue/skin bleed:** this is not often a huge problem in birds unless they are self-mutilating. Pressure should be applied and, if this is ineffective, cornflour and a gauze pad. The bird should be prevented from picking at the area. Uncontrolled haemorrhage necessitates a clinic visit and would merit an emergency admission.
- **Cloacal bleed:** this may be due to a number of factors; for example, cloacal damage, papilloma or haematuria/melaena, or a damaged prolapsed organ such as the oviduct or intestine. Local pressure with a moist gauze pad may suffice. Other cases will need investigating. In the case of a prolapsed organ, the area must be kept moist and professional assistance obtained (see 'Cloacal prolapse').

In all cases, the bird should be kept warm and, if bleeding continues, then urgent assistance is needed.

Burns

- **Skin burns:** these are usually as a result of coming into contact with boiling water, although occasionally burns from naked flames or electrocution do occur. Cold water or saline should be run over the area for a few minutes, then it should be covered with a sterile pad and veterinary help sought.
- **Crop burns:** these usually occur as a result of feeding hand-rearing food that is too hot, especially formula that has been heated in a microwave. If the mistake is spotted immediately, cold water should be used to dilute the crop contents down and the crop gently massaged. However, in the majority of cases, the damage has occurred already and a crop fistula has appeared (Figure 8.17). This should be covered with a pad and an appointment made for remedial surgery on the crop. These birds can become dehydrated and hypoglycaemic quite quickly.

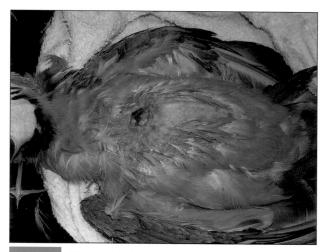

8.17   Blue and Gold Macaw chick with a crop fistula.

Cloacal prolapse

This may be a simple protrusion of part of the cloacal mucosa (e.g. cloacal papillomatosis) or as serious as prolapse of internal organs (e.g. intestine or oviduct) (Figure 8.18). In all cases, further trauma should be prevented. If possible, the bird is restrained gently in a towel and the prolapsed area kept moist with dampened gauze swabs or KY® jelly. With some nervous birds, any attempt at catching and first aid may make the situation worse by inadvertently causing the bird to traumatize the prolapsed tissue on perches or cage bars. In these cases immediate transport to the clinic in its cage is the preferable option if it is possible to do so.

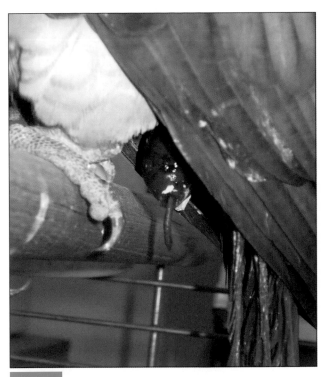

8.18   African Grey Parrot with cloacal prolapse.

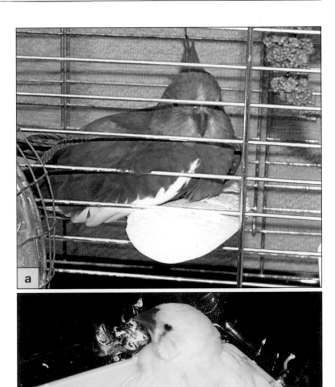

8.19   (a) Egg-bound Cockatiel that has collapsed.
(b) Zebra Finch collapsed with hypocalcaemia and requiring emergency attention.

Collapse

A bird may be 'collapsed' for a number of reasons ranging from severe shock to egg binding (Figure 8.19). First aid for all cases involves ensuring that there is no respiratory obstruction and then placing the bird in a heated cage or under a heat lamp (26.7–29.4°C), making sure that it does not overheat due to an inability to move away. Judicious use of a warm hairdryer (with the cage covered in towels) may help to effect an increase in the environmental temperature in the immediate area if there are no other options, but this can potentially cause dehydration by dessicating the bird. If the bird is still able to sit up and swallow then energy-providing warm oral fluids should be administered (e.g. a critical care formula, if available, or glucose or honey diluted with water). The crop must not be overfilled. Any female bird that could possibly have reproductive-related issues (e.g. egg binding) should also be given oral calcium.

Further treatment, handling or investigation should be limited until the bird is more stable. Hot water bottles, 'hot hands' (sealed surgical gloves containing warmed water), or other methods of maintaining a satisfactory environmental temperature (e.g. within clothing) whilst the patient is being transported should be used. Care must be taken to limit the risk of iatrogenic burns when using these warming methods.

Contamination of feathers with oil

Oil can be cleaned off with dilute detergent (e.g. washing up liquid) but multiple washes may be needed, and extreme care must be taken to ensure that the bird does not become hypothermic. A heated cage is an absolute necessity to dry the bird after washing. Oral fluids and food may need to be given as supportive treatments, and gastrointestinal protectants if anything other than vegetable oil has been ingested. If the contamination is as a result of a bird coming into contact with hot fat in the kitchen then thermal burns may have occurred.

Convulsions/seizures

Convulsions and seizures have many possible aetiologies, and certain circumstances may indicate the likelihood of a particular reason (e.g. paramyxovirus infection (PMV3) in aviary birds; trauma, contact with toxins or a stroke in Budgerigars).

Immediate first aid advice is to keep the bird in a dimly lit or dark container, with all perches and water dishes (risk of drowning) removed. It should be ensured that there is no vomiting or regurgitation and that the airways are clear. The bird should be gently wrapped in a light towel and placed on the padded floor of the cage. Owners should be extremely quiet and gentle when handling their bird so that more seizures are not triggered.

It is impossible to make a telephone diagnosis due to the wide range of possible causes (including hypocalcaemia, hypoglycaemia, toxins, cardiac problems and heavy metal poisoning). If hypocalcaemia is suspected based on circumstantial evidence, such as an African Grey Parrot on an unsupplemented diet (Figure 8.20), the administration of oral calcium can be recommended. Similarly, a raptor that is of low bodyweight and has been flying in adverse weather conditions should be given oral glucose, as hypoglycaemia would be likely. Other patients should be kept as warm and quiet as possible and treated as emergency admissions. If there is an obvious cause of toxicity, then it is

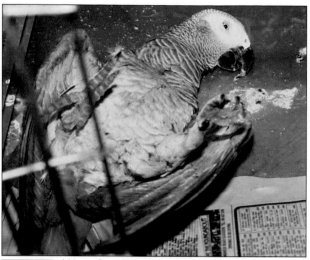

8.20 African Grey Parrot with hypocalcaemic tetany. Orally administered calcium can be advised in this case.

imperative that the bird be removed from the source. Bathing off any topically applied medication (e.g. insecticidal sprays) might be possible, but is difficult if the patient is continuously fitting (see Chapter 32).

Crop stasis

The clinical signs of crop stasis are delayed emptying of the crop between feeds in young birds and impaction or 'sour crop' in adult birds (Figure 8.21).

In cases of delayed emptying in an adult raptor that is otherwise well, gently syringing water or administering electrolyte solutions by tube will often stimulate emptying of the crop. Owners should be wary that the contents of the already full crop do not overflow into the trachea. A raptor keeper may be able to massage some of the crop contents from the distended crop up the oesophagus and out of the mouth. If the bird is obviously unwell and the contents of the crop have a putrid smell then emergency veterinary examination is

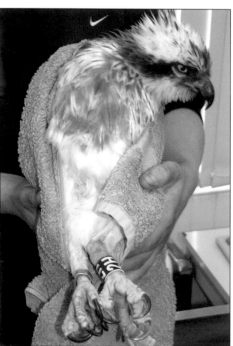

8.21 Osprey requiring emergency treatment for sour crop, toxaemia and a fractured tibiotarsus.

essential. These birds can be quite toxaemic and occasionally the crop will even rupture.

Crop stasis in young birds has many causes but cold feeds or a cold environment will make the situation worse. First aid advice is to administer warm, dilute fluids (electrolyte replacers or critical care formula) and massage the crop contents to disperse any impaction. Continue with diluted feeds until the bird can be examined.

Dehydration

If the bird is mildly dehydrated then it should be kept warm and electrolyte-replacing fluids administered orally. If there is no rapid improvement then parenteral fluids will be needed. Dehydration and chilling/shock may lead to irreversible renal tubule blockage with urates.

Diarrhoea

Acute, severe diarrhoea can result in dehydration, so first aid actions are aimed at rehydration with oral electrolytes, keeping the bird warm and possibly administering anti-diarrhoea agents and/or gastro-protectants such as kaolin or Pepto-Bismol™. If the bird is frugivorous then fruit should be removed and a very basic diet offered (e.g. boiled rice, peanut butter or baby food). Extreme care must be taken when handling small birds that are dehydrated and debilitated from the effects of diarrhoea because they are extremely weak and hypoglycaemic.

Eye problems/trauma

If a foreign body is seen in the eye, gentle flushing with saline or artificial tears may resolve the problem. If the eyelids are stuck together then gentle bathing should enable them to be opened. Bilateral blepharitis/conjunctivitis is likely to be part of a systemic condition and is not an acute problem, but the bird still needs to be seen with some degree of urgency so that a diagnosis can be made. Birds with eye problems should be kept in subdued lighting (see Chapter 21).

Feather destructive disorder

Feather loss is always concerning to an owner but, more often than not, it is a chronic condition that does not need same-day attention (Figure 8.22). It has many possible causes and will generally need a complete medical examination to diagnose. Some cases of feather loss may be due to viral infections (e.g. psittacine beak and feather disease), whilst other cases may be due to other diseases or psychological problems. In the unusual situation of a bird losing lots of feathers very quickly (i.e. within a few hours) or that is obsessively attacking its skin and feathers, the best advice to give the owners is to keep the bird in dim light, keep it warm and to spray it with warm water or saline if there are any self-inflicted skin wounds. With these birds, veterinary attention is warranted sooner rather than later, and sedatives or behaviour-modifying drugs may be needed. A last resort is fitting the bird with a foam collar, but this should be applied by a veterinary surgeon since there can be many problems associated with using this. Birds will quite commonly throw themselves about the cage until they get used to the collar, and are therefore at risk of causing themselves traumatic injury. It can be extremely distressing for both the bird and its owner (see Chapter 30).

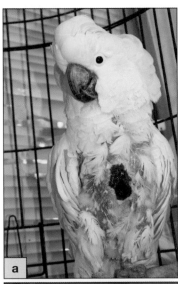

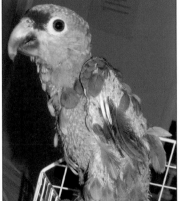

8.22 **(a)** This self-mutilating Moluccan Cockatoo can wait for a routine appointment; non-changing levels of mutilation are not emergencies but an increasing level of mutilation may require a more urgent appointment. **(b)** Psittacine beak and feather disease in a Red-lored Amazon.

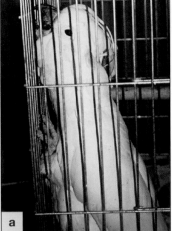

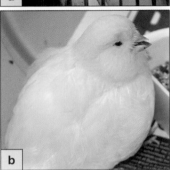

8.23 **(a)** This Moluccan Cockatoo is hanging from its cage, signalling extreme respiratory distress. **(b)** Border Canary in severe respiratory distress with cyanosis of the beak and open-beak breathing.

Respiratory distress

Respiratory distress may be either tachypnoea, as seen in a pneumonic bird, or dyspnoea seen in a bird with some sort of airway obstruction. Both are serious and the aim of first aid is to help oxygen exchange and alleviate the distress of the patient. Open-beak breathing and hanging vertically from the bars of the cage by the beak are signs of severe distress, as are cyanosis of the feet, beak or facial skin (Figure 8.23). Handling in these situations may make the distress worse and have fatal results. Providing fresh air and seeking veterinary attention as soon as possible is the best plan of action. Obvious blockages of the nares or discharges in the mouth may be removable by gentle bathing with cotton buds.

- **Acute dyspnoea:** the veterinary surgeon must be contacted for advice because immediate air sac tube placement may be needed (see Chapter 17). Some clinical signs may be alleviated by providing a more humid environment, for example by taking the bird into a shower room or boiling a kettle in the room near the bird. Nebulizing the bird may also help if the equipment is available. The bird should be kept warm and in an area with subdued lighting. Cage perches should be lowered.
- **Tachypnoea:** this may be as life-threatening as dyspnoea (e.g. if due to inhalation of Teflon® fumes or if pneumonic). The bird should be provided with a good air supply, stress-free environment and warmth, and not handled unless absolutely necessary. Fans and hairdryers may help to provide a slightly improved air supply.

Treatment as outlined above may stabilize the patient so that it can be more safely transported to the clinic. One would normally expect to see some sort of improvement within 30–60 minutes. A definitive diagnosis needs to be quickly established so that appropriate therapy may be initiated (see also Chapters 20 and 22).

Vomiting

First aid for birds that are vomiting frequently, apart from the general nursing advice of warmth and quietness, can be difficult because the patient is unable to retain any oral fluids. Administering electrolyte replacers in small volumes is worth trying, but most birds need to be admitted for a proper diagnosis to be made (see Chapter 27).

Wing tip oedema

This condition in raptors definitely requires urgent first aid if the distal parts of the wing are to be saved from avascular necrosis. It is most often seen in cold weather. First aid consists of removing the bird from an outside environment and trying to re-establish the blood supply to the extremities with a combination of vigorous massage of the affected areas with or without the use of Preparation H® (haemorrhoid cream), use of a hairdryer on a warm setting to heat up the carpal area, and encouraging the bird to flap its wings on the fist. All cases are serious until they improve and thus veterinary attention is imperative.

Handling and transporting birds

Kevin Eatwell

Parrots, raptors and passerines have different anatomical conformations and therefore present different challenges when it comes to handling and transport. Therefore, this chapter will consider each group of birds separately. There is a small risk of mortality with handling, particularly of small or diseased birds, or if handling is prolonged. This can be due to the restriction of breathing or to the bird overheating. Thus, preparation is vital; getting all materials ready and close to hand before capturing the bird is important.

It is worth warning the owner about the risks prior to restraint and having a brief visual inspection of the bird's condition prior to handling. Even if a bird appears amenable to handling, caution is still required, as a bird with apparently mild clinical signs could be harbouring severe systemic disease. If an owner refuses to allow handling of the bird they should be advised that this impairs the clinician's ability to effectively diagnose and treat the bird.

Basic equipment

Birds are generally restrained using freshly laundered towels of an appropriate size and the clinic will require a large number of these. For small birds, paper towels can be used as an alternative. Recommended sizes for parrots include:

- Budgerigar – flannel
- Parakeet – tea towel
- Parrot – hand towel
- Macaw – small bath towel.

Thin examination gloves should be worn to reduce the risk of transmission of disease between avian patients; larger gauntlets or gloves should not be used as they reduce the dexterity of the clinician. A gauntlet will be required for handling birds of prey that are on the glove prior to restraint. Hoods (Figure 9.1) and restraint jackets can be used for birds of prey but, ideally, owners should be encouraged to bring their own falconry equipment as it is difficult to sterilize practice equipment between cases. Padded nets are essential for controlling escaped birds in the clinic (Figure 9.2). These must be easy to clean and sterilize between patients.

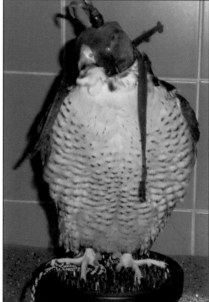

9.1 This Peregrine Falcon has been hooded and the bird is much calmer as a result.

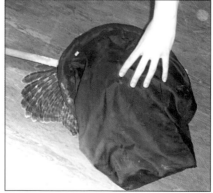

9.2 A padded net is invaluable for capturing escaped birds. However, caution should be exercised as there is a risk of injury to the bird.

Parrots and parakeets

These range from small Budgerigars to larger parrots such as the African Grey. Some owners can find catching their bird at home difficult. Many owners require advice on how to catch, handle and transport their bird safely to the clinic. This is generally not a problem for the small parrots as they can be brought into the clinic in their cages, but larger parrots should be transferred to a suitable carrier; if this is not possible, a home visit may be required. These owners are also bonded to their pets and will want to minimize the distress to their birds; certain methods such as using heavyweight gloves and just grabbing the bird may adversely affect the pet–owner bond. In addition, gloves reduce the dexterity of the handler and it is very difficult to gauge the amount of pressure being applied to the bird.

The author recommends that the owner change their clothing to a brightly coloured jumper or wear a hat so the birds is able to distinguish between an owner about to pet the bird *versus* an owner about to catch the bird and maybe do something unpleasant. Parrots living as aviary birds are usually captured using a net by their owner and veterinary advice is generally not required for the capture process.

Handling of small parakeets in the home environment

Catching a parakeet can be performed single-handedly. The bird should ideally be contained in their cage at home; these cages are usually small with small entrance doors. If multiple birds are contained in one cage it is often best to use the smallest entrance to minimize the risk of other birds escaping. Doors and windows should be closed and curtains/blinds drawn (to produce a visual barrier over the glass) and any fans or ventilation turned off. Cages are often overfilled with perches, toys and food items, all of which can complicate the capture process. These should be removed as much as possible, particularly if the person catching the bird is inexperienced. In addition, the light can be turned off or reduced, which may calm the bird. In some cases the bird can be identified on its perch, the light turned off completely, and the bird simply picked off the perch. A torch can be used to pinpoint the exact location of the bird if the room is totally dark.

If the bird is going to be transferred into a transport box or smaller cage then this should be ready and close by, to facilitate a speedy transfer. For parakeets, a cardboard carrier or wooden carry box with ventilation holes is suitable. The entrance hole to the box should be of just sufficient size to fit in a hand to grasp the bird. Breeders may have a carry cage or a show cage.

A bird presented in a box or travelling cage does provide limited immediate husbandry information; the clinician will need to ask supplementary questions about the bird's home environment. Videos or images of the home set-up are particularly useful in this situation, and in many cases are often volunteered by the owner. If possible, it would be preferable to transport the bird in its usual cage.

Once everything is ready then the bird can be caught. Small paper towels, flannels or tea towels (washed prior to use) can be used to aid in the capture of parakeets. Using a towel also reduces the risk of direct contamination of the bird's feathers with oils from human skin, and reduces the risk of making the bird hand shy. A bird-catching net can be useful, but most owners are unlikely to possess one. Assessing the bird prior to capture is important, as severely weakened or dyspnoeic birds are at a greater risk from handling, particularly if small (see also Chapter 11). All avian species can overheat quickly during handling, so

performing the task quickly, but competently, is important. Rough handling can lead to damaged wings, legs or toes if the bird panics, as limbs can easily become trapped in cage bars. Beak damage is possible if the bird is forcibly pulled off the cage bars.

Parakeets will bite if given the chance. All species are capable of drawing blood (although a Budgerigar has to be quite determined) and can cause bruising at the site of the bite. The feet can also have sharp nails but rarely do any significant damage. As a result, control of the head and beak is the main priority to avoid injury to the handler.

The towel used is draped over the hand. Ideally, the bird should be allowed to grasp on to the side of the cage and then the forefinger and thumb are used to restrain the head with the rest of the hand supporting the bodyweight and restraining the wings gently around the bird (Figure 9.3). An alternative to this is to place the head between the first and second finger with the palm of the hand being used to restrain the wings and body.

When ready to release the bird, it should be gently lowered into the carry box or fed through the door and, if possible, allowed to grip on the floor or side bars of the carrier prior to release. The hand and towel are then promptly removed and the door closed, being careful to ensure no feathers or parts of the bird are going to become trapped. Birds with long claws can get tangled in the towel and feet may have to be gently removed from the towel prior to releasing the bird. A bird trapped by its nails can be easily injured as it tries to escape.

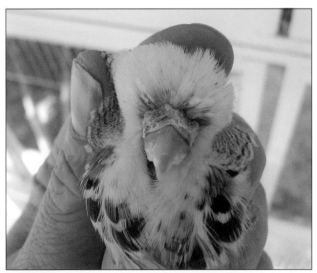

9.3 The head of this Budgerigar is being restrained between the thumb and first finger.

Handling of parrots in the home environment

Catching parrots requires two hands and an assistant who can help stabilize the cage and remove the bird. Birds should ideally be caught from a confined space, such as their usual cage, but, depending on the cage size (which may be too large to reach all the corners at full arm length), capture from within a room of the house may be more practical. The general approach is identical to that outlined for parakeets.

If the bird is going to be transferred into a carry box (Figure 9.4), it is important to get that ready and close by. Cardboard boxes are not suitable for any

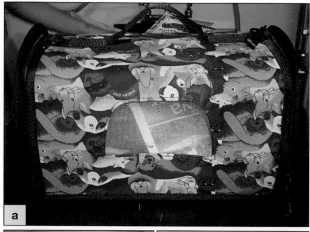

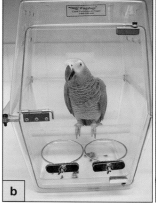
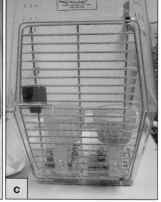

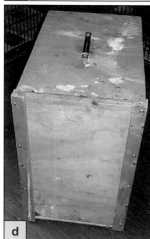

9.4 (a) A commercially available pet carrier, suitable for birds. (b) Commercially available carrier for birds. There is no newspaper in this carrier, which allows for collection of urine if needed, but increases the risk of soiling. (c) Commercially available carrier for birds. There is newspaper on the floor, but the addition of food and water containers is likely to cause mess during transit. (d) Homemade box carrier with poor hygiene and no ventilation.

A suitably sized towel should be selected; a large parrot will need something more like a bath towel. It is advisable to put a fold along the top of the towel and have this thicker area in hand, to give greater protection to the hand and offer good support to the bird's head. The aim here is to restrain the bird without getting bitten, and avoid causing trauma to the bird (Figure 9.5).

If the bird is being caught from a cage then all the cage clutter should be removed. There is usually at least one larger cage opening to allow entry of both hands and a towel. If this is not the case (usually with a smaller, less expensive cage), the top can be lifted off the base and then access gained via the bottom to catch the bird. This should be performed by an assistant. The towel-covered hand should be placed inside the carrier or cage and the bird's response observed. It is common for them to flap about initially, and it is worth waiting for a short time to see if they settle. Many birds will respond positively if spoken to soothingly; harsh shouting should be avoided. The bird should then be grasped quickly, but gently, from behind with the thumb and fingers supporting the neck or lower beak and the towel engulfing the wings and body (Figure 9.6). The bird needs to be fully immobilized before removing it from the cage or carrier, as thrashing wings and legs could easily be caught and damaged in the cage bars. For larger birds, a second hand may be required to restrain the bird's wings and legs within the towel. The claws and beak may also be hanging on to the side of the cage and require an assistant to remove them. The bird's legs are then wrapped inside the towel and the bird lifted out of the cage. If the bird is fractious, the room can be darkened to facilitate capture.

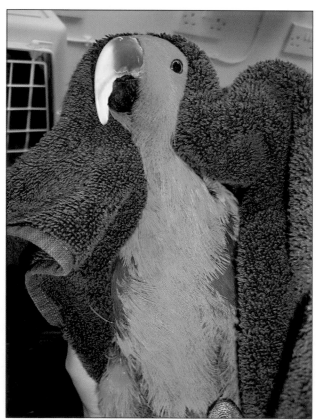

9.5 This male Eclectus Parrot has his wings restrained by the towel and his head is controlled by the thumb and first finger.

bird bigger than a Cockatiel as they can easily destroy them and escape. Wooden boxes (with suitable ventilation holes and a larger entrance hole) can be used, and a modified cat carrier is a good alternative. Cat carriers can vary in size, and a suitably sized container should be chosen. A perch can be fixed in the cage if the owner wishes; dowelling is usually sufficient. Other owners use a low-level perch to give the bird some grip, which can be screwed through the plastic at either end. Some owners like to cable tie or wire a two-hook feeder to the front of the carrier (for food or water), but this is not required for a short journey and just creates mess. Cat carriers will ultimately require replacing due to the destructive nature of parrots. Dedicated parrot carriers are also commercially available and can include holders for food and water and perching. Whilst these appeal to many owners, they are probably not required.

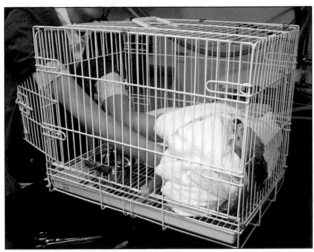

9.6   A towel-covered hand is used to restrain this parrot.

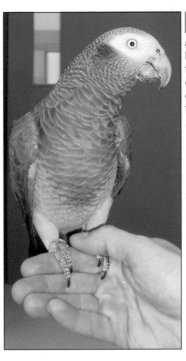

9.7   This parrot has been allowed to perch on the hand but the handler's thumb is being used to control the digits to discourage the bird from flying off.

If the bird is to be caught from the room, extra care has to be taken. All the doors and windows must be shut and curtains and blinds drawn. Where possible the room should be small with minimal furniture. Ornaments and pictures are additional hazards that can be damaged in the process or lead to injury of the bird, as the bird can fly away easily, leading to a fraught chase around the room, risking injuries such as broken feathers, fractures, keel wounds and beak tip damage. The risk of injury is increased with wing-clipped birds, as they often climb to escape and may fall.

If the bird is tame, then it may be possible to capture whilst it is gently held by another person; however, there is a risk that the 'cuddle' may expose the person to being bitten, depending on the nature of the bird.

If the bird is on a play perch or on top of the cage, then the room could be darkened, allowing the bird to be gently wrapped in the towel as before.

If the bird does fly, the priority is to get it to settle quickly on to a secure surface, preferably the floor of the room. Once it settles, the room can be darkened and the towel wrapped around the bird. If the bird is on the floor, the approach is from above with the towel dropped over the bird. Having done this, the bird is gently pushed down until the head is secured and the feet can be wrapped into the towel and the bird lifted. Recapture in essence is the same as before but the bird may be a little wiser to the process and a little more problematic to capture. Parrots can do significant damage with their beak. Many will hopefully release their grip quickly. If they do not, securing the room and releasing the bird over a surface will generally result in the bird releasing the handler.

It is possible to train parrots to accept restraint in a towel as part of their routine daily activities (see Chapter 5). This should be encouraged as rough handling can lead to phobic behaviours. It is not uncommon for an owner to report marked behavioural changes as a result of handling their pet parrot if it has had an intensive period of treatment at the clinic. In this case, a tame bird is encouraged to engage with the handler by stepping on to their hand. The handler then talks to the bird to settle it down. At this point the handler firmly but gently pins the bird's feet with the thumb (Figure 9.7). A corner of the towel is held between two fingers on the same hand and introduced calmly to the bird. The other hand is then used to slowly and calmly bring the rest of the towel around the back of the bird. Should the bird flip backwards, the towel can simply be wrapped around the bird in that position.

When the bird is ready to be released it is important for it not to be dropped, but lowered gently back into its carrier or cage. The bird should be allowed to get a foothold and, even better, a beak hold on the bars or perch, before the towel is removed gently again to avoid flapping.

Transporting parrots and small parakeets to the clinic

It is important to remove any water sources during transport as these can easily leak over the cage base and in some cases get the bird wet (and consequently cold). Owners should make sure that any clips or flaps over the holes for the feeders are secured to prevent escape in transit. Parrots can be transported in their cage if it is small enough to be placed in a vehicle. Most parakeets are transported in their usual cage.

It is preferable to bring them in a front- or top-opening cat carrier, into which a perch can be placed. If their normal cage is being used, advise the clients to remove all toys and have only one perch in. This will facilitate capture and reduce the chance of injury on the journey. Owners must not transport their parrots on their shoulder or hand, even if the bird is well trained or has clipped wings. Owners should also be discouraged from removing the bird from its cage until instructed to do so. If a bird is identified as being distressed in the waiting area, it may be best to take it to a quieter area of the practice in its carrier and darken the lighting, provided suitable hygiene control measures are in place. In emergency cases (such as severe collapse), a quick visual subjective assessment of the bird upon arrival will suffice to determine that the bird should be taken straight through to the clinical areas for emergency treatment (see Chapter 11). Care must be taken in such cases; handling should be brief enough to only obtain salient information that will affect the clinical management of the case (e.g. it is important to identify if dyspnoea is caused by coelomic fluid or a mass as this alters the differential diagnosis list and prognosis).

Taking a full clinical history prior to handling is important in every case and may yield useful information about the health status of the bird as well as the clinical problem being presented to the clinician. It makes logical sense for the bird to be restrianed for a brief period and there are a number of simple clinical techniques that can be performed whilst the bird is restrained. These include weighing the bird, providing oral or parenteral medications, and performing a crop wash or a nail trim. Getting all items required for these procedures and having them close to hand is important to reduce the restraint time. Birds can also be weighed in small plastic pet carriers or their carry boxes.

Handling of parrots in the clinic

The bird should be presented in a front-opening carrier. If not, and if the cage is full of clutter, it is advisable to remove as much as possible before attempting to handle the bird. Capture in the clinic is not that dissimilar to the methods used at home; it may be easiest for the owner to restrain the bird initially and pass it to the veterinary surgeon (veterinarian) for physical examination. The method for catching a parrot from a pet carrier is described in Figures 9.6 and 9.8.

Some owners may wish to handle their bird themselves, and this can be particularly helpful when a less experienced clinician is examining fractious aviary birds (for which the pet–owner bond is less important). Owners of companion birds may also wish to handle their bird, and some clinicians prefer this for keeping the bird calm. This works best for birds that are habituated to human contact, and there are a number of techniques described to facilitate examination whilst minimizing stress to the bird (Wilson, 2001; Doneley, 2011).

In cases where the veterinary surgeon must perform a physical examination, it should be considered whether the owner should remain in the room. Many owners are unlikely to have seen a bird physically examined before and many birds will object to a full clinical examination by being vocal. This can cause anxiety both for the bird and the owner. Anxious owners may try to intervene and be injured by their bird. Even if the owner is not involved in handling, the bird may associate the experience with the owner, which may upset the pet–owner bond. To avoid this, many practitioners either ask the client to leave the consulting room or take the bird into the preparation area for assessment. For veterinary surgeons who are less experienced at handling birds, it may be preferable to not have the owner watching; however, experienced handlers should take the opportunity to allow the owner to witness good avian handling techniques. The best set-up allows the owner to remotely observe the process with the parrot being unaware; for example, by having the client out of the room viewing through an observation window or recording the examination. This is quite a sensible option, particularly if anything unexpected occurs or the bird sustains any trauma.

If the bird has been presented loose on the owner's shoulder, then it is difficult for the owner to safely restrain it without the risk of the bird biting them either to aid its balance or to try to evade restraint. An alternative is for the veterinary surgeon or an assistant to take the bird on their hand instead. The bird may be a little more flighty in these cases and restraining a digit may be helpful by allowing the bird to rest on the index finger and using the thumb to gently keep a little pressure on the bird's toes; then, an assistant can restrain the bird. However, this technique is very quickly learned by the bird and will work on only one or two occasions.

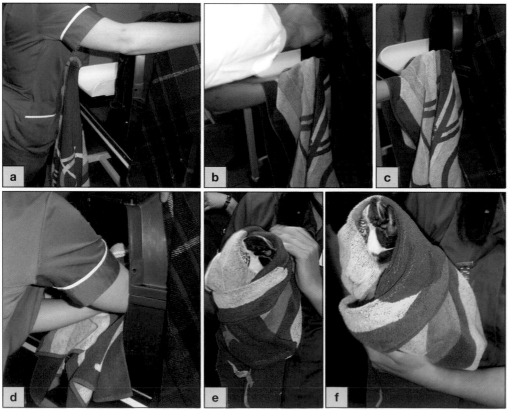

9.8 Catching a parrot from a pet carrier. **(a)** The carrier is placed on a suitable surface and the door is opened. **(b)** A second person will be required to stabilize the carrier. **(c)** A towel of a suitable size is used to fill the open space. **(d)** The parrot is driven to the back of the carrier and the towel used to engulf the bird, with the head being restrained first. The towel is then wrapped around the bird's wings. **(e)** The bird is then withdrawn from the carrier. **(f)** The towel can then be adjusted to enable examination of the bird.

Passerine birds

These are usually presented as aviary birds or caged birds kept in small groups or pairs. As a result they may be tame, but are usually not used to being handled. There is minimal risk of damage to the handler and the only real defence a passerine has is to peck the handler, although some of the larger species (e.g. barbets) do have a significant bite. Restraint and capture is often stressful for these birds; there is an adrenergic response that can lead to the shedding of a large number of both primary and contour feathers, an escape mechanism that is used to evade capture by predators in the wild. This, although cosmetic and harmless, can render a bird temporarily flightless until there is new feather growth. In some species the loss of feathers can be quite marked.

Handling of passerine birds in the home environment

Passerines kept in an aviary are often captured using a padded bird net. The bird can be restrained in the net and transferred to a transport box, or a flannel or paper towel can be used to handle it. Caged birds are often captured by hand. It is important to remove all clutter from the cage prior to capture, as passerines are quick and able to evade capture much more easily than a parrot. Prolonged pursuit increases the risk of injury further and hyperthermia is a risk. There is a risk of death when handling critically sick passerines, and in these cases clinical examination should be brief after a period of visual assessment from a distance. The wings require restraint in the same way as for parrots, but there is no requirement to hold the head, unless they are a large species where the beak is a significant size. Generally a single-handed hold is required. The fingers and thumb are used to control the wings.

Transporting passerines to the clinic

Passerines are typically transported in their own cage or in a small carry box. This may be custom made or a cardboard box.

Handling of passerines in the clinic

Capture must be prompt and handling minimized. Given their size it is very easy for an escaped passerine to find any small space in the consulting room and evade capture. There is a greater risk of trauma to passerines as even the smallest of items can cause injury. Clearing the surfaces and putting items away into cupboards is wise.

Raptors

Birds of prey can be seen as wildlife casualties, zoological specimens or birds owned by private falconers. These may be used for breeding, display or hunting. Falconers are generally well used to handling their birds, including physical restraint for examination or treatments (known as casting the bird).

Handling of raptors in the home environment

Raptors are typically restrained on a gauntlet on the left hand of the falconer. They are tethered to this via anklets, which join on to jesses (thin leather straps) and link into a swivel through which a leash is threaded. This leash is typically held between the third and fourth digits, preventing the bird from walking up the falconer's arm and off the glove or flying off (bating) the glove. Some birds may be hooded whilst on the glove, typically falcons. Hawks may not be used to wearing a hood. Birds being free lofted will usually come to a gloved hand but may lack anklets and jesses and may simply be placed into a travel box. Birds from zoological collections may require netting and restraining through the net with a towel. Wildlife casualties are best restrained with a towel from above to prevent injury to the handler (see the *BSAVA Manual of Wildlife Casualties*). The method for getting a raptor on to the glove is described in Figure 9.9.

Transporting raptors to the clinic

Captive raptors will probably be used to travelling, and therefore the falconer should have an appropriate set-up for this, usually a travel box or cadge (an open box with a perch used for transport) in the car. Sometimes the bird may be kept on the glove of a passenger throughout the journey. It is good practice to ask falconers who do not have a box to keep their birds in their vehicle until they are to be seen, for their own and the bird's safety. Transport boxes are often homemade but are also available commercially. It is important to consider design carefully, as these birds can spend a considerable amount of time in their travel boxes.

There are a number of points to consider when selecting a travel box for a raptor. Firstly, the risk of trauma has to be considered. Generally the bird's owners are aware of this and boxes should be large enough to allow the bird to perch, without the risk of any feather damage, but not oversized to allow excessive movement. Boxes are often of a solid construction and keep the bird in a dark environment. Ventilation holes are required and should be placed at a low level. This allows air flow but reduces the risk of the bird being able to see out easily or having flashing lights startling it. Birds may be hooded in transport, which will further calm them. In addition, many birds are transported with a tail guard in place to reduce the risk of damage to tail feathers in transport (Figure 9.10). Tail guards are commercially available but can also be made easily. Typically, radiographic film, sheet plastic or stiff cardboard is used. This is gently folded around the tail feathers and taped in place using surgical tape adhered to the contour feathers distal to the vent. Many of the commercial designs are intended to fit around the bell or radiotransmitter aerial on the bird's tail.

Handling of raptors in the clinic

All raptors have the potential to bite, but the main danger to a handler from a bird of prey is from its talons. The feet and talons are designed to lock on to prey and could cause a very nasty injury if handled incorrectly (Figure 9.11). Feet should be controlled throughout any handling procedure. All species will bite, particularly owls, eagles and vultures, but usually this is annoying more than harmful. However, for larger species caution is advised, and some clinicians prefer to wear gauntlets with larger species.

Prior to handling, observing the bird as it stands is useful to determine its demeanour and likely response to casting. Casting involves wrapping the bird in a towel of a suitable size and securing the feet and talons. If a bird of prey is presented in a travel box and it is not wearing

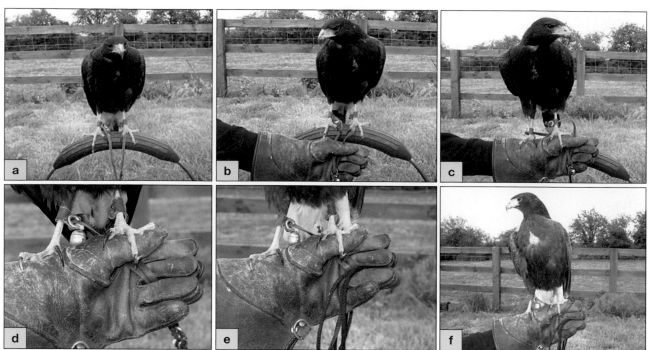

9.9 Getting a raptor on to the glove. **(a)** The handler needs to approach the bird calmly, presenting the gloved hand. **(b)** The jesses are grasped between the thumb and the fingers. **(c)** The bird is gently approached with the gloved hand placed under the bird's chest. The bird should instinctively step on to the glove. **(d)** The leash is then passed through the fingers and tightened to prevent the bird moving up the arm of the handler. **(e)** The leash is then looped around the fingers. **(f)** The bird is then securely held on the glove.

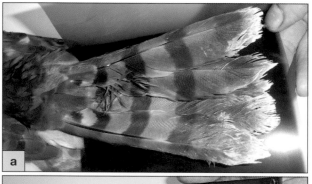

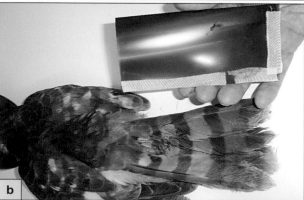

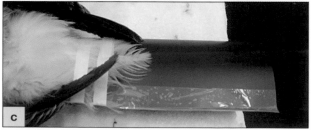

9.10 **(a)** Tail feathers can be damaged without proper protection. **(b)** A tail guard, prior to attachment. **(c)** A tail guard appropriately attached.

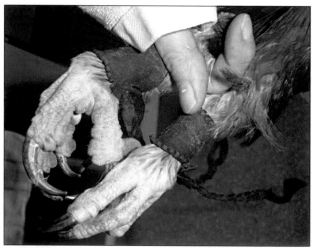

9.11 This Martial Eagle could still inflict damage with its talons and these are being appropriately restrained.

jesses, it will need to be cast from the box. This might be the case if it is a wildlife casualty or if it has been taken straight from an aviary (typically out of the falconry season). If the bird is presented with anklets, jesses and a leash, it will be presented either already on the glove or will go on to a glove from its box. Many birds will come on to a gloved hand even if it is not the owner's. Most falconers are competent at handling their own birds and will be able to hood them more easily (birds are usually less suspicious of a familiar individual; Figure 9.12). However, sending the owner out of the room and getting an assistant to get the bird out of the box will help to prevent a loss of trust between the bird and falconer, especially if it is a young bird new to training. To get a bird up on to the fist, the handler needs to grasp the jesses between the thumb and finger with a gloved hand, and then lift the hand up in front of the bird's legs.

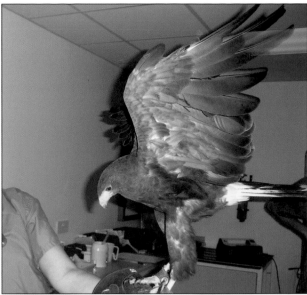

9.12 This Harris' Hawk is reluctant to settle on the glove of a stranger.

It should step forward willingly up on to the raised glove. The leash can then be secured by passing it between the third and fourth fingers and then wrapping it around the bottom two (see Figure 9.9). The bird can be hooded with its own hood at this point.

To cast the bird, allow it to settle and stand at ease with its wings resting against its body. This is relatively easy if the bird can be hooded, but a non-hooded bird may be suspicious and it may be difficult to get it to keep its wings down. The gloved hand should be slightly lowered to make casting the bird easier. The person casting the bird needs to approach it from behind, holding out a suitably sized towel in both hands with them held apart. This needs to be wrapped quickly but gently around the bird's shoulders, wings and body with the handler ending up with one of the bird's legs securely in each hand and the bird's back cradled into the handler's chest. The legs should be promptly secured one in each hand, with the tarso-metatarsus held between the third and fourth fingers. This can be through the towel or the hands can be slipped just around the edge of the towel so there is direct contact and control. It is possible to transfer both legs to one hand with a single digit positioned between the tarsometatarsi to reduce the risk of damage. If the bird is resistant to casting, the jesses can be held at a short distance and the handler can grasp the tarsometatarsi of the bird (one in each hand) whilst the bird is quickly wrapped in a towel by another assistant. The wings will require careful folding in to avoid feather damage. If the bird bates off the glove, then the handler can grasp the tarsometatarsi of the bird (one in each hand) with the bird suspended upside down. The wings are folded in and the bird wrapped in the towel as before prior to examination or manipulation (Figure 9.13). Dimming the lighting can help to steady a diurnal bird, but provides an advantage for nocturnal species. If the bird is presented in a box then a towel can be used to cover the top and lowered over the bird. It can then be gently pushed to the floor. The shoulders and wings are controlled and then the hands are slid laterally to control the limbs before the bird is lifted from the box. Some species will flip on to their backs and can be difficult to restrain. In

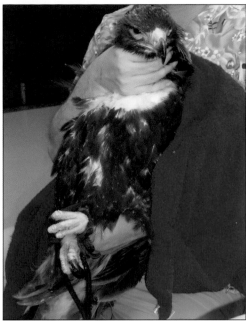

9.13 Appropriate restraint of a raptor. The feet are being restrained, the wings are protected in a blanket, and the head is being restrained.

these cases, allow the bird to bind with the towel, then it can be lifted out of the box (or the legs simply elevated) and then the tarsometatarsi can be restrained and the bird's wings gently folded into the towel.

Restraint jackets (Figure 9.14) can also be used for owned raptors and serve to immobilize the bird and restrain the wings and legs: in essence they consist of material with (usually hook and loop) fastening straps used to restrain the bird. They should only be used for a short time period to prevent overheating. Care is still needed as the bird may have sufficient limb function to cause injury to handlers. They are, however, very useful

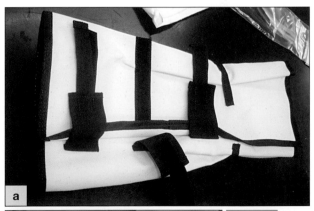

9.14

(a) A restraint jacket for raptors. (b) A Harris' Hawk in a raptor restraint jacket.

in emergency situations, for example, if a bird has sustained a fracture. Other simple restraint devices such as the sleeve of a shirt can be used.

With the bird's feet and wings restrained and contained, the bird can now be safely examined. When it is time to release the bird it should be held over the glove or perch and allowed to get a foothold before the towel is gently unwrapped. This will help to prevent unwanted flapping that could damage feathers.

References and further reading

Doneley B (2011) The physical examination. In: *Avian Medicine and Surgery in Practice*, ed. B Doneley, pp. 40–54. Manson Publishing, London

Mullineaux E and Keeble E (2016) *BSAVA Manual of Wildlife Casualties, 2nd edn*. BSAVA Publications, Gloucester

Raftery A (2008) Handling and transport. In: *BSAVA Manual of Raptors, Pigeons and Passerine Birds*, ed. J Chitty and M Lierz, pp. 42–47. BSAVA Publications, Gloucester

Wilson L (2001) Psittacine restraint in the examination room. In: *Veterinary Clinics of North America: Exotic Animal Practice*, ed. TL Lightfoot, pp. 633–639. Saunders, Philadelphia

History taking and examination

Craig Hunt

Birds have a tendency to hide signs of illness until disease is well advanced. As a result, many birds are presented to the veterinary clinic in an advanced stage of ill health, and may present with one or more life-threatening conditions. Similarly, birds presented in the early stages of illness may often appear normal to the inexperienced owner or veterinary surgeon (veterinarian). In both scenarios, a thorough history is essential to aid the veterinary surgeon in formulating a differential diagnosis list, investigation and treatment plan. A good history, it may be argued, is at least as informative as the clinical examination itself. If an owner believes the bird to be ill or behaving abnormally, then it is wise to believe them, even if the patient appears to be healthy and normal during the consultation. Many patients will outwardly improve upon arrival at the veterinary clinic and owners may apologize for apparently wasting the veterinary surgeon's time. It is prudent to emphasize to the client that this is a normal and common response to the stress of travel and a strange environment, and that they should never feel their concerns are a waste of time. Indeed, waiting until the avian patient is clearly ill and in need of medical intervention may be leaving it too late and significantly increase the risk of patient death.

Whether the patient is severely ill or being presented for a 'well bird' consultation, a thorough history can be very informative; many birds, especially parrots, are provided with an inadequate diet, housing and/or environment. A good history will enable the veterinary surgeon to identify deficiencies and advise the owner on improvements and prevention accordingly.

The avian consultation is often significantly longer compared with the average dog or cat consultation, and appropriate time should be allocated. Trying to accomplish a thorough history, clinical examination and give appropriate advice in a 5–10 minute consultation is impossible. In non-urgent cases, history forms may be filled out by the owner prior to the consultation, which can help to save time and allow the veterinary surgeon to focus on the pertinent points during the consultation.

Examples of history forms are shown in Figures 10.1–10.3. Figure 10.4 provides an overview of clinical examination.

History

In most cases a clinical history is gathered prior to physical examination. This gives the clinician time to evaluate the patient from a distance and to ascertain whether the bird is able to cope with restraint and physical examination or whether it should be first stabilized in a heated oxygen cage. During history taking, the owner and veterinary surgeon should refrain from interacting with the bird to allow time for it to settle and be more likely to display normal behaviours and any abnormal clinical signs.

The current complaint should be ascertained early on in the consultation to allow questioning to be targeted and detailed, but care should be taken not to narrow the focus too much as this risks missing vital clues.

The length of time the bird has been in the current owner's possession and its contact (current and historical) with other birds may help narrow the list of differentials; a singly housed bird that has been in the owner's possession for several years is less likely to be suffering from an infectious disease and more likely to be suffering from nutritional disease and/or organ dysfunction. If the bird has been recently acquired and/or is one of a group of individuals with similar signs then infectious disease is more likely.

Following history taking, any items brought along by the owner may be examined. Items that are most useful include a sample of fresh droppings, castings (raptors), moulted feathers, seed/pelleted foods offered, any recent medications and any toys with which the bird plays; small cage birds are ideally brought with their cage, where practical. Digital photographs of the patient's housing arrangements are very useful when it is impractical to transport an enclosure; similarly, digital recordings (including sound) of a patient's behaviour at home can prove invaluable since patients commonly do not display described behaviours in the consulting room.

Dietary causes of disease, particularly in parrots, are considered a major factor, if not the major underlying factor, in many ill birds brought to veterinary practice. Time should be spent ascertaining what the bird is offered to eat and, more importantly, what it actually eats; many parrots will selectively feed when offered

Raptor history form

Date:...   Patient ID:...

Species:...   Age:...

Sex:...   Visual/DNA/surgical/laid an egg:...

Captive-bred/wild-caught:...   Hand-reared/crèche-reared/parent-reared:...

Length of time owned:...

Current activity (e.g. display/hunting/breeding):...

Flying weight:.....................   Moulting weight:.....................   Current weight:.....................

Aviary type and approximate size:...

Perching (e.g. block/bow/indoors/free flight):...

Perch surface material:...

Flooring material:...

Heating supplied:...

Cleaning and disinfection frequency and agent(s):...

Other birds kept (same enclosure/adjacent enclosures):...

Appearance of mutes:...

When were mutes last passed?...

Appearance of casts:...

When did the bird last cast?...

How often is the bird flown?.....................   When did the bird last fly?.....................

What quarry is the bird flown at?.....................   Is quarry eaten?.....................

Flight performance:...

Diet (type/quantity/frequency):...

Diet storage:.....................   Diet supplier:.....................

How is frozen food thawed?...

Is whole prey offered?.....................   Is all food offered eaten?.....................

Supplements:.....................   Frequency:.....................

Describe the current problem:...

....

....

When were signs first noted?...

Have any treatments been administered?...

Any previous illnesses in this bird?...

Are any other birds affected?...

Any unexplained deaths?...

Any previous tests (e.g. mutes/blood/post-mortem)?...

Additional comments:...

....

....

....

10.1   Example of a history form for raptors.

Psittacine history form

Date:...   Patient ID:...

Species:...   Age:..

Sex:...   Visual/DNA/surgical/laid an egg:..................................

Captive-bred/wild-caught:..   Hand-reared/parent-reared:...

Length of time owned:...   Source: breeder/show/pet shop/home-bred:...............

Current activity (e.g. companion/breeding/display):...

Normal weight:...   Current weight:..

Leg ring/microchip number:..

Enclosure type and approximate size:...

Where is enclosure located:...

Indoor/outdoor: ....   Heating supplied?...

Perch type:..

Flooring material:...

Cleaning and disinfection frequency and agent(s):...

Air filtration:...

Companions:...

Other species of birds kept:..

How long does the bird spend in a cage/out of a cage?..

How long is the bird allowed to sleep?...

Hours exposed to natural sunlight:...

Hours exposed to ultraviolet lamp:.........................   Make of lamp:..

Distance of lamp from the bird:................................   When was the lamp last changed?................................

Diet (list items eaten and their relative proportions in a typical week):...

....

Items offered but refused:...

Treats:...

Supplements:...   Frequency:...

How is drinking water offered?...

Are any supplements added to the water?..

How often does the bird bath or shower?..

Is the bird's wing clipped?...

How and at what age?...

Is the bird exposed to cigarette smoke, candles, cooking fumes, Teflon™? Please specify:................................

....

Describe the current problem:...

....

When were signs first noted?...

Have any treatments been administered?..

Any previous illnesses in this bird?...

Are any other birds affected?...

Any unexplained deaths?..

Any previous tests (e.g. faecal/blood/post-mortem)?..

Additional comments:...

....

10.2   Example of a history form for psittacine birds.

Passerine history form

Date:... Patient ID:...

Species/breed:.................................. Age:..

Sex:.. Visual/DNA/surgical/laid an egg:.......................

Captive-bred/wild-caught:............... Hand-reared/fostered/parent-reared:..............

Purpose of stock (e.g. display/breeding/showing):...

Length of time owned:..

Source: Breeder/show/pet shop/home-bred:..

Enclosure type and approximate size:..

Indoor/outdoor..

Heating supplied:...

Perch type:..

Perch surface material:...

Flooring material:..

Cleaning and disinfection frequency and agent(s):...

Companions?..

Other species of birds kept:..

Diet:...

Supplements:...

Frequency:..

Describe the current problem:...

....

....

....

....

When were signs first noted?..

Have any treatments been administered?..

Any previous illnesses in this bird?...

Are any other birds affected?..

Any unexplained deaths?...

Any previous tests (e.g. faecal/blood/post-mortem)?..

Additional comments:..

....

....

....

....

10.3 Example of a history form for passerine birds.

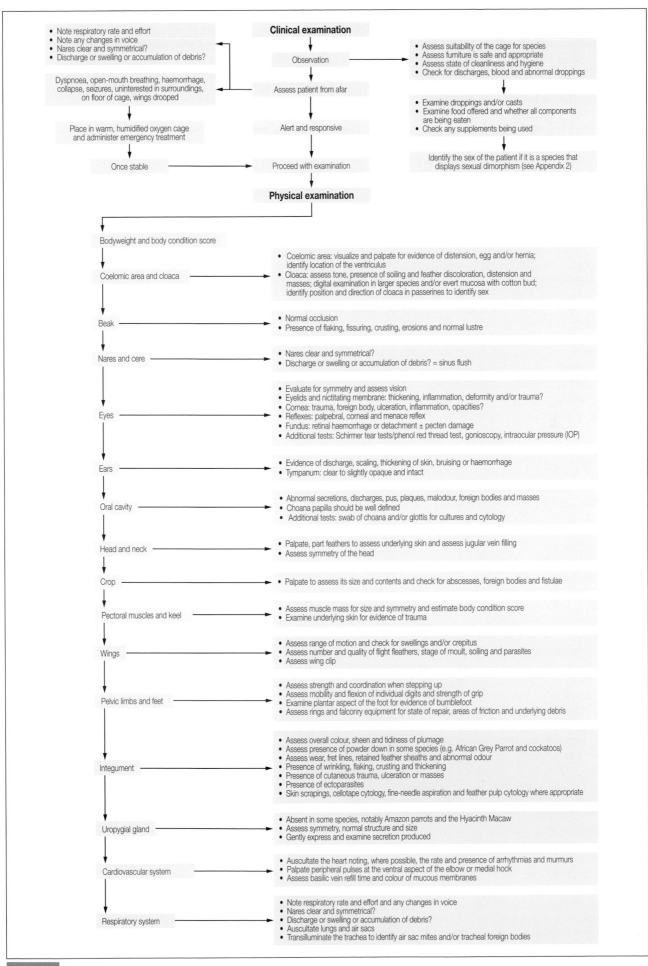

- Note respiratory rate and effort
- Note any changes in voice
- Nares clear and symmetrical?
- Discharge or swelling or accumulation of debris?

Clinical examination

Observation

- Assess suitability of the cage for species
- Assess furniture is safe and appropriate
- Assess state of cleanliness and hygiene
- Check for discharges, blood and abnormal droppings

Dyspnoea, open-mouth breathing, haemorrhage, collapse, seizures, uninterested in surroundings, on floor of cage, wings drooped

Assess patient from afar

- Examine droppings and/or casts
- Examine food offered and whether all components are being eaten
- Check any supplements being used

Place in warm, humidified oxygen cage and administer emergency treatment

Alert and responsive

Identify the sex of the patient if it is a species that displays sexual dimorphism (see Appendix 2)

Once stable

Proceed with examination

Physical examination

Bodyweight and body condition score

Coelomic area and cloaca
- Coelomic area: visualize and palpate for evidence of distension, egg and/or hernia; identify location of the ventriculus
- Cloaca: assess tone, presence of soiling and feather discoloration, distension and masses; digital examination in larger species and/or evert mucosa with cotton bud; identify position and direction of cloaca in passerines to identify sex

Beak
- Normal occlusion
- Presence of flaking, fissuring, crusting, erosions and normal lustre

Nares and cere
- Nares clear and symmetrical?
- Discharge or swelling or accumulation of debris? = sinus flush

Eyes
- Evaluate for symmetry and assess vision
- Eyelids and nictitating membrane: thickening, inflammation, deformity and/or trauma?
- Cornea: trauma, foreign body, ulceration, inflammation, opacities?
- Reflexes: palpebral, corneal and menace reflex
- Fundus: retinal haemorrhage or detachment ± pecten damage
- Additional tests: Schirmer tear tests/phenol red thread test, gonioscopy, intraocular pressure (IOP)

Ears
- Evidence of discharge, scaling, thickening of skin, bruising or haemorrhage
- Tympanum: clear to slightly opaque and intact

Oral cavity
- Abnormal secretions, discharges, pus, plaques, malodour, foreign bodies and masses
- Choana papilla should be well defined
- Additional tests: swab of choana and/or glottis for cultures and cytology

Head and neck
- Palpate, part feathers to assess underlying skin and assess jugular vein filling
- Assess symmetry of the head

Crop
- Palpate to assess its size and contents and check for abscesses, foreign bodies and fistulae

Pectoral muscles and keel
- Assess muscle mass for size and symmetry and estimate body condition score
- Examine underlying skin for evidence of trauma

Wings
- Assess range of motion and check for swellings and/or crepitus
- Assess number and quality of flight fleathers, stage of moult, soiling and parasites
- Assess wing clip

Pelvic limbs and feet
- Assess strength and coordination when stepping up
- Assess mobility and flexion of individual digits and strength of grip
- Examine plantar aspect of the foot for evidence of bumblefoot
- Assess rings and falconry equipment for state of repair, areas of friction and underlying debris

Integument
- Assess overall colour, sheen and tidiness of plumage
- Assess presence of powder down in some species (e.g. African Grey Parrot and cockatoos)
- Assess wear, fret lines, retained feather sheaths and abnormal odour
- Presence of wrinkling, flaking, crusting and thickening
- Presence of cutaneous trauma, ulceration or masses
- Presence of ectoparasites
- Skin scrapings, cellotape cytology, fine-needle aspiration and feather pulp cytology where appropriate

Uropygial gland
- Absent in some species, notably Amazon parrots and the Hyacinth Macaw
- Assess symmetry, normal structure and size
- Gently express and examine secretion produced

Cardiovascular system
- Auscultate the heart noting, where possible, the rate and presence of arrhythmias and murmurs
- Palpate peripheral pulses at the ventral aspect of the elbow or medial hock
- Assess basilic vein refill time and colour of mucous membranes

Respiratory system
- Note respiratory rate and effort and any changes in voice
- Nares clear and symmetrical?
- Discharge or swelling or accumulation of debris?
- Auscultate lungs and air sacs
- Transilluminate the trachea to identify air sac mites and/or tracheal foreign bodies

10.4 Clinical examination flowchart.

mixed seed and will commonly cherry pick the sun-flower seeds and/or peanuts. Owners may say they give vegetables and fruit to their birds but, upon more detailed questioning, many will admit that these are not offered very often and, when they are, they may be ignored by the parrot.

With raptors, it is important to ascertain that they are offered and eat whole prey items rather than just lean meat, as the latter will lead to calcium deficiency and metabolic bone disease. Lead toxicity is always a possibility when raptors are fed wild prey (particularly pheasant, rabbit and pigeon) which may have been previously shot, even if the owner is adamant the items were examined and found to be shot-free. Several infectious diseases, including trichomonosis, salmonellosis, falcon and owl herpesviruses, are commonly carried by wild pigeons and may be transmitted to the raptor to which they are fed. Poultry adenovirus has been implicated in several disease outbreaks in raptors, particularly Peregrine Falcons fed quail or day-old chicks. Asking the owner to describe their method of storage and defrosting of frozen foods may be helpful.

The manufacturer, quantity, frequency and method of administration of any vitamin and mineral supplements should be determined and, ideally, the container examined during the consultation. How much access to ultraviolet radiation (UVA and UVB light) in the form of natural sunshine and/or avian lamps should be ascertained, and whether it is unfiltered (i.e. it does not pass through glass or plastic before reaching the bird, since most plastics and glass filter out much of the useful UVB radiation). If a lamp is used, the age of the bulb should be determined; bulbs that have been used for 6 months or more may not be providing adequate UVB light.

The frequency with which the bird is offered the opportunity to bathe or have a shower, and how often it actually participates in these activities, is important. How the bird reacts to the activity is of particular interest in behavioural cases – it is quite common that owners will force pet parrots to have a shower or bath rather than train them to enjoy the activity; the stress caused by forced bathing may be a significant factor in feather picking, aggressive and phobic behaviours.

The owner should be asked to describe their cleaning routine for the enclosure and food/water bowls, including the frequency and detergents/disinfectants used. If the cage is presented, examining it may give additional clues.

It is routine for trained (hunting and display) raptors to be weighed daily, and the author encourages owners of tame pet birds to also weigh their birds daily. Weight fluctuations, in particular sudden weight loss, can alert the owner to early signs of disease and help the veterinary surgeon identify a timeline for the disease process or deficiencies in management and put the current body condition score into context.

The likelihood of ingestion of, or exposure to, toxins should be ascertained; in birds displaying gastrointestinal signs or presented 'fluffed up', the owner should be asked if the bird may have had the opportunity to ingest toxins such as heavy metals (e.g. lead and zinc) or some house plants (e.g. many bulbs, peace lilies). In birds presented with respiratory signs, exposure to aerosols, such as cigarette smoke, cooking fumes, polytetrafluoroethylene (Teflon™) and scented candles, should be determined. Certain ingested toxins (e.g. avocado) may

also present with respiratory signs. Figure 10.5 is a useful resource for identifying common toxicities.

Additional important questions to ask about birds presented with apparent respiratory disease include whether there is a recent history of anaesthesia, which should alert the clinician to the possibility of a tracheal stricture (most common in macaws). A recent stressful event, such as a move or training, in some species of raptors (especially Goshawks and Golden Eagles) may suggest aspergillosis; if there is a change in voice or loss of voice it is likely that the syrinx is affected. Evidence of yawning, coughing, sneezing, head shaking or picking at the nares are all suggestive of respiratory disease.

The reproductive history and current status of the patient should be ascertained; egg binding, egg yolk coelomitis, hypocalcaemia and 'stroke' (caused by egg yolk emboli) often occur in patients with a recent history of egg laying, although the clinician should be aware that a lack of apparent reproductive activity does not rule out these conditions being present. Certain conditions such as aggression, regurgitation, feather destructive disorder and cloacal prolapse may be triggered by reproductive activity or they may have a non-sexual cause. Ascertaining the reproductive status (see Chapter 4) allows the clinician to advise the owner on appropriate treatment and (where necessary) behavioural training and environmental manipulation.

Birds with underlying disease such as hepatopathies, nephritis, atherosclerosis and air sacculitis often display signs of discomfort, and the clinician should enquire as to whether the bird is displaying any suspect behaviour such as pruritus, yawning, nose picking, picking at feathers and/or skin over specific areas, self-trauma and/or signs of non-specific irritation. The bird may pick or traumatize a specific area in cases of nephritis (synsacrum and/or flank) and musculoskeletal disease (over affected bones or joints), or signs of irritation may be more generalized, such as in the case of hepatitis and air sacculitis.

Behavioural problems

In addition to the history described above, birds presented with behavioural problems, such as feather picking, aggression and excessive screaming, require additional and more in-depth questioning of the owner and thus longer consulting times; follow-up consultations are to be recommended to assess response to, and to ensure client compliance with, any recommendations.

Provision of digital images of the layout of the house and the bird's cage position within the house can yield useful information. Through images and questioning, the following information should be ascertained:

- Proximity of the cage to the kitchen, windows, doors, lights, televisions and people traffic
- Photoperiod, type and intensity of light to which the bird is exposed and where the bird sleeps at night should be determined, since excessive day length and disturbed sleep (e.g. the bird sleeps in the living room with the television on) and lack of appropriate UV light can be significant causes of stress
- Day and night routine should be evaluated for potential stressors, such as the bird being left on its own and/or the presence of cats and dogs
- Time allowed out of the cage and time interacting with the owners and whether the bird reacts badly to any members of the family

Toxins	Source	Comments
Ingested		
Lead	Curtain weights, leaded windows, old paint (pre-1960s), lead shot, solder, electrical and plumbing clips	Weakness, anorexia, regurgitation, diarrhoea, polyuria, polydipsia, biliverdinuria, haemoglobinuria, seizures, neurological signs, death
Zinc	Galvanized materials (including cage), wire, nails, screws, washers, jewellery	Similar to lead
Alpha-chloralose	Pesticide used primarily against gulls, crows, pigeons and rodents	Raptors – eating contaminated prey; incoordination, hyperaesthesia, ptyalism
Coumarin	Rodenticides	Haemorrhage (internal and external)
Mycotoxins	Contaminated feed	Renal and hepatotoxicity, immunosuppression and neurological signs
Nicotine	Tobacco, cigarettes, cigars	Tachypnoea, emesis, neurological signs, excitation, collapse, coma and death
Persin	Avocado (*Persea* spp.)	Respiratory distress, death
Plants	Lily of the valley (*Convallaria majalis*), oleander (*Nerium oleander*), rhododendron and azalea (*Rhododendron* spp.), yew (*Taxus* spp.), foxglove (*Digitalis purpurea*), kalanchoe (*Kalanchoe* spp.)	Cardiotoxic
	Rhubarb (*Rheum* spp.)	Leaves only; renotoxicity
	Cycad, sago, zamia palms (*Cycad* spp.), mushrooms *Amanita* spp.)	Hepatotoxicity
	Autumn crocus (*Colchicum* spp.), castor bean (*Ricinus* spp.)	Multisystemic effects
	Peace lilies (*Spathiphyllum* spp.), calla lilies (*Zantedeschia aethiopica*), philodendrons (*Philodendron* sp.), dumb cane (*Dieffenbachia* sp.), mother-in-law's tongue (*Sansevieria trifasciata*), pothos (*Epipremnum* spp.)	Irritation of tongue and oral cavity, dysphagia, regurgitation, anorexia, oral pain; rarely life-threatening
Inhaled		
Aerosol sprays	Furniture polish, hairspray	Respiratory signs
Carbon monoxide	Faulty household heating, car exhaust	Dyspnoea, stupor, sudden death
Solvents	Glue fumes, paint fumes	Respiratory tract irritation, dyspnoea, death
Polytetrafluoroethylene (PTFE/Teflon™)	Overheated non-stick pans and cooking utensils, hair dryers, ironing boards, irons, heat lamps	Respiratory signs and death
Smoke	Tobacco, cooking, candles, incense sticks, open fires	Respiratory tract irritation, conjunctivitis, cough, sneeze, feather plucking/mutilation
Other		
Nicotine	Skin (especially hands) and clothing of smokers	Contact dermatitis, self-mutilation usually of the feet
Ivermectin	Injection and topical preparations	Blindness, seizures, death; propylene glycol carrier may be toxic especially in small birds
Metronidazole toxicity	Oral and injectable preparations	Tremor, seizures, death
Aminoglycosides, cephalosporins, tetracyclines, amphotericin-B	Toxic effects exacerbated in dehydrated patients and patients with renal dysfunction	Nephrotoxicity

10.5 Common toxins of avian species.

- Recent changes to the living quarters and surrounding environment or change in the owners' routine may all cause stress
- Whether the bird is wing clipped and by who and how it was performed should be ascertained; the author has seen a number of parrots develop severe fear responses and/or feather destructive disorders and self-mutilation immediately following wing clipping.

The same question may need to be asked several times in different ways, as some owners may be selective about the information they give and may not volunteer information freely. The owner should also be questioned as to how they react when the bird displays abnormal or unwanted behaviours; in many instances the owners are unknowingly reinforcing the bird's behaviour. Examples of reinforcement include owners laughing at a parrot's aggression towards another family member or reprimanding a bird for pulling its feathers.

Clinical examination: observation

Upon arrival, it is prudent to quickly observe and triage the patient for signs of obvious distress and/or conditions that may require immediate treatment including collapse, dyspnoea and haemorrhage (see Chapter 11). Such patients should be immediately placed into a hospital cage and humidified oxygen administered.

Analgesia, sedation and/or fluids should be administered as deemed appropriate.

Rushing in to catch and examine the patient may cause important information to be lost or at worst may lead the patient to decompensate. This should be carefully explained to the client; many owners are keen to have the bird physically examined immediately and do not appreciate the importance of the bird's history, and may even question the clinician's competence or confidence with birds.

Whilst observing from a distance, the clinician should pay attention to the bird's interest in its surroundings, its posture, respiratory effort, limb carriage, and the quality and position of the feathers. Tail bobbing, open-mouthed breathing and/or audible respiration indicate significant respiratory compromise and necessitate a period of stabilization prior to full examination. Many sick birds have problems maintaining body temperature and will fluff out their feathers in an attempt to conserve body heat – a generally abnormal sign in a strange, potentially stressful, environment.

If the cage has been brought in, it too should be examined. Clinicians should check the following:

- Suitability for purpose (size, design and materials)
- State of cleanliness in which the cage is presented (this may give insight into hygiene precautions taken by the owner)
- Cage furniture for potential toxic substances, for example, toxic woods and heavy metal components (such as lead in bells), and sharp edges and/or inappropriate perches, which could predispose to injury
- Relationship of perches to the food and water bowls, especially to ensure that droppings are not able to contaminate food/water bowls from perches placed above
- Contents of the food bowls and cage floor, to gauge the type and quantity of food provided (and eaten)
- Number and appearance of the droppings (may indicate recent anorexia, diarrhoea or polyuria); birds with reduced activity due to illness or injury may accumulate droppings under the perch. If the owner brings a sample of paper from the cage floor from the previous day(s), then this should also be examined (see Appendix 4)
- Evidence of vomiting or regurgitation, often indicated by hulled seeds stuck to the bars of the cage and/or furniture; regurgitation may be indicative of disease, but may also be a result of motion sickness (often in macaws) or courtship display, in which case it is often directed towards a reflective surface such as a mirror (most commonly seen in Budgerigars).

The recently regurgitated pellet (casting) of a raptor may also be examined, if available, and should be assessed for evidence of foreign material, parasites, blood and maldigestion (Figure 10.6).

Sexing

Identifying the sex of the bird may be requested by the owner and can be helpful in formulating a differential diagnosis list; for example, a female bird lying on the floor of an enclosure may be attempting to lay eggs. Many parrot owners have an opinion of the bird's

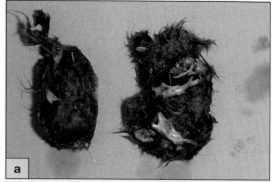
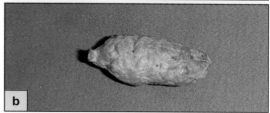
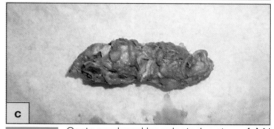

10.6 Casts produced by selected raptors. **(a)** Normal cast from a wild Tawny Owl, consisting of bone and fur (left) and broken open to demonstrate the presence of bone (right). The colour of the cast reflects the pelage of the prey item: a shrew, in this case. **(b)** Normal cast from a captive Harris' Hawk fed day-old chicks. Only the indigestible feather is present as non-owl raptors fully digest the bone. **(c)** Abnormal cast from a Harris' Hawk fed day-old chicks. In this case, the presence of flesh and bone in the cast suggests maldigestion, which might occur with gastroenteritis, endoparasitism and heavy metal toxicosis. Occasionally, such a pellet may be produced as a result of motion sickness, particularly in birds not accustomed to travel (i.e. non-falconry birds).

gender but this is often based on observation of the bird's size and preference rather than science. Most raptors, parrots and some commonly kept passerines are not easily sexed by external characteristics, although there are some exceptions (see Appendix 2). Definitive determination of sex will require DNA analysis or endoscopic examination in most cases, unless the bird has laid an egg (see also Chapter 4).

Physical examination

If the bird is deemed fit enough to tolerate handling, after assessment of the clinical history and distant observation, the patient should then be subjected to a thorough, but not protracted, physical examination. Handling technique should minimize stress and not disrupt the human–bird bond (particularly important in bonded parrots and falconry birds). Prior to handling the bird, ensure that everything that may be required is to hand to avoid unnecessary delays. Commonly required items are listed below; additional items may include a falconry glove for handling trained falconry birds, although most falconers are likely to bring their own, and a net is useful to capture small passerines.

Recommended equipment for physical examination of birds

- Clean towel for capture and restraint
- Paediatric stethoscope
- Source of illumination and magnification (e.g. ophthalmoscope/otoscope)
- Sample pots and microbiology swabs
- An assistant may be helpful

WARNING

At all times veterinary surgeons must be aware of the bird's tolerance for a procedure. If at any time the bird appears not to be coping with the procedure, it should be placed back in its cage or returned to its owner. Warning signs include tachypnoea, open-mouthed breathing, loss of interest, a reluctance to hold on to objects or no longer attempting to bite the restraining towel or examiner

Potential dangers such as windows, ceiling fans and air-conditioning units should be suitably covered or turned off as appropriate, and all windows and doors firmly closed. Members of staff should be trained to not enter without permission once a bird is in the consulting room – an observation window is very useful. Ideally, the clinician should be able to darken the consulting room and use a red light, which allows them to see and approach the bird whilst restricting the bird's ability to see and escape, minimizing stress caused by chasing the patient around its cage or the consulting room.

Once the bird is suitably restrained, the examination should proceed in an orderly fashion to avoid missing important clues.

Bodyweight and condition

Bodyweight should be ascertained using accurate gram scales; tame parrots and trained falconry birds will usually stand on a T-perch on adapted scales (others may be weighed in a carrier or wrapped in a towel and the carrier/towel weight subtracted). Weight ranges across a species, and especially between sexes; the range can be wide and weight alone may not indicate the physical status. Body condition score (BCS) is a more useful indicator of health and may be estimated by palpation of the pectoral muscle mass; reduced muscle mass may indicate weight loss and/or atrophy due to lack of use, such as may occur in cage birds. Many healthy falconry birds may appear leaner when compared with cage or aviary birds due to their athletic nature and reduced body fat. Subcutaneous fat, which tends to accumulate over the shoulders and inguinal regions, may be palpated in particularly obese birds and may help differentiate an obese bird from a particularly fit and active bird.

Coelomic area and cloaca

In most healthy individuals much of the coelom is protected by the large keel, ribs and pelvic bones, leaving a relatively small area of the ventral coelom accessible for visualization and palpation. The coelomic area is normally flat to moderately concave in outline. The ventriculus may be palpated on the left side of the coelom and can be confused with an egg, particularly in larger parrots. In many species, female birds in breeding condition will naturally lose feathers over the ventral coelomic area, forming a 'brood patch'.

Distension of the coelom, indicated by a convex outline, indicates intracoelomic organ enlargement, a recent meal in raptors, ascites, or the presence of an egg and/or hernia. Birds with a distended coelom often present with dyspnoea due to compression of the air sacs. Ideally, the coelomic area and body condition are assessed at the commencement of the physical examination; birds with ascites and/or those in poor body condition are less likely to withstand prolonged examination. It is also important to ensure that the patient with ascites is held in a vertical position during examination, to reduce compression of the air sacs.

The cloaca is often obscured by the plumage and may be parted by gently blowing the feathers or wetting with water. The normal cloaca is tightly closed and kept scrupulously clean through regular preening and bathing. A flaccid cloaca, perineal soiling and stained feathers may all indicate disease due to compromised cloacal function or an inability and/or lack of energy to preen the area. Digital examination of the cloaca is possible in larger species, whilst a moistened cotton bud may be used to evert the cloacal mucosa in smaller species. The mucosa is generally pink, though it may be pigmented in some species, such as cockatoos, and should be smooth and moist. Irregularities of the cloacal mucosa may occur with papillomas, neoplasia and inflammation (cloacitis). Cloacaliths are sometimes encountered, particularly in brooding females and in birds with neurological deficits.

During the breeding season it may be possible to identify the sex of some passerines from the appearance of the cloaca. In male passerines a cloacal promontory develops as a result of swelling of the caudal ductus deferens and the cloaca points in a direction perpendicular to the tail. Female passerines have a less pronounced cloaca, which points in the same direction as the tail.

Beak

Signs of poor beak health include flaking, fissuring, crusting, erosions and malocclusions. In species that possess large numbers of powder down feathers, such as Grey Parrots and cockatoos, a glossy appearance to the beak may indicate disease such as psittacine beak and feather disease (PBFD) caused by a circovirus. Underlying nutritional deficiencies are often the cause of poor beak quality, in particular hypovitaminosis A in psittacines. Beak overgrowth may be an indicator of hepatic disease and/or lack of normal wear due to inappropriate food provision and/or lack of suitable environmental enrichment. *Cnemidocoptes* mites are a common cause of crusting lesions, particularly in Budgerigars, and in severe cases may result in abnormal beak growth. Trauma from collision injuries and fighting, particularly in parrots, is common.

Sinus inflammation/infection may sometimes result in a line of abnormal keratin growth along the beak. This may be permanent or persist until the abnormality grows out, which could take up to 1 year or more.

Nares and cere

The nares should appear clear and symmetrical. The normal parrot possesses an operculum that acts as a barrier to foreign bodies, whilst in falcons the naris contains a specialized tubercle, which is an adaptation for high-speed flying/diving, helping to divert air flow. Signs of disease include discharge and/or swelling indicative of upper respiratory tract (URT) infection and/or sinusitis. Rhinoliths are common in parrots, especially Grey Parrots, and are the result of accumulated keratin, environmental dust and often secondary inflammatory debris, which expands within the nares causing obvious distortion. In patients with suspected nasal and/or sinus disease, the nares (and to some degree the sinuses) may be flushed with sterile saline in the conscious patient to obtain diagnostic samples and to establish the presence of obstructive disease. The nares in parrots communicate such that fluid entering one naris should exit the opposite naris; in all species fluid flushed into the nares should exit the choana. Solid rhinoliths are generally not amenable to flushing, and need to be manually removed.

The prominence of the cere, a thickened fleshy area at the base of the maxillary beak, varies amongst species. The cere is generally prominent in raptors, but is variably prominent in parrots. Cere colour may be used to identify sex in Budgerigars, being blue in most males and brown in females; cere hypertrophy in female Budgerigars may indicate excessive levels of circulating oestrogens. Changes to the colour of the cere in adult Budgerigars from brown to blue in females and blue to brown in males may occur as a result of increased circulating levels of testosterone and oestrogen, respectively, and is usually a result of neoplasia of the gonads.

Eyes

Adnexa

The eyes are relatively large in birds compared with mammals but, in many avian species, due to the small patient size, the corneal surface is generally small (<10 mm) and examination using good illumination and magnification is essential. Avian patients with visual impairment of one eye tend to look at onlookers with the good eye, which can make examination of the diseased eye difficult without manual restraint. Distant examination should evaluate symmetry and the presence of swellings and discharges; an attempt to evaluate the patient's vision should be made.

Chronic sinusitis may result in the globe sinking into the orbit and most commonly occurs in macaws. In birds the lower eyelid is considerably more mobile than the upper eyelid. A nictitating membrane is present, and is normally thin and almost clear, coursing across the cornea from a mediolateral or dorsomedial to ventrolateral direction. Eyelids and the nictitating membrane should be examined for signs of thickening, inflammation, discharge and irregularities and/or wounds; in cases of ocular irritation or inflammation, the ocular surfaces of the eyelids and nictitans should be examined for the presence of trauma or foreign bodies – this will require general anaesthesia in most cases.

Palpebral and corneal reflexes may be assessed by gentle touch using a damp cotton bud tip rolled to a fine point.

Cornea, iris and lens

The avian cornea is significantly thinner compared with that of mammals, which has important consequences relating to traumatic injuries and foreign bodies. Traumatic injuries to the cornea are frequently seen in wild casualties and in psittacine birds maintained in flocks, often as a result of fighting. Examination should evaluate for evidence of trauma, inflammation and opacities. Fluorescein may be used to delineate corneal ulceration as in other species.

In some species the colour of the iris may give an indicator of the age or sex of the individual. For example, the juvenile African Grey Parrot has grey irides that turn yellow from around 6–9 months of age and in many adult Umbrella Cockatoos the iris of the male is usually dark brown whereas that of the female is red.

The lens should be evaluated for clarity and the presence of cataract. The pupillary light reflex (PLR) in birds may be elicited but, because the pupillary musculature is striated muscle and under conscious control, the reflex may be overridden by birds, particularly under the stress of an examination. The consensual PLR is absent in birds due to the lack of decussation at the optic chiasm; however, pupil constriction of the contralateral eye may be observed due to light passing through the very thin bone between the eyes and stimulating the retina directly. Note that the avian pupil does not dilate under the influence of atropine, due to the pupillary musculature being striated muscle. Pupil dilation is best achieved by placing the patient under inhalation anaesthesia (and preferably ventilated and maintained via an air sac tube), during which the pupil will usually dilate sufficiently for a thorough examination. Other techniques described include intracameral and systemic injection of muscle relaxants, such as D-tubocurarine and vecuronium, respectively, but these are more invasive and associated with a significant risk of blindness and potentially death and are best performed by an experienced avian ophthalmic specialist.

Retina

The avian retina differs markedly from that of mammals: the normal fundic examination reveals a large pecten (which provides a vascular supply of oxygen and nutrients to the photoreceptors), choroidal vasculature and pigmentation, and one or two foveae. The optic disc is at least partially obscured by the pecten. Direct and indirect ophthalmoscopy may be used to examine the fundus of birds but is more difficult due to the small pupil size of many species. Pupil dilation under anaesthesia, as described above, greatly facilitates fundic examination.

Retinal haemorrhage and detachment with or without pecten damage are common in avian trauma cases. The retina should be assessed in all cases of trauma and in any wild bird presented for assessment for potential re-release; failure to do so may be considered negligent.

Specific eye tests

A more detailed ophthalmic examination, when deemed appropriate, may include the Schirmer tear test (STT) or the phenol red thread test (PRTT), intraocular pressure and gonioscopy. Consultation with and/or referral to a specialist ophthalmologist with experience in birds may be advisable in many cases at an early stage. STT may be evaluated in larger species such as raptors, although it has not been evaluated for most species and normal results do appear to differ between species; the PRTT may be more appropriate to assess tear production in avian species, but there are currently few published normal values and the test may be difficult to acquire in some countries, including the UK (see Chapter 21).

Ears

Normally, the ears are covered by feathers and are invisible to the observer. Matting of the overlying feathers with discharge may be seen in cases of otitis externa but, in most cases, disease is not noticed until the overlying feathers are moved by gently blowing or using a cotton bud. The normal ear is covered in a thin epithelium with no discharge and minimal to no scaling of the skin; the tympanum should be clear to slightly opaque. Note that in some species of owl, such as the Barn Owl, the ears are positioned asymmetrically, an adaptation that allows these birds to accurately locate prey by sound.

Thickening and oedema of the skin as a result of squamous metaplasia is occasionally seen in parrots and in particular the Cockatiel. Purulent discharge may indicate an infection secondary to changes in the skin (similar to dogs) or infection with a primary pathogen, such as *Trichomonas* spp. Bruising and haemorrhage are indicative of blunt force trauma, such as occurs when birds fly into mirrors or windows or are struck by a vehicle. This is often an indicator of a significant trauma and, in many instances, the eye(s) will have been damaged in the process; a thorough ocular examination of such cases is mandatory, especially in the wild casualty.

Oral cavity

In birds with relatively weak beaks (such as passerines and many of the smaller raptors), the oral cavity may be examined by gently opening the beak and placing an index finger in the commissure, thus preventing its closure. Examination of parrot beaks generally requires some form of pliable gag (e.g. a suitably sized piece of rubber tubing or hose) to maintain the oral cavity open, taking care not to damage the beak, although with care and experience the index finger may be placed in the commissure of the beak as described for other species.

Once the beak is open the oral cavity should be checked for malodour, which may indicate inflammation and/or infection, or upper gastrointestinal disease such as sour crop, although halitosis in some Amazon parrots may be normal. The oral cavity should be examined for the presence of abnormal secretions, pus and plaques, foreign bodies and masses. The tongue should be manipulated using a cotton bud or similar and examined on all sides for the presence of foreign bodies or abscesses. The glottis at the base of the tongue and the proximal trachea are easily visualized in passerines and raptors, although they are often obscured by the fleshy tongue in parrots, and should be clear of mucus and discharges.

The choana should be examined for evidence of discharge; the papillae surrounding the choanal slit are normally well defined and pointed. Evidence of blunting of the papillae or absence of the papillae is suggestive of disease (especially hypovitaminosis A) and is seen most commonly in the seed-fed parrot.

Additional oral cavity tests

A swab may be taken from the choanal slit for cytology and culture. Additionally, at this point a swab may be passed into the crop or a crop wash performed (see Chapters 12 and 15).

Head and neck

The head and neck should be observed and palpated for asymmetry. Feathers are parted by brushing against the direction of growth or by gently blowing to assess the underlying skin. It is normal in most birds to have, on either side of the neck, large areas of bare skin without feather tracts (apterae); the jugular vein is often easily identified on the right side but is generally markedly smaller on the left in most species. Assessing the extent and rate of jugular filling can give a crude estimate of hydration and/or circulatory pressure and is easily performed by gentle occlusion at the base of the neck.

Crop

The crop is a dilatation of the lower cervical oesophagus situated at the base of the neck over the thoracic inlet. The crop is well developed in psittacids and raptors (with the exception of owls, which lack a crop) and is less prominent in most passerines. The crop is palpated to assess its size and contents, and the oral cavity may be checked for malodour at the same time. The crop of most healthy parrots tends to contain varying amounts of food during normal waking hours, reflecting periods of ingestion throughout the day, whilst in raptors the crop tends to fill after a single daily meal and subsequently decreases in size as the contents are 'passed over' to the stomach. As a rough guide, the crop of raptors should empty within 4 hours of a normal-sized meal – distension of the crop after this time may indicate crop stasis and risks spoiling of the food (sour crop), which is easily detected by smelling the oral cavity.

Occasionally, abscesses and foreign bodies may be palpated in the crop, the latter tending to comprise hair or manmade fibres in pet psittacids and occasionally pieces of falconry furniture such as jesses and leashes in trained raptors.

Crop fistulae, often the result of feeding inappropriately hot formulae to hand-reared parrots, are occasionally encountered and appear as matted feathers in the area of the crop as a result of leaked crop contents.

Pectoral muscles and keel

After palpating the neck and (where applicable) the crop, palpation proceeds over the pectoral muscles and central keel bone to assess muscle mass and body condition score (see 'Bodyweight and condition'). The area should be examined for evidence of trauma and asymmetry of the muscle mass, and the feathers should be gently parted to examine the underlying skin.

Wings

With the bird (including the wing not being examined) suitably restrained, each wing is gently extended in full and palpated along its length, looking for evidence of reduced range of motion, swellings and/or crepitus. Each individual joint (shoulder, elbow and carpus) may then be individually extended, flexed and palpated. The flight feathers are examined for their presence, damage (e.g. through self-trauma, caging or wing clipping), stage of moult, and for soiling, discharges and/or parasites. Following examination, the bird should quickly retract and fold the wing into the normal resting position; failure to do so indicates pathology. Care should be taken to avoid the bird's wing striking personnel and surrounding objects such as examination tables and cages, which can result in significant injury to both parties. Older birds, especially female parrots and cockatoos, may suffer from osteoporosis and are thus at increased risk of sustaining fractures.

Pelvic limbs and feet

Tame parrots and trained raptors are initially assessed whilst standing on the hand (gloved hand for raptors). If possible, the bird is requested to 'step up' from its perch to assess strength and coordination since, in order to step up, the bird is temporarily standing on one foot and transfers weight to the other foot (some parrots will initially steady themselves with their beak by holding on to or resting their beak on the outstretched hand; a bite may be inadvertently elicited by the inexperienced or unconfident handler at this time if they react as if a bite were about to take place). Once the bird is standing on the hand it may be gently unbalanced by rocking the hand to and fro to alter weight-bearing and to assess the strength of grip in each foot. With the bird steady on the hand, each digit may be gently lifted dorsally to assess flexion and mobility (care needs to be exercised with some trained raptors, which can strike out at the approaching hand at this point; some parrots may attempt to bite). The foot may then be completely lifted up to expose the plantar aspect and examined for evidence of ulcerative pododermatitis (bumblefoot). Some patients are best restrained in a towel to safely examine their feet: an assistant holds each leg above the foot, taking care to avoid the legs rubbing together or the bird grabbing itself and causing injury.

Any leg rings or falconry equipment should be examined for their suitability for purpose, state of repair and for areas of friction or keratin build-up on the legs; the ring number (if visible) should be noted at this time.

Some birds may allow palpation of the limbs whilst standing on the hand/fist but most will require restraining at this point to examine the limb in more detail by flexing and extending the individual joints, palpating them, and to trim the claws if required.

Integument

Most healthy birds have smooth supple skin over the wings, upper limbs and body, forming scales of varying size and thickness over the feet and up to the intertarsal joint in most species. In some birds, such as owls and eagles, feathers may replace the scaly skin to varying degrees and may cover all but the plantar aspect of the feet.

Signs of disease include wrinkling, flaking, crusting and thickening; increased skin fragility is commonly observed, particularly over areas of increased motion such as the propatagium and inguinal areas, and is commonly an indication of poor nutrition. Cutaneous masses including neoplasms, feather cysts, granulomas and abscesses may be seen. Useful diagnostic tests include skin scrapings, tape strip cytology, fine-needle aspiration and feather pulp cytology.

The plumage should be initially observed from a distance to assess its overall appearance; the plumage of a healthy bird should be perfectly neat and tidy and closely knitted together with a glossy sheen. Ruffled and unkempt feathers are an indication of disease either as a result of poor feather quality and growth (such as occurs in malnutrition and circovirus infection),

or a lack of normal preening activity. Lack of normal preening may be due to inability to reach the affected area, such as may occur with musculoskeletal pain or confinement to inappropriately sized enclosures, or may reflect weakness and lethargy.

Closer examination of the feathers and underlying skin is conducted during the course of the clinical examination. Transillumination of the feathers in a dimly lit room is a useful technique to reveal some parasites and more subtle lesions. Damage to the extremities of the flight and tail feathers is generally an indication that the bird is housed in an inappropriate enclosure; damage to the feathers may otherwise be caused by ectoparasites or be self-induced in feather pickers. The extent and style of any wing clip should be noted.

Some species, notably macaws and raptors, may have a distinctive natural odour to their plumage, whilst feathers from all species may absorb odours such as cigarette smoke and cooking fumes from the environment.

Abnormal coloration of the feathers may be a result of malnutrition, liver disease or PBFD; typically, green feathers will discolour yellow, blue to white, and grey feathers to red. Green, blue and grey feathers may all develop black discoloration if time between moults is prolonged or as a result of contact with oils from the owner's hands.

Developmental abnormalities may include retained feather sheaths, strictures, a failure to grow, absence of powder down, formation of feather cysts and fret lines, and have multiple aetiologies including malnutrition, liver disease, viral infections (e.g. polyoma and circovirus) and stress.

Uropygial gland

The uropygial gland is absent in some species (see Chapter 2). Its appearance varies, but it is generally a bilobed structure at the base of the tail with a terminal papilla, which is sometimes surrounded by a small tuft of feathers. The gland should be inspected for symmetry, normal structure and size; upon gentle pressure an oily substance should be produced from the papilla. Blockage of the uropygial gland is relatively common, especially in malnourished parrots and older birds, and results in an enlarged gland that fails to produce secretion when pressure is applied. Secondary infection may be a consequence of obstruction, and self-trauma around the pelvic region can sometimes be attributed to an obstruction or inflammation of the uropygial gland. Neoplasia may occur, with the Budgerigar overrepresented.

Cardiovascular system

The heart is best auscultated with the bird unrestrained to minimize stress-induced tachycardia and arrhythmias but, in practice, this is only feasible in some well socialized parrots, falconry birds and in severely debilitated birds. The point of maximal intensity (i.e. where the heart sounds loudest) can vary depending on the species and the patient's body condition, but is generally loudest on the left and right caudal sternal borders; in some birds the heart may be easier to auscultate over the thoracic inlet below the crop. The rapid heart rate of most birds can hamper identification of murmurs and arrhythmias. Heart sounds may be muffled due to pericardial effusion, ascites, hepatomegaly and obesity.

Peripheral pulses can be difficult to palpate but this should be attempted and is most often achieved over the ventral aspect of the elbow or medial hock. An estimate of perfusion may be made by assessment of the basilic vein or jugular vein refill time.

Pallor of the mucous membranes may be assessed in species with naturally pink mucous membranes (most raptors and passerines), but can be difficult to impossible in species with pigmented mucous membranes (many parrots). As for other species, pallor is an indicator of poor tissue perfusion and/or anaemia. In some species, most notably the Grey Parrots, cardiovascular compromise and poor perfusion can cause a bluish hue to the periorbital skin, and the eye may have a sunken appearance.

Respiratory system

Respiration is initially assessed from a distance; respiratory compromise may be indicated by tachypnoea, open-mouthed breathing, a tail bob or audible respiratory sounds. If respiration is deemed to be compromised, the bird will benefit from a period of rest in an oxygen cage and a mild sedative (e.g. midazolam 0.25–1 mg/kg + butorphanol 1–3 mg/kg) and/or a bronchodilator (e.g. terbutaline 0.01 mg/kg i.m. or nebulized with 9 ml saline) administered as deemed appropriate before commencement of the physical examination. A brief examination involving palpation of the keel and coelom to assess body condition and the presence of ascites is useful and may be accomplished in the process of transferring the patient from its carrier to the oxygen cage.

Respiration is barely noticeable in the relaxed, normal bird; stressed birds may display tachypnoea and even open-mouthed breathing, and may be difficult to differentiate from a bird with a truly compromised respiratory system – caution is warranted and such birds should be treated as per compromised patients. Due to the avian lung being fixed, normal lung sounds are very quiet to inaudible and, when detectable, consist of a very mild blowing sound. Audible respiratory noises are abnormal and may include wheezes, clicks and crackles; alterations in voice are relatively common and help locate pathology to the syrinx.

> **WARNING**
>
> Stressed birds may display signs of a compromised respiratory system, such as tachypnoea and open-mouthed breathing, and therefore should be treated as birds with a compromised respiratory system

The upper respiratory tract (nares and infraorbital sinus) and, in some species, the proximal trachea may be assessed whilst examining the head and oral cavity, taking note of any swellings, discharges and asymmetry. Disease of the upper respiratory tract may produce an audible soft, snuffling sound and may result in a moderate tachypnoea; dyspnoea may occasionally be seen if both nares are obstructed, causing the bird to open-mouth breathe. Examination of the trachea and syrinx is limited and generally requires endoscopy under general anaesthetic, but in conscious birds the trachea can be transilluminated with a bright, focal light source such as a Finoff transilluminator after gently wetting the feathers over the neck; this is particularly useful in canaries and finches to identify air sac mites (*Sternostoma tracheacolum*), which may be seen as small, mobile, black dots.

Obstructive diseases of the trachea include strictures, trauma and parasites (e.g. *Syngamus trachea* and air sac mites). Clinical signs may be subtle in mild cases but typically result in an obviously dyspnoeic bird with an outstretched neck and increased inspiratory effort. Compression of the trachea from goitre is common in the seed-fed Budgerigar, a result of iodine deficiency, and commonly produces a distinct click or wheeze. In severe cases overt dyspnoea may be seen.

Disease of the syrinx may produce a change in pitch or tone of voice (often sounds husky) or may result in a complete loss of voice; if the syrinx is significantly obstructed, clinical signs are similar to that of tracheal obstruction.

Occasionally a bird will be seen with a generalized or, more commonly, a localized area in the neck region, of feather elevation, associated with an accumulation of air under the skin; this is often a result of the escape of air from a ruptured air sac.

QRG 10.1: Observation

Normal appearance

A healthy looking Scaly-breasted Lorikeet in a large aviary in its native Australia. The plumage appeared immaculate, the claws were short and the beak was shiny, smooth and normally occluded.

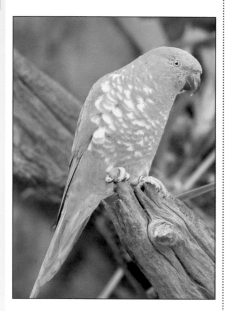

A normal, healthy looking, tame White-faced Scops Owl presented for a well bird examination. The plumage was ruffled (normal appearance for this species) but otherwise neat and tidy, and the eyes wide and bright.

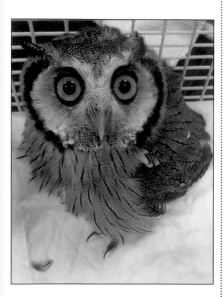

A captive-bred adult Peregrine Falcon used for falconry. This bird looked very healthy, bright, alert and responsive. The plumage was immaculate; the feet and talons were of good conformation and bright in colour and smooth. The beak had good conformation and the eyes were bright and wide.

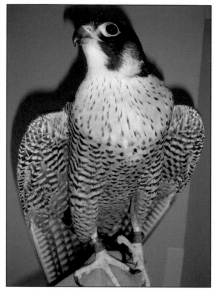

A juvenile wild Peregrine Falcon that was picked up by a member of the public after falling out of its nest. This bird appeared in very good health but was acting as if it were a tame falconry bird, which can be normal in some wild raptors when they are a few weeks old. Care and experience are required to differentiate wild birds suitable for release and escaped falconry birds. This bird also had a blue cere, which is a normal variation in juvenile wild Peregrines (the other colour being yellow) and is not a sign of ill health.

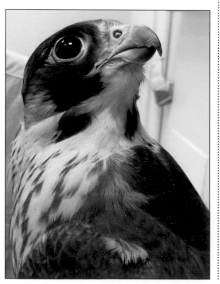

General signs of illness

A pair of Zebra Finches; the male bird on the right can be distinguished from the female on the left by the bold er markings and orange cheek patches. The male appears larger than the female due to the feathers being fluffed up. In this case, the bird had subcutaneous emphysema as a result of trauma to one of the air sacs, but was otherwise well. Many diseases may result in a bird being fluffed up, and a careful history and examination are required to help identify the cause.

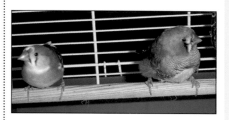

A captive-bred European Goldfinch was presented with a 1-week history of lethargy, weakness, weight loss and sitting next to the food bowl. Healthy small passerines are generally not tame and should appear bright and alert, and usually utilize a perch in their carrying cage. The patient displayed several signs of major concern: the bird was sat on the floor of the cage with its plumage fluffed up and its wings drooped; and its eyes were not completely open, despite being in the presence of onlookers. These signs are suggestive of severe disease. There was evidence that the bird has been eating from the food bowl, but on closer examination much of the seed was uneaten, suggesting that the bird was sham-eating, which is commonly observed in sick small passerines and Budgerigars. Droppings were visible on the cage floor, many of which had reduced faecal content, consistent with reduced food intake, intestinal obstruction or, more rarely, ileus.

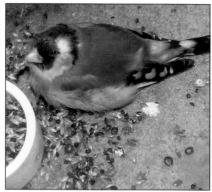

QRG 10.1 *continued*

A Cockatiel with a recent history of lethargy, anorexia and malaise was presented in the cage in which it is housed for the majority of each day. The bird was fluffed up and hunched in a strange environment, indicative of severe illness. There was a significant amount of faecal soiling to the perches and cage bottom; perches were placed directly over the food bowl, resulting in faecal soiling of the food. The food itself comprised mostly sunflower seeds. The bird was diagnosed with coliform enteritis, almost certainly a result of malnutrition and the unhygienic conditions.

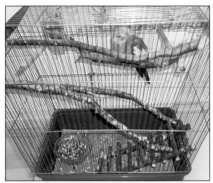

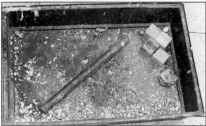

An aged Blue-fronted Amazon was presented with a 5-day history of lethargy and reduced appetite. The patient displayed several signs of major concern: the bird appeared too weak to support its own weight and was holding on to the cage bars with its beak; its eyes were lemon-shaped rather than being wide and round; and its plumage was fluffed up. Such a patient is potentially suffering from multi-organ disease and is likely to decompensate with handling. Before being examined further, the patient was placed in a humidified and warmed oxygen cage.

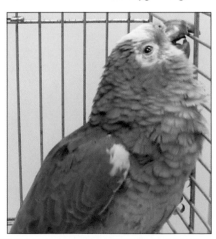

A Red-masked Conure was presented outwardly bright and alert, but lying on the cage floor. This could indicate a fear response but other differential diagnoses include hindlimb weakness and/or paralysis, egg binding and generalized weakness due to systemic disease and organ failure.

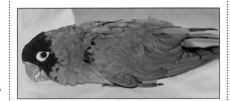

A female White-fronted Amazon sleeping in the consulting room; a sure sign of underlying illness. The plumage was neat and tidy and of normal colour, which suggests that the illness may be of recent onset. This species is one of the few Amazon parrots that display sexual dimorphism; males have red covert feathers over the alula, whereas in females these feathers are green.

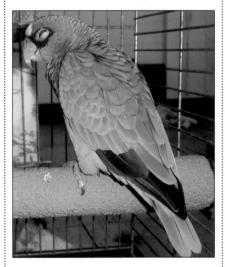

A 15-year-old African Grey Parrot was presented displaying signs that should alert the clinician to the presence of severe underlying illness. Despite being in a strange environment and the cage top being removed from around the bird, it remained fluffed up, hunched and with its eyes closed. There was evidence of feather picking behaviour over the wings and there was a number of red covert feathers, which can be associated with malnutrition or circovirus infection.

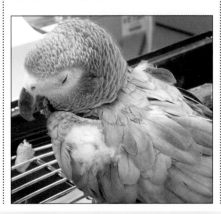

An elderly African Grey Parrot was presented in a state of collapse. A blue discoloration of the face, particularly around the periorbital area, and the sunken appearance to the eye were noted. This is a typical finding in African Greys with severe cardiovascular compromise. Such patients need to be handled with great care after first being rested in an oxygen-enriched, humidified hospital cage.

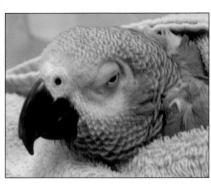

Overgrown beak

A tame, healthy Double Yellow-headed Amazon appeared relaxed on presentation, exploring and interacting with its surroundings. Its plumage was neat and tidy and of normal coloration; the eyes were bright and wide open. The beak was slightly overgrown with some flaking, which is most likely a result of lack of normal wear. In this case, the beak improved with the provision of non-toxic branches to chew. Malnutrition may also result in similar beak changes, but was considered unlikely in this case since the bird was offered, and ate, a suitable balanced diet, including pellets, fresh fruit and vegetables.

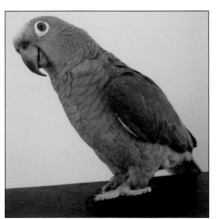

QRG 10.1 *continued*

Sour crop

A Harris' Hawk was presented with sour crop. Its eyes were lemon-shaped, the crop was visibly distended and there was soiling of the feathers over the head and neck as a result of regurgitation.

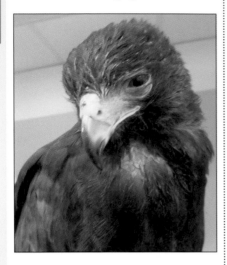

Respiratory distress

A juvenile Snowy Owl was presented in respiratory distress following several days of inappetence and lethargy. The bird was placed in an oxygen cage and nebulized with saline. The wings were obviously drooped and the eyes almost closed. Palpation of the keel and pectoral mass, as the bird was transferred to the hospital cage, revealed a body condition score of 1/5. Differential diagnosis include aspergillosis, severe endoparasitism and foreign body ingestion.

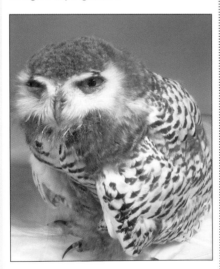

Drooping wing

An 18-year-old captive Common Buzzard was presented with its wing held in abduction and drooping, indicating wing trauma or inflammation.

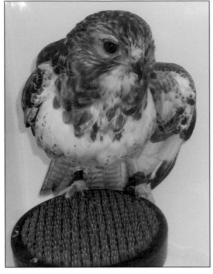

Feather plucking

A 3-year-old African Grey Parrot was presented with a history of feather plucking for several months. There was normal feathering to the head, which is typical of feather pluckers as they are unable to pick at the feathers on the head and upper neck. Otherwise, this parrot was displaying normal, active behaviours, aware of its surroundings and interacting with onlookers.

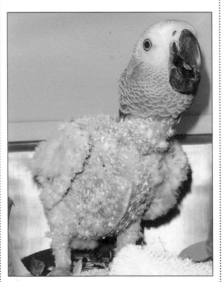

Excessive egg laying

A female lovebird with a recent history of excessive egg laying was presented in her own cage. The bird was found hiding under the floor covering, but looked very alert and responsive, with wide open eyes and neat plumage. However, the cage floor was soiled and covered in a deep layer of seed, indicating inadequate husbandry. Causes of excessive egg laying are often multifactorial; *ad libitum* feeding of a seed-based diet is a significant factor in many cases.

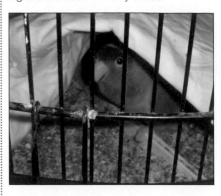

Legs and feet

A male Budgerigar was noted not to be fully weight-bearing on the right leg. This is a common, albeit often quite subtle, sign in Budgerigars that may be easily missed without distant observation after allowing the bird to relax. Common causes include limb trauma, testicular tumours and renal inflammation or neoplasia.

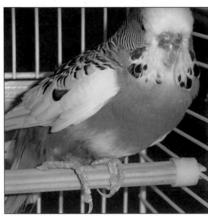

A Green-winged Macaw was presented as an emergency having sustained an injury to its foot, which had led to significant blood loss. Despite the macaw appearing outwardly well, the amount of blood loss suggested that the bird may be in a critical condition and could decompensate with excessive handling. The bird was placed in an oxygen cage and given mild sedation (midazolam ± butorphanol) 10 minutes before handling to apply a dressing.

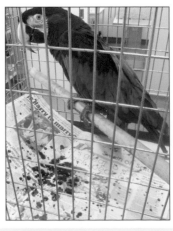

▶

QRG 10.1 *continued*

A Harris' Hawk with a recent history of ulcerative pododermatitis (bumblefoot) was presented to the author's practice in a carrier in a poor state of cleanliness. There was old faecal material and castings, and growing mould on the floor of the carrier. Such environmental conditions may predispose to respiratory conditions such as aspergillosis.

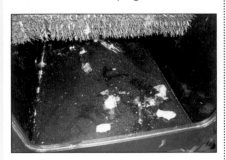

A wild Kestrel was found by the side of the road by a member of the public and was initially unable to fly. Following first aid and care at a rescue facility, it was noted that the bird was able to fly but was lame. Distant observation revealed the bird to be very alert and responsive, as would be expected of a wild Kestrel, but the right foot was knuckled over as a result of extensor tendon damage. The bird was euthanased due to being unfit for release into the wild.

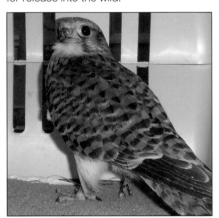

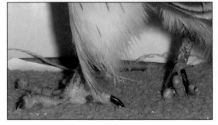

Cage furniture

A toy bell removed from the cage of a parrot displaying neurological signs, anorexia and biliverdinuria with an elevated blood lead level. The clapper is made of lead and fragments were ingested as the parrot played with the toy.

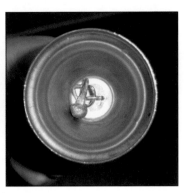

Diet

Specially formulated pelleted foods are ideal for parrots.

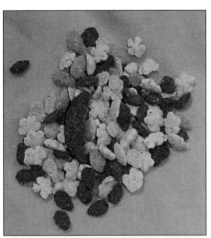

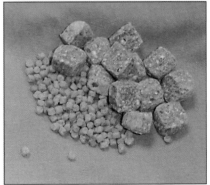

A suitable seed ration for a medium-sized parrot if used as part of a balanced diet with a variety of vegetables and fruits. Some seeds and peanuts are restricted. In addition, the seeds are hulled, which reduces mess and the risk of fungal contamination.

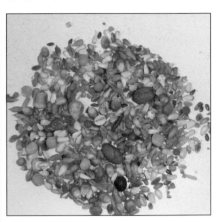

A sample of seed that was the sole food offered to a parrot displaying signs of lethargy, inappentence and increased respiration. The seed mix was composed predominantly of sunflower seeds and peanuts. The latter had been dyed to appeal to owners.

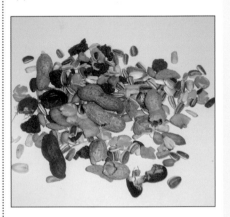

QRG 10.2: Body condition scoring

Assessment of body condition in birds is achieved by pectoral muscle palpation and prominence of the keel bone. There are various scoring systems that can be used, but the one shown here is a 5-point scale where:

- 1 = very thin
- 2 = thin
- 3 = ideal
- 4 = overweight
- 5 = obese

Gouldian Finch with a body condition score of 2/5.

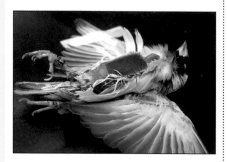

Peregrine Falcon with a body condition score of 2/5.

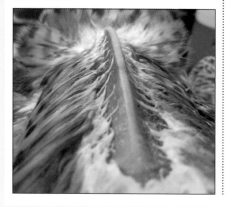

Long-eared Owl with a body condition score of 3/5.

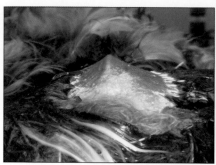
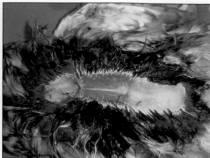

Kestrel with a body condition score of 5/5. Note the large amounts of lipoid deposits visible through the skin.

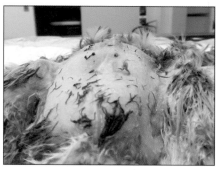
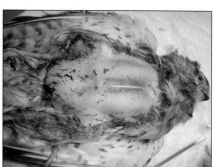

QRG 10.3: Examination of the coelom and cloaca

Ascites

A Budgerigar with marked ascites as a result of liver disease. Note also the reduced pectoral muscle mass. Body condition score was 2/5.

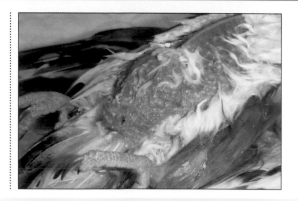

QRG 10.3 *continued*

Enteritis

A female Eclectus Parrot with soiling of the feathers surrounding the cloaca and ventral coelom due to enteritis.

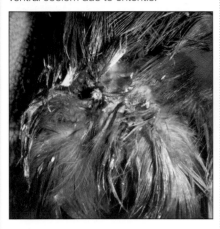

Cloacal prolapse

Moderate soiling of the flaccid cloaca in an African Grey Parrot with a chronic history of behavioural cloacal organ prolapse.

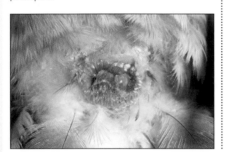

Excessive egg laying

Ventral coelomic area of a lovebird with a recent history of egg laying. There was mild distention of the coelomic area consistent with organomely, in this case the oviduct and ovary.

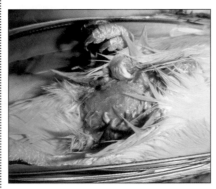

A 5-year-old female Cockatiel with a history of lethargy and anorexia following a period of excessive egg laying. A large hernia containing accumulations of fat and bowel was evident. There was also excessive scaling of the skin of the legs and coelomic area and bilateral bumblefoot.

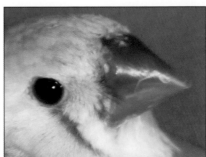

Prolapsed oviduct in a Budgerigar with a recent history of excessive egg laying.

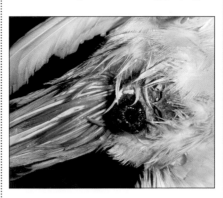

QRG 10.4: Examination of the beak

Normal appearance

Most passerines have a simple pointed beak, as seen in this Goldfinch, although the thickness of the beak varies between species.

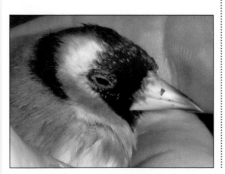

Note the variation in normal appearance of the beak of this Zebra Finch with the Goldfinch. Both birds are passerines and predominantly seed-eaters.

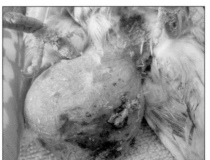

The beak of this Sulphur-crested Cockatoo appears dull due to a fine covering of powder down. This is normal in cockatoos and Grey Parrots.

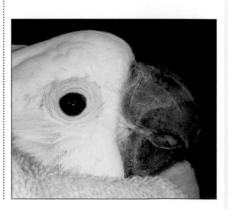

QRG 10.4 continued

Hyacinth Macaws have the largest beak of all parrots. The beak in this healthy bird has normal occlusion, a glossy sheen and minimal flaking of keratin.

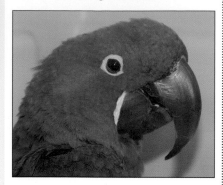

Typical appearance of the beak in a healthy hawk. Note that the beak is hooked but lacks the tomial tooth present in falcons.

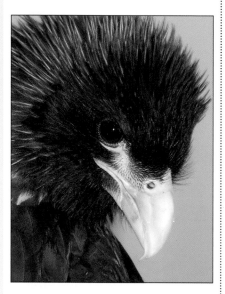

Typical appearance of the beak in falcons. The tomial tooth visible in this Kestrel aids in breaking the neck of its prey.

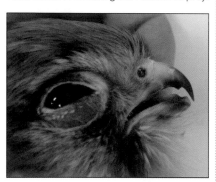

Prognathism

Ducorps' Cockatoo displaying mandibular prognathism.

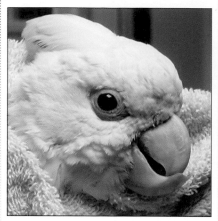

Overgrowth

A healthy male Eclectus Parrot with a slightly overgrown beak. This species shows obvious sexual dimorphism: the males are predominantly green, and the females are predominantly purple and red.

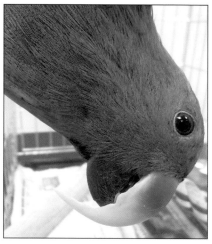

Overgrown beak in an elderly Harris' Hawk. In raptors, beak overgrowth is typically the result of being fed soft foods, such as day-old chicks. Note the debris occluding the nares, which may be due to poor health, infection and/or reduced mobility affecting the ability of the bird to groom.

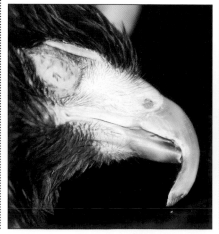

Keratin flaking

Marked flaking of the keratin of the beak in an Orange-winged Amazon. This is commonly caused by poor nutrition or lack of normal wear.

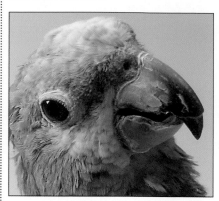

Necrosis

Orange-winged Amazon with necrosis of the distal maxillary beak. This was a result of a bite wound from a conspecific.

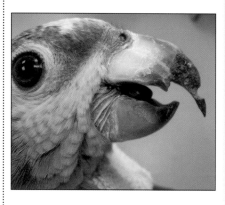

Psittacine beak and feather disorder

Psittacine beak and feather disorder (PBFD) is caused by chronic circovirus infection. Note the glossy appearance to the beak in this Sulphur-crested Cockatoo, signifying the lack of feathers, which is typical of this disease. There is feather loss over the head, as well as the body, which distinguishes such cases from feather pluckers that have normal plumage on the head.

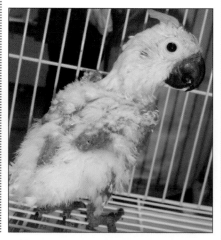

QRG 10.5: Examination of the nares and cere

Normal appearance

Normal appearance of the naris in an African Grey Parrot.

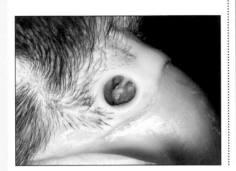

Typical appearance of the naris in falcons, in this case a Peregrine Falcon. There is a prominent tubercle that allows improved air flow during high-speed aerial dives. This individual has a large vertical split in the upper beak.

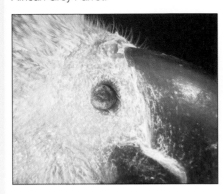

Typical appearance of the naris in a Turkey Vulture. It is possible to see right through the nares, which is normal for this species. (Note: the specimen is deceased).

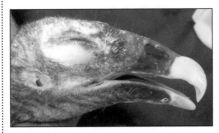

Nasal discharge

A juvenile African Grey Parrot with a mucopurulent nasal discharge as a result of a congenital deformity (choanal atresia).

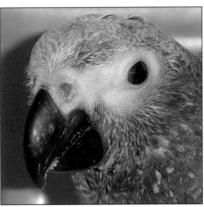

Rhinolith

A Double Yellow-headed Amazon with a rhinolith: an accumulation of keratin and inflammatory exudate within the naris. Common causes are poor nutrition and dusty environments.

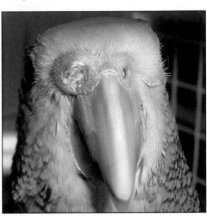

Hypertrophic cere

A mature female Budgerigar with brown, roughened and slightly hypertrophic cere. Mature males of this species typically have smooth, deep blue cere.

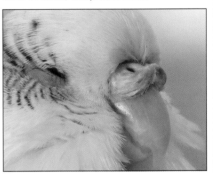

QRG 10.6: Examination of the eyes

Normal appearance

A juvenile African Spotted Eagle Owl with opacity of the lens. This is a normal finding in pre-fledgling raptors and should not be mistaken for pathology.

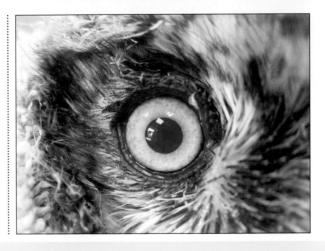

QRG 10.6 *continued*

Sinusitis

Sinusitis in an African Grey Parrot. Note the swelling rostromedial to the orbit and the purulent ocular discharge.

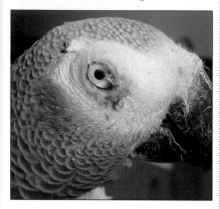

Chronic sinusitis in a Corella.

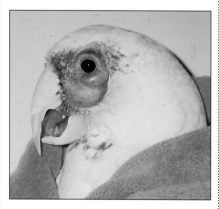

Harris' Hawk with a periorbital swelling due to sinusitis. There is also evidence of dried discharge on the feathers around the head. Note that the beak has been trimmed too short.

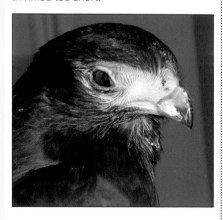

Ocular discharge

An aged European Eagle Owl with purulent ocular discharge, marked inflammation and swelling of the conjunctiva. There was also a reduced Schirmer tear test reading. The cause was attributed to distichiasis.

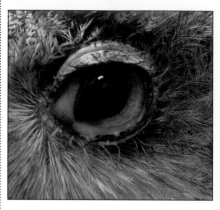

Blepharospasm

A Tawny Eagle presented with a history of chronic blepharospasm and apparent ocular irritation. Closer examination revealed distichiasis.

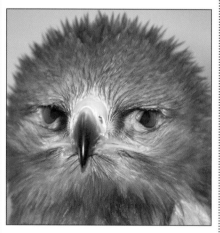

Cataracts

An aged African Grey Parrot with a mature cataract.

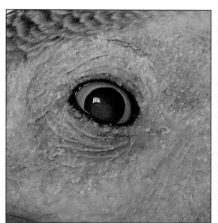

An aged Eagle Owl with a mature cataract in the right eye and an early cataract in the left eye.

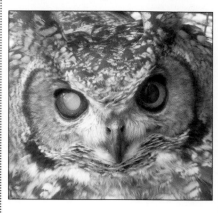

Corneal ulcer

An Eagle Owl with an area of corneal mineralization and a large corneal ulcer. Fluorescein was used to delineate the ulcer and can be seen underrunning the corneal epithelium around the edges of the ulcer. This is consistent with an indolent ulcer.

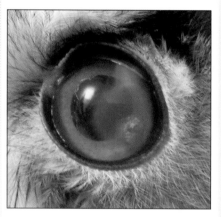

Conjunctival swelling

Orange-winged Amazon with a firm swelling of the lower conjunctiva. Mycobacteriosis was confirmed on histology of a biopsy sample.

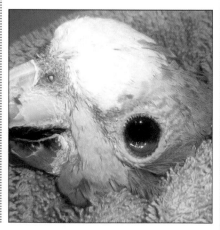

QRG 10.6 *continued*

Red iris

A mature female Umbrella Cockatoo with a red iris.

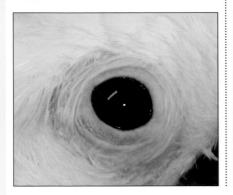

Ocular trauma

A Gyrfalcon hybrid with a large tear in the nictitating membrane following a tussle with a pheasant. Note the obvious asymmetry of the eyes.

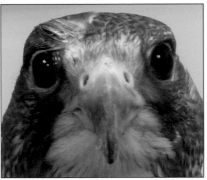

Hyphaema in a wild Common Buzzard that was hit by a car. Ocular trauma occurs in up to 30% of all impact injuries. Many lesions will be missed unless a thorough ocular examination, including the fundus, is undertaken.

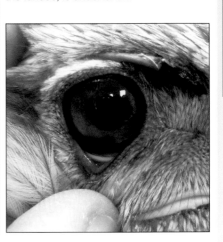

QRG 10.7: Examination of the ears

Normal appearance

Crimson-bellied Conure with ear coverts parted to reveal the normal ear opening typical of psittacine birds and passerines.

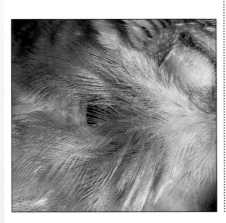

A Long-eared Owl with the ear coverts parted to reveal the extent of the normal owl ear.

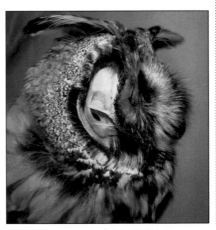

Otitis

A wild Short-eared Owl presented collapsed and emaciated. Bilateral purulent otitis is evident.

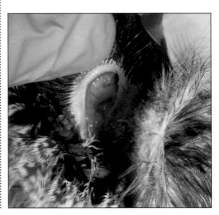

QRG 10.8: Examination of the oral cavity

Normal appearance

Oral cavity in a normal Red-tailed Hawk.

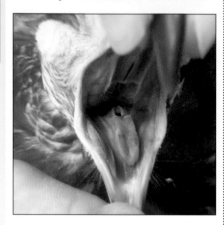

Oral view of the choana of a healthy Cockatiel. Note the prominent and sharply pointed papillae surrounding the choanal cleft.

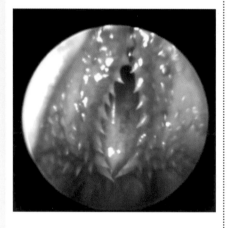

Abnormal appearance

Oral cavity of a Blue-fronted Amazon that had been fed a seed-only diet for several years (left). Compare this with the normal appearance of the oral cavity (right). Note the lack of papillae around the choanal cleft. Hypovitaminosis A is the most likely cause.

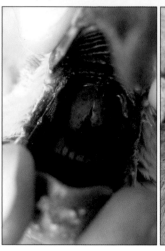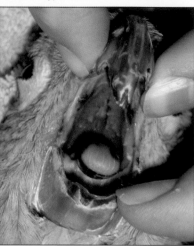

Tongue lacerations

A Harris' Hawk presented with evidence of oral pain. Closer examination revealed two lacerations on the dorsal surface of the tongue consistent with the bird having bitten its own tongue. This is most often observed in hawks with overgrown beaks secondary to a predominantly soft food diet (e.g. day-old chicks).

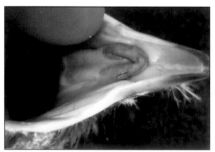

Ulcerative lesions

A Ferruginous Hawk presented with an idiopathic ulcerative lesion affecting the hard palate. The lesion appeared self-limiting and was monitored over a number of years without change. Differential diagnoses include neoplasia, infection and trauma.

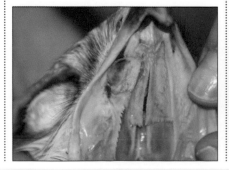

Caseous plaques

An Indian Eagle Owl with caseous plaques over the oral mucosa. These are typical of trichomonosis but the differential diagnoses include capillariasis, candidiasis and bacterial stomatitis (often *Pseudomonas* spp.).

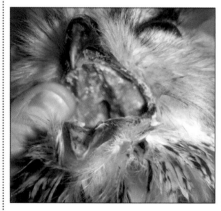

Nematodes

African Spotted Eagle Owl with a nematode attached to the pharynx.

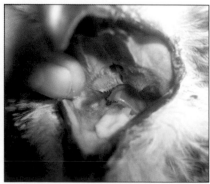

QRG 10.9: Examination of the head and neck

Normal appearance

A featherless area just caudal to the lower mandibular beak is normal in psittacine birds such as this African Grey Parrot. Note the flaking of the skin and bruising under the keratin of the beak, which is a result of malnutrition.

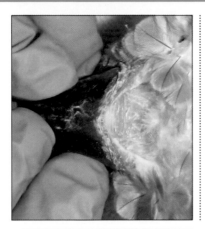

Swellings

Swellings of the ventral neck are relatively common. The differential diagnoses include sterile abscesses due to hypovitaminosis A, true abscesses, foreign body reactions following penetration through the oral mucosa, and neoplasia.

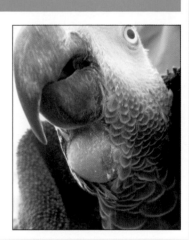

QRG 10.10: Examination of the crop

Normal appearance

Seed-filled crop in a healthy Zebra Finch. The crop may be examined by gently blowing the feathers or wetting the feathers to expose the underlying skin, through which the crop can be visualized and palpated.

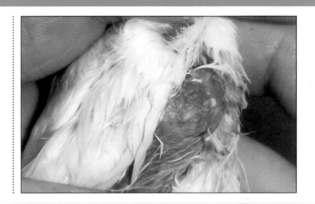

QRG 10.11: Examination of the pectoral muscles and keel

Subcutaneous masses

A Budgerigar with a large subcutaneous mass over the pectoral area. This is a frequent finding in Budgerigars and is often associated with a seed-only diet and/or obesity.

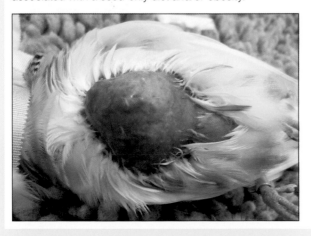

Trauma

Traumatic injuries to the thin tissues overlying the keel are common in heavy-bodied parrots such as African Greys that have been improperly wing clipped and crash land on solid floors. In some species, especially cockatoos, this area may also be a target for self-mutilation. If wing clipping is to be performed, it is essential that it is tailored to the individual bird (see Chapter 15).

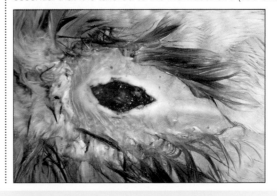

QRG 10.12: Examination of the wings

Normal appearance

Dorsal view of a normal, healthy wing of a captive-bred European Goldfinch. Note the immaculate plumage.

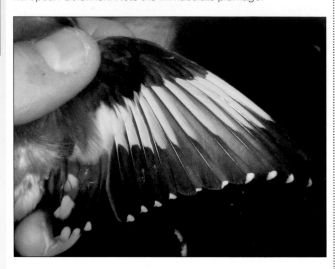

Ventral view of a normal, healthy wing of a Ringnecked Parakeet. Note the immaculate plumage.

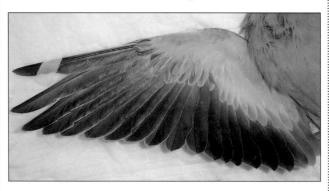

Normal appearance of the wing of a wild Long-eared Owl.

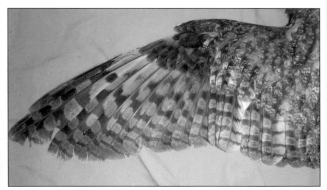

Drooping wing

A wild Little Owl presented with a drooped wing as a result of severe bruising to the shoulder, most likely due to collision with a vehicle. Such injuries generally carry a good prognosis, although it is essential that the patient be examined thoroughly to rule out other injuries (especially ocular-related) and that it is monitored closely and re-evaluated on a regular basis.

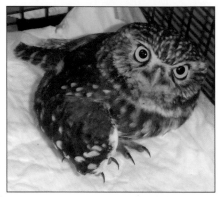

A Harris' Hawk presented with a slightly drooped left wing. A clear swelling is visible on the dorsal aspect of the metacarpal and there is wetting of the surrounding feathers from a discharge. The whole length of the wing should be palpated, checking for swelling, crepitus and pain. Palpation revealed cold pitting oedema of the wing, which is characteristic of wing tip oedema.

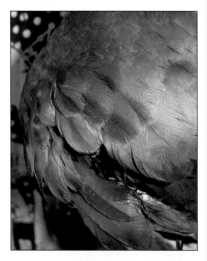

Trauma

A juvenile wild Peregrine Falcon presented with a wing injury. In a healthy bird at rest, the tail feathers and primary feathers are folded together and held symmetrically. Any asymmetry is likely due to injury; the affected wing may be held higher or lower than the opposite wing, depending on the location of the injury.

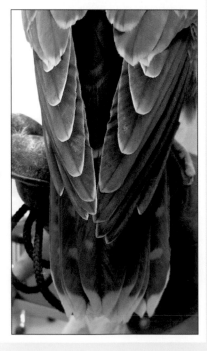

QRG 10.13: Examination of the pelvic limbs and feet

Normal appearance

Healthy Zebra Finch feet showing smooth, shiny scales and short, sharp claws.

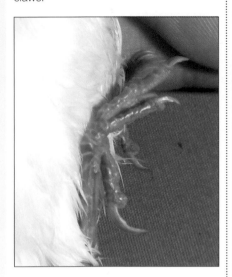

Normal plantar aspect of the foot of an African Grey Parrot. Note the prominent papillae with no evidence of ulceration or erythema.

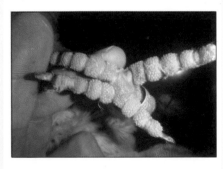

Normal foot of a wild Long-eared Owl. Note the prominent dermal papillae and size of the talons. Feathering extends as far as the foot in most owls, and in some species the toes are also covered in feathers.

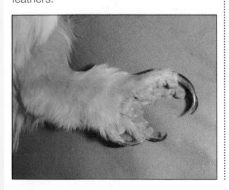

Equipment injuries

The accumulation of keratin and debris beneath the leg ring in this Mealy Amazon has resulted in a tourniquet effect, causing deep and extensive wounds to the underlying soft tissues and restricting blood supply to the foot.

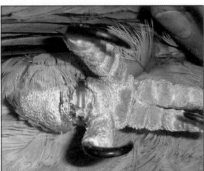

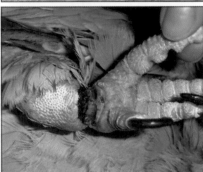

Harris' Hawk with a misplaced anklet. It is important to examine leg rings and other furniture in falconry birds. The leather anklets should always be placed below the leg ring. If the anklet is misplaced, the leg ring may be forced downward and injure the foot when the bird pulls against the anklets. In this case, the impression the ring has made at the top of the foot can be clearly seen.

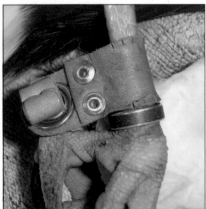

Old or badly maintained leather falconry furniture tends to become hard and unforgiving and may cause abrasions and contusions to the legs, as seen in this Harris' Hawk.

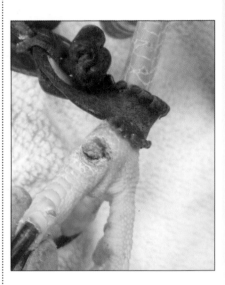

Scaling, crusting and ulceration

A 7-year-old Canary presented with roughened and thickened leg scales. This condition may be attributable to mite infection, poor nutrition or possibly age-related. Note that the claws are also significantly overgrown.

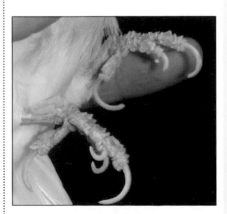

QRG 10.13 *continued*

Cnemidocoptes infection in this Budgerigar has caused swelling and the accumulation of crusts beneath the leg ring, resulting in ischaemic necrosis of the underlying skin and soft tissues.

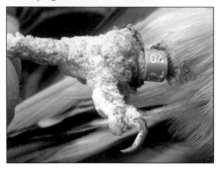

A Blue-fronted Amazon presented with generalized ulceration and scaling of the feet as a result of malnutrition and multisystemic disease.

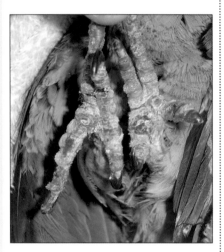

Swelling

Swelling at the base of the talons is a relatively common finding in captive raptors. The most common cause is infection due to excessive pressure at the base of the talon. This can be the result of overgrown talons and/or the accumulation of food debris underneath the talon. Rupture of the underlying tendons may result in untreated cases.

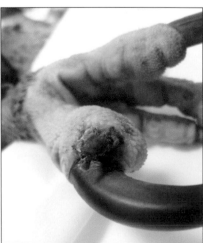

Pododermatitis

Plantar aspect of the foot of a Green-winged Macaw with early signs of pododermatitis. Note the flattening of the papillae and ulceration of the hock.

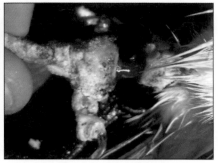

A Harris' Hawk with a grade 2 pododermatitis lesion. The underside of the foot may be examined by carefully lifting the foot off the perch or glove. If the bird is not tame or there is the potential to be grabbed by a raptor, then the bird should be restrained to examine the plantar surface of the foot.

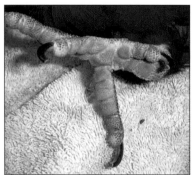

A Gyrfalcon hybrid with a grade 4 pododermatitis lesion.

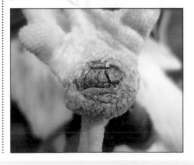

Femoral fracture repair

In order to fully examine the limbs, most birds require anaesthesia. This wild Buzzard showed significant shortening of the right leg following surgical repair of a comminuted femoral fracture. Such shortening of one leg is likely to increase the weight-bearing load on the other leg, which predisposes to pododermatitis.

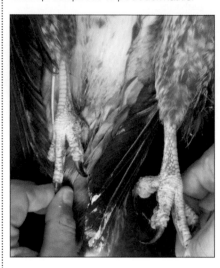

Trauma

A female Harris' Hawk was presented 8 weeks after sustaining an injury during hunting. Note the swelling and erythema of the second digit on the left foot and the pus discharge at the base of the talon. A general assessment of flexor tendon function may be ascertained by feeling the grip whilst the bird is held on a falconry glove. Individual digits may be assessed by lifting the digit off the glove and evaluating the bird's ability to flex the digit.

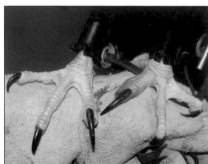

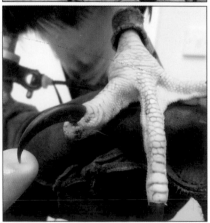

QRG 10.14: Examination of the integument

Feathers

Normal appearance

Blood feathers (pin feathers) represent the growing stage of the feather. During the growth phase, feathers have a substantial blood supply and can be easily identified due to their much thicker, greyish structure. When damaged, these feathers are a source of discomfort and have a tendency to haemorrhage substantially.

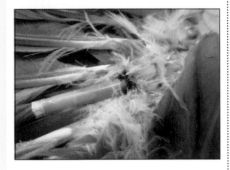

A serrated appearance to the leading edge of the flight feathers is normal in owls and functions to reduce air turbulence and thus noise during flight.

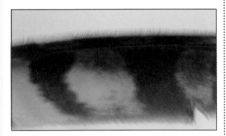

Fret marks

Fret marks, sometimes referred to as stress or hunger lines, are an indicator of interruption to the growth of the feather during its development. Fret marks may be found in small or large numbers and are particularly common in birds during their first year.

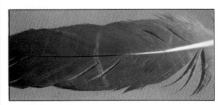

Discoloration

An 11-year-old Timneh Grey Parrot presented with black feathers over much of its body. The bird was kept in a dark corner of the kitchen, fed only sunflower seeds and exposed to cooking fumes. The bird had not moulted for at least 3 years. Abnormal changes to feather coloration occur due to malnutrition, prolonged moulting intervals, hepatopathies, viral infections (e.g.

psittacine beak and feather disease) and soiling of the feathers with substances such as oils.

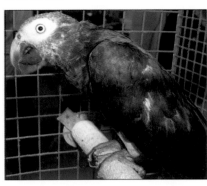

Yellow discoloration of green feathers, such as in this Blue-fronted Amazon, can be an indicator of underlying hepatic disease and/or malnutrition.

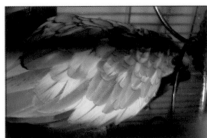

Poor quality

This male Harris' Hawk suffered from several bouts of severe illness, including pyoderma, over a period of 5 years. In this instance, the owner had noticed that its feathers did not knit together neatly as normal. The uropygial gland was enlarged and appeared to be blocked, which resulted in a lack of conditioning to the feathers from the preen gland oil, and the quality of the feathers subsequently deteriorated.

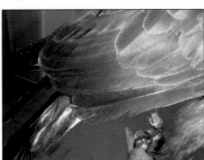

A Blue and Gold Macaw presented after sustaining a fractured wing as a result of crash landing, which was caused by an inability to fly due to poor feather quality. Where present, a number of tail and flight feathers had failed to be unsheathed by the bird. Failing to unsheathe newly formed feathers is generally an indicator of poor health and/ or husbandry. Common causes include

an inability to preen as a result of debilitating disease or a lack of suitable space in which to manoeuvre. Malnutrition is often an underlying cause.

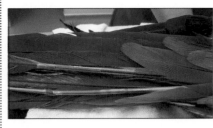

Cysts

Feather cysts are common in Canaries (top) and may occur singly or in multiple numbers. Cysts also occur sporadically in other species such as on the wing of this Harris' Hawk (bottom).

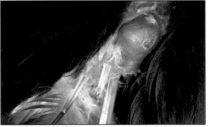

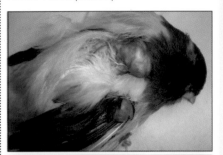

Loss

A Sulphur-crested Cockatoo presented with generalized feather loss, including the head. This presentation is classic for psittacine beak and feather disease. Note the glossy beak due to loss of the dust-producing feathers.

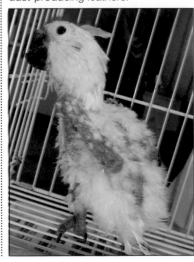

QRG 10.14 *continued*

Young African Grey Parrots are typical feather pickers. All the feathers, except those covering the head and downy body feathers, have been removed. The bird otherwise appears healthy. Such cases are very challenging to treat and require an in-depth history, clinical examination, imaging and laboratory testing to try to achieve a diagnosis and suitable therapy. In a large proportion of cases the bird continues to pluck to at least some degree.

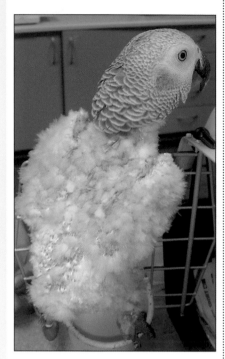

Chronic feather plucking in an African Grey Parrot. All feathers, except those on the head, have been removed. Generalized pyoderma (most likely a result of the feather plucking) is also present, and is most severe in the axillae.

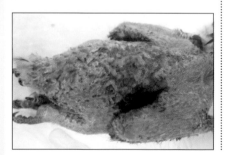

An African Grey Parrot presented with a recent history of feather plucking, which had progressed to extensive self-mutilation over the flank and pelvic area. When self-mutilation is focused over a particular area, there is often an underlying lesion. In this case, the bird had an aspergilloma adjacent to the right kidney.

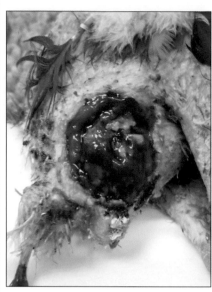

Skin
Bruising

A Kestrel presented with bruising. Bruising is evidenced by green discoloration of the skin and tends to appear 3–4 days after an injury has been sustained. This may be used to provide an estimate of the time of injury.

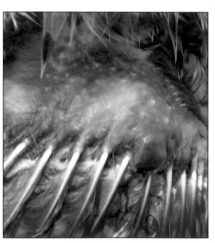

Thickening and scaling

Severe generalized thickening and scaling of the skin associated with feather loss in a Yellow-fronted Amazon. This was the result of chronic malnutrition and secondary pyoderma. The bird appeared hyperaesthetic and examination required anaesthesia.

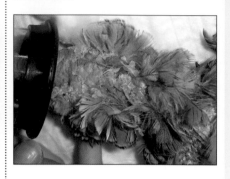

Pyoderma

Focal pyoderma in the inguinal region of an African Grey Parrot as a result of accidentally flying into a bowl of dirty kitchen water.

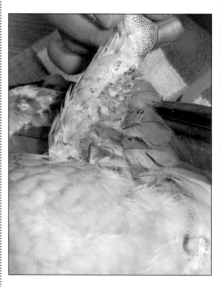

Cutaneous mass

A Harris' Hawk presented with a large cutaneous mass in the inguinal region (subcutaneous cell carcinoma). This site appears predilected for neoplastic changes in a number of avian species, most notably the Harris' Hawk and Peregrine Falcon.

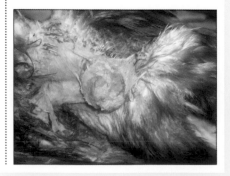

QRG 10.15: Examination of the uropygial gland

Normal appearance

Normal appearance of the uropygial gland of an African Grey Parrot. The gland has been squeezed gently to express preen gland oil.

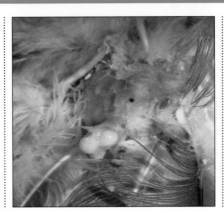

Normal appearance of the uropygial gland in a Short-eared Owl. The shape and size of the gland vary between species.

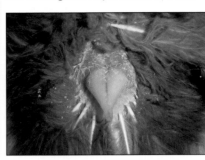

Hospitalization and basic critical care

11

Alex Rosenwax

Hospital setup for birds

Emergency and hospital equipment

Many avian cases presented to veterinary surgeons (veterinarians) are emergencies (Figure 11.1) and, usually, the only wildlife cases admitted to the hospital are emergencies. For veterinary surgeons wishing to consult on birds, it is important to have the veterinary clinic setup for avian patients, in terms of both the treatment room and the hospital. Admitting a bird without having the appropriate avian-specific equipment in place can have serious consequences, both in an emergency and during hospitalization (see also Chapters 7 and 8).

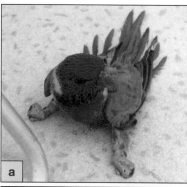
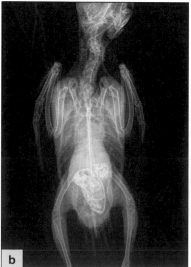

11.1
Emergency presentations.
(a) Bilateral peripheral paralysis in a lorikeet with confirmed lead poisoning. **(b)** Dystocia in a Monk Parakeet with a collapsed retained egg.
(© Deborah Monks)

Checklist of emergency and hospitalization equipment

- Cages
- Heat source
- Pharmaceuticals
- Foods
- Crop needles
- Oxygen delivery masks and chambers
- Biosecure area
- Bandages and casting material
- Needles, syringes and catheters

Pharmacy

Medications should be available as suspensions for oral and in-water use, and as injectables. Dropper bottles and a mortar and pestle are required to convert tablets into liquid or paste for oral medications. It is useful to have the medication already formulated in dropper bottles for ease of use. Larger non-psittacine birds (e.g. chickens, ducks and some raptors) are regularly given tablets.

Checklist of emergency kit medications

- Fluoroquinolones (enrofloxacin) for Gram-negative infections
- Co-amoxiclav for skin and Gram-positive infections and bite wounds
- Metronidazole oral suspension or ronidazole powder for gastrointestinal motile protozoa
- Doxycyline powder, tablets, paste and injectable (when available) for *Chlamydia* infections
- Various wormers and mite treatments, including moxidectin, ivermectin, levamisole, fenbendazole and oxfendazole
- Itraconazole, fluconazole and ketoconazole suspensions for fungal infections
- Calcium EDTA or D-penicillamine for heavy metal poisoning
- Meloxicam for analgesia and inflammation
- Butorphanol and buprenorphine for analgesia
- Diazepam for seizures

▶

BSAVA Manual of Avian Practice: A Foundation Manual. Edited by John Chitty and Deborah Monks. ©BSAVA 2018

Checklist of emergency kit medications *continued*

- Vitamin K for coagulopathies
- Stainless steel crop needles (Figure 11.2) with rounded metal tips of varying sizes (10–18 G width with longest crop needle 16–20 cm long) to collect samples and administer oral fluids and drugs
- Small-gauge needles and catheters (as small as 25–27 G needles)
- Small-sized syringes (0.3 ml and 1 ml) for administering minute quantities of drugs accurately, with or without attached needles

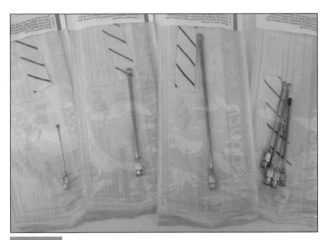

11.2 Autoclaved crop needles.

Many birds are in a critical condition on presentation and require non-invasive diagnostic tests suitable for immediate therapeutic decisions. Simple special stains are commonly used for emergency non-invasive diagnostics in birds. Cytology stains (such as Diff-Quik®) are readily available in most small animal clinics and are regularly used for a quick indirect haematology or cytology examination in birds. Gram stains are used by most avian clinicians to diagnose and qualitatively assess gastrointestinal bacterial and yeast infections. To examine these slides, a decent quality bifocal microscope is essential, as critically ill avian patients often suffer from common parasitic, fungal and bacterial complaints that can be easily diagnosed at the time of initial examination (see Chapter 12).

For blood collection, small tubes of 0.5–1 ml need to be available. Heparinized tubes are suitable for most diagnostic blood tests, both biochemical and haematological. Clotted tubes can also be used. Fluoride oxalate tubes are not necessary as avian blood glucose does not decrease significantly in heparinized tubes.

Small weighing scales are also a necessity, with accuracy of 0.1 g for birds <130 g. For larger birds, human paediatric scales are useful. Birds should be weighed on arrival and then (at minimum) daily, preferably in the morning to avoid any variations related to food intake and faecal output.

Cages for hospitalized birds

Parrots

Cages of various sizes need to be available for the housing of different species of birds. For short-term hospitalization, the cage can be relatively small to allow easy heating and access. However, it should still be large enough for the bird to stand on a perch, and the ceiling height should be high enough for the bird to stand upright with good clearance for the head and crest, with the tail not touching on the floor, sides or wire of the cage. Many of the macaws and some of the *Polytelis* spp. (e.g. Princess Parrots) have very long tails relative to their body size and thus require larger cages.

It is preferable to use hospital cages with three solid sides and an enclosed roof. This allows the heat to be retained, there is less wire to potentially shred the feathers and it provides more security for the bird. Hospital cages can be purchased (Figure 11.3) or, if the need arises, a standard commercially available bird cage, with towels or sheets covering three of the sides and the roof, can be used.

It is important that the cage has a small door to safely move birds into and out of it, as well as a larger door for cleaning access. If no specific bird cages are available for larger birds, collapsible dog cages or standard hospital cages can be useful. A standard bird cage can also be placed within a dog or cat hospital cage for added biosecurity (Figure 11.4).

Birds should be housed in cages with wire diameters and spacing appropriate for their species (Figure 11.5; see Chapter 3). Larger parrots (>150 g) require a thick-gauge wire, preferably made of stainless steel or powder baked. Parrots will chew and ingest the cage wire, so zinc and rusty metals must not be used.

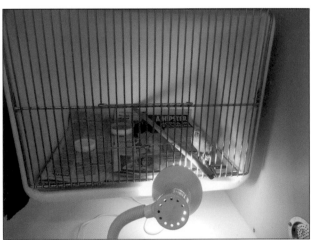

11.3 This Budgerigar is being warmed by a heat lamp placed outside the cage.

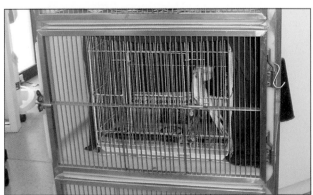

11.4 Cockatiel in a standard bird cage placed inside a hospital cage, providing extra protection and biosecurity.

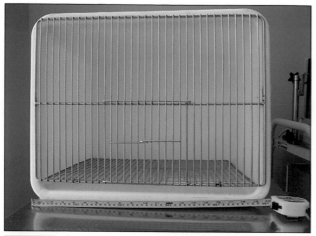

11.5 Cage with enclosed sides and small door with removable front, suitable for Budgerigars and Cockatiels.

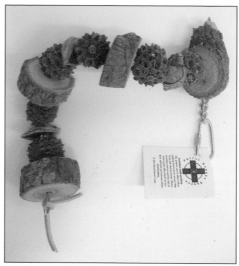

11.7 Small natural 'boing'.

The floor can be made of similar gauge wire to the walls, to allow droppings to fall through for easy cleaning. Paper can be placed over the wire to prevent small or weak birds sustaining injuries if their feet slip through the wires. Plain white paper is best as it allows the colour of the droppings to be examined, but newspaper can also be used. If birds shred the paper or a urine sample is required, the paper should be removed to allow the droppings to fall through the wire for collection on the cage floor or a plastic sheet.

Towels and sheets can be used on the floor to prop up neonates, collapsed birds or those recovering from anaesthesia (Figure 11.6). The towel can be fashioned into a 'doughnut' shape, encircling the body to prevent the bird rolling over while, at the same time, propping the bird's head up. However, towelling as a floor covering is not appropriate for active adult birds, which may pick at and ingest fibres, risking gastrointestinal obstruction. Birds may also catch their nails or talons in the towelling. Hot water bottles should not be left in the cages of active parrots as they will chew and ingest the rubber.

Clients may want to leave toys and paraphernalia for their birds (Figure 11.7). These may be useful comforting items but must be made of non-metallic, non-toxic materials and be easily cleaned. Rope perches and other fibrous material can be used only with caution as psittacine birds may ingest the material, leading to the formation of gastrointestinal foreign bodies.

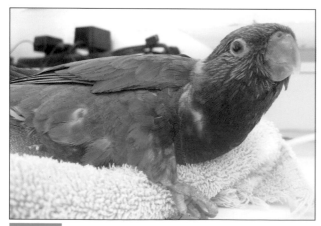

11.6 Lorikeet propped up on a towel.

Easily cleaned perches of various sizes need to be provided. Plastic or stainless steel food and water containers that can either be clipped to the cage side or sit securely on the floor should be used; ceramic bowls can be placed on the floor for larger birds. Large water bowls must not be used for small birds, as weak birds may fall in the water and become hypothermic or drown. In general, the placement of bowls needs to be versatile. Unwell birds need the food and water to be adjacent to them or they will ignore it. Food may also be scattered on the floor or placed high up near or on the perches.

> **PRACTICAL TIP**
>
> Foods appropriate to the species seen, as well as high-energy replacement food sources, need to be stored at the clinic. Birds have fast metabolisms and need food readily available. Placing a bird in hospital with no familiar food or no easy access to food can be fatal. The client should bring some of their own food with them, both to check that the food is appropriate and to have familiar food available

> **PRACTICAL TIP**
>
> It is a common misconception that pet birds should be kept in dark quiet areas. Many pet birds do better around people in a well lit area, even when unwell, with enclosed walls and a roof to give some sense of security. Most wild birds, some raptors (non-falconry birds) and passerines should be kept away from humans, in dimmed light

Raptors

Raptors can usually be hospitalized in relatively small cages, provided a curtain or sacking is placed inside the wire to avoid the birds damaging themselves. Tail guards need to be fitted to hospitalized raptors (Figure 11.8). The cage should be kept in a semi-dark quiet area of the hospital. Hoods (Figure 11.9) can be applied for examination and during cage cleaning; medications may be given in food to avoid the stress associated with handling. To decrease stress for raptors unaccustomed to humans, the cage can have a slatted floor

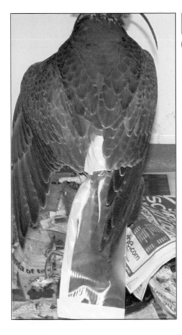

11.8 Tail guard on a raptor.
(© John Chitty)

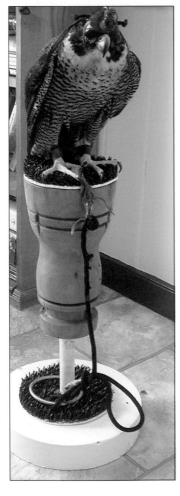

11.9 Peregrine Falcon tethered and hooded on a soft perch. (Courtesy of R J Doneley)

with a tray underneath to allow easy cleaning. Alternatively, the cage floor can be tiled or covered with heavy-duty linoleum. Perching areas should have soft, easily disinfected covers in cases where 'bumble-foot' (ulcerative pododermatitis; pressure sores on the ventral foot surface) may develop (Figure 11.9). The perches need to be of an appropriate diameter to avoid the raptor's talons piercing their own foot or the toes being overextended, which causes increased pressure on the ventral surface of the foot.

Passerines

Passerines (e.g. finches, canaries and Mynah birds) can be kept in light-gauge wire cages as they do not commonly chew the cage wire. Unlike pet parrots, many smaller passerines are uncomfortable with human contact. They are more likely to injure themselves if sudden movements are made near their cages and should not be kept in high-traffic areas in the veterinary hospital.

Biosecurity

In many countries there are no effective vaccinations available for pet caged parrots. Depending on the country, a paramyxovirus vaccine may be available for Columbiformes. Common parasites, viruses and bacteria (including *Chlamydia*) can be harboured in hard-to-clean cages. Aerosol transmission between hospitalized birds can also occur. Thus, it is inappropriate to keep a systemically unwell wild bird suffering from unknown disease next to a comparatively healthy bird.

Many infectious agents are found in saliva and faeces. These can lodge on the feathers, and this is another reason why birds should be kept apart from each other. This quarantine can be achieved by keeping birds a suggested minimum distance of 1 m apart, or by using the protective shape of the cage design. Neonates are particularly susceptible to diseases such as psittacine circovirus (psittacine beak and feather disease) and polyomavirus. Do not house individual birds, especially neonates, next to other birds untested for contagious diseases. Birds with suspected contagious disease should be kept in isolation and young birds should be kept in a separate low-traffic area with the airflow not in contact with the main area of the clinic.

Emergency cases may involve zoonotic diseases. *Chlamydia* bacteria are more likely to be excreted from stressed or unwell birds. The bird may not be showing classic clinical signs of *Chlamydia* infection. If possible, tests for contagious or zoonotic diseases should be included in the diagnostic panel. Until results are known, all birds admitted to the hospital with an unknown health status should be assumed to have a contagious or zoonotic disease. Appropriate occupational health and safety precautions should be taken in any emergency case, including staff wearing masks and gloves. All staff should be briefed on how to avoid and detect the classical clinical signs of avian *Chlamydia* in the workplace (Figure 11.10; see Chapter 19).

Receptionists should be trained to recognize the obvious signs of contagious or zoonotic diseases and inform the hospital staff at the time of appointment scheduling or when bringing birds through to the treatment area (see Chapter 8). This will minimize the exposure of other birds and staff to zoonotic and contagious diseases during an emergency.

Checklist for the common clinical signs of *Chlamydia* infection

- Watery green droppings (see Figure 11.10b)
- Dyspnoea that may or may not include sneezing
- Conjunctivitis and sinusitis (see Figure 11.10a)
- 'Fluffed up' posture or lethargy
- Death

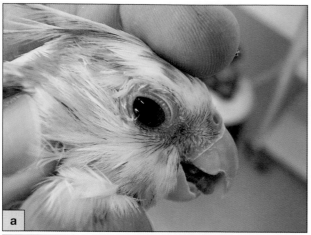

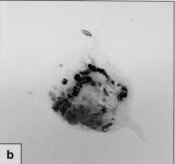

11.10 **(a)** Cockatiel with conjunctivitis caused by *Chlamydia* infection. **(b)** Green watery faeces from a bird with *Chlamydia* infection; the red area indicates that the bird may also be passing blood.

Heating for hospitalized birds

Birds have a high surface area and a fast metabolism; they utilize a large part of their energy keeping warm. 'Fluffing up' is the method a bird uses to insulate itself from the cold, trapping air between its feathers. Most hospitalized birds require a heat source. This can be provided in several forms. There are commercially available brooders (Figure 11.11) and emergency cages that have inbuilt heat sources. These are useful, although some brooders have the disadvantage of being hard to clean. The large areas of transparent acrylic or glass in some brooders may also give the bird a poor sense of security.

Simpler methods to keep birds warm include using heaters or desk lamps with a 40-watt pearl lightbulb adjacent to the bird in its cage. Fan-forced heaters should not be used as they may dry the air (see 'Emergency and critical care').

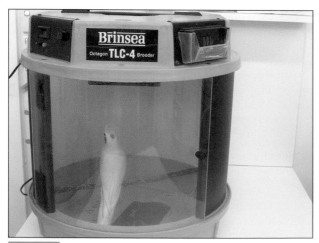

11.11 Cockatiel in a brooder.

Hospital treatment room setup for birds

The hospital examination room should have few or no windows; any windows must be securely locked. There should be no potential predator species in close proximity. The room should be small, able to be darkened, and have no places for the bird to hide or roost, so any escaped bird can be recaptured easily (Figure 11.12). If the treatment room is not appropriate, the bird should be moved to another room, such as a consultation room, for its routine daily hospital examination and treatment. Birds should have several easily disinfected perches available to sit on, both in the treatment room and in their cage, to allow them to display natural perching behaviour. This assists in determining the health of the bird. Birds unable to perch (e.g. due to ataxia, bandaged or cast legs or bumblefoot) should not be examined on slippery surfaces such as metal tables.

Towels of varying sizes need to be kept available to assist in catching birds. Caution should be exercised when gripping passerines and parrots with thick protective gloves, to avoid accidental pressure on a bird's chest, which can lead to stress and possibly asphyxiation.

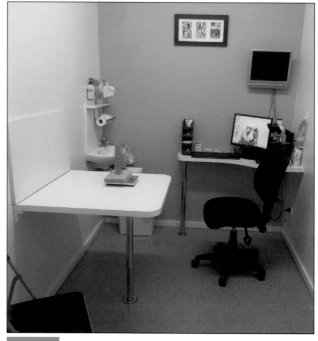

11.12 Appropriate examination room for birds.

Feeding

Parrots and seed-eating birds

The most common companion birds are primarily seed-eaters or birds that are treated as seed-eaters when kept as pets. In the wild these birds usually eat native fresh seed, not the dried processed seed provided by many keepers, and encouraging a transition to pelleted foods is recommended for the long term (see Chapter 6). However, familiar foods that may not be appropriate may still need to be offered initially in hospital to encourage a bird to eat.

It is important to determine which nutritional strategy group a bird belongs to.

Seed-eaters: These are birds primarily fed seed and some vegetables in the hospital environment, and include:

- Small seed-eaters (e.g. Budgerigars, doves, canaries and finches)
- Medium-sized seed-eaters (e.g. Cockatiels, Princess Parrots, African lovebirds and rosellas)
- Larger seed-eaters (e.g. Galahs and cockatoos).

Hospitalized small birds being fed on a seed diet should be offered a mix of seed to allow them to select the seed variety they prefer. Bird pellets or crumble should also be available at all times, although many birds in hospital will not eat them. Birds fed on a Budgerigar or Canary seed mix may not be being fed a fully balanced diet (see Chapter 6); however, it is still preferable to offer seed to anorexic birds in hospital to encourage sick or nervous birds to eat than risk starvation. Other plants and vegetables (mentioned below) should also be offered, especially fresh grass and grass seeds.

A selection of fresh vegetables, such as spinach, beans, parsley, broccoli, carrots, chard and corn, should be fed. Grass should be provided daily for all non-fruit-eating parrots. Household foods, such as cooked pasta, rice, toast, eggs, mashed potato, chicken bones and other meats, may be offered in small amounts if it encourages the bird to eat. In general, fruit can also be offered; however, many small seed-eating birds will not eat fruit.

Medium to larger seed-eating birds eat the same diet as small birds but can also have 10–15 sunflower or safflower seeds added per day.

Seed- and fruit- and/or nut-eaters: These birds will eat seeds in hospital as well as fruit and/or nuts:

- For fruit- and seed-eaters, add fruit to the large seed-eater diet. This diet suits Asiatic birds such as Moustached, Alexandrine and Indian Ringnecked Parakeets, as well as South American and African birds such as conures, Senegal Parrots, Grey Parrots, Amazons and Eclectus Parrots
- For larger nut and fruit and seed-eating parrots, nuts, fruit and vegetables should be given. This diet suits various types of macaws from Central and South America.

In addition to the seed diet described above, for fruit-eating birds, banana, papaya, melon, oranges, apples, grapes and kiwi fruit can be provided. For macaws, more vegetables and fruit and some nuts should be added to the seed diet.

Nectarivorous birds

These species, including lories and lorikeets, should have fruit and vegetables but not seed.

There are several lorikeet commercial food preparations available. The wet foods are palatable and are useful for getting anorexic birds to eat. Some poorly formulated wet foods may cause yeast infections (e.g. thrush and sour crop), especially in smaller birds. Dry food powders are also available, but many unwell lories and lorikeets will not eat them. There are also lorikeet pellets. Commercial lorikeet nectars can be offered as an additive but cannot be used as the base diet.

Plants and flowers, particularly those from their native habitat, can be used to supplement the diet of lorikeets and lories. They are not grass-eaters. Fruit and vegetables should be regularly supplied.

Insectivorous birds

Insectivorous or partially insectivorous birds are more likely to be wild birds or part of softbill collections in aviculture. Inappropriately formulated insectivore foods may lead to malnutrition and the accumulation of iron in the liver. There are commercially available feeds for insectivorous birds (Figure 11.13), comprising small semi-dry round balls or oval-shaped pellets. In some cases, the food may also be presented as a slurry in a bowl. Live food can be offered, but care must be taken to monitor the health and storage of the live food as well as preventing it escaping into the hospital environment.

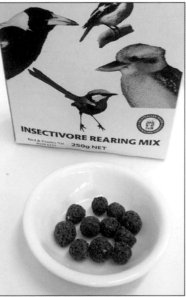

11.13 Commercial insectivore food pellets.

Natural foods for Australian and Asiatic species

Some native Australian plants are found worldwide in gardens and can be fed regularly to Australian and Asiatic native birds in hospital, including *Polytelis* spp., *Neophema* spp., *Platycercus* spp., rosellas, Budgerigars, Cockatiels and cockatoos. Natural plants can be offered to all birds, as parrots like to chew the plants up as 'toys' and this may also encourage birds to eat.

Natural foods are available seasonally. They include:

- Insects (including grubs and wood-boring larvae)
- Tree leaves and blossoms
  - Banksia
  - Eucalyptus, acacia
  - Grevilleas (Figure 11.14a)

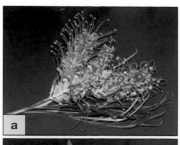
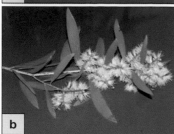

11.14 **(a)** Grevillea plant for nectar-eating birds. **(b)** Melaleuca plant for native Australian species.

- Mallees, casuarina
- Melaleuca (Figure 11.14b)
- Hakia
- Nectar, pollen and wild fruits in season
- Grass roots
- Wild grasses and their seeds.

PRACTICAL TIP

Most Australian seed-eating parrots do not drink large quantities of water

---

Raptors

Raptors eat various foods, including day-old chicks, mice, rabbits, and feathered and unfeathered quails. Raptors regurgitate the indigestible part of the meal, including the hair and feathers; some owls also regurgitate parts of the skeleton. This is called casting. Normal raptors will produce a cast within 8–16 hours of a meal. A bird should not be fed again until it has cast the previous meal. Foods that involve casting should not be fed to chicks <12 days of age or to raptors with gastrointestinal problems. Some breeding females may have trouble with casting due to the lack of space in the abdominal cavity caused by the ovarian follicles and active oviduct.

Many raptors refuse to eat in hospital and will require force-feeding. In these cases, nutritional supplementation will also be necessary. For short-term simple supplementation, the standard emergency critical care diets suitable for cats may be used.

Nutrition of hospitalized birds

Determining whether a hospitalized bird is eating is not always straightforward. Birds may appear to be eating but not be ingesting the food: food may be shifted around in the bowl by the bird searching for the preferred seed; fruit and vegetables may have been shredded but not eaten. A lack of regular droppings in seed-, nectar- and fruit-eating birds indicates that the bird is not eating, but droppings may also be absent if the bird is unable to pass faeces due to gastrointestinal stasis or blockage. In some cases, the faeces may be adhered to the feathers surrounding the cloaca. Urates (the white portion of the droppings)

will often still be passed when the bird is not eating. The presence of faeces should not be used as the only indicator of eating if the bird is being force-fed supplementary food. In these cases, immediately prior to supplementary feeding, the crop can be palpated for the presence of food.

There are species-specific habits that need to be taken into account when assessing whether a bird is eating.

- Most seed-eating parrots will hull their seed, leaving the lighter husks in the cage and food bowl (Figure 11.15). Birds may still hull seeds but produce no droppings if they are vomiting or unable to ingest the seeds.
- Seed-eating passerines (such as canaries) may eat the whole seed, leaving no husks.
- Nectarivorous birds (such as lories and lorikeets) will need to be observed drinking liquid food or eating dry food.
- Raptors should be observed eating. They will cast the indigestible food and pass faeces after they have eaten. Anorexic birds may still defecate but their faeces will be sparse, green and tacky.

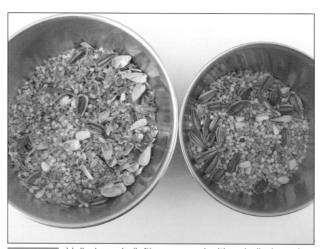

11.15 Hulled seeds (left) compared with unhulled seeds (right).

Many birds live and feed in social flocks; therefore, social interaction will often stimulate the bird to eat. If a tame pet bird continues to be anorexic, it is important to have the client visit and encourage the bird to eat. A consultation room or equivalent space is a useful private room for the client's visits. Prior to the bird being brought into the room, it is important to check that any food and/or treats brought by the client are safe and suitable, and to discuss with them appropriate handling of their bird. The client should be left alone with the bird and the clinician should check in at least once mid-visit to assess the bird's response to the food offered.

Wild and non-tame birds may prefer to eat in isolated areas. Unless directly affecting a bird's ability to recover, a selection of foods that the bird prefers should also be provided to stimulate the initial desire of the bird to eat. In the longer term, once the bird is eating, it will be important to attempt to transition the bird on to the appropriate nutritious food, if this is not already being eaten (see Chapter 6).

Emergency and critical care

A high proportion of avian veterinary cases are considered, at minimum, minor emergencies. Any cases with an unclear health status should be hospitalized (see Chapter 8).

The most common presenting signs of an emergency are being 'fluffed up', sleeping all the time, laboured breathing, vomiting, diarrhoea, poor ability to stand or walk and seizures. Other obvious emergency signs are wounds on the bird or blood in the cage.

Triage steps for the collapsed bird

1. Bird taken through to treatment area for immediate warming and oxygen.
2. Client in waiting room completes admittance forms.
3. Emergency medications and fluids are prepared.
4. Discuss with client the history, options and tests available, as well as advising them on the limited information that can be gathered as the bird may be too weak to be handled.
5. Assess whether the patient is stable enough for examination.
6. Brief examination.
7. If stable enough, administer emergency medications and collect limited samples for appropriate tests.
8. Once stable and able to be handled, conduct in-depth physical examination and collect samples for appropriate testing.

WARNING

It is important to handle a collapsed bird as little as possible. It is best to pick up a very ill bird in a towel to avoid any problems during handling. A bird that is too unwell should not be handled at all but simply warmed up

---

Five-point checklist for hospital support

- Safe cage
- Heat
- Fluid therapy
- Oxygen
- Nutritional support

Hypothermia

All birds presented should be assumed to be at least mildly hypothermic, especially if 'fluffed up', a typical sign that a bird is cold and ill. Being 'fluffed up' is the most common noticeable sign of a bird emergency.

Unwell birds are usually hypothermic and need to be placed in a heated environment. A commercial brooder or incubator can be used if available; fully feathered birds should be kept at 29°C and 70% humidity. A shallow dish of water can be placed in the cage or brooder if it does not have a humidity source. If the bird is seizuring or ataxic, the dish must not be placed on the ground or in any other position that the bird could fall into and then either become wet and hypothermic or drown. For these birds, humidity may be achieved with a moist towel or by lightly spraying the walls of the enclosure with water.

Radiating heat is the most effective heat source. When no commercial brooder is available, a radiating heat lamp can be used. In these cases, a normal desk lamp with a 40-watt pearl lightbulb placed outside the cage directly adjacent to the 'fluffed up' bird is effective, otherwise a porcelain or red heat lamp can be used. The incandescent lightbulb can be left on 24 hours a day for up to 48 hours continuously, but after this time should be replaced with infrared lights or a heated room at night to ensure an adequate diurnal rhythm. To insulate the cage, cover the other three sides and roof of the cage with a towel or blanket. Towels must be placed away from the heat source to avoid them being a fire hazard. The continual light encourages birds to eat when unwell. The heat lamp also gives an indication of a bird's ability to thermoregulate, as the bird will move away from the lamp when improving.

Alternatively, a heated room or a heater, preferably with a thermostat, can be used. Electric oil heaters are ideal as they give off a slow heat and have a thermostat. Fan heaters can be used but they move dry heated air around, which many birds cannot tolerate. Hot water bottles give only temporary relief, need to be changed often and usually will not heat the ambient air appropriately. When no heat source is available, covering the bird's cage can at least minimize heat loss but is not effective in heating the bird. Note that handling birds cools them down, as their normal temperature is over 40°C.

If anaesthetized or collapsed, a bird's cloacal temperature can be taken. Cloacal temperature readings in active birds are difficult to obtain and often of little practical value.

Fluid therapy

Fluid therapy at the hospital can be administered either by injection or orally. Many birds will initially be started on fluid therapy by injection and progress to oral fluids at a later stage. Oral fluids are preferred in birds with mild dehydration, that are not vomiting and do not have crop stasis. Fluid therapy is often given via subcutaneous injections. Intravenous fluids are also used but can be problematic as their administration may involve heavy restraint or anaesthesia of the bird. Indwelling catheters are not tolerated by many smaller birds but are still used on occasion. For these reasons, intravenous fluids may be given as a one-off bolus or used as a continuous infusion in an anaesthetized bird (Figure 11.16). Many collapsed or severely weakened

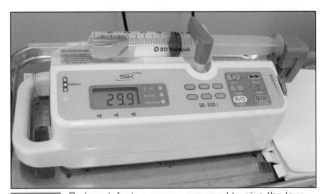

11.16 Syringe infusion pumps are used to give the low and precise flow rates required for continuous intravenous fluid therapy in birds.

birds cannot tolerate the handling needed for a one-off intravenous bolus or even, in some cases, intraosseous fluids; however, these birds are the ones most in need of intravenous fluids. These birds should be placed in a warm humid environment and, if possible, subcutaneous fluids administered.

Oral fluids

There are various commercially available avian oral rehydration products. These products or lactated Ringer's solution can be delivered by crop needle or tube. Rigid crop needles made of stainless steel with a ball on the tip should be used. Sizes vary from 18 G for a Budgerigar and 16 G for a Cockatiel to 10–12 G and 16–20 cm long for macaws and cockatoos. For birds such as raptors, a crop tube or a plastic or rubber flexible tube can be used.

In most non-psittacine birds the tube passes relatively easily over the tongue and into the crop (Figure 11.17a). In psittacine birds it is more difficult to pass the rigid crop needle through the side of the beak and into the oesophagus without inadvertently entering the trachea (see Chapter 15).

Some birds will clamp down quite hard on the crop needle. If this happens, slowly rotate the crop needle back and forth while gently continuing to insert it. If an attempt is made to insert the crop needle at the tip of the beak, the bird will simply bite down on the crop needle and press its tongue upwards, precluding insertion. Once through the beak commissures, the crop needle is passed over the tongue, down the cervical oesophagus and into the crop. To confirm that the crop needle is not in the trachea, palpate the tip of the needle in the crop using the thumb or finger against the crop wall. Gently press the inserted crop needle against the skin. If the crop needle has been inadvertently placed in the trachea it will not freely move around in the crop, will not be palpable when pressed against the skin of the crop, and the tracheal rings may also be palpated around the crop needle. A small amount of fluid can be injected to assess the bird's reaction prior to injecting all the fluid through the crop needle. Once the crop needle is confirmed to be in the crop, fluids should be injected quite firmly (Figure 11.17b) and the crop needle removed from the crop as soon as the syringe is empty (Figure 11.17c).

Regurgitation of fluid back into the pharynx suggests that the crop has been overfilled, the tube is in the trachea or the operator's hand is pressing on the crop during the restraint process. If this occurs, the bird should be placed immediately in its cage or, preferably, in an oxygenated cage. As a general rule, 2–3% of an adult bird's bodyweight per oral feeding should be given. This may be built up to as high as 5–8% of bodyweight. In hand-fed juveniles, volumes greater than 5–10% of bodyweight can be used per feed. For all birds, the food or fluids should be fed warmed (around 38°C for neonates).

Oral to beak fluids and nutritional support

Smaller passerines, such as canaries and finches, may not tolerate the handling for administration of injectable fluids or crop tubing. These birds may have oral fluid therapy administered directly on to the beak, where it will be siphoned into the oral cavity. Some hand-reared parrots tolerate being fed or given oral fluid therapy by syringe directly to the mouth or beak.

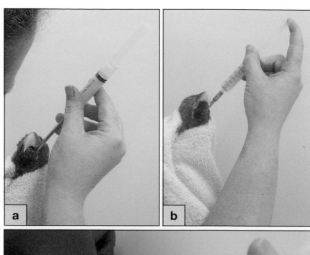
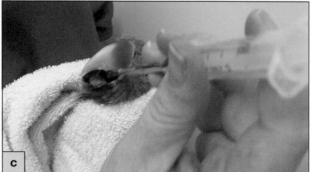

11.17   Administration of oral fluids. **(a)** Inserting the crop needle into the oral cavity. **(b)** Injection of the fluids into the crop. **(c)** Removal of the now empty crop needle.

Subcutaneous fluids

Subcutaneous fluids are given in the inguinal area, into the flap of skin between the medial upper femur and abdomen (Figure 11.18). This is usually the best location for psittacine birds as it allows greater volumes to be given (Figure 11.19). The subscapular region is an alternative site for subcutaneous fluid therapy. Higher doses of subcutaneous fluids may lead to the development of oedema, if poor circulation is present. Warmed lactated Ringer's solution is the preferred solution for subcutaneous fluid therapy. Occasionally, glucose is added to this, but caution should be exercised as the solution will become hypertonic, possibly resulting in the pooling of the fluids in the subcutaneous space (see Chapter 15 for technique).

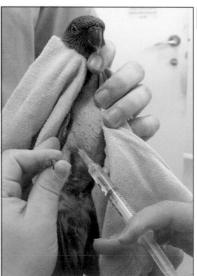

11.18

Administration of subcutaneous fluids.

Bird species	Volume (ml) dose given
Budgerigar	1–1.5
Cockatiel	2–3
Canary	0.2–0.5
Princess Parrot	2–3
Eclectus Parrot	8–10
Galah	8–10
Sulphur-crested Cockatoo	15–20
Rainbow Lorikeet	3
Peach-faced Lovebird	1–1.5
Finch	0.1–0.5

11.19 Volume of subcutaneous fluids that can be given in the inguinal area.

Intravenous fluids

The use of intravenous fluids during hypovolaemic shock or in collapsed patients is considered the most efficient method of administering fluid therapy. Intravenous fluids are given in the jugular, basilic (wing) (Figure 11.20) and medial metatarsal veins. The fluids

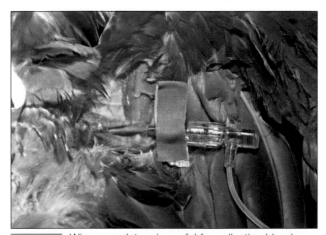

11.20 Wing vasculature is useful for collecting blood samples for measurement of packed cell volume and as an alternative site for fluid therapy.

may be given as a slow bolus (Figure 11.21) or a catheter may be placed in the vein for continuous infusion. The medial metatarsal vein is useful in larger birds and for continuous fluid administration. The basilic vein is useful for continuous fluid infusions in anaesthetized birds or for a single bolus of fluids. The jugular vein can be used for both boluses and continuous fluid infusions, although conscious birds may find the catheter uncomfortable and quickly remove it or chew the giving set (see below). Intravenous fluids are useful as a bolus perioperatively or as a constant-rate infusion during surgery. For constant-rate infusion, the catheter is attached to a syringe pump (see Figure 11.16). This will allow accurate fluid rates at very low-flow rates. The fluids should also be warmed to minimize hypothermia.

There are several complicating factors associated with the use of intravenous fluids in birds. The lack of ability to safely restrain severely debilitated birds to give fluids or place a catheter, especially in smaller birds, may preclude the use of intravenous fluids. In many cases, the bird must be anaesthetized to allow catheter placement. Haematomas at the site of venepuncture are very common, especially with the basilic vein. In small severely debilitated birds, the need for anaesthesia and risk of haematoma formation may preclude the use of catheters and constant infusion. Many birds, in particular parrots, are quite adept at removing catheters and giving sets. To avoid these problems, a slow bolus of fluids may be administered to smaller birds via a 25–27 G needle. The disadvantage of bolus fluids is the possibility of hypervolaemia, which may lead to polyuria and fluid loss. If a catheter and giving set are left in place in conscious birds, Elizabethan collars are required to avoid the birds chewing the giving set.

Intraosseous fluids

Intraosseous fluids have been advocated as a simpler method of administering fluid therapy to birds compared with intravenous fluids. This advantage must be weighed against the possibility of limb fracture during catheter placement, the pain associated with its placement and the lower fluid rates that can be given. The results are similar to intravenous administration, with

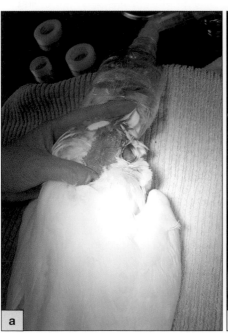

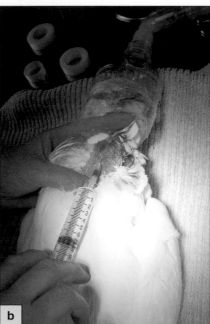

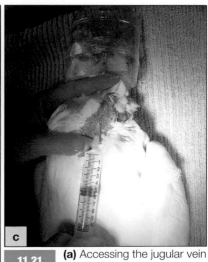

11.21 (a) Accessing the jugular vein for a bolus of intravenous fluids. (b) Checking the needle is in the jugular vein prior to administration of the fluid bolus. (c) Slow injection of the bolus of warmed intravenous fluids.

50% of the fluid appearing in the circulation within 30 seconds. Intraosseus fluids are advocated for longer surgical procedures and for the first 1–2 days of hypovolaemic shock. Except in moribund birds, an anaesthetic is required as there is pain associated with the placement of the catheter (see Chapter 15 for technique).

Fluid rates for intraosseous and intravenous fluids

Isotonic fluids are regularly used in birds. Fluids are administered at 3–10 ml/kg/hour. Fluid boluses can be given slowly over 2 minutes at 20–30 ml/kg. Higher rates of continuous intravenous infusion, of up to 100 ml/kg/hour, have been reported but are rarely used as they can cause fluid overload. The intraosseous space, unlike veins, does not expand. This limits the speed at which intraosseous fluids can be administered. Crystalloids, colloids and whole blood are also used, as in mammals.

Nutritional support

Assisted feeding is one of the mainstays of hospital care for sick and injured birds. Birds have a large surface area to bodyweight ratio and a high metabolic rate. Unwell birds will be in a catabolic state even if eating moderately. Many sick birds are anorexic in hospital. Assisted feeding should be considered in all but the healthiest of hospitalized birds, as long as they are not vomiting, regurgitating or collapsed. For nutritional support, foods are given in a similar manner to oral fluids (Figure 11.22). Hand-rearing formulas are often given via crop gavage, as many other foods do not easily pass through a rigid crop needle. If possible, commercial crumble or pellets can be dissolved and fed through the crop needle to adult birds. Nasogastric tubes cannot be placed in birds. If crop tubing is not possible, an oesophageal tube may need to be placed.

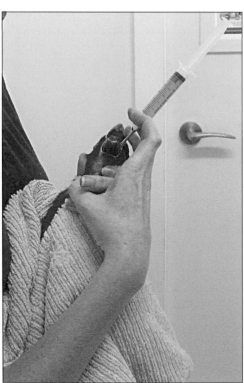

11.22 Oral nutritional support being given via a crop needle.

Levels of nutritional support

Level 1: Severely debilitated bird suffering starvation or sepsis

Glucose should be added to the fluid therapy regime. Treatment can involve intravenous 25% dextrose given slowly to effect at 1–2 ml/kg. In dehydrated patients, add glucose at a 5% solution to lactated Ringer's by adding 1 ml of 50% glucose to every 9 ml of lactated Ringer's. It is advisable to check the blood glucose level prior to instituting the fluid therapy.

Level 2: Upright with severe beak, oral or crop lesion present

Continue fluid therapy and glucose. If vomiting continues for more than 48–72 hours and no gastrointestinal blockage is present, consider placing an oesophageal tube. A soft oesophageal tube can be placed through an incision at the base of the mandible. Enteral feeding has also been described for larger birds by surgically implanting a Foley catheter into the proximal duodenum, with the catheter exiting through the lower abdominal wall.

Level 3: Able to stand upright, semi-stable, not vomiting or regurgitating

The bird should initially start on a commercial electrolyte solution or an emergency avian replacement supplement. These contain electrolytes, vitamins and carbohydrates, with some also having protein supplements. The supplement should be used in the first 24 hours to provide a highly metabolizable source of energy, although after 24–48 hours (earlier in birds less than 100 g) further nutritional support will be required. Once fluid deficits have been replaced and the bird requires only maintenance fluids (usually after 48–72 hours), then appropriate doses of oral electrolyte solution can replace subcutaneous fluids. This can be in the form of neonatal hand-rearing formulas or an adult commercial formulated diet added as partial supplements to the commercial avian emergency replacement supplement. The food must be crushed and dissolved adequately to pass through a crop needle or tube. These birds should be crop fed 3–5 times per day.

Level 4: Nutritional support for birds in a catabolic state in hospital

These birds may be eating moderately or not at all. The amount and type of food supplements will be determined in part by how much the bird is eating. Non-carnivorous birds should be fed 2–4 times daily by crop tube. Some passerines and smaller psittacine birds may be fed by inserting a syringe into the oral cavity. Once stabilized, adult hand-reared birds may revert to juvenile behaviour and be fed by syringe or spoon fed into the oral cavity. Longer-term food support (depending on the species) should be similar to the bird's normal adult nutritional maintenance food (e.g. dissolved commercial pellets, lorikeet wet mixes and insectivore mixes). This may not easily pass through smaller crop needles, and may require the addition of a small pinch of commercially available pancreatic enzymes to help dissolve the food. In some circumstances, a larger crop needle may need to be used, but with caution, as this may irritate the oral cavity and pharynx, affecting the bird's desire to eat on its own.

Calculating daily fluid requirements

Total fluids per day are calculated by a method similar to that used for mammals. Maintenance fluid therapy is based upon 5% of bodyweight. However, different bird species in different physiological states may have higher than 5% maintenance levels; for example, layer chickens consume 13.5% of their bodyweight per day and growing chickens 18–20% of their bodyweight. Birds eating pelleted foods in hospital will usually require higher fluid maintenance levels than those on seed diets. Once the maintenance fluids have been estimated, the additional replacement fluid level needs to be calculated.

Various methods have been described to determine the degree of dehydration (e.g. skin and eyelid tenting, packed cell volume (PCV), mucous membrane colour and capillary refill time). However, in the clinical situation, and in fully feathered birds, the level of dehydration is quite difficult to assess. Therefore, it is best to assume that a bird is at least 5–10% dehydrated. The standard formula for calculating the total daily fluid requirement is:

Maintenance fluids (x) + assessed dehydration (y) = total (z)

On a practical level, fluids are given as 10% of bodyweight daily (100 ml/kg bodyweight/day) for 3 days and then at a maintenance rate of 5% thereafter. To achieve this level of fluid therapy over 3 days, fluids may be divided into 2–4 doses per day at approximately 2–3 ml/100 g bodyweight (20–30 ml/kg per dose). This makes a total daily dose of approximately 50–100 ml/kg/day.

Packed cell volume as an indicator of deydration

The PCV is normally 35–55%. It varies between species, as well as with age and breeding status. An increased PCV may be an indicator of dehydration. Dehydration can also be indicated when there is a combined increase in PCV, total solids/total protein and urea (see Chapter 12).

Emergency medications

The use of antibiotics and antitoxins (such as calcium EDTA) may be warranted if the history indicates they are necessary for immediate treatment of a life-threatening condition. However, it is preferable to wait for a diagnosis prior to administering any medications. When administering emergency medications, it should be borne in mind that some birds will have, at least, a secondary bacterial infection. Emergency medications can obscure a definitive diagnosis, but this is a secondary consideration in such cases.

Diazepam (at 0.5 mg/kg i.v., i.m. or s.c.) can be administered in cases of seizuring birds.

Corticosteroid use is controversial as it may lead to extreme immunosuppression, adrenal suppression and poor wound healing. Its use should be limited to birds with cranial tumours and, debatably, for immediate use in some patients with head trauma, tick bite reactions and other acute inflammatory conditions (e.g. those that may lead to acute airway problems), as well as spinal cases. For cranial tumours, dexamethasone sodium phosphate (2 mg/kg i.v. or i.m. once) has been used in birds. For more acute cases it is preferable to use ultra-short-acting intravenous preparations.

Oxygen supplementation

Oxygen therapy is required for dyspnoeic birds. Dyspnoeic birds may have simple infections, aerosol toxicosis, tracheal obstruction or pressure in the coelomic cavity affecting the air sacs. Common signs of dyspnoea include open-beak breathing, respiratory noise and tail bobbing.

Most semi-active non-collapsed birds will not tolerate manual restraint and an oxygen mask placed on their face; birds will usually need to be placed in some form of oxygen chamber. An enclosed space such as an incubator or oxygen box can be used. A simple method, when no other option is available, is to place cling wrap around a small cage and pipe oxygen into the cage (Figure 11.23). A large facemask can be placed completely over a smaller bird to provide high levels of oxygen immediately. Studies show that birds cannot tolerate continual long periods of 100% oxygen therapy as they may suffer 'oxygen toxicosis', possibly from perivascular oedema. The aim is to provide an oxygen concentration of 40–50% for 1–2 hours, and then reassess. If a bird is unable to cope without oxygen supplementation, it will need to continue. Severely dyspnoeic birds cannot be handled immediately and should be placed in an oxygen chamber. Any examination or procedures must be performed in small steps, returning the bird to the oxygen chamber between each stage.

Air sac tube placement

If a tracheal obstruction is present, inserting a catheter into the left caudal thoracic air sac will give immediate relief from dyspnoea. These birds will exhibit open-beak breathing, usually with an outstretched neck, and a 'squeaking' sound on respiration. Tracheal or syringeal obstruction is commonly caused by inhaled foreign

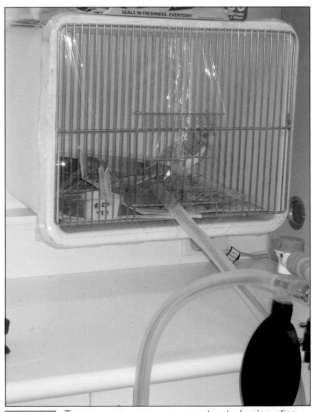

11.23 Temporary oxygen cage constructed using cling wrap.

bodies (such as seeds), *Aspergillus* granulomas and plaques from bacterial infections. Air sac tubes are contraindicated in birds with lower respiratory tract disorders due to ascites or organomegaly. Birds affected by airborne toxins from smoke and polytetraflouroethylene (from non-stick pans) will show no improvement with placement of air sac tubes. See Chapter 16 for placement technique.

As with the insertion of an endotracheal tube into the trachea, patency is determined by observing air movements or vapour in the tube on expiration. It is not uncommon for the tube to move or lie against the internal organs or air sac walls. If patency seems to disappear, retract the tube slightly to avoid contact with internal coelomic structures. Once the tube is correctly placed, suture the tube to the skin incision using the finger trap method or butterfly tape and suture around the tube (Figure 11.24). The external end of the tube should be long enough to extend past and be secured to the bird's tail. The tube can be left in place for several days. Often, as the bird's dyspnoea improves, its movements around the cage will lead to shifting of the tube within the coelomic cavity, compromising the patency of the air sac tube. If this is the case, the tube may need to be reinserted or slightly shifted manually.

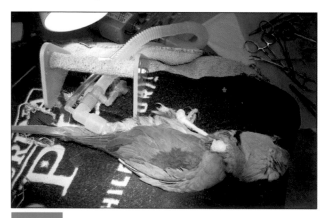

11.24 Air sac tube in place.

Specific emergencies

Burns

Burns may occur because a flying bird has accidentally landed in boiling water or cooking oil, or because the owner has placed the bird too close to a heat lamp or heater. Liquid burns are mostly confined to the feet and legs if the bird is removed quickly, whereas heat lamp burns are more commonly seen on the upper half of the body.

Initially, a burn may not appear to be severe. Wounds should be cleaned with cool water and dilute chlorhexidine, and standard fluid therapy commenced. These birds, despite their heat-related burns, may become hypothermic and so, once treated, need access to a heat source. After cleaning, the affected unfeathered areas should be covered with silver sulfadiazine. If oil is involved, it should be removed using very dilute washing-up liquid (see 'Oil contamination'). Appropriate antibiotic cover for *Pseudomonas* spp. and Gram-positive cocci, as well as analgesics, should be prescribed. The bird needs to be monitored for a minimum of 3 days to assess the seriousness of the burns,

as blisters may take this long to form. If severe necrosis appears, debriding the area may be warranted. In severe cases, the wounds may also need regular bandaging for 1–3 weeks, as per standard burn wound healing treatments.

> **WARNING**
>
> DO NOT use corticosteroid or oil-based creams on burns, as these affect feather integrity and, if ingested, potentially cause immunosuppression

Oil contamination

Pet and wild birds are inquisitive and may land in unheated oil or be iatrogenically coated with oily medications and other compounds. Wild birds may present with commercial oil contamination (Figure 11.25). Oily feathers cannot insulate the bird, thus all birds should be treated for hypothermia. The safest and simplest way to remove the oil is with a dilute dish-washing detergent. The oil will need to be removed in stages, alternating between washing, cleaning and drying (in a heated room or with a hair dryer) and resting in a heated environment.

Hyperthermia

Birds do not have sweat glands and therefore cannot dissipate heat easily, although they are insulated from moderate heat exposure by their feathers. As a bird progresses to hyperthermia, it will exhibit open-beak

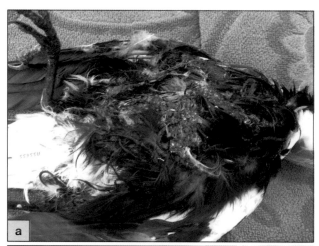

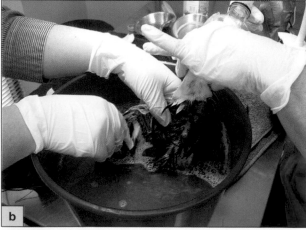

11.25 **(a)** Magpie covered in tar and oil. **(b)** The tar and oil are removed in stages by warm bathing in dilute detergent, with the magpie under anaesthetic.

breathing and usually hold its wings away from its body. Hyperthermia can be distinguished from respiratory distress by the fact that in patients with hyperthermia the feathers are not 'fluffed up' and there is rarely any audible respiratory whistle or click. There is also a history of heat exposure, especially related to hot days, usually with direct sunlight exposure.

Untreated overheated birds will progress to hyperthermia, ataxia and seizures. Cool the bird by misting or, if severe, wetting the feathers with water. Subcutaneous fluids are administered in milder cases or combined with small doses of intravenous fluids in severe cases. The bird must not be overcooled.

Haemorrhage

Acute haemorrhage is often related to trauma from beak injuries, flight-related misadventures and bleeding nails, as well as fight and/or bite-related injuries. Blood loss may also be related to self-trauma, bleeding subcutaneous lipomas and coagulopathies related to poor liver function (Figure 11.26). Although birds appear to lose large volumes of blood, they are able to withstand comparatively higher blood volume losses per unit bodyweight in comparison with small animal patients. Birds can lose 30% of their blood volume with only moderate clinical signs. This may be due to their ability to mobilize immature red blood cells and the absence of an autonomic response to haemorrhage that in mammals contributes to haemorrhagic shock. Blood loss is more serious in malnourished and/or unwell birds. These birds may have coagulopathies related to high-fat diets and liver problems.

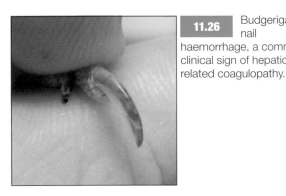

11.26 Budgerigar with nail haemorrhage, a common clinical sign of hepatic-related coagulopathy.

The clinical signs of severe anaemia from blood loss in birds are pale mucous membranes and pale skin on the feet and nares. The birds will often be tachypnoeic and, although hard to determine in small birds, tachycardic.

Oxygen therapy is required to increase the efficiency of the remaining red blood cells. Stemming the haemorrhage is of primary importance.

Haemostasis for specific haemorrhage sites

For cases of self-trauma, or if the bird continues to cause haemorrhage by picking or biting at the site of blood loss, an Elizabethan collar may need to be placed on the bird. This should be used only if the bird continues to irritate the area, as collars are generally too cumbersome and heavy for the already weakened bird.

Blood loss from broken nails often appears more serious than it is, with the apparent large volumes of blood seen in the cage caused by the bird hopping around the cage, spreading what is actually a small volume of blood much further (Figure 11.27). Applying

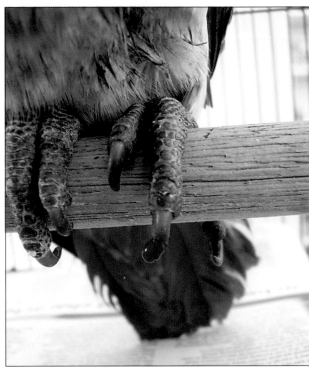

11.27 The volume of blood associated with bleeding nail tips may, on first appearance, seem to be large relative to the bird's bodyweight. Birds can spread a small amount of blood widely in their cage.

pressure at the site of haemorrhage rarely stops the bleeding. Many simple nail haemorrhages can be stemmed with standard chemical cauterization. If bleeding continues, clipping the bleeding area and cauterizing the tip under anaesthesia will arrest the bleeding. In some cases, each time the bird moves or attempts to clean the cauterizing material off the nail, the haemorrhage returns. In these cases, the two adjacent toes may need to be bandaged together for a short period or an Elizabethan collar may be placed. Rarely is electrocautery, under anaesthesia, necessary to achieve haemostasis. Clients at home can be advised to press plain flour or corn starch on to the site of haemorrhage until they can access veterinary care.

Beaks may bleed after bite wounds from other birds, as a result of getting caught in a door and after beak trimming. As with nails, pressure on the site of haemorrhage rarely stops the bleeding. Chemical cauterization should be used with caution as the bird may inhale the dry cauterizing material. In some cases, electrocautery under anaesthesia is necessary to achieve haemostasis. Following haemostasis, many birds will need at least 1–7 days of analgesic and nutritional support, in addition to fluid therapy, as the pain may decrease the bird's use of its beak for prehension (Figure 11.28). At home, as with nail haemorrhage, corn starch or flour can be placed on the beak tip to stem the bleeding until the client can access veterinary care.

Feathers are usually broken due to trauma after a bird flies into the cage sides when frightened or during a 'night fright'. Feather haemorrhage is more common in birds that have had wing clips, especially if the clip is severe. The shaft of growing feathers has a vascular supply. Once the feather has fully grown the blood vessels recede. The immature feathers, or blood feathers, on the wings and tail rely on the surrounding feathers to splint and protect them until they are fully grown

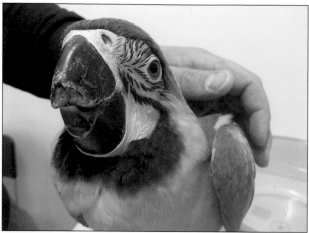

11.28 This macaw still requires some nutritional support several weeks after severe beak trauma.

and the blood vessels recede. If the wing is clipped, the growing blood feather may be exposed to traumatic incidents.

The bird may be presented with multiple wing or tail feathers covered in blood but with only one bleeding feather (Figure 11.29). The complete removal of the broken blood feather(s), including the base, will significantly decrease the bleeding. To remove it, the base of the feather should be grasped and pulled with a haemostat, forceps or thumb and finger, whilst the base of the skin around the feather is held with the other thumb and finger. If the bleeding continues, apply gentle pressure to the area. Birds may also catch their wing tip in the cage wire, losing multiple blood feathers and large areas of the wing tip skin. If multiple feathers have been lost, a bandage will need to be applied to the wing tip to decrease further trauma and haemorrhage.

Wounds resulting from trauma, self-trauma and bleeding lesions may need to be bandaged to avoid further blood loss. If on a wing or a leg, a simple pressure bandage can be applied (Figure 11.30). For wounds involving the thorax or the abdomen, a full body bandage is required. Care must be taken to apply enough pressure for haemostasis but without compromising respiratory effort.

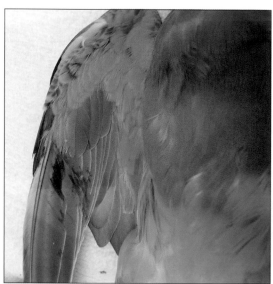

11.29 One broken feather may result in blood across the wing.

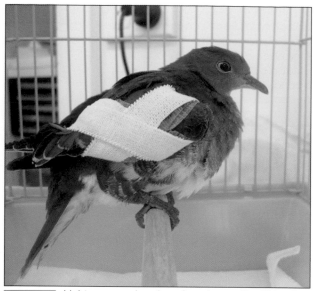

11.30 Light pressure bandage for a traumatized bleeding wing.

Blood transfusions

Birds with a PCV of less than 20%, or when there has been more than 3 ml/100 g bodyweight blood loss following haemorrhage, may benefit from a blood transfusion or use of synthetic replacements (e.g. Oxyglobin®) (Figure 11.31). Less serious problems can be dealt with via intravenous or intraosseous crystalloids or standard fluids. In cases where there is no alternative available, subcutaneous fluids should be used and the bird placed in a heated environment (although this is not ideal, as poor circulation affects fluid uptake from the subcutaneous tissues). Fortunately, birds mobilize immature red blood cells quite quickly and, as long as the fluids maintain adequate vascular pressure, the PCV should return to normal within 7 days.

It is important to assess the likelihood of the bird surviving the transfusion procedure (likely requiring general anaesthesia and/or restraint) in comparison to the benefits of the transfusion.

Animal bites

Birds are commonly presented with animal bites. Smaller wild passerines may be presented for cat bites, and larger captive birds for dog and, occasionally, cat bites. Smaller birds that are placed in cages outside in the

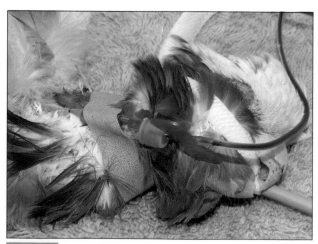

11.31 Blood transfusion. (Courtesy of RJ Doneley)

daytime may be attacked by wild carnivorous birds and, if left outside at night, attacked by rats. Feathers can act as a cushion to prevent some damage, but may also mask smaller penetrating wounds from cats. If a cat has been seen attacking the bird, even when no wounds are visible, a short course of antibiotics should be considered.

If a parrot attacks another parrot there are usually two bite wounds, often with a deeper one from the upper maxilla. The wounds are usually on the feet or on the beak. Occasionally, other birds will bite the dorsal head caudal to the crest (Figure 11.32).

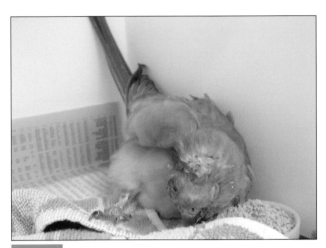

11.32 Head trauma following attack by a cage mate.

Rats often bite the bird's toes and are the usual cause of a bird presented missing the whole or part of its leg. Dog bites will usually have two entry points and the wound may be on any part of the body. Some dogs will hold the bird in their mouth without biting through the feathers or penetrating the skin. Wild birds may spear smaller birds, such as canaries, through the cage wire, leaving deep wounds or fractured limbs.

Penicillin antibiotics, such as co-amoxiclav, are the drugs of choice for traumatic bite wounds. Fluoroquinolones alone, such as enrofloxacin, do not have the appropriate broad spectrum of action to be effective in treating bite wounds. Analgesia and fluid therapy should also be provided. Many small to moderate wounds may require some debriding, but suturing the wound closed is often unnecessary as avian skin migrates quite quickly to cover comparatively large wound areas. The exception is areas of high movement, for example on wing joints, where sutures may be required.

Cardiopulmonary resuscitation

Cardiopulmonary resuscitation (CPR) of birds follows similar routines to those for mammalian species. It is rarely successful in severely debilitated birds but should be attempted in all healthy birds that have suffered a sudden misadventure, including anaesthetic problems (see Chapter 16).

Seizures

For information on seizures, see Chapter 32.

Sample taking and basic clinical pathology

12

John Chitty

Clinical examination and history taking are the mainstays of any clinical investigation. However, in birds, these are rarely sufficient to result in a complete diagnosis. Many diseases present with similar clinical signs, so it is therefore necessary in most investigations to take clinical samples for laboratory analysis (Figure 12.1). There are many options available to clinicians and this chapter will describe some of the more commonly performed tests. Obtaining a good quality sample, and the correct handling and storage of that sample, are vital in order to gain accurate clinically useful results (Figure 12.2).

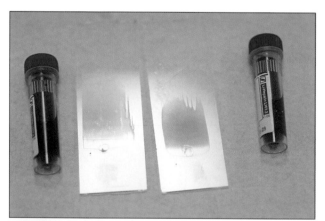

12.1 Typical sample: two x 1.3 ml heparinized blood samples and two air-dried smears. This is sufficient to allow electrolyte analysis plus a full profile and electrophoresis. (© John Chitty)

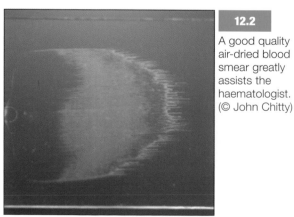

12.2 A good quality air-dried blood smear greatly assists the haematologist. (© John Chitty)

Internal *versus* external laboratory

There is often a debate about the benefits of performing laboratory tests in-house or via an external laboratory (Figure 12.3). To a large extent, the answer depends on which external laboratory and also which facilities (and staffing) are available in-house. Before using a particular external laboratory, its experience in avian clinical pathology should be ascertained, as well as its test availability and requirements in terms of sample quality and handling, and turnaround time for urgent samples.

External laboratory
- Minimum 24-hour delay in results unless close to hand
- No outlay on equipment, staff or disposables
- Minimal profit
- Access to clinical pathology specialists and specialized technicians
- Not all laboratories experienced with avian samples
- Equipment maintained and regular internal and external verification procedures

In-house laboratory
- Almost immediate results
- Expensive to run
- Potentially profitable
- Dependent on interest, ability and time constraints of staff
- Opportunity to gain experience through caseload
- Often issues with maintenance and irregular verification procedures

12.3 Considerations when deciding between in-house and external laboratories.

With respect to in-house laboratories, the experience of laboratory technicians is of great importance, as is the type of equipment available and whether or not it is validated for avian samples. For some biochemistry analysers, it is also important to ascertain whether or not 'standard' normal values are applicable (Johnston *et al.*, 2007).

In summary, the need for fast results must be balanced with the production of accurate verifiable results. Therefore, when establishing a practice laboratory, it can be helpful to identify which tests are essential to have immediately for the critical patient and which are not (Figure 12.4).

Important to have immediate results

- Haematocrit
- Plasma glucose
- Plasma electrolytes
- Acid–base balance
- Cytology

Desirable to have immediate results

- Renal parameters
- Plasma protein analysis
- Liver parameters
- Fluid analysis
- Haematology counts

Not vital to have immediately

- Bacteriology
- Hormone assays
- Serology
- Electrophoresis

12.4 Importance of rapid results for various laboratory tests.

Sampling methods

Blood sampling

Indications
Given the difficulties in diagnosing disease on the basis of clinical signs, blood sampling for haematological, biochemical and/or serological analyses is extremely useful in the investigation of most sick birds presented. As with all sampling, a good quality sample is vital in order to gain good results; blood samples are easily damaged by poor sampling technique or poor sample handling.

Sampling
A surprisingly large volume of blood may be taken from a bird for sampling (Figure 12.5), from various sites (Figures 12.6–12.10). As in mammals, blood volume may be calculated as 10% of bodyweight (i.e. a 500 g bird has 50 ml circulating blood volume), and healthy

Species	Approximate 'normal' bodyweight	Blood volume that can be safely taken in sick birds (that have not already lost blood or body fluids)*
Canary	20 g	0.1–0.2 ml
Budgerigar	30 g	0.3–0.4 ml
Cockatiel	100–120 g	1 ml
African Grey Parrot	400 g	5 ml
Moluccan Cockatoo	1 kg	10 ml
Harris' Hawk	700–1400 g	7–15 ml

12.5 Blood volumes that may be collected in various species. *Do not take full amount unless imperative.

Site	Restraint	Advantages	Disadvantages	Recommended species	Tips
Right jugular vein (Figure 12.7) (see QRG 12.1)	▪ The bird should be restrained or anaesthetized and the neck extended ▪ Parting of the feathers reveals the vein running under a large apterium ▪ Placement of a digit at the base of the neck raises the vein	▪ Easy ▪ Large volumes can be taken ▪ Haemostasis relatively simple	▪ Very difficult for left-handed operators, although the left jugular vein may be utilized in larger species ▪ Handling may be difficult in larger raptors or macaws ▪ Struggling birds may cause laceration of the vein and fatal subcutaneous haemorrhage; general anaesthesia may therefore be appropriate, especially if inexperienced. Restraint may be stressful to sensitive or dyspnoeic birds	▪ Route of choice in passerines, raptors and parrots	▪ Anaesthesia may be recommended for this technique ▪ Gentle digital pressure is applied afterwards to avoid haematoma formation, which can be significant on occasion, especially in hepatopathies
Superficial ulnar/basilic vein (Figure 12.8) (see QRG 12.2)	▪ The bird should be restrained or anaesthetized and placed on its back ▪ One wing is extended and the vein visualized ▪ The operator raises the vein with their free hand	▪ Easier for left-handed operators ▪ Restraint relatively simple, especially in larger species	▪ Fragile vein and may be hard to draw large volumes, especially in smaller birds ▪ Haemostasis can be hard to achieve and the bird should be replaced in the cage to allow it to calm down and its blood pressure to drop (this is preferable to prolonged handling) ▪ Unlike jugular venepuncture, haemorrhage from this vein is unlikely to be fatal and is readily visible; however, small losses may cause a lot of mess and distress to owners ▪ Occasionally, a haematoma may form along with a slight wing drop that may last a day or two	▪ All, barring very small passerines/ psittacine birds	▪ To facilitate haemostasis a drop of tissue glue may be helpful

12.6 Venepuncture sites in birds. (continues)

Site	Restraint	Advantages	Disadvantages	Recommended species	Tips
Superficial plantar metatarsal/ caudal tibial vein (Figure 12.9) (see QRG 12.3)	■ The bird should be restrained and the leg extended ■ The operator can raise the vein with their free hand ■ Restraint is normally minimal	■ Superficial, simple to visualize and raise ■ In passerines, can be pricked to allow collection of blood drops ■ Useful to have haemostatic agents to hand to control bleeding	■ Haemostasis difficult, though short-term bandaging can be applied	■ The short tarsometatarsal bone of psittacine birds makes this vein difficult to access and use ■ In adult raptors it may be difficult to work close to the feet, but it is useful in juveniles and vultures of all ages	■ Tissue glue may facilitate haemostasis or a light temporary dressing may be applied
Toe clip		■ Traditionally, it has been felt that blood from nail clips would be contaminated with tissue fluid and urates. However, Bennett *et al.* (2015) showed this not to be the case	■ In raptors, damage to talons is generally undesirable. In all species it is likely that cutting nails to the quick would cause pain and thus compromise welfare ■ Clinically useful volumes are hard to obtain in this manner		■ In all species: not recommended due to potential contamination of collected blood with urates and tissue fluid, as well as welfare concerns

12.6 (continued) Venepuncture sites in birds.

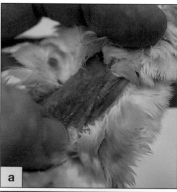

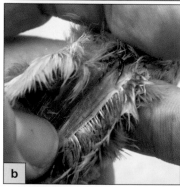

12.7 **(a)** Right jugular vein in a Cockatiel. **(b)** A modified ringer's grip allows access to the jugular vein in this Greenfinch. (© John Chitty)

12.8 Ulnar (basilic) vein in a Senegal Parrot. (© John Chitty)

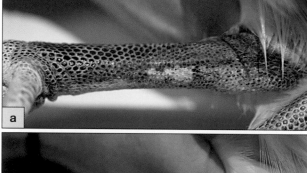

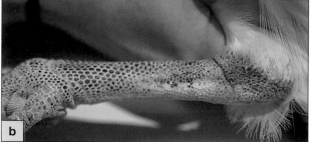

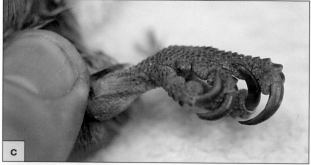

12.9 Caudal tibial vein. **(a)** King Vulture. **(b)** The same region in a King Vulture before vigorous cleaning. (Note the urates on the skin: this is a feature of New World vultures and the skin must be cleaned before venepuncture.) **(c)** Conure. The vein is short and tortuous, and hard to utilize. (Note: green staining on the feet is from perch pigment.) (© John Chitty)

12.10 **(a–b)** Arterial blood sampling in parrots. The arrows indicate the brachial artery. (Courtesy of A Montesinos)

birds have been shown capable of 40–50% blood volume loss before entering hypovolaemic shock. Even though sick birds are more likely to be less tolerant of blood loss, it is safe to presume that up to 2–3% bodyweight may be taken in sampling.

Even very small volumes of blood can impart considerable information on the bird's clinical condition; for example, 0.1 ml from a Canary can be used for:

- Blood smear (Figure 12.11)
- Haematocrit tube (Figure 12.12):
  - Packed cell volume
  - Buffy coat
  - Total solids

Many in-house analysers can assess a range of parameters on 0.1 ml blood, in some cases full biochemistry panels, but certainly essential critical care parameters including electrolytes, glucose and haematocrit

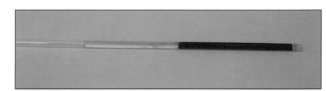

12.12 Haematocrit tube. This test allows packed cell volume measurement, analysis of total solids from the plasma, and assessment of the buffy layer (between red cells and plasma) which gives a rough estimation of white cells. (© John Chitty)

Samples should be taken into heparin for both haematology and biochemistry; EDTA appears to lyse cells in many species. In addition, fresh air-dried smears should always be made whenever blood is taken to negate any effects of the anticoagulant.

When analysing in-house, smears may be stained with routine commercial trichrome stains. While not producing as good quality staining as traditional stains, such as Wright's or Giemsa, the commercial products are much simpler to use and produce reasonable

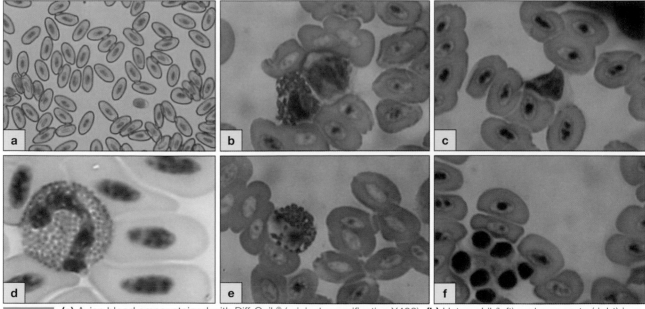

12.11 **(a)** Avian blood smear stained with Diff-Quik® (original magnification X400). **(b)** Heterophil (left) and monocyte (right) in a blood smear (original magnification X1000). **(c)** Avian lymphocyte (original magnification X1000). **(d)** Avian eosinophil (original magnification X1000). **(e)** Avian basophil (original magnification X1000). **(f)** Clump of thrombocytes with normal morphology (original magnification X1000). (a, d, © John Chitty; b, c, e, f, © Nick Carmichael)

quality repeatable results. Good quality references are available to aid the recognition of cells (e.g. Campbell *et al.*, 2007; Clark *et al.*, 2009; Latimer, 2011).

Interpretation

Interpretation is not always straightforward. Finding accurate normal values is a major problem in many of the species seen in practice. Whether using laboratory or machine normal ranges or tables of reference ranges from textbooks, it is important to know the details of the animals used to create these values. These details include the number of animals, whether wild-caught or captive, whether healthy or sick at the time of sampling, and whether the samples were opportunistic or planned. See Appendix 3 for tables of selected normal values.

Haematology

Absolute counts can be very useful; however, relative counts may also provide important information (e.g. a relative monocytosis with normal cell counts may still indicate a chronic inflammatory reaction).

Knowledge of species-specific responses is also essential; for example, most birds utilize the heterophil as the primary cell in inflammatory responses. However, some species (e.g. cockatoos) are more likely to show lymphocytosis in inflammation, and healthy birds may even exhibit a reversed differential. Similarly, age-related and sex-related variations should always be taken into account.

Even more important than the cell count is cell morphology, and it is for this reason in particular that an experienced avian cytologist is imperative in the interpretation of haematological samples. Evidence of toxicity in cell lines is indicative of an active inflammatory response regardless of white cell counts.

In anaemic birds, it is essential to type the anaemia as regenerative or non-regenerative using cell morphology in order to determine the appropriate clinical approach. Additionally, blood parasites are much more common in birds than other domestic pets, and their accurate identification is required in order to determine their likely clinical significance (many species are not significant unless in large numbers and/or in young birds).

Figure 12.13 provides guidelines for interpreting haematological parameters in birds.

Biochemistry

Biochemical interpretation can be difficult and has the potential to raise more questions than it answers. As in other species, it is better used to confirm or deny differentials than to achieve definitive diagnosis in isolation. As with haematology, there are variations between species, ages and sexes.

Testing methodology can impact results. For example, the presence of a pre-albumin fraction in the protein spectrum means that standard wet and dry chemistry measurement of albumin and total protein to produce an estimated globulin level (and hence albumin:globulin ratio) is not accurate. Wherever possible, protein estimation should be via plasma or serum electrophoresis.

A guide to interpretation is provided in Figure 12.14.

Parameter	Conditions associated with a raised count	Conditions associated with a lowered count

Haematocrit/packed cell volume	■ Haemoconcentration (typically dehydration)
	■ Polycythaemia (extremely rare)
		■ Regenerative anaemia:
		  - Blood loss
		  - Haemolysis
		  - Blood parasites
		  - Lead toxicosis
		■ Non-regenerative anaemia:
		  - Bone marrow disease
		  - Renal disease
		  - Chronic debility and/or disease
		  - Lead toxicosis

Total white cell count	■ Inflammation and/or infection ■ Lymphoproliferative disease ■ Stress	■ Stress ■ Debility ■ Sequestration (especially in debilitated bird) ■ Toxicity
Heterophils (see Figure 12.11b)	■ Inflammation and/or infection (acute or chronic) ■ Stress	■ Debility ■ Sequestration (especially in debilitated bird)
Lymphocytes (see Figure 12.11c)	■ Inflammation/infection ■ Lymphoproliferative disease (rare)	■ Stress ■ Infection ■ Debility and/or chronic disease ■ Toxicity
Monocytes (see Figure 12.11b)	■ Chronic inflammatory response	Not applicable
Eosinophils (see Figure 12.11d)	■ Inflammatory response in mast cell-rich tissues (e.g. gut, lung, skin or reproductive system)	Not applicable
Basophils (see Figure 12.11e)	■ Inflammation and/or infection (an unusual finding and significance often unclear. Some authors (e.g. Fudge, 2000) state that basophilia may be seen in chlamydiosis)	Not applicable
Thrombocytes (see Figure 12.11f)	■ Platelet equivalent. Numbers less relevant than morphology. Can be seen phagocytosing bacteria in very intense immune reaction or septicaemia	■ Very rare; may indicate depletion or absolute lack

12.13   Interpretation of haematological parameters in birds.

Parameter	Conditions associated with a raised value	Conditions associated with a lowered value
Total protein	▪ Haemoconcentration ▪ Inflammatory disease	▪ Malnutrition ▪ Malabsorption ▪ Parasitism ▪ Liver disease ▪ Renal disease ▪ Gut disease ▪ Skin losses (extensive damage)
Albumin	▪ Haemoconcentration	▪ Malnutrition ▪ Malabsorption ▪ Parasitism ▪ Liver disease ▪ Renal disease ▪ Gut disease ▪ Skin losses (extensive damage)
Pre-albumin	▪ Early inflammatory response	See Albumin (above)
Alpha-globulin	▪ Acute inflammation ▪ Reproductively active female	▪ May reduce in later stages of inflammatory response
Beta-globulin	▪ Acute inflammation ▪ Acute or chronic responses in certain infections, e.g. aspergillosis (with rise in gamma-globulins)	Not applicable
Gamma-globulin	▪ Chronic inflammatory response (especially polyclonal) ▪ Monoclonal gammopathy seen rarely in lymphoproliferative disease	Not applicable
Uric acid	▪ Renal disease ▪ Postprandial (to be of value, uric acid testing must be performed after food has been withheld for 12–24 hours in raptors) ▪ Dehydration ▪ May be raised after a long journey	▪ Malnutrition/malabsorption ▪ Liver disease
Urea	▪ May rise with dehydration, otherwise of little value	Not applicable
Creatinine	No value	No value
Aspartate aminotransferase (AST)	▪ Hepatocellular damage ▪ Tissue damage ▪ Important to assess with CK; if CK is raised too then AST rise is likely due to tissue damage	Not applicable
Creatine kinase (CK)	▪ Tissue damage: rises possible even with difficult venepuncture ▪ Large rises seen in muscle damage and/or necrosis	Not applicable
Glutamate dehydrogenase (GLDH)	▪ Hepatocellular damage ▪ Specific but quite insensitive	Not applicable
Gamma-glutamyl transferase (GGT)	▪ Biliary stasis	Not applicable
Lactate dehydrogenase (LDH)	▪ Hepatocellular damage ▪ Tissue damage	Not applicable
Sodium	▪ Water deprivation ▪ Dehydration ▪ Salt poisoning	▪ Renal disease ▪ Iatrogenic (over-rehydration) ▪ Enteritis
Potassium	▪ Dehydration ▪ Renal disease ▪ Acidosis ▪ Easily raised artefactually by haemolysis; should always be measured patient-side or on separate sample	▪ Renal disease ▪ Alkalosis ▪ Diuresis
Ionized calcium	▪ Overdosage of calcium and/or activated vitamin D_3 supplements ▪ May be elevated in breeding females (and certainly should be at higher end of normal range), though ionized calcium is generally more tightly regulated than total calcium levels	▪ Malnutrition ▪ Malabsorption ▪ Lack of ultraviolet light exposure ▪ Renal disease ▪ Possibly idiopathic in Grey Parrots
Total calcium	▪ Consists of ionized (active) calcium and protein-bound (inactive) calcium, hence protein levels will affect total calcium levels with the result that some 'true' hypocalcaemic birds may appear normocalcaemic on total calcium. Similarly, apparent hypercalcaemia may simply reflect high protein levels	
Bile acids	▪ Liver dysfunction. Potentially of great use, but there are difficulties in interpretation, especially in continuously feeding granivores where marginal elevations may be questionable	Not applicable

12.14 Interpretation of biochemical parameters in birds. (continues) ▶

Parameter	Conditions associated with a raised value	Conditions associated with a lowered value
Cholesterol	▪ Excess dietary intake ▪ Hepatic lipidosis ▪ Breeding females ▪ Hypothyroidism ▪ May be linked to atherosclerosis	▪ Malnutrition and/or malabsorption
Triglycerides	▪ Excess dietary intake ▪ Hepatic lipidosis ▪ Breeding females ▪ May be linked to atherosclerosis	▪ Malnutrition and/or malabsorption

12.14 (continued) Interpretation of biochemical parameters in birds.

Arterial sampling

Although not commonly performed, arterial sampling can be very useful in blood gas assessment, especially during anaesthetic monitoring (see Figure 12.10).

Serology

As in other species, positive serology only indicates exposure to an agent. However, in conjunction with clinical signs and other clinical pathology or imaging, 'smoking gun' evidence of active infection may be provided. Serology is also a useful tool in screening healthy or in-contact birds for disease exposure.

The most common serological tests are for:

- *Chlamydia psittaci*
- Avian bornavirus
- *Aspergillus* spp.

See Chapter 19 for information on interpretation of results.

Toxicology

When investigating suspected toxicoses, it is vital to contact the testing laboratory before sampling, as different anticoagulants may be required.

Tests for heavy metals (lead and zinc) are most commonly performed. Blood lead levels are highly relevant, whereas plasma zinc levels correlate poorly with tissue levels and so may not prove diagnostic. Samples for zinc measurement should be taken in plastic syringes and transported in plastic-capped heparin tubes, as rubber plungers and caps may affect results.

Suggested avian blood screening 'panel'

- Full haematology
- Protein electrophoresis
- Total protein
- Uric acid
- Electrolytes
- Calcium (total and ionized)
- Enzymes:
  - Aspartate aminotransferase (AST)
  - Creatine kinase (CK)
  - Glutamate dehydrogenase (GLDH)
  - Gamma-glutamyl transferase (GGT)
- Bile acids
- Cholesterol
- Triglycerides

Faecal sampling

A lot of information can be gained from the gross appearance of the droppings (or 'mute' in raptors). The droppings consist of faeces, soluble and insoluble

urine, and so 'loose droppings' may represent diarrhoea or polyuria (see Appendix 4).

In caged birds, substrates, such as sandpaper or grit, contaminate the droppings, making microscopic analysis impossible. Therefore, owners should be advised to collect a day's droppings on newspaper or kitchen roll, thus allowing proper examination of the relative constituents of the droppings and the appearance of each. It is important to remember that droppings produced during travelling may be a lot looser (stress polyuria) than normal and that there is a great difference between species and feeding groups (e.g. seed-eating parrots have a smaller 'drier' dropping than raptors and nectar-feeding parrots such as lories and lorikeets).

Indications

Faecal examinations should be performed whenever there is evidence of true diarrhoea. In general, three different types of test should be considered:

- **Parasitology:** indicated in cases of weight loss; poor doing; loose or haemorrhagic faeces; or respiratory signs where gapeworm is suspected. Appropriate for birds kept in outdoor aviaries or those with access to soil or invertebrates periodically. Most indoor-kept caged birds are unlikely to suffer gut parasitism
- **Faecal cytology:** indicated in all cases of loose faeces in parrots. This test is not appropriate for raptors. Some texts recommend it as a health screening tool for parrots; however, there is little evidence to show that the morphology of the faecal bacterial flora is a sign of underlying poor health in an overtly healthy bird. Use of collected samples for this test will further reduce its effectiveness. Either very freshly voided samples, or cloacal swabs (Figure 12.15), should be used
- **Faecal culture:** indicated in cases of true diarrhoea in all species.

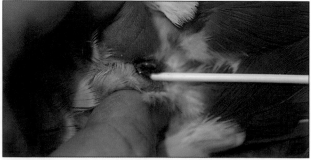

12.15 Cloacal swabbing is more likely to give meaningful cytology and culture results than use of voided samples. (© John Chitty)

For some parasitic (e.g. *Giardia*) or bacterial (e.g. *Chlamydia*) infections, where there is intermittent shedding of organisms, it may be appropriate to collect 3 days' droppings for testing. However, freshly voided samples are usually preferred.

Parasitology: Standard faecal flotation methods are appropriate for birds, as for conventional species. Where lungworm is suspected, Baermann techniques should be used; however, lungworm is unusual in the species covered in this manual.

Where only small amounts of faeces can be obtained, a simple wet preparation may be more appropriate than flotation, as this will at least give an indication of whether parasites are present and some qualitative guide to numbers. Clinicians should be aware of the parasite species likely to be found in each of these species and their relative pathogenicity. In raptors, it is important to recognize secondary parasitism (parasites that had infected prey and are simply passing through the predator).

Faecal cytology: In the 'normal' parrot, there should be a moderate number of organisms consisting of approximately 70% Gram-positive rods, 25% Gram-positive cocci and a few yeasts and Gram-negative rods (Figure 12.16). Departures from this (especially excessive or budding yeasts, large numbers of Gram-negative rods or the presence of large spore-forming Gram-positive rods) may indicate an unbalanced gut flora and the cause of the diarrhoea (Figure 12.17). This enables rapid and more appropriate 'first guess' antimicrobial use.

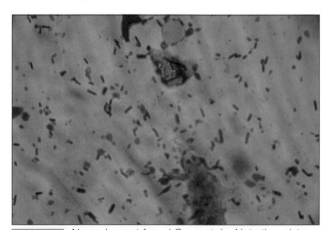

12.16   Normal parrot faecal Gram stain. Note the mixture of mainly Gram-positive cocci and rods. (© John Chitty)

Faecal culture: Interpretation of culture can be difficult and should be compared with cytology wherever possible. Isolation of *Salmonella* or *Campylobacter* spp. is relatively common (especially in raptors) and these may be part of a normal bacterial flora or can be pathogenic. Otherwise, all culture results must be interpreted in relation to the clinical signs (see Chapter 19).

Faecal wet smears

This is a quick and inexpensive way to identify a number of potential abnormalities in droppings. A small amount of faeces is diluted in either saline or a coloured counterstain (such as Diff-Quik® 2), and examined after applying a cover slip (Figure 12.18). Motile organisms (protozoa and bacteria) are easily identified. *Macrorhabdus* are also easily identified as large, cigar-shaped organisms with slightly mottled interiors. After some experience is gained, it is also possible to make a rough assessment of the bacterial level, and the morphology, which can dictate whether the clinician progresses to a Gram stain.

12.18   Faecal smear. It is important that the smears are not too thick. (© John Chitty)

Interpretation
For information on results interpretation, see Chapter 19.

Skin and feather sampling

Indications
Sampling of feathers and skin is indicated in all cases of dermatological disease or feather destructive disorders (see Chapter 30). The technique used should be appropriate to the lesions found. For a fuller discussion see Chitty (2005).

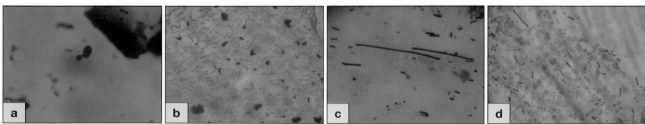

12.17   Abnormal parrot faecal Gram stains (original magnification X100). **(a)** Budding yeast cell indicates active yeast growth. This is a significant finding even if found in small numbers, as is development of pseudohyphae. **(b)** Overgrowth of Gram-negative rods is usually a sign of gut imbalance and is normally only seen in parrots with enteritis (it is normal in raptors). **(c)** Avian gastric yeast (*Macrorhabdus ornithogaster*, previously known as 'Megabacterium'). A few may be found in normal birds. However, large numbers in thin birds are likely very significant. **(d)** Gram-positive sporulating rods are likely to be *Clostridium* spp. and are not a normal finding. This parrot had acute enteritis. (© John Chitty)

Techniques

Skin scrape: This is performed where there are crusts or hyperkeratotic lesions suggestive of parasitism. The procedure is performed as in dogs or cats with the scraping being taken into 10% potassium hydroxide or liquid paraffin. Unlike in mammals, the cells are often present as 'rafts' or 'sheets'.

Lesions are most commonly found on the scaled areas of skin, with *Cnemidocoptes* mites being frequently implicated. Lesions on feathered skin (often around the head) may be associated with epidermoptid mites.

Feather digest: This is performed where there is evidence of feather damage but no parasites are found on gross examination. It is also useful where changes in the calamus (colour or increased opacity) indicate possible quill mite infestation. An erupting or damaged feather is digested in warmed 10% potassium hydroxide for 2 hours before centrifugation and microscopic examination.

Pulp cytology: Two techniques are described for different types of feather.

- For remiges and rectrices, the feather may be removed and the calamus cleaned and incised. Clear fluid forming along the cut may be collected for cytology; bloodstained fluid should be discarded. The rest of the feather pulp may be utilized for bacteriology (by inserting a small swab) and/or preserved for histopathology by placing the whole feather in formal saline.
- The other technique is indicated when birds are plucking body feathers and blood feathers are present. Here, the feather is removed and the sample obtained by gently squeezing the pulp, forcing fluid from the proximal end (Figure 12.19). The first drop is discarded, but subsequent clear fluid used to make a stained smear. Alternatively, the feather may be left *in situ* and fluid aspirated using a 1 ml syringe and 25 G 16 mm needle via the superior umbilicus (Figure 12.20).

Skin acetate: This technique is indicated where there is excessive scale, the skin appears 'dry' or where there are exudative, crusting or hyperkeratotic lesions. It is performed by placing acetate tape strips over the lesions. The tape is then placed on a microscope slide and stained.

Staining and examination of cytological specimens is similar to routine cytology (see below), with commercial trichrome stains being extremely useful.

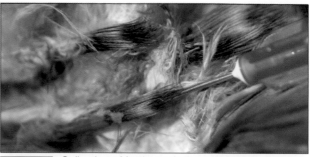

12.20 Collection of feather pulp from a blood feather. (© John Chitty)

Skin biopsy: In dermatological disease in other species, biopsy is most likely to give meaningful results. In birds this largely holds true, though lesions are unusual. Biopsy is indicated in all feather and/or skin disorders where there are obvious skin lesions or where there is apparent pruritus.

The technique of skin biopsy is similar to that in other species, though the elasticity of bird skin tends to result in a small curling sample and a large hole. To increase its usefulness, the following may help:

- Never prepare the biopsy site as per normal aseptic surgery
- Always include a blood feather in the biopsy sample (and request sectioning of this along with the skin)
- Remember that avian skin is very thin and it is easy to enter deeper structures, especially if using a biopsy punch; excisional surgery is usually safer
- Take samples from both affected and unaffected skin
- To improve orientation, place fresh biopsy specimens on plain kitchen roll, then place the specimen and paper together in formal saline (Figure 12.21)
- When performing biopsy in parrots (especially plucking birds), warn owners that the bird is very likely to remove the sutures. In these cases, biopsy sites can be managed as open wounds and allowed to granulate.

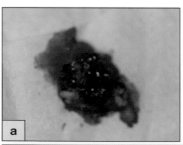

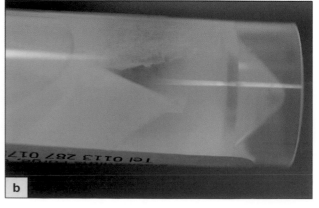

12.21 **(a)** Fresh skin biopsy specimen placed on paper. **(b)** Paper and biopsy sample in formal saline pot for submission. (© John Chitty)

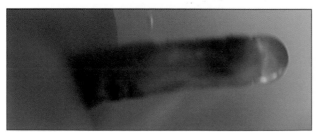

12.19 A drop of clear fluid is extruded from the tip of a feather. The initial blood-tinged portion is discarded and the second drop used to make a smear. (© John Chitty)

Interpretation

Cytological interpretation is similar to that of other organs (see below). It is important to be able to recognize parasites. Otherwise, inflammatory reactions are those most commonly encountered (Figure 12.22); neoplasia is unusual (though squamous cell carcinoma of the skin is common, it is often poorly exfoliative and biopsy is usually more diagnostic). There are a number of excellent guides for cytology (e.g. Campbell and Ellis, 2007; Samour, 2008; Doneley, 2011).

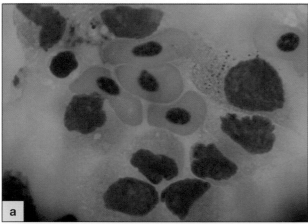

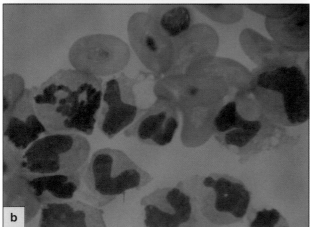

12.22 **(a–b)** Aspirates taken from feather pulp showing large numbers of mixed inflammatory cells (heterophils and monocytes) in a case of pulpitis. (© John Chitty)

Crop and proventricular washing and/or aspiration

Indications

Crop washing is indicated in all cases of regurgitation, especially in the smaller species (e.g. Budgerigars and Cockatiels) where crop infections are relatively common.

Proventricular washing is more useful in larger species where there is evidence of maldigestion (e.g. passing undigested seed), melaena, or proventricular enlargement on radiographs. In these cases it may also be combined with proventricular endoscopy and insertion of barium for contrast studies. While this is a relatively simple technique, it is possible to perforate the gut wall when passing a tube from the beak direct to the proventriculus. For this reason, proventricular washing should not be performed unless some experience has been gained in either cadavers or the wet lab situation. See the BSAVA Manual of Psittacine Birds for technique.

Interpretation

When crop washing (see QRG 12.4), a small sample is usually obtained and this should be examined immediately as a wet preparation, looking for trichomonads (Figure 12.23) and avian gastric yeast. If these are not obvious then slides should be air-dried and stained with a trichrome or Gram stain to assess the presence of bacteria and/or yeasts.

The presence of large numbers or budding yeasts or heavy monocultures of bacteria imply overgrowth and will help to direct antimicrobial therapy.

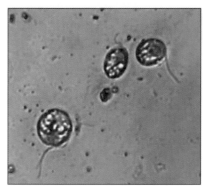

12.23 Trichomonads from a Budgerigar crop wash. These parasites may also be found in faecal samples. (© John Chitty)

Virological and mycoplasmal sampling

Indications

Viral isolation is rarely performed. Instead, polymerase chain reaction (PCR) and/or serological investigations are performed, with sampling directed by clinical signs. Mycoplasmal culture may be performed, (though specialized laboratories, sampling and transport materials are required), but has been largely superseded in practice by PCR tests. As these investigations are performed quite commonly, it is worth contacting the diagnostic laboratory to ascertain their requirements for each test (see Chapter 19).

Bacteriology

Antibiotic 'failure' is a common occurrence in avian practice. There may be a number of causes, including incorrect dose rate and/or drug, incorrect diagnosis or, potentially, failure of the bacteriology testing to show the pathogenic bacterial species and, therefore, the correct sensitivity pattern.

Effective sample taking can work towards avoiding these failures. The following questions should always be asked when taking bacteriology samples:

- **Are pathogens likely to be found?** Is this likely to be a bacterial lesion? Is there a particular pathogen it is likely to be associated with? Some lesions are not associated with bacteria at all or there may be sufficient inhibitory factors (e.g. sampling from the centre of an abscess) that there is little chance of any bacterial growth from a swab
- **Are commensals likely to be found?** All areas of the body are likely to be associated with commensal bacterial species. These may invade damaged tissue, or may be facultative pathogens or just normal 'passengers' in sampling
- **Is contamination likely to occur?** When internal areas are sampled, contamination from more superficial regions is common (Figure 12.24).

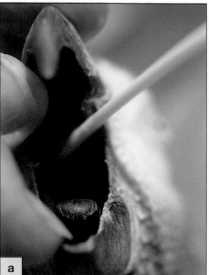

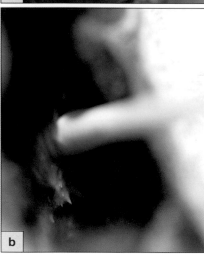

12.24 **(a–b)** When sampling the upper respiratory tract, use of the cranial portion of the choana is less likely to result in contamination than use of the nostril. However, screening of healthy birds via choanal swabbing is unlikely to achieve meaningful results. (© John Chitty)

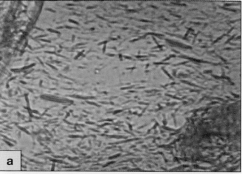

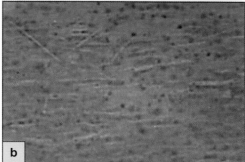

12.25 **(a)** Plain preparation of a joint aspirate showing urate crystals (gout) (original magnification X400). **(b)** The stained preparation. Staining will wash out crystals, though 'negative staining' may remain (original magnification X1000). Therefore joint aspirates should always be air-dried and examined as plain preparations before staining. (© John Chitty)

Urine sampling

Indications

Urine testing is less useful in birds because droppings are a mix of urine and faeces. Therefore, finding glucose in urine is not necessarily glucosuria unless there are very high levels. As with faeces, gross appearance of the droppings (see Chapter 10) may be more useful than laboratory testing. Excessive amounts may indicate polyuria. Blood may be seen through the liquid part of the dropping. It should be determined whether this is throughout the urine (and therefore of renal origin indicating conditions such as lead toxicosis in parrots) or as distinct haemorrhage (cloacal mixing, often of cloacal or reproductive tract origin, and the finding of biliverdinuria is an indicator of liver disease or the presence of green lead salts in lead toxicoses).

Droppings may be collected on paper and, if very quick, urine may be aspirated and checked for specific gravity and cytology (useful with respect to inflammatory cells and renal casts).

Cytological sampling

As in small animal practice, cytology is a very useful tool because it is quick, easy and cheap to perform and does not necessitate expensive analytical equipment.

Most techniques utilized in small animal medicine are also appropriate in birds (e.g. fine-needle aspirates, impression smears, washes) (Figure 12.26). Standard trichrome stains are most useful in practice, though Gram and modified Ziehl–Nielsen stains are also useful for assessment of bacterial, mycobacterial and protozoal infections.

There are several excellent guides to avian cytological techniques and interpretation available (e.g. Echols, 1999; Campbell and Ellis, 2007; Doneley, 2011).

Tips to obtain more meaningful bacteriology results

- Swab from deeper lesions, after superficial debris and contamination has been cleaned away
- Submit biopsy specimens for culture (e.g. infected bone or abscess wall)
- Utilize anaerobic and aerobic culture, especially in abscess specimens
- Cytological analysis. Aspirates (Figure 12.25) can be smeared on slides or direct impression smears of open lesions can be examined. Ideally, both a Gram stain and a trichrome stain (e.g. Diff-Quik®) should be used. The finding of inflammatory cells is always suggestive of infection (especially with mixed cell populations) and bacteria may be directly visualized. A sparse mixed population of bacteria suggests contamination or commensal organisms, whereas the presence of many monomorphic forms is of greater significance. This enables a rapid provisional diagnosis and prompt 'first guess' antibiosis based on bacterial morphology
- Histopathology. This will reveal organisms and cellular responses to them, which may help distinguish infection from contamination

Clinical sign	Appropriate sample
Ascites or pericardial effusion	Needle aspiration of fluid (Figure 12.27); ultrasound guidance useful
Organomegaly (especially liver, but any palpable mass)	Fine-needle aspirate; ultrasound guidance useful
Masses	Fine-needle aspirate
Neurological signs (e.g. seizures, torticollis, tremor)	Cerebrospinal fluid (Echols, 1999); it should be noted that this is extremely difficult in birds and sample harvest is very small. This should be attempted in the live patient only after extensive cadaver practice
Osteomyelitis	Intraosseous lavage; care should be taken with pneumatized bones
Upper respiratory disease (e.g. rhinoliths, nasal discharge, sneezing, head shaking)	Swabbing of the choanal slit (see Figure 12.24), or collection of nasal flush material via the choanal slit
Joint swelling	Joint aspirates to distinguish septic arthritis (Figure 12.28), osteoarthritis and gout (see Figure 12.25)

12.26 Clinical signs and appropriate samples for cytology. (Note: some sampling techniques will require anaesthesia to immobilize the bird.)

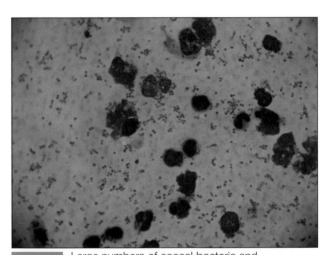

12.27 Large numbers of coccal bacteria and inflammatory cells indicate septic peritonitis and coccal infection. (© John Chitty)

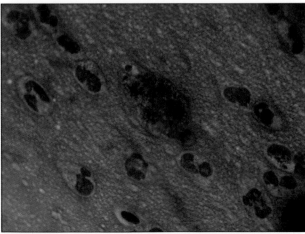

12.28 Joint aspirate in septic arthritis. Note the highly proteinaceous background and inflammatory cells. (© John Chitty)

Assessment of the 'normal' bird

Regular health checks of pet or falconry birds is recommended. In addition to a physical examination and faecal screening of birds kept outside, further laboratory testing may be requested, though in all cases it is most appropriate to assess an individual bird's need based on its signalment, husbandry and previous disease history.

Sampling recommended for newly acquired birds

- Full haematology
- Biochemistry panel (as described earlier)
- Infectious diseases:
  - *Chlamydia* serology and circovirus PCR in psittacine birds
  - Atoxoplasmosis (peripheral blood smear or buffy coat examination) in passerines. (Note this does not replace the need for adequate quarantine arrangements for birds entering collections.)

Routine health check

Healthy birds presented for routine health checks, which do not have a previous disease history either individually or in their collection, and have not been exposed to any other birds, do not require further laboratory testing on a regular basis. Regular monitoring of plasma ionized calcium may be appropriate for some indoor-housed Grey Parrots. Where owners are concerned, full haematology will likely provide the most appropriate test for general health monitoring.

Acknowledgements and declaration of interest

The author is a paid consultant to CTDS Lab Ltd and is grateful to Nick Carmichael MRCVS for pictures of blood cells.

References and further reading

Bennett TD, Lejnieks DV, Koepke H et al. (2015) Comparison of haematologic and biochemical test results in blood samples obtained by jugular venipuncture versus nail clip in Moluccan Cockatoos (*Cacatua moluccensis*). *Journal of Avian Medicine and Surgery* **29**, 303–312
Campbell TW and Ellis CK (2007) *Avian and Exotic Animal Hematology and Cytology, 3rd edn*. Blackwell Publishing, Ames
Chitty JR (2005) Feather and skin disorders. In: *BSAVA Manual of Psittacine Birds, 2nd edn*, ed. N Harcourt-Brown and J Chitty. BSAVA Publications, Gloucester
Chitty JR and Lierz M (2008) *BSAVA Manual of Raptors, Pigeons and Passerine Birds*. BSAVA Publications, Gloucester
Clark P, Boardman W and Raidal S (2009) *Atlas of Clinical Avian Hematology*. Wiley-Blackwell, Ames
Doneley B (2011) *Avian Medicine and Surgery in Practice: Companion and Aviary Birds*. Manson Publishing, London
Echols S (1999) Collecting diagnostic samples in avian patients. *Veterinary Clinics of North America: Exotic Animal Practice* **2**, 621–649
Fudge A (2000) *Laboratory Animal Medicine*. Saunders, Philadelphia
Harcourt-Brown N and Chitty JR (2005) *BSAVA Manual of Psittacine Birds, 2nd edn*. BSAVA Publications, Gloucester
Harrison G and Lightfoot T (2006) *Clinical Avian Medicine*. Spix Publishing, Palm Beach
Hawkey CM and Dennett TB (1989) *Comparative Veterinary Haematology*. Wolfe, London
Johnston MS, Rosenthal KL and Shofer FS (2007) Asessment of a point-of-care analyser and comparison with a commercial laboratory for the measurement of total protein and albumin concentrations in psittacines. *American Journal of Veterinary Research* **68**, 1348–1353
Latimer KS (2011) *Duncan and Prasse's Veterinary Laboratory Medicine: Clinical Pathology, 5th edn*. Wiley-Blackwell, Ames
Mayer J and Donnelly TM (2013) *Clinical Veterinary Advisor: Birds and Exotic Pets*. Saunders, St Louis
Melillo A (2013) *Clinical and Diagnostic Pathology. Veterinary Clinics of North America: Exotic Animal Practice, Vol 16*. Elsevier, Philadelphia
Samour J (2008) *Avian Medicine, 2nd edn*. Mosby Elsevier, Philadelphia

QRG 12.1: Blood sampling – jugular vein

Equipment

- Appropriately sized needles and syringes
- Cotton wool swabs
- Surgical spirit

> **PRACTICAL TIP**
> - Other than for very small birds, an assistant will be required

Patient preparation

The bird is anaesthetized or sedated or caught and wrapped in a towel.

Technique

1 The assistant should hold the bird in a towel.

2 Stand on the bird's right side, hold its head and 'stretch' the neck cranially and slightly to the left. Should the bird become distressed, the procedure should be abandoned and oxygen provided.

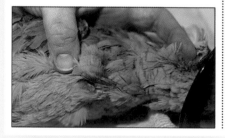

3 The vein is raised by placing the thumb of the hand holding the head across the right side of the neck.

4 The apterium on the right side of the neck is located.

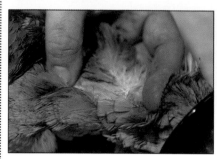

5 The skin and feathers are moistened with a spirit-soaked swab (avoid excessive soaking to reduce hypothermia and preening of spirit).

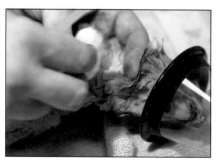

6 The vein is exposed and the needle entered into the vein, passing cranially. The vein is very superficial.

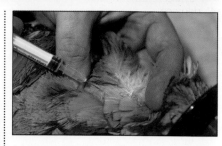

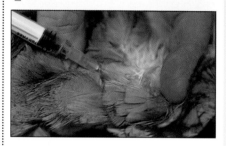

7 Blood is withdrawn.

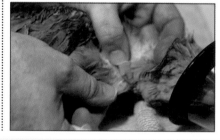

8 Pressure is placed on the venepuncture site for 20–30 seconds. If there is no haematoma formation the bird can be released.

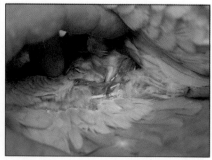

QRG 12.2: Blood sampling – brachial vein

Equipment

- Appropriately sized needles and syringes
- Cotton wool swabs
- Surgical spirit
- Tissue glue

> **PRACTICAL TIP**
> - Other than for very small birds, an assistant will be required

Patient preparation

The bird is anaesthetized or sedated or caught and wrapped in a towel.

Technique

1 The bird is laid in dorsal recumbency. Should the bird become distressed, the procedure should be abandoned and oxygen provided.

2 Stretch out one wing and, holding it by the distal part, gently press the wing such that the dorsal surface is flat on the table.

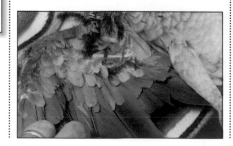

3 If the vein requires raising, a finger may be placed on the ventral wing just distal to the shoulder joint.

QRG 12.2 *continued*

4 The hypodermic needle is fixed to the syringe and, using the guard, bent at 45 degrees.

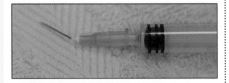

5 The brachial vein is located where it runs along the humerus, and the feathers parted and moistened with a spirit-soaked swab (Note, avoid excessive soaking to reduce hypothermia and preening of spirit). Sometimes it is necessary to pluck a minimal number of feathers.

6 The vein is exposed and the needle entered, passing cranially. The vein is very superficial and fragile; avoid excessive pressure when withdrawing blood.

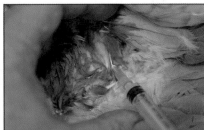

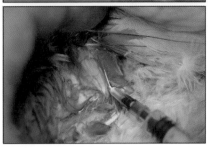

7 The needle is withdrawn and pressure is placed on the venepuncture site for 30–60 seconds.

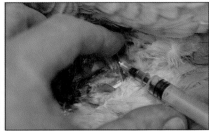

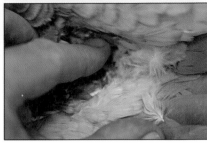

8 If there is no haematoma formation the bird can be released. If there is haemorrhage from the site, tissue glue may be applied. If haemorrhage is minimal, the bird may be released and placed in a warm dark place for 5 minutes; the resultant drop in blood pressure will usually aid haemostasis.

QRG 12.3: Blood sampling – caudal tibial vein

Equipment

- Appropriately sized needles and syringes
- Cotton wool swabs
- Surgical spirit
- Tissue glue

Patient preparation

The bird is held in a towel by an assistant, who presents one foot for sampling, whilst securely holding the other foot.

Technique

1 The vein is located on the medial surface of the tarsometatarsus. To raise the vein, the assistant should grip just proximal to the intertarsal joint.

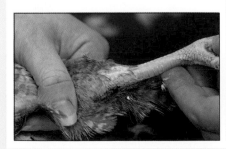

2 The skin is rubbed vigorously with a spirit-soaked swab.

3 The vein is exposed and the needle entered, passing cranially. The vein is very superficial and fragile; avoid excessive pressure when withdrawing blood.

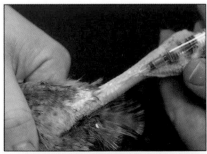

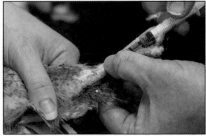

4 Pressure is placed on the venepuncture site for 30–60 seconds.

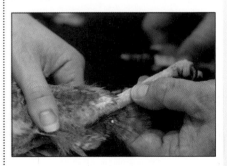

5 If there is no haematoma formation the bird can be released. If there is haemorrhage from the site, tissue glue may be applied. If haemorrhage is minimal the bird may be released and placed in a warm dark place for 5 minutes; the resultant drop in blood pressure will usually aid haemostasis.

QRG 12.4: Crop wash

Equipment

- Metal crop tube (or Spruells needle)
- Syringe
- Warmed saline (0.5–1 ml/30 g bodyweight)

Patient preparation

The bird should be conscious to reduce reflux. The bird is restrained in a towel and held 'vertically' with the head uppermost. Should the bird become distressed, the procedure should be abandoned and oxygen provided.

Technique

1 The neck is straightened, the beak opened and fingers placed in the fleshy part of the mouth commissures. In large raptors or macaws a mouth gag may be used.

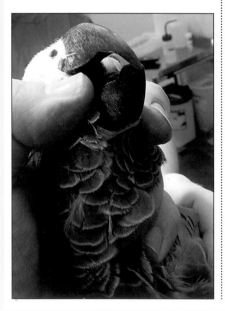

2 The tube is entered into the oesophagus by passing it down the right side of the mouth and pharynx.

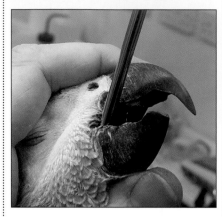

3 Once in the crop, the end of the tube should be palpated.

4 Warmed saline is gently passed into the crop and the crop is massaged.

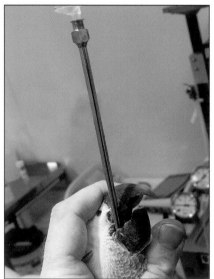

5 Fluid is withdrawn and the process repeated two or three times.

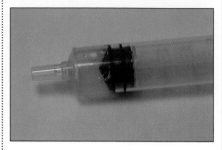

6 The bird is released and the sample taken immediately for examination as a wet preparation and as stained air-dried smears.

Euthanasia: grief and bereavement

13

James M. Harris

Given the relatively short lifespan of most avian patients, the terminal bird is a daily presentation. In published studies, 4% of cases involve loss, meaning an average of 1.4 cases per workday in an average practice (Harris, 1983). This is sufficient to justify spending time and effort to provide a good euthanasia service. Ending the life of a patient in a humane manner is not a difficult procedure (see Chapter 15). However, understanding the attachment of clients to their companion animal, the position the bird has within the family, possible family politics related to the pet, history of prior losses, and human emotions and responses to loss is complicated at best. All aspects of this complex situation must be considered and understood for the veterinary surgeon (veterinarian) to be successful in providing a good service. The aim of this chapter is to help all readers have a better grasp of the complexities surrounding euthanasia, to be better prepared to assist clients and to care for themselves. Caring for the veterinary team is just as important as caring for the patient and client.

Attachment

There are many reasons for keeping birds as pets, including a desire to breed them, intellectual interest, attraction to their decoration, beauty and vocalizations (Figure 13.1), companionship, sport (falconry) (Figure 13.2) and emotional fulfilment. It is helpful for the practitioner to have an understanding of the nature of the bond between the client and their bird. For some clients, the bond is casual or practical in nature. For others, especially where the bird occupies a surrogate position within the family, the bond may be extremely strong and a significant emotional reaction to loss should be expected. Keddie (1977), a British psychiatrist, stated 'Those who insist on a special relationship with their dog or cat put themselves at risk from a mental health point of view. In cases where such over-dependence on a pet does exist, there is likely to be a sharp reaction on the part of the owner when the pet dies or has to be "put to sleep".' This statement also applies to pets of other species such as birds.

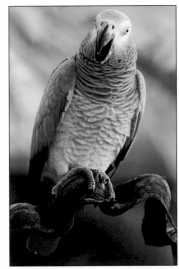

13.1 African Grey Parrots are a commonly kept companion bird species, renowned for their talking abilities.

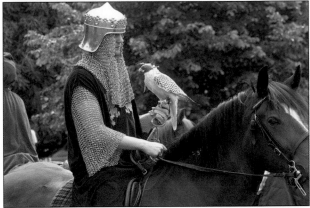

13.2 Although ostensibly 'performance' birds, raptors are often highly valued on an emotional level by their owners. (© John Chitty)

Loss

There are many different types of loss: death from natural causes, death from trauma, disasters, lost animals, theft and death via euthanasia. Client decisions regarding euthanasia are often accompanied by feelings of guilt, and the veterinary surgeon needs to provide the owner with support and validation for the

13

decision reached. When working with families, it can be helpful for the veterinary surgeon to have an understanding of the dynamics of the family unit, including the number (and age) of the adults and children, the number of pets, who is attached to the bird and what role the bird occupies within the family. There may be warning signs that a severe response to the loss of a pet may occur. For example, clients may say that they 'rescued' the bird, that the bird is or was a 'last link' pet (i.e. the pet of a deceased family member), or indicate that the bird is a child substitute (i.e. the client speaks 'motherese' to or about the bird – 'he/she is like a child to me'). These situations could indicate the possibility of an extreme grief response or the onset of pathological grieving. Numerous losses within a short period of time (also known as 'piggyback losses') can also affect the response of the client to death.

Grief

Grief is a natural response to loss and has a number of stages: denial, anger, bargaining, depression and acceptance.

The five stages of grief

When a bird dies at the veterinary practice and the client is contacted, the types of response that may be seen in relation to the different stages of grief include:

- Denial – 'You must be incorrect. It is someone else's bird'
- Anger – The client may swear. 'I know it's your fault. I'm contacting my attorney'
- Bargaining – 'If Sweetie recovers, I promise I will donate money to charity each month'
- Depression – 'I feel suicidal. I cannot live without Joey'
- Acceptance – 'I have great memories of Petie and his funny antics. I will contact you for advice on a new bird'.

It should also be recognized that for clients with missing birds, whether they have flown away or been stolen, establishing 'closure' and accepting the situation is very difficult when there is hope that the bird will be found or will return

---

There is no set time for each stage and the grieving client may move forward and backward through the stages. The time taken to move through all five stages of grief depends on the level of attachment of the individual family member to the bird. Prior losses may also affect the response. Pathological grief occurs when an individual gets 'stuck' in one stage and cannot move forward. It is appropriate for the veterinary practice to provide relevant literature to clients (Figure 13.3), as well as maintain a list of registered professional mental health and/or grief counsellors to whom clients can be referred if required.

Legally, veterinary surgeons are responsible for only animal health and welfare, but it must be remembered that in order to achieve this goal, practitioners must engage with owners and understand the human–animal bond, which at times can be complex. Thus,

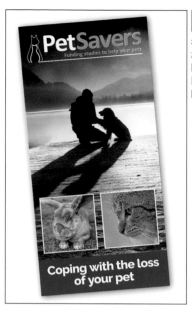

13.3 Support paperwork, such as this *Coping with the loss of your pet* brochure produced by PetSavers, may be beneficial to clients.

whilst there is no legal imperative, it could be argued that veterinary surgeons have a moral obligation to assist their clients in dealing with significant stressors related to animal care. With the recognition that veterinary surgeons have no formal training in human counselling, in these situations it is reasonable that a clinician could offer immediate support and subsequent referral to a healthcare professional to clients who are clearly struggling to come to terms with the loss of their pet.

Euthanasia consultations

An astute practice consultant once said: 'the first and last visits of a client with the patient are the most important two visits.' On the first visit to the veterinary practice, a large amount of information is given to the client. It would be appropriate to include within this material information on the average life expectancy of the species presented for examination. Mentioning the average life expectancy of the bird on the first visit can help on the last (Figure 13.4).

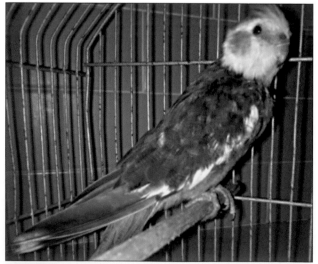

13.4 A geriatric Cockatiel. Owners who are aware of the expected lifespan of their bird can more effectively manage their expectations of pet ownership. (Courtesy of Dr Melinda Cowan)

Inpatients

When a patient is admitted to the veterinary practice for diagnostic procedures, treatment or nursing care, the contact telephone number(s) of a responsible adult should be verified and added to the patient's medical record prior to hospitalization. Clients need to be advised that they must be available at all times at the given telephone number(s) whilst the patient is under the care of the practice.

Sudden death should be reported to the client immediately in a sensitive telephone call. It is not appropriate to tell a client who arrives at the practice at the end of surgery to collect their bird that it died earlier that morning. If a bird dies whilst it is under veterinary care, clients need to be allowed time to view the remains. This can be particularly helpful for children. If the client and their family are unable to view and spend time with the remains immediately after euthanasia, the bird can be refrigerated or frozen until a convenient time. Clients need to be advised if the remains are to be frozen.

Outpatients

If a terminal illness is suspected during a consultation, the client should be advised of this fact as well as the prognosis for the outcome (i.e. not favourable, poor or grave). Giving the client time to prepare for the loss of their pet will help to soften the blow.

For a scheduled euthanasia appointment, there are considerations in terms of time and use of the facility. Where possible, appointments should be scheduled before the practice lunch break or at the end of the day. It is not appropriate to schedule appointments on the morning following a long weekend, when there is a busy surgery and cases being transferred from the emergency practice. If a euthanasia appointment has been scheduled, the practice staff should be made aware. The staff should present a serious but compassionate posture to the arriving client(s), who should be taken into a private waiting area. It is not appropriate for grieving clients to have to sit in a busy reception area. The waiting area should be furnished with comfortable chairs, soft lighting and non-medical pictures, and lots of facial tissues should be available.

Prior to euthanasia

Any relevant paperwork, including consent forms, should be completed prior to the consultation. The different options should be discussed with the client prior to the consultation, including:

- Does the client wish to be present during the euthanasia procedure?
- If not, does the client or any family member wish to view and spend time with the remains?
- How does the client wish to care for the remains? There are many choices, depending on what is available in the area and local legislation (Figure 13.5).

It is imperative that any special requests from the client (e.g. placing a few feathers in an envelope as a keepsake) are understood and can be complied with. In addition, it may be appropriate to collect fees for the euthanasia consultation at this time to reduce the anguish of clients receiving an invoice for the fee at a later date.

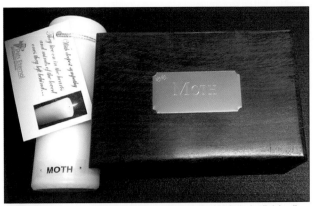

13.5 Some owners elect to have their birds individually cremated and the ashes returned.
(© Deborah Monks)

Following euthanasia

Following euthanasia, clients should be allowed to spend time with the remains if they wish. If the remains are to be taken home for burial, a suitable box should be provided if the client has not brought one with them.

The veterinary practice should follow up with the client after the euthanasia consultation. A telephone call in the evening to check on the client and let them know that the veterinary surgeon or nurse is thinking about them, is often appreciated. A personally written condolence card (Figure 13.6) can also be sent. The author writes the following: 'Thank you for your unselfish kindness. (Name of bird) was very fortunate to have you as its special friend'. Computer-generated condolence letters are impersonal and inappropriate. A note should be added to the client record so that the same card and message are not sent a second time if future losses occur.

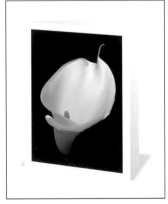

13.6 PetSavers sympathy card. A condolence card sent to clients following euthanasia of their pet bird is often appreciated.

It should be remembered that the death of a patient does not terminate the veterinary practice's contract with the client. Veterinary staff should still be available to provide a service to the client, which may include answering follow-up questions, dealing with the response of family members and other pets to the loss of the deceased animal, and assisting with the selection of a new pet, if that is what the client desires.

Special considerations for children

Children are often the primary members of the family attached to the bird. The death of a pet is often the first loss experienced by a child, and encouraging them to express their feelings allows them to practice grieving, which is helpful in preparing them for other losses they will encounter throughout their lives. Parents should be encouraged to be honest with their children regarding euthanasia.

A number of years ago, the author was lecturing at a veterinary school on this subject and realized that one of the students was quite upset. After the lecture, the student stated that when they were 5 years old and at school, their pet budgerigar had become unwell and died at the local veterinary practice. Not wanting to have a dead bird in the house, the parents pretended to have a burial service, but instead actually buried a small rock. However, the student found out and years later the effects of this deception were still clearly visible, and the student was still angry

Caring for the veterinary team

The impact of euthanasia on the veterinary surgeon and the practice team needs to be considered. It should be remembered that due to the complexities of family life, for each individual patient, the veterinary team often has to deal with multiple family members trying to reach a unanimous decision, which can increase emotional load. Feelings of professional failure, personal attachment to the patient and the process of empathizing with the client can cause additional stress. To be successful in dealing with clients and patients at a time of terminal illness and death, staff must be comfortable with these issues themselves. Unresolved personal problems need to be worked through and there is a variety of professional services available to assist with this process if required.

References and further reading

Doyle P (1980) *Grief Counselling and Sudden Death*. Thomas, Springfield

Harris J (1983) A study of client grief responses to death or loss in a companion animal practice. In: *New Perspectives on our Lives with Companion Animals*, ed. AH Katcher and A Beck, pp. 370–376. University of Pennsylvania Press, Philadelphia

Harris J (1984) Non-conventional human/companion animal bonds, pet loss and human bereavement. In: *Pet Loss and Human Bereavement*, ed. W Kay *et al.*, pp. 31–36. Iowa University Press, Ames

Harris J (1984) The veterinarian's role in the human/animal bond. In: *Dynamic Relationships in Practice: Animals in the Helping Professions*, ed. P Arkow, pp. 271–283. Latham Foundation, Alameda

Harris J (1984) Understanding animal death: bereavement, grief and euthanasia. In: *The Pet Connection*, ed. RK Anderson *et al.*, pp. 261–275. University of Minnesota Press, Minneapolis

Keddie KM (1977) Pathological mourning after the death of a domestic pet. *British Journal of Psychiatry* **131**, 21–25

Kay W, Cohen S, Fudin C *et al.* (1988) *Euthanasia of the Companion Animal*. Charles Press, Philadelphia

Lagoni L, Butler C and Hetts S (1994) *The Human–Animal Bond and Grief*. WB Saunders, Philadelphia

Nieburg H (1982) *Pet Loss: A Thoughtful Guide for Adults and Children*. Harper and Row, New York

Post-mortem examination

Mike Cannon

A post-mortem examination is an extremely important part of the service a veterinary surgeon (veterinarian) can offer to wildlife carers, aviculturists and pet bird owners. For those new to avian medicine, a post-mortem examination can be a daunting prospect; training received prior to this point is likely to have been focused on mammalian issues and veterinary surgeons may feel outside their comfort zone when treating birds. However, the veterinary principles previously studied in the context of mammals can be adapted to any new species encountered. Prospective avian practitioners will need to research the anatomy, physiology, common diseases and normal behaviour of bird species, and then apply the familiar veterinary principles. In many instances, species are more similar than they are different, and this extends to pathological changes detected during a post-mortem examination (Harrigan, 1981).

The services of an experienced avian veterinary pathologist are often not available, and it therefore becomes the role of the practitioner to carry out post-mortem examinations. In the author's experience, the most common requests for post-mortem examinations come from aviculturists who are not only interested in the cause of death but are concerned that it may be a contagious disease and want to protect the rest of their collection.

It is important to discuss the post-mortem procedure with the client beforehand, so they understand what will happen to their bird and will be able to give informed consent. It is also important to discuss if they wish to have the bird returned after the procedure, as this may alter how the examination is performed. It is important to ensure that the bird remains in an acceptable state to be returned to the owner, as this may assist with closure over the death of their cherished pet.

Every post-mortem examination should be treated as a valuable learning exercise that greatly increases knowledge and understanding of avian anatomy and physiology. Thorough examination and note-taking are recommended; the benefits of this learning are also carried over to surgery, endoscopy and many other aspects of avian medicine. Clinicians new to avian post-mortem examinations should take every opportunity to examine and record 'normal' birds in order to become familiar with anatomy as well as the normal variations in size, texture and colour of the organs.

The value of the information received from an examination will depend upon the quality of the technique used, and clinicians should use the bird's history, previous examination notes and the results of other diagnostic tests for reference (Orosz, 2008). A thorough post-mortem examination will often provide more information than diagnostic procedures performed on the live bird.

A consistent, organized and systematic method of making and storing good records is mandatory. Occasionally, the post-mortem examination may be important evidence in a legal case and lead to the veterinary surgeon being called into court as an expert witness. The careful collection, submission, processing and storage of specimens is crucial in legal cases (Cooper and Cooper, 2008), and it is therefore good practice to perform every post-mortem examination with this in mind, taking multiple images of normal and abnormal organs to corroborate notes.

Maintaining a high standard of good records is mandatory. All stages of the examination, from the initial discussion with the client to a tentative or definitive diagnosis, should be recorded. These notes should accompany specimens sent out to an external laboratory.

A separate set of instruments for post-mortem examination, sterilized between cases, is recommended and clinicians should have the facilities to carry out most of the simple stains and clinical pathology tests in-house. However, the services of an experienced avian veterinary histopathologist are invaluable, as many times organs will appear to be grossly normal yet reveal pathology when samples are submitted for histopathological examination.

Whilst the examination is being carried out, a veterinary assistant or nurse should complete a form as per the clinician's instructions. Forms that itemize the organs and body systems are preferable, to ensure that no part is overlooked (Figure 14.1). This should be stored digitally with the bird's records.

The author recommends a shorthand system of up and down arrows to indicate 'increased' or 'decreased' and a subjective system of '+' and '−' signs to indicate changes in quantity or size. This system can be modified to suit an individual's needs so that '+', '++', '+++', etc. will have relevance to the individual operator. This is a simple and quick method, and overcomes the tendency in a busy practice to put off compiling accurate records. It is also much easier to quickly scan the examination sheet at a later date.

Avian post-mortem examination

Date: ....

Name: ....

Street: ....

Town: .... Postcode: ....

Phone: ....

Species: .... Age: .... Sex: (please circle) M   F

Length of ownership: .... New/Old; Pet/Aviary

Animal ID: ....

Medications: ....

Diet: ....

Recent deaths: (please circle) Y   N   Species involved: ....

History: ....

....

....

Examination: (circle any abnormal features/organs and give details in comments section)

External:	Pectoral muscle	Weight loss	Dehydration	Fat deposits
	Wounds	Skin	Claws	Feathers
	Eyes	Ears	Soiling	
Internal:	Subcutaneous tissues			
Respiratory:	Nares	Sinuses	Choana	Trachea
	Upper airway	Syrinx	Air sacs	Lungs
Cardiovascular:	Heart	Blood vessels	Pericardium	
Haematopoietic:	Spleen	Bursa	Thymus	Bone marrow
Digestive:	Oral cavity	Beak	Tongue	Oropharynx
	Crop	Oesophagus	Proventriculus	Ventriculus
	Small intestine	Caecum	Large intestine	Cloaca
	Liver	Bile duct	Gall bladder	Pancreas
Musculoskeletal:	Muscles	Bones	Joints	
Urinary:	Kidney	Ureter	Cloaca	
Reproductive:	Gonads	Reproductive tract	Yolk sac	
Endocrine:	Pituitary	Thyroid	Parathyroid	Adrenal glands
Nervous:	Brain	Spinal cord	Peripheral nervous system	

Pathology: (circle)

Crop wash	Faecal float	Faecal smear	Intestinal scrape	Impression smear
Gram stain	MZN	Macchiavello	Diff-Quik	Clearview
Culture:	Heart blood	Faeces/GIT	Other (specify)	

Histopathology: (specify tissues) ....

Diagnosis: (please circle)   Definitive   Tentative

Comments: ....

....

....

....

14.1 Example of a post-mortem examination form. GIT = gastrointestinal tract; MZN = modified Ziehl-Naelsen stain.

Preparation

Aims of post-mortem examinations

The aim of a post-mortem examination is not only to diagnose the cause of death. Conclusions can also be drawn regarding the progress of the disease as well as any other disease processes that may have been affecting the bird. This allows the examination to be a useful tool to monitor concurrent diseases or problems that may also affect other birds in a collection. This helps to provide information on the effectiveness of any preventive medicine programme that is being undertaken and allows recommendations to be made regarding other preventive steps that may need to be included, as well as the modification of present techniques.

The primary aim should be to use the information gleaned from the post-mortem examination to design management procedures that will prevent further problems.

History

All post-mortem examinations begin with as detailed a history as possible. Ideally, the practitioner conducting the post-mortem examination should also discuss the case directly with the owner. The following information must be recorded prior to the examination:

- Contact details of the veterinary surgeon making the submission
- Bird species:
  - Flock or aviary details of other species kept at this location
  - Age groups and numbers
- Presenting signs
  - Are the signs confined to a particular group, variety, age or sex?
  - Is this bird typical of the current problem?
- Any recent introductions of birds or other animals
- Number of dead birds
- How long the bird has been dead
- How the cadaver has been stored
- Description of housing and feeding
- Any recent changes to the bird's environment
- Recent medication history (antibiotics, particularly chlortetracycline or oxytetracycline, may interfere with microbial flora).

A good history will allow the examiner to begin to develop a differential diagnosis, which helps in planning for any tests that may be required, before the examination begins.

Autolysis

Client education is an important factor in receiving a bird in a useful state. It is preferable to receive a bird that is still alive (sometimes appropriate in avicultural circumstances) or (more likely) one that has only recently died. The smaller the bird and the longer it has been dead, the more likely it will be that autolysis has begun. This can markedly reduce the value of the post-mortem examination.

The onset of autolysis can be delayed by instructing the client to thoroughly soak the bird in soapy water or alcohol/methylated spirits. The cadaver should be wrapped in cling-wrap or similar and kept chilled at around 5°C until the examination can be performed.

This allows a useful post-mortem examination to be carried out up to 72 hours after death. Examination can still be performed after this time but some organs, such as the intestines, cannot be examined with confidence.

It is most important to instruct the client to not freeze the bird unless it cannot be examined within 72 hours of death. Freezing has been found to cause variable tissue damage in canine patients (Baraibar and Schoning, 1985) and it is likely that similar changes occur in avian patients. The more subtle pathological tissue changes are likely to be missed at post-mortem examination, if the animal has been frozen (D Phalen, personal communication).

Histopathological changes in frozen tissues (Baraibar and Schoning, 1985)

- Extracellular fluid accumulation
- Cellular shrinkage in all tissues
- Loss of staining
- Fractures in tissue, particularly brain and small intestine
- Haemolysis
- Increased amounts of haematin in lungs, liver and kidneys
- Some areas of bronchi lost cilia
- The most affected organs were the brain (fractures and neuronal degeneration) and liver (loss of architecture, shrunken hepatocytes, diluted sinusoids)
- Small intestinal changes were intermediate
- The lungs and kidneys were least affected

Equipment

It is important to be aware of zoonoses and take steps to minimize exposure to potential pathogens; gloves should always be worn and a separate set of instruments reserved for avian post-mortem examination should be used.

Use of a facemask and other appropriate personal protective equipment, if available, is strongly recommended. Inhalation of pathogens is a definite risk, particularly when examining Australian parrots and birds with suspected *Chlamydia* infection. Most large pathology laboratories will have a vented dissection hood to overcome this problem. This is unlikely to be available in a small animal practice, so a number of precautions should be taken:

- Thoroughly wet the cadaver with a detergent-based disinfectant or soapy water (Figure 14.2)
- Be aware of the pattern of air flow in the area where the examination is being conducted
- Examiners should stand with the air flow coming from behind them so that it flows across the cadaver.

WARNING

The most dangerous time for inhalation is immediately after the coelomic cavity is opened and the sternum removed, when a fine cloud of contaminated air and aerosols rises towards the examiner. This can be minimized by wetting the cadaver or temporarily covering the cadaver, with a damp cloth or similar, during the opening procedure

---

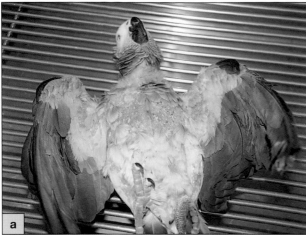

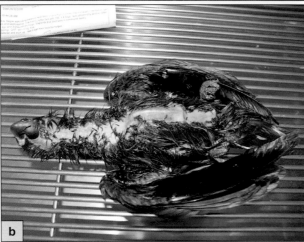

14.2 (a) Deceased African Grey Parrot ready to be wetted for examination. (b) Deceased female Eclectus Parrot that has been wet down and laid out for external examination, prior to dissection. Feathers are parted to allow the initial incision.

Instruments recommended for avian post-mortem examination (Figure 14.3)

- Scalpel blades and handle
- Glass microscope slides
- Cover slips (22 x 50 mm; 1 box)
- Plastic glass slide transporters (x 10)
- Leak-proof zip-lock bags
- Dispenser bottle containing disinfectant (e.g. chlorhexidine, alcohol, F10)
- Adson rat-toothed forceps
- 15 cm sharp/sharp scissors
- Iris scissors (curved and/or straight)
- Large utility scissors or bone-cutting forceps (for larger birds)
- Sterile swabs and transport media
- Buffered 10% formalin and a range of suitable containers
- Sterile containers
- Weighing scales
- Preservative for parasites (e.g. absolute alcohol 70 ml + glycerine 5 ml + water 25 ml)
- Camera (operated by an assistant) for collecting high-resolution images

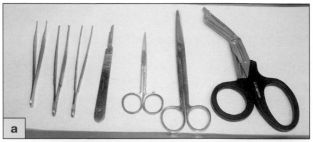

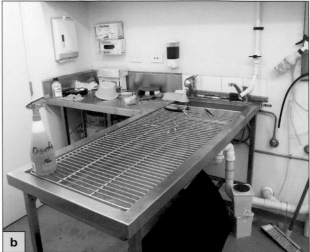

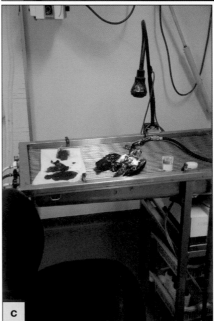

14.3 (a) Typical set of post-mortem examination instruments. (b) A typical stainless steel table and equipment used for post-mortem examinations. Stainless steel tables like these are easy to clean, which is very important. (c) A typical workstation ready for a post-mortem examination includes good lighting, gloves, water, paper towels, post-mortem instruments, formalin, specimen jars and a chair.

Live bird examination

If presented with a live bird, the veterinary surgeon should do a thorough clinical examination prior to euthanasia (see Chapter 10). A relatively small amount of time spent making these observations can point towards which areas may have pathology and provide guidance for areas of focus during the post-mortem examination. Many simple clinical pathology tests can be performed in-house for timely results; more complex tests (or tests for those cases which may have a legal element attached) can be sent to an external accredited pathology laboratory (see Chapter 12).

- **Blood samples** may be collected from the wing vein or jugular vein, depending on the species and the signs displayed, and measured for packed cell volume (PCV) and haemoglobin levels. A blood smear may also be used to detect haemoparasites.
- **Swabs** of any discharges, for culture and sensitivity or cytology, should be taken.
- **Fresh faecal samples** should be collected for Gram staining, a warm saline smear or Diff-Quik® stain for cytology.
- **Skin scrapes and obvious parasites** are taken for cytology or fungal cultures.

Euthanasia

Pathologists need to be aware of what method of euthanasia has been used so that they can take this into consideration when looking at tissue changes. If oral barbiturate is aspirated it will cause changes to the lungs; similarly, intramuscular injection of barbiturate can cause local necrosis that may be mistaken for pathological change. Preferred methods of euthanasia that cause minimal known side effects or artefacts that disrupt post-mortem examination are:

- Inhalation of neat isoflurane or halothane (use a small chamber with rubber from a surgical glove as a cover that fits snugly around the bird's neck and allows it to inhale the anaesthetic)
- Vertebral crushing of an anaesthetized bird (place the cervical vertebrae between the handles of a pair of scissors and close them quickly, to crush the vertebrae; preferable to decapitation)
- Intramuscular (pectoral) or intravenous (jugular or wing vein) injection of a small volume of pentobarbital euthanasia solution, diluted 1:10 in saline (oral administration or intracoelomic injection can be used if these routes are not possible).

Full-strength pentobarbital euthanasia solution will cause artefacts in the tissues, especially the lungs, and large doses may cause artefacts from chemical necrosis that continues well after the bird has died. See Chapter 15 for more information about euthanasia and client communication.

Specimen preparation and transport

The veterinary surgeon has a duty (and usually legal requirement) to protect the environment and humans from contamination during the transport of the tissue to an external laboratory. Legal requirements and guidelines differ between countries, and it is the veterinary surgeon's responsibility to become familiar with what is required in their area. The external laboratory can also supply relevant information and directions.

- Bird carcasses must be wrapped in several layers of plastic, with good sealing to trap any discharges, and, in most instances, ice packs to minimize autolysis. Ectoparasites should be checked for, as they will abandon the body when it cools.

- Specimens for histopathology should be fixed in buffered 10% formalin for 24 hours, using 10 times the volume of formalin to that of the tissue. Prior to sending the samples to the laboratory, 90% of the fluid should be decanted and replaced with surgical gauze swabs placed over the tissues to absorb the remaining fluid and keep them moist during the trip. These precautions will minimize impact, should the container become damaged and leak formalin (a significant hazard) into the environment during transportation.
- Blood should always be collected into heparinized blood transport vials; ethylenediaminetetraacetic acid (EDTA) is not recommended. It is important to note that blood smears should be made prior to the sample being placed in anticoagulant, and as soon as possible after the blood is collected.
- Serum specimens need to be allowed to coagulate before centrifuging and the serum harvested.
- Faeces should be transported in small containers with a secure lid, with 2–3 drops of saline added to keep the sample moist.
- Parasites:
  - Helminths are initially placed in 0.9% saline or water to relax for several hours, then fixed in 10% formalin or 70% alcohol. They should be placed in a secure container and several layers of plastic to capture any leaks
  - Ectoparasites: for example, mites, lice and ticks are best transported in 10% formalin or 70–90% alcohol.
- Bacteriology swabs are transported as normal or as directed by the external laboratory.

PRACTICAL TIP

It is a good idea to check with the external pathology laboratory, prior to collecting blood samples, what volumes of serum should be collected for the tests required

PRACTICAL TIP

If heavy metal toxicity is suspected, obtain a survey radiograph of the patient before beginning the post-mortem examination. The acid environment in the ventriculus makes it extremely difficult to identify metal particles grossly – they look just like small stones that are normally present. A survey radiograph of the bird in ventrodorsal or lateral recumbency is the best means of detecting heavy metal particles

In addition to samples collected in formalin, the following should also be considered (St Leger, 2010):

- Serum for biochemistry, hormone assays and immunoglobin titres for infectious agents
- Cytological preparations (impression smears) of blood, body fluids, bone marrow or tissues
- Sterile collection and ultralow freezing or filter paper collection of faeces and tissue samples (e.g. skin, skeletal muscle, liver, spleen, brain) for molecular or genetic testing
- Swabs for bacterial, mycoplasmal or fungal culture

- Double sets of samples (e.g. fat, kidney, liver, brain, stomach contents, eye) in glass and foil for toxicological testing
- Liths for content analysis
- Collection of faeces for flotation
- Collection of ecto- and endoparasites for identification.

Post-mortem examination

External examination

Initially, record the owner's name, and the species, age and sex of the bird(s). Species identification is important for records and establishing how commonly some diseases are found in certain species. Accurate identification is important, so access to a reliable avian field guide is recommended. Do not rely on initial history for identification as clients and others can be mistaken.

Before dissection begins, a complete external examination should be performed.

1. The bird should be weighed (and weight recorded).
2. Scan for a microchip transponder identification number and record this on the bird's file, along with any leg ring number (Figure 14.4).

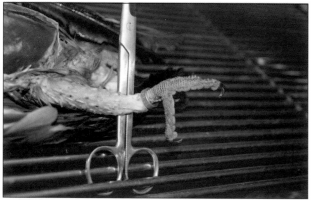

14.4 Check for individual identification. Record leg ring number or microchip transponder number.

3. Examine for any discharges, vomitus, tumours, fractures (old or new), skin or feather lesions, and ectoparasites.
4. Note any swellings, particularly in the abdominal region or the joints.
5. Palpate the crop and its contents.
   - If it is empty, suspect:
     - Anorexia
     - Lack of food due to competition with other birds or poor feeding strategies from the owner.
   - If it is full, suspect:
     - The bird had been eating well until just prior to death; consider sudden events such as toxicity (inhaled or consumed) or trauma
     - This can be confusing as some chronically ill birds will still eat well and have a full crop at death.
     - Ask more questions of the owner to try to support or deny these suspicions.
6. Make an estimate of the bird's nutritional and hydration status by palpating the pectoral muscle mass (Figures 14.5 and 14.6).

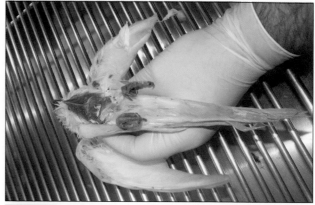

14.5 A prominent keel bone and loss of pectoral muscle mass are common findings in many birds that have been masking disease.

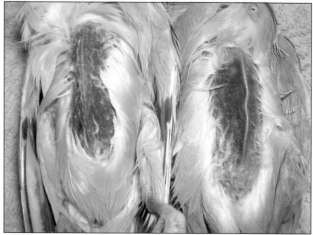

14.6 Inspection of the keel bone. Note the bent keel bone in the bird on the right. This is a sign that the bird may have suffered with metabolic bone disease in the past. The bird on the left is normal.

   - Record the bird's body condition score (BCS). The author prefers a score of cachexic (1/5) through to obese (5/5), with normal being 3/5.
   - Any system may be used as long as it is reliably repeatable.
7. Examine the eyes.
   - Erythema of the conjunctiva is often associated with infection (bacteria (*Chlamydia* spp.) or viruses) or trauma from fighting with cage mates – particularly during the breeding season.
     - In parrots the most common cause of conjunctivitis is *Chlamydia psittaci*. It is important to be aware of this organism's zoonotic potential and practise good hygiene during the examination, to avoid transmission.
     - Common environmental causes include ammonia that builds up in aged substrate and dust from inappropriate or aged cage substrate that is disintegrating from wear and tear.
   - Any ocular abnormalities should be thoroughly examined with good lighting and an ophthalmoscope.
     - If blood is detected in the anterior chamber, consider coagulopathy or trauma.
     - Pus or fibrin tags in the anterior chamber are often associated with panophthalmitis from septicaemic diseases such as salmonellosis (Harrigan, 1981).

8. Examine the beak.
   - Beak deformity can be associated with:
     - Inappropriate food; for example, food that is too soft to wear the beak normally
     - Congenital problems
     - Psittacine circovirus (psittacine beak and feather disease)
     - Tumours
     - *Cryptococcus* spp. infection
     - Trauma and fractures.
   - Hyperkeratotic changes in Budgerigars are usually associated with infestation with the *Cnemidocoptes* mite.
     - Microscopically examine a portion of the hyperkeratotic material, crushed in a drop of immersion oil, to confirm the mite's presence.
9. Examine the feathers and plumage.
   - Note any soiling or pasting of faeces or urates on the vent or surrounding feathers. This may indicate diarrhoea or polyurates/polyuria.
   - Soiled feathers around the face and head may suggest vomiting.
     - There may also be stains on the wings where the bird had wiped their face and beak.
     - Budgerigars with *Trichomonas* spp. infestation will vomit; seeds may be found stuck to the cage bars or other parts of the bird's environment.
   - Assess the general condition of the feathers, looking for damaged and ragged feathers that may indicate chronic disease or may be due to skin irritation.
   - Transilluminate the wings and tail feathers by holding them up to a window or bright light source. Look for ectoparasites or other evidence of infestation such as lice eggs attached to the rachis of these long feathers.
   - For close examination, pluck a feather and examine under the microscope. Look for:
     - Empty feather follicles
     - Retained feather sheaths on developing feathers
     - Dystrophy/damage to feathers.
   - Feathers are usually arranged in lines or tracts called pterygia. In cases of alopecia the pattern of loss may affect this distribution.
10. Examine the skin.
   - Thick scabs on the bare skin areas (cere, wattles, combs, eyelids and legs/feet) may be a sign of mosquito bites or poxvirus.
   - Trauma can be seen as contusions, lacerations and excoriation.
   - Areas with moist or dry exudation can be seen with chronic and acute bacterial dermatitis.
   - Swellings of the skin may be examined by fine-needle aspiration and cytology. Differential diagnoses for skin swellings include:
     - Neoplasia:
       * Malignant: fibrosarcoma and osteosarcoma are not uncommon causes of masses
       * Benign: lipomas are a common finding in Cockatiels, Budgerigars, Galahs and cockatoos.
     - Poxvirus infection
     - Haematoma
     - Feather cysts (particularly in Canaries and Budgerigars).
   - Examine the bilobed uropygial gland on the dorsal sacral area as this is prone to neoplasia and cystic hyperplasia.
11. Examine the pelvic limbs and feet.
   - Overgrown claws can be a sign of lameness or unwillingness to ambulate.
   - Examine the plantar surface of both feet, looking for inflammation or erosion of papillae.
     - This is often associated with poor diets, particularly vitamin A deficiency (e.g. where birds have been fed diets with a high seed component).
     - Discuss size and material used for perches with the owner. Do the perches have sandpaper coverings?
     - Discuss chemicals or cleaning products that the bird may have been exposed to in the environment.
   - A fine white powdery material present in or adjacent to a joint may be a sign of synovial gout. To confirm this diagnosis, use a small-bore hypodermic needle (25–27 G) to prick the area. Express some of the material to examine microscopically; urate crystals have a distinctive shape.
   - Finches and Canaries can develop hyperkeratosis, protruding from the posterior and plantar surfaces of the feet. Always check these lesions microscopically for *Cnemidocoptes* mites.
   - Raptors may develop large, painful and inflamed swellings and draining sinuses from abscesses that have formed in the plantar pad or extended into the tendon sheaths. This is often associated with inappropriate perching and infection by opportunistic bacteria. This is often referred to as bumblefoot (pododermatitis).
   - Nodular scabby lesions of the feet and digits may be associated with poxvirus (in pigeons, magpies and gallinaceous birds) or herpesvirus (in raptors) infection.
   - Swelling of individual digits is often associated with fine thread material (e.g. cotton or nylon) that has encircled the digit and caused distal ischaemia.
   - If a leg ring is present, examine it to be sure it was not too tight and causing a constriction. This is a good opportunity to confirm and record identification numbers.

The examiner should record all observations and findings, even if they are not immediately applicable to the differential diagnosis.

Internal examination

Prior to dissection, the carcass must be soaked thoroughly to minimize the amount of aerosols rising from the patient, as discussed earlier. The author uses 70% alcohol (methylated spirits) or chlorhexidine solution to thoroughly wet all the plumage down to the skin.

The dissection must be a systematic examination of all the body systems, performed in an orderly routine that will guarantee nothing is missed. There are as many methods of dissection as there are examiners performing them. Excellent discussions of methods of dissection and tissue colours, consistency, shape, etc. can be found in Harrigan (1981) and the Australian Government's *Hygiene Protocols for the Prevention and Control of Diseases (Particularly Beak and Feather Disease) in Australian Birds* (see 'References and further reading').

The examination must be thorough; it should not stop when an obvious lesion is found. Selected samples of any obvious lesion or lesions should be taken to be submitted for histopathology and the examination completed with tissue specimens being selected as indicated.

1. Place the bird in dorsal recumbency.
2. Pluck all the feathers on the ventral surface of the body, so that the skin can be examined more closely before the incision is made. The feathers are plucked so that the whole ventral surface of the body is exposed, from the vent to the base of the beak.
3. The initial incision is started at the base of the keel bone and only penetrates the skin. The incision is continued proximally to expose the pectoral muscle and then up along the ventral aspect of the neck (Figure 14.7a).
4. Use blunt dissection with scissors or tips of fingers to reflect the skin and reveal the crop, oesophagus and underlying structures (Figure 14.7b–f).
   - Assess the amount of subcutaneous fat present.

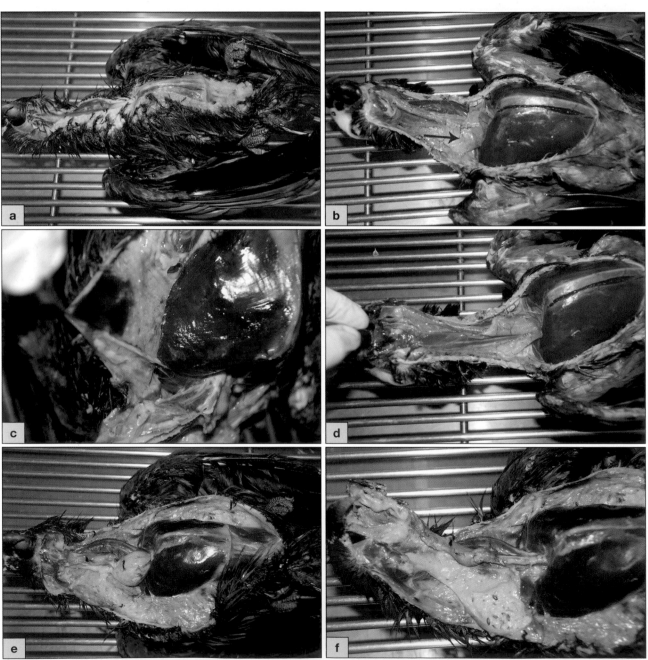

14.7 **(a)** Initial incision in the skin of the cervical area down to the caudal aspect of the keel bone. **(b)** The incision is extended to reveal cervical structures and the crop (arrowed). **(c)** Subcutaneous and intramuscular haemorrhage from injections just prior to death are visible in this bird. **(d)** Extend the incision to expose subcutaneous structures as well as the pharynx and mouth. **(e)** Bird with the skin removed to reveal the underlying structures. **(f)** Bird with incision to expose crop contents continued through the right mandible to reveal the underlying structures.

- Assess the pectoral muscle mass. Ill birds mobilize the fluids, fat and protein components of their muscles to maintain their body when compromised. The pectoral muscles are the largest muscle mass in birds, so any loss of condition is more obvious here.
  - Reassess the BCS assigned during the external examination (Figure 14.8).
  - Haemorrhage within the pectoral mass may be a sign of recent injection, trauma or coagulopathy (see Figure 14.7c).
  - White flecks within the pectoral mass may be a sign of haemoparasites such as *Plasmodium* spp.
- Note the other underlying cervical structures such as vagus nerves, jugular veins and other blood vessels.
- In young birds, search for the thymus or its remnants. This organ is seen as firm, grey-pink lobulated masses of lymphoid tissue, extending from the thoracic inlet cranially and bilaterally on the lateral aspect of the trachea. This is an indirect assessment of age as it is obvious in juveniles but gradually undergoes atrophy as the bird approaches puberty.
- Once the crop is exposed it is opened with scissors (see Figure 14.7f).
  - Record any presence of food – has the bird been eating appropriately?
  - Note the presence of any lesions and/or foreign bodies.
    * Ingluvioliths have been reported and have a firm mineral consistency.
    * Cotton, fur and other material-based foreign bodies are becoming more common in birds that groom the dogs and/or cats in the family, sleep in cloth hammocks and/or chew rope toys and perches.
    * Crop lacerations, perforations or burns that slough may be seen in hand-raised birds fed inappropriately by novice owners.
    * Crop material that leaks into surrounding tissues causes significant cellulitis.
- The incision is continued from the lumen of the crop into the proximal oesophagus and continued up through the pharynx into the oral cavity. The beak is incised at the lateral aspect and laid across to expose the dorsal pharynx, glottis and choana.

5. Samples may also be taken from the crop, oesophagus, pharynx and oral cavity as indicated.
   - Within the mouth or crop mucosa, white plaques or diphtheritic membranes that are tightly adhered to the mucosa and cause bleeding when removed may be due to a range of causes. Collect samples and perform the following tests for differentiation:
     - Warm saline smear:
       * *Capillaria* spp. – bilobed ovoid eggs
       * *Candida* spp. – large ovoid yeasts, may have budding
       * *Trichomonas* spp. – large motile protozoans. Motility is obvious only when the sample is fresh. These organisms are heat labile and lose motility as the host cools.
     - Gram stain:
       * *Candida* spp. – large Gram-positive ovoid yeasts. May have budding and/or pseudohyphae. Often, the crop mucosa is thickened and rough (often described as having a 'Turkish-towel appearance' (Figure 14.9))
       * Bacterial flora – it is normal for bacteria to be present. High levels of Gram-negative rods may be a concern. Take care with interpretation as some of the bacteria present in the mouth, oesophagus or crop may simply be transient contaminants carried on food.

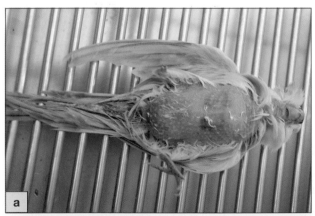

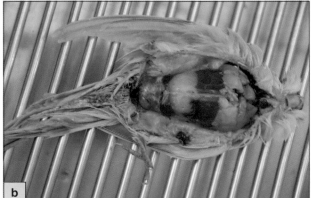

14.8 An obese Budgerigar **(a)** before and **(b)** after skin removed to reveal excessive fat stores.

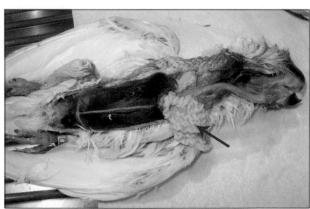

14.9 'Turkish towel' changes to the lining of the crop (arrowed) in an Indian Ringnecked Parakeet. This is a common finding with candidiasis infection of the crop and/or oesophagus. A warm saline smear of a scraping of the crop mucosa will confirm the diagnosis.

- Virology and histopathology:
  * Avian poxvirus – prior to sending off samples, consider if there are additional clinical signs elsewhere in this bird or other birds in the collection, to support this as a cause.

6. If the external examination revealed any signs of respiratory disease, perform a more thorough examination of the upper respiratory region.
   - To examine the turbinates and periorbital sinuses, use a pair of sturdy scissors to cut across the base of the beak to enable sight into the turbinates and ventral aspect of the periorbital sinus on each side.
   - The incision is continued into the periorbital sinus surrounding each orbit.
   - The contents of all areas are examined. Any suspicious contents are swabbed for culture and sensitivity as well as cytology or other tests as indicated.
   - Vitamin A deficiency can cause a build-up of keratinous debris in the sinuses, as a result of squamous metaplasia.

7. To examine the trachea, two incisions may be required because the tracheal rings are complete. Using iris scissors, make an incision along each lateral aspect of the trachea (Figure 14.10).
   - Begin the incision at the glottis and continue down to the syrinx (the distal trachea and syrinx cannot be examined thoroughly until the keel bone has been removed).
   - Remove the ventral section of the trachea to allow a thorough inspection of the mucosa.
   - The normal tracheal mucosa has a dull, dry appearance with no sign of congestion, excess fluid or haemorrhage.
     - Inflammation of the mucosa is often seen as erythema, an increased seromucus discharge that makes it quite moist.
     - Inspect the syrinx closely for mycotic plaques or small seeds.
     - Note any mites, helminths, foreign bodies, lesions or discharges (microscopic examination of a warm saline smear of a sample of mucus will help differentiate these causes).

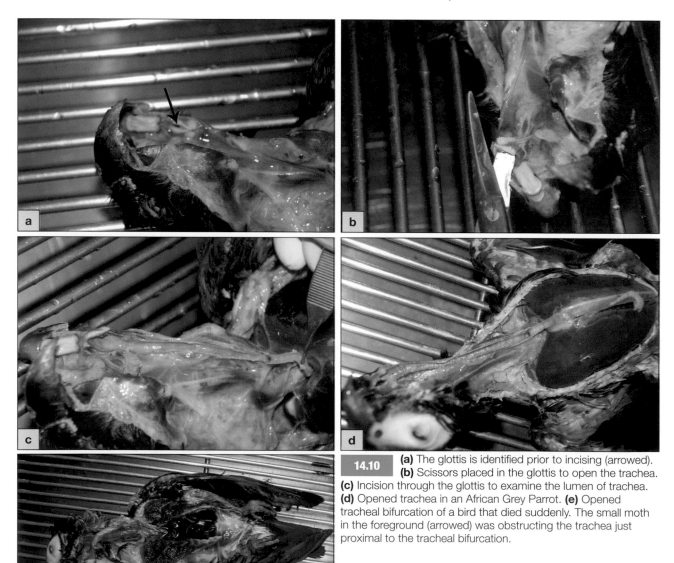

14.10 **(a)** The glottis is identified prior to incising (arrowed). **(b)** Scissors placed in the glottis to open the trachea. **(c)** Incision through the glottis to examine the lumen of trachea. **(d)** Opened trachea in an African Grey Parrot. **(e)** Opened tracheal bifurcation of a bird that died suddenly. The small moth in the foreground (arrowed) was obstructing the trachea just proximal to the tracheal bifurcation.

- Collect samples in as aseptic a manner as possible for bacteriology, virology or other tests as indicated.
8. Once the head and cervical areas have been thoroughly examined, focus on the coelomic cavity (Figure 14.11).
    - The initial incision in the muscular wall is made just caudal to the xiphoid process of the keel bone in the mid-ventral area.
    - This incision is extended to the lateral aspects of the keel bone while elevating the xiphoid process of the keel bone, to visualize the heart and surrounding viscera and avoid incising these structures. The pericardium will need to be dissected free from its attachments to the keel bone.
9. The ribs are transected laterally with robust scissors. This incision is continued bilaterally to allow cutting through each of the coracoid bones, so that the keel bone can be raised cranially and laid to one side (see Figure 14.11f).
    - If there is trouble locating the coracoid and thoracic inlet, use a little finger (in large birds) or an appropriately sized probe (in small birds) to enter via the thoracic inlet so that it may be visualized in the anterior coelomic cavity; from the caudal aspect, the finger or probe can be seen and this allows easier location of the thoracic inlet.

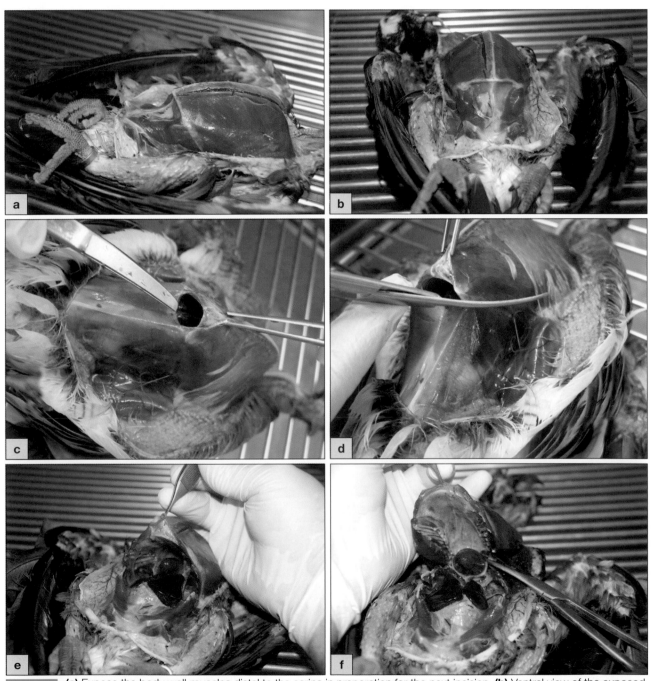

14.11 **(a)** Expose the body wall muscles distal to the carina in preparation for the next incision. **(b)** Ventral view of the exposed body wall muscles. **(c)** Once the abdomen is opened, the liver and other coelomic structures are visible; these should be avoided during the dissection. **(d)** Use scissors to cut through the lateral body wall and ribs, aiming towards the coracoid. **(e)** Extend the incision, elevating the carina. **(f)** Having cut the lateral body wall bilaterally, the carina can be raised to reveal coelomic structures *in situ*. Use large scissors to cut the coracoid bones.

10. Examine all the coelomic organs *in situ*, before removing anything (Figure 14.12).
   - Gently displace the viscera slightly to one side and then the other, to view and examine the air sacs without breaking them.
   - Any lesions or discharges should be noted and samples collected for culture and sensitivity testing.
   - Impression smears from the air sacs, liver, pericardium or other organs may be indicated.
   - Examine the liver closely.
      - The liver is normally similar to that of mammals with a reddish-brown colour and sharp edges.
      - Green discoloration may be seen with excessive production of bile pigments or obstruction of their outflow via the bile duct. The bile pigment of birds is the green biliverdin compared with the yellow-brown bilirubin seen in mammals.
      - Young birds that are still metabolizing the fat from their yolk may have a yellow coloration.
      - A pale liver (excess fat deposited in the liver) may be a sign of hepatic lipidosis or debilitation/starvation.
      - An enlarged liver with edges that are blunt is a sign of inflammation.
      - Petechiation and areas of haemorrhage suggest hepatitis.
      - A pale enlarged liver with a waxy cut surface is indicative of amyloidosis.
      - Pin-point white foci throughout the liver are usually areas of focal necrosis. Possible causes include *Salmonella* infection, Pacheco's disease/herpesvirus (in parrots) and *Yersinia* infection.
      - Other bacteria, mycotic infection or helminth migration may be indicated by spots that are abscesses, so they are often larger than the pin-point foci seen with necrosis.

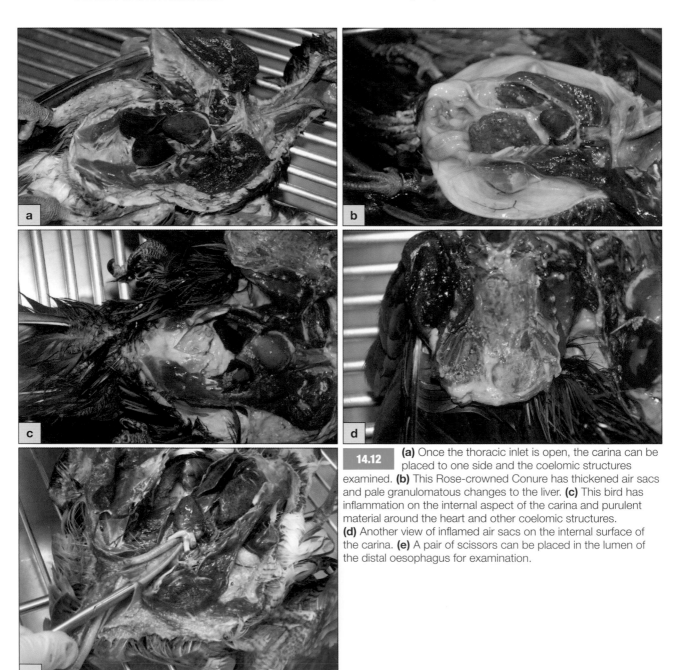

14.12 (a) Once the thoracic inlet is open, the carina can be placed to one side and the coelomic structures examined. (b) This Rose-crowned Conure has thickened air sacs and pale granulomatous changes to the liver. (c) This bird has inflammation on the internal aspect of the carina and purulent material around the heart and other coelomic structures. (d) Another view of inflamed air sacs on the internal surface of the carina. (e) A pair of scissors can be placed in the lumen of the distal oesophagus for examination.

- Haemorrhagic or caseous tracts may be signs of helminth migration.
  - Circular areas of white necrosis are often associated with *Histomonas* spp. or other protozoan organisms.
- Where atrophy, reduced size and fibrosis or deformation of the liver are present, toxicosis causing hepatopathy, congestive heart failure and chronic hepatitis should be considered.
- Diffuse enlargement may indicate neoplasia, *Chlamydia* infection or viral hepatitis.
- Infection with *Chlamydia* or other causes of septicaemia may cause a fibrin film or cast on the serosa of the liver. Collect samples of this aseptically, as soon as possible, to avoid contamination when opening other organs.
- Visceral gout will be seen as a powdery white film on the serosa of the liver and may extend to other organs such as the pericardium.

11. Once the carina has been removed, inspect the area of the thoracic inlet and identify structures. Important structures to inspect are the:
- Distal oesophagus
  - Use scissor points to open the lumen and examine for any lesions, foreign bodies, etc.
  - *Trichomonas* plaques are sometimes seen here in raptors, Budgerigars and pigeons.
- Thyroid and parathyroid glands bilaterally
  - Thyroid glands in birds are not associated with the larynx as in mammals. They are small glands, usually ovoid in shape, found near the junction of the brachial and carotid arteries at the thoracic inlet (Harrigan, 1981). In Budgerigars they are pin-head sized and not normally visible, but if the birds have goitre (from an iodine-deficient diet), they can be up to 10 mm in diameter.
  - Parathyroid glands are found adjacent and posterior to the thyroid glands. Normally they are not visible. If the bird has nutritional secondary hyperparathyroidism from an inappropriate diet, they can become enlarged enough to be visualized. This is seen more often in Grey Parrots than in other species.

12. Examine the air sacs.
- Normal air sacs are thin and transparent.
- Many of the thoracic air sacs will have been damaged when removing the keel bone, but the abdominal air sacs should be present and the viscera easily visualized through them.
- Adult birds may have small amounts of fibrosis or fat present on the surface of the air sacs. Excessive fibrosis or opacity is abnormal, as is the presence of plaques or caseous material within the lumen of the air sac. These changes are indicative of a disease process.
- Fibrin is indicative of inflammation and is often associated with septicaemia or viral, bacterial, mycoplasmal or fungal infection.
  - *Chlamydia* infection causes thickening and significant coating of the membrane, and there may be foamy fibrin fluid present.
  - *Aspergillus* spp. cause a thick caseous discharge on the surface of the membrane, and mycelia that are grey-green, white or yellow in colour may be present.

- Large volumes of clear fluid in the air sacs may be water and are a sign that the bird may have been:
  - Drowned
  - Given intraperitoneal fluids that missed and accidentally went into the air sac
  - Euthanased by intracoelomic injection (if the fluid is green or pink/purple, this may be the euthanasia solution).
- Helminths may be present within the air sacs. They can be quite numerous in falcons and other birds of prey but do not seem to cause pathology. This is a common presentation in raptors in the Middle East and occasionally in Australia but not in the UK or USA.
- Finches may have air sac mites (*Sternostoma tracheacolum*) present. Mites cause a strong inflammatory response and the birds can be quite ill. In freshly deceased birds, these mites are seen as very small pin-head sized dots that are motile. In cool or longer deceased animals they are not motile. Microscopic examination will help with identification of any dots.
- A simple way to collect the air sac membrane for histopathology is to strip the air sac material on the internal aspect of the carina, once it has been displaced cranially.

13. Once the viscera have been examined *in situ*, each organ must be examined individually, starting with the heart (Figure 14.13).
- Identify the great vessels and sever their attachments, removing the heart.
- Assess the level of epicardial fat and compare with dietary components. It is normal for fat to be present around the coronary groove and at the apex.
- Starvation may be suspected if there is serous atrophy of the epicardial fat deposits. This is seen as gelatinous brown mucoid-like material in many of the fat deposits, but is more easily visualized in the epicardial fat reserves.
- Examine the pericardium.
- Pericardial fluid is normally of small volume and clear.
  - Pericardium distended with blood may indicate cardiac tamponade, severe external blunt trauma or intracardiac euthanasia.
  - Excessive clear or mildly blood-stained pericardial fluid is often associated with heart failure.
  - Pericarditis with thickening of the pericardium and a fibrin film covering the epicardium (this makes the pericardium appear white) may be associated with septicaemia or viral vasculitis.
  - Fibrinous pericardial fluid may be seen in *Chlamydia* infection.
  - White powdery film covering the pericardium is associated with visceral gout. Microscopic examination will reveal uric acid crystals.
  - Increased pericardial fluid with white mineralized plaques on the pericardium may indicate intracardiac or intravenous euthanasia with undiluted barbiturate solution.

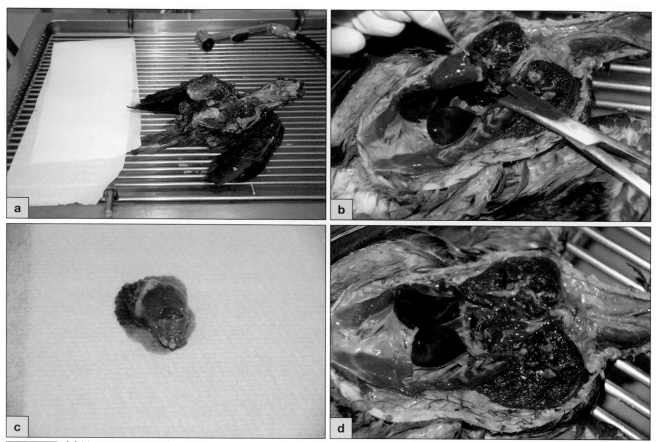

14.13 (a) Use a paper towel to place specimens collected from the patient and absorb any discharges. (b) Grasp the heart and cut through the great vessels at the base of the heart. (c) Heart removed from body. Note the thickened pericardium and inflammatory material present. (d) Once the heart has been removed, the syrinx and surrounding structures can be examined.

- Pericardial or heart contents can be useful for culture and should be sampled at this point if required. Open the pericardium with a scalpel or scissors, identify the great vessels and use them to enter the atria, incising the atrial walls and finally the myocardium. If required, use a swab to collect a sterile sample.
- A blood smear from the ventricle contents may show blood parasites and a Gram stain may demonstrate bacteraemia.
- Thoroughly examine the heart (this may be performed later in the post-mortem examination).
    - Assess the cardiac conformation.
        * Is the heart enlarged unilaterally or bilaterally?
        * Are the major vessels normal?
    - Assess the time of death.
        * Recent or sudden death will present with the ventricles in diastole and expanded.
        * If the bird has been dead for some time, the ventricles will be in systole and contracted.
    - Cardiac failure will present with single- or double-sided ventricular dilatation, and so an enlarged myocardium.
    - Open the right ventricle, beginning at the pulmonary artery, through the ventricular wall down to the apex and then continue around to the other side. Pass through the atrioventricular (AV) valve and into the right atrium and vena cava. This exposes the

entire ventricle, both AV valves and the pulmonary artery semilunar valves (Harrigan, 1981). Examine the interventricular septum for any abnormalities. Repeat this form of incision for the left ventricle and atrium.
    - Open the AV valve leading to the aorta and note any mineralization of the wall. Palpate for thickening that may be a sign of atherosclerosis or arteriosclerosis. This is more commonly seen in parrots (Harrison and Lightfoot, 2006).
    - In small birds, this level of dissection of the heart is not possible, so the whole heart should be submitted for histopathology.
14. Once the heart has been removed, the distal oesophagus can be grasped with forceps and elevated so that the distal attachment of the oesophagus to the proventriculus can be severed, allowing the proventriculus to be elevated out of the body. By snipping the adjacent air sac membranes, the gastrointestinal tract and liver can be removed as a whole unit (Figure 14.14).
- Identify the spleen at the isthmus (junction of the proventriculus and ventriculus) and close to the posterior aspect of the liver.
    - There is considerable species variability in the shape of the spleen. It is spherical in parrots and elongated and tubular in finches and Canaries.
    - Take note of its size (in mm) because in many septicaemic diseases the spleen becomes greatly enlarged – particularly *Chlamydia*

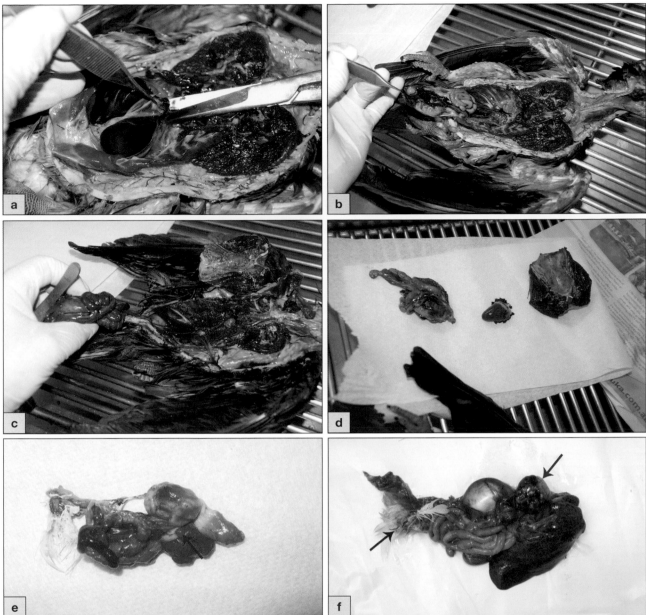

14.14 (a) Use a pair of scissors to identify and elevate the distal oesophagus as it connects to the proventriculus. (b) Continue to elevate the oesophagus and draw it up caudally to allow removal of the whole gastrointestinal tract. (c) Once the gastrointestinal tract has been removed, incise around the vent to ensure the bursa of Fabricius is included in the structures removed (important in any bird under 1 year old). (d) The tissues are placed to the side for more thorough examination. (e) Note the relative size of the spleen (arrowed). This is a normal size and shape for parrots. (f) The gastrointestinal tract is laid to one side for closer examination and dissection. Note the enlarged haemorrhagic spleen (red arrow) and feathers at the vent (black arrow). This bird was diagnosed with mycobacteriosis on histopathology.

infection in parrots and *Yersinia* infection in finches. Small white spots visible on the serosa may be micro-abscesses and indicate that swabs should be collected for bacteriology.

- Dissect out the spleen and retain for histopathology or microbiology as indicated.
- Continue to raise and dissect out the gastrointestinal tract as a whole. Continue the incision and dissect the surrounding tissues to emerge through the skin lateral to the vent and allow the cloaca to be removed intact.
- Take care that food material, debris or blood does not spill out and contaminate the kidneys.
- Examine the external serosa of the cloaca to see if there is a bursa of Fabricius on the dorsal surface of the cloaca. This is laid to one side and the remaining organs examined *in situ*.
- When all the gastrointestinal tract has been removed, examine the peritoneum for:
  - Signs of fibrin, indicative of inflammation/septicaemia, foreign bodies and ventriculus/intestinal perforation
  - Neoplasia
  - Plaques of *Aspergillus* spp.
  - Excess fluid from heart failure.
15. With the gastrointestinal tract removed, the gonads, kidneys and adrenal glands (and lungs) can be visualized (Figure 14.15).
  - The normal kidney is a red/brown lobular structure, extending from just caudal to the lungs down towards close to the cloaca.

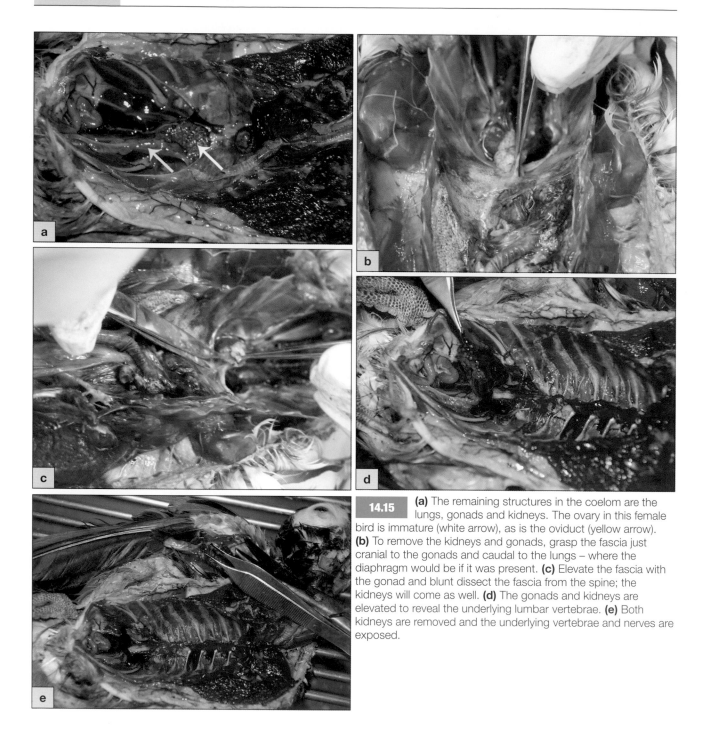

14.15 **(a)** The remaining structures in the coelom are the lungs, gonads and kidneys. The ovary in this female bird is immature (white arrow), as is the oviduct (yellow arrow). **(b)** To remove the kidneys and gonads, grasp the fascia just cranial to the gonads and caudal to the lungs – where the diaphragm would be if it was present. **(c)** Elevate the fascia with the gonad and blunt dissect the fascia from the spine; the kidneys will come as well. **(d)** The gonads and kidneys are elevated to reveal the underlying lumbar vertebrae. **(e)** Both kidneys are removed and the underlying vertebrae and nerves are exposed.

- There are three lobes bilaterally and they are buried in indentations within the caudal vertebrae and sacrum.
- Only the ventral surface is easily visualized. This is usually smooth with very fine lobulations visible.
- The whole kidney must be dissected out of the indentations for a full examination.
  * The kidneys, gonads and adrenal glands are usually dissected out as a group.
  * Begin by elevating the anterior poles of the kidneys as well as the gonads and dissecting the fascial attachments to the bony spine.
- Examine the ureter.
  - The ureter runs along the ventral surface of the kidney, on the ventromedial aspect, from the middle of the kidney down to the cloaca.

- White urates are not normally visualized within the stroma of the kidney or the proximal part of the ureter.
- Examine the kidneys.
  - Congestion, swelling, the presence of urates and pale coloration are the common signs of kidney disease.
  - Close examination may reveal white tubules, full of urates, in the body of the kidney.
  - The most common renal problems are:
    * Neoplasia (e.g. renal adenocarcinoma in Budgerigars, nephroblastoma in chickens). A common sign seen with neoplasia is lameness on the affected side as the tumour mass places pressure on the femoral nerves and spine
    * Nephrosis from toxins and metabolic disorders

* Nephritis from infections (viral, coccidian and flukes). Collect any material to examine oocysts (coccidia) and eggs (flukes) microscopically.
* Examine the adrenal glands.
    - These are usually small, yellow to orange, triangular-shaped glands, anterodorsal to the kidneys, close to the midline on each side.
    - There can be variation in the size, colour and shape of the adrenal glands between species.
    - In breeding birds, the enlarged gonad will obscure the adrenal gland, making it hard to evaluate.
16. Examine the gonads and reproductive tract.
    * Are they quiescent or active?
        - Does this match the stage of the breeding season that is currently present?
    * Female birds.
        - With a few exceptions (some falcons and the Brown Kiwi) most birds have only the left ovary and left oviduct present. The right oviduct is present during the embryonic stage but usually regresses before, or soon after, the egg hatches.
        - The ovary in juvenile birds is in a quiescent state. It is a flat, mostly triangular structure found at the anteroventral aspect of the left kidney. It extends across the midline and is often found overlying the adrenal gland as well. The undeveloped follicles give it a granular appearance that is usually creamy-grey in colour.
        - In adult birds out of the breeding season, the ovary is in a quiescent state and covered by small yellow-golden spherical yolks. The oviduct is smaller and not well developed.
        - During the breeding season the yolks are more developed. Yellow-golden yolks at many different stages of development may be seen and the oviduct is enlarged.
        - In some birds the ovary may have a dark colour from melanin pigmentation. This is normal.
        - In some egg-laying chickens, the oviduct and ovary can be quite enlarged and need to be dissected out with care.
        - Common problems:
            * Underdeveloped state when should be cycling
            * Neoplasia is commonly seen in Budgerigars and Cockatiels. Lymphomatosis, adenocarcinomas, leiomyosarcomas, leiomyomas, adenomas and granulosa cell tumours have been reported (Harrison and Lightfoot, 2006)
            * Degeneration and rupture or involution of follicles are seen with infection or excessive stress. Ruptured follicles release yolk material into the coelom, potentially causing yolk-related peritonitis. Many birds can tolerate yolk material well but opportunistic infectious agents (particularly *Escherichia coli* in parrots and *Salmonella pullorum* in chickens) can use the yolk material and develop into a bacteraemia/septicaemia
            * Impaction of eggs and inflammatory material in the lumen of the oviduct, causing it to be greatly distended

* The oviduct may experience motility issues. Yolks or partially formed eggs deposited in the coelomic cavity from reverse peristalsis of the oviduct, cause prolapse of the oviduct through the cloaca.
* Male birds.
    - Males have two bean-shaped testes, one each side of the midline at the cranioventral aspect of the kidneys.
    - It is normal for the testes to be different in shape and size compared with each other. The left testis is usually larger than the right testis in juvenile birds but at maturity this changes and the right testis often grows larger than the left testis (King and McLelland, 1984).
    - The testes are usually cream coloured but can also have melanin pigmentation.
    - In juvenile birds, the testes are thin and small.
    - In an adult breeding bird they can be quite large, but undergo development and regression during the annual breeding cycle.
    - Common problems:
        * Underdeveloped state when should be breeding
        * Orchitis (*Chlamydia* infection secondary to infection in adjacent structures such as air sacs and kidneys)
        * Neoplasia: Sertoli cell tumour, seminoma, interstitial cell tumour and lymphosarcoma have been reported (Harrison and Lightfoot, 2006).
* Samples of these tissues are collected as indicated.
17. The lungs are embedded in the ribs, anterior to the kidneys (Figure 14.16).
    * Normal lungs are pink and similar to the lungs of mammals but denser, as they do not inflate. They are embedded into the rib cage and vertebrae on their dorsal surface.
    * Use blunt dissection with the tips of scissors to remove one or preferably both lungs and examine the dorsal and cut surfaces.
    * Palpate and examine for any masses (e.g. abscesses, foreign bodies).
    * Pneumonia is less common than air sacculitis as a manifestation of lower respiratory tract disease.
    * Common problems:
        - Mycotic or bacterial infections
            * Fibrinous exudate on the lung surface or dark red areas of congestion and inflammation
            * Granulomas
            * Focal abscesses (infiltration from emboli)
        - Neoplasia (diffuse, nodules) is more easily identified during palpation.
18. Return to the gastrointestinal tract that was removed earlier and placed to the side (Figure 14.17).
    * If not already done, samples can be taken from the liver and spleen (e.g. impression smears, swabs).
    * Tease out the mesentery from the intestines and arrange the intestines on the table in a shape that allows visualization of all parts.

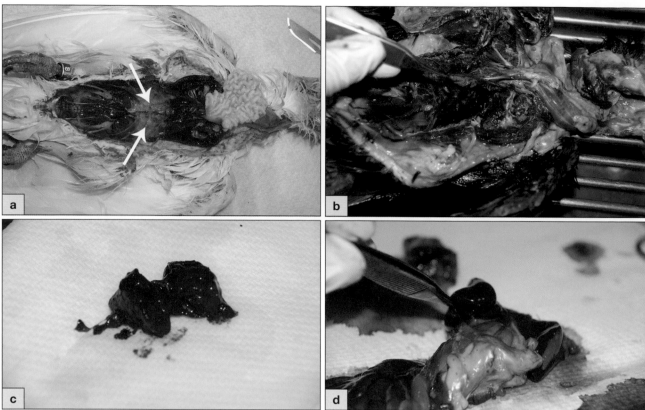

14.16 **(a)** The lungs (arrowed) of this Indian Ringnecked Parakeet are a normal pink colour. **(b)** Use blunt dissection to remove the lung lobes. **(c)** Lungs are removed for examination and sampling. Note the fibrin tags on the external surface. **(d)** Select and harvest samples with typical lesions.

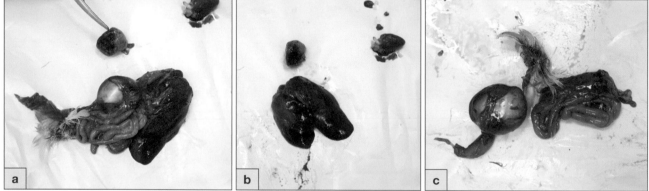

14.17 **(a)** This enlarged spleen has been removed; impression smears can be collected for cytology and the spleen sent for histopathology. **(b)** The liver is removed so the proventriculus, ventriculus and intestines can be dissected and examined. **(c)** Proventriculus, ventriculus and intestines are removed after the liver, to allow examination.

- Look for signs of:
  - Intestinal obstruction from a foreign body, intussusception or similar changes
  - Focal peritonitis from a perforation or lesion in the gastrointestinal tract.
- Examine the mesentery that is present.
  - In young birds there may be a brown nodule of what appears to be inspissated material, attached to the mesentery, intestines or floating in the coelomic cavity. This is the yolk remnant.
- Birds have two stomachs – the proventriculus and the ventriculus.
- Open the gastrointestinal tract, beginning at the proventriculus, continuing through the isthmus to the ventriculus.

19. Examine the proventriculus (Figure 14.18).
    - The proventriculus is the softer, glandular component of the stomach system.
      - In birds that eat digestively resistant foods (e.g. granivorous, herbivorous and insectivorous birds), there is a distinct boundary between the proventriculus and ventriculus.
      - In birds that eat relatively soft foods (e.g. carnivorous or piscivorous birds) this margin is less distinct and the proventriculus is relatively larger and the ventriculus smaller.
    - The proventriculus usually has a muscular wall and a glandular mucosa that is a grey-white colour. There are small openings of these glands spread over the mucosa, adjacent to dense lymphoid tissue.

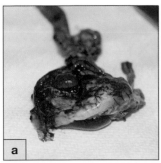
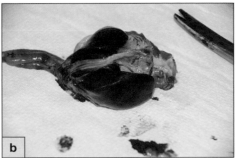
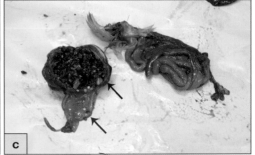

14.18 Examine the **(a)** gastrointestinal tract and **(b)** spleen. **(c)** The proventriculus (red arrow) and ventriculus (black arrow) are opened and the contents examined.

- Helminth parasites may be found in the proventricular lumen, or they may form small nodules in the mucosa.
- Mild congestion of the mucosa may be a sign of mycotic or bacterial infection.
- The isthmus that connects the proventriculus to the ventriculus is a common site for lesions caused by the avian gastric yeast *Macrorhabdus ornithogaster* (previously called Megabacteria). It is present as a thick paste-like material that causes a blockage of the proventricular outflow.

20. Examine the ventriculus (Figure 14.19).
- The ventriculus is the large muscular component of the stomach system in most common bird species.
    - Examine the serosa prior to cutting into the lumen.
    - Perforations of the ventriculus wall may lead to focal peritonitis in the adjacent tissues.
- The lining of the ventriculus in granivores is a thick layer of keratin called the koilin layer (Figure 14.19c). This is resistant to the grinding that is required for the hard seeds these birds consume. Suitable grit should be present in these birds to assist grinding.
    - If small grit is provided, it does not remain in the ventriculus long enough to be useful.
    - If large grit is provided, it may cause a foreign body obstruction or impaction.
    - Raptors form a cast of fur, feathers, bones and other indigestible components that is regurgitated. This may be present at post-mortem examination.

- Grit may not be required for granivores on a pelleted diet, as the food is more easily digested.
- Collect the contents of the ventriculus and examine the components to assess if they are digestible and appropriate for the species. Identify any foreign bodies that may be present.
    - Metallic foreign bodies, especially lead, zinc or copper, can be toxic.
    - If toxicosis is suspected, collect a sample of liver, kidney and brain and freeze for toxicology analysis.
    - Alternatively, if this is suspected before the post-mortem examination is commenced, a whole-body radiograph can be useful for diagnosis. It should be noted that not all radiopaque materials are metal and not all metal opacities are toxic. Use the history to assist in identifying possible sources of any radiopacities.
    - If only the ventriculus is available, radiography can be performed to assess its contents.
- Peel the koilin layer from the interior of the ventriculus and examine for parasites underneath.
    - A range of spiruroids, mainly *Cheilospirura* spp. and *Acuaria* spp. in Australian finches, have been reported.
        * They can be visualized under the koilin layer (Harrigan, 1981).
        * These parasites can be difficult to see and magnification may be required.
        * Infection may be associated with ulcerative changes in the mucosa.
    - Ulceration of the ventriculus mucosa is common but often the cause is not identified.

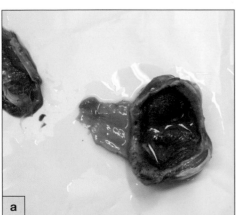
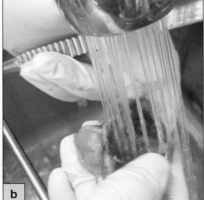
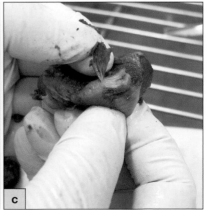

14.19 **(a)** Once the contents have been examined, **(b)** the ventriculus can be washed to reveal the koilin layer. **(c)** Peel the koilin layer away to examine for parasites or other lesions.

21. Examine the small intestine (Figure 14.20).
    - Carnivorous and piscivorous birds have a short small intestine.
    - Examine the serosal surface of the length of the intestine.
        - Look for any signs of inflammation, indicative of petechiae, haemorrhage or congestion.
        - Fibrin or caseous purulent material on the serosa is indicative of peritonitis.
        - A white powdery coating is indicative of visceral gout.
        - Perforations, plaques and red or white areas of necrosis may indicate pathology that has penetrated from the mucosal surface.
    - Look for a uniform diameter throughout the intestines.
        - Areas of ballooning, dilatation or flaccidity should be examined more closely.
        - Look for the presence of helminths such as *Ascaridia* spp. in parrots and tapeworms in finches.
    - Use sharp pointed scissors to open the lumen. If possible, open the entire intestine and examine the mucosa.
    - Use a scalpel blade to perform a scraping of the lining of the intestine from at least three separate positions:
        - The anterior segment (duodenum), identified easily as it forms a loop with the fleshy pancreas in the centre of the loop
        - The middle segment, found adjacent to the yolk sac diverticulum
        - The posterior segment, proximal to the caecum (if it is present)
        - Examine each of these scrapings under a microscope as a wet saline smear and/or a Gram stain, looking for helminth eggs, protozoan oocysts and abnormal bacteria.
    - Examine the intestinal contents.
        - The anterior segment contains a thick fluid of freshly mixed and digested material from the ventriculus. It can resemble, and be mistaken for, exudate.
        - In the middle and posterior segments it is not uncommon to have minimal contents present.
    - The normal mucosa should be a yellow creamy colour.
    - Look for pathological changes.
        - Mild enteritis (e.g. bacterial):
            * Excessive serous fluid contents
            * Mild flaccidity present
            * Perform a Gram stain.
        - Coccidia or capillaria:
            * More significant flaccidity
            * More voluminous mucoid fluid present.
        - Protozoa and migrating helminth parasites:
            * More extensive and focal haemorrhage
            * Ulcers present on mucosa
            * May have diphtheritic membranes present on mucosa.
        - Careful examination and consideration of the signs should help differentiate between necrosis and autolysis.
    - Take representative sections for histopathology and cytology. Specimens for histopathology are best opened and flattened to allow fixation in this position, for consistent results.
    - Collect any parasite specimens encountered for identification.

22. Perform a similar examination as for the small intestine on the colon, caeca (if present) and cloaca (Figure 14.21). This area has similar signs to those seen in the small intestine.
    - The presence of paired caeca identifies the end of the small intestine.
    - Mesentery attaches the caeca to the lateral aspect of the small intestine for most of their length. Peel away this attachment, to allow better visualization of each caecum.
    - Some commonly encountered birds (e.g. parrots) do not have caeca – in these birds the termination of the small intestine is not easily identified.
    - In pigeons the caeca are greatly reduced to small, vestigial, nodular structures.

23. Examine the pancreas.
    - The pancreas is situated within the loop of intestine formed by the duodenum. It is fleshy in appearance and has sharp edges.
    - Selenium deficiency has been reported to cause atrophy and fibrosis of the pancreas.
    - Complete atrophy may be a result of paramyxovirus type 3 (PMV-3).
    - Neoplasia:
        - Primary pancreatic tumours are rare
        - Metastatic tumours from lymphosarcoma and oviductal (magnum) carcinoma have been reported (Harrigan, 1981).

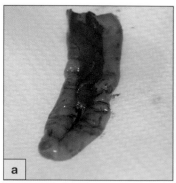
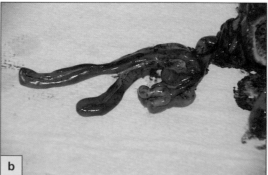
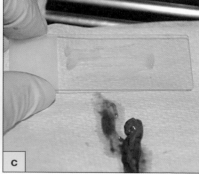

14.20   **(a)** Tissue samples of duodenal loop and pancreas can be selected for submission for histopathology and other tests as indicated. **(b)** Samples of the contents of the intestines can also be taken for **(c)** microscopic examination in warm saline smears or stains such as Diff-Quik® or Gram.

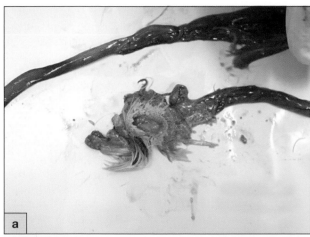

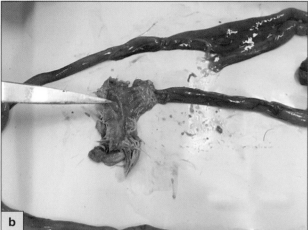

14.21 **(a)** The vent should be opened and dissected to reveal the **(b)** mucosa of the cloaca.

24. Open each caecum (in those species that have them) using scissors placed in the lumen.
   - Small nodules protruding into the lumen at the junction with the intestine are composed of lymphoid tissue (the caecal tonsils).
     - Normal contents will vary depending on the dietary components. Their colour can vary from yellow to dark brown.
     - The normal mucosa is clear and smooth with a small number of folds on the surface.
     - Normal caecal contents are easily removed from the mucosa. If the contents are thickened, laminated or attached to the mucosa, pathology should be considered:
       * Previous haemorrhage that has dehydrated will form a cast of caseous exudate (sometimes laminated and attached to ulcerated mucosa) that has a friable and granular consistency
       * Infection with organisms such as *Salmonella* spp. or *Histomonas* spp. may be seen as a fibrinous coating on the caecal mucosa
       * Fresh haemorrhage may be associated with euthanasia by cracking the cervical vertebrae.
     - Perform a mucosal scrape with a scalpel blade and examine microscopically for evidence of protozoan or helminth infestation.

25. The large intestine/colon/rectum is normally quite short.
   - Collect a faecal sample from here to examine for helminth eggs and protozoan oocysts.
   - Retain specimens for histopathology as indicated.
26. Examine the bones and joints (Figure 14.22).
   - Check the joints for swelling and accumulation of white material; these are signs of articular gout, seen particularly in Budgerigars, lovebirds and *Neophema* spp.
   - After palpation to assess swelling, open the major joints of the long bones (shoulder, elbow, stifle, hock, tarsal and metatarsal joints). The hock in particular should be examined, to rule out bending and dystrophy seen with perosis (slipping of the Achilles tendon).
   - Check for signs of arthritis and tenosynovitis.
     - Acute cases have swollen joints, full of exudate, with obvious signs of inflammation.
     - Chronic cases often have ankylosis and lameness.
     - Common causes include *Mycoplasma*, viruses, bacteria (e.g. *Staphylococcus* spp. in aviary birds) and helminths.
     - Select appropriate samples to differentiate these causes.

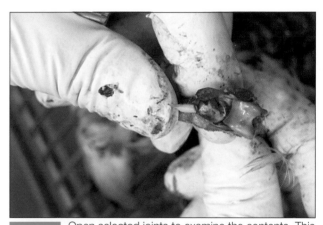

14.22 Open selected joints to examine the contents. This is a stifle.

   - Examine the long bones and assess for pliability, fractures and osteomyelitis.
   - For close examination of a bone, it is best to fix it in formalin, demineralize it and examine histologically.
   - Open a couple of long bones and examine the bone marrow (with fresh cytology smears), if any is visible. Bone marrow can be harvested from either the tibiotarsus, femur or tarsometatarsus and placed in 10% buffered formalin.
   - In adult birds the medullary cavity of the tibiotarsus is filled with adipose tissue that may be depleted to a gelatinous consistency in starvation (Harrigan, 1981).
27. Examine the ribs once the lungs have been removed.
   - Metabolic bone disease or osteodystrophy may be seen as healed fractures where the bone has been bent or changed degree of angulation.
   - Rickets may cause swelling of the attachment of the ribs to the vertebrae. This appears as a string of beads, beneath the lungs.

28. Remove the skin and muscles from the skull in preparation for examination.
   - To examine the skull, some practitioners find it easier to remove the head at the atlanto-occipital joint, but the author prefers to leave the head attached, particularly in small birds, as the body gives some stability when manipulating the skull.
   - Examine the bones of the skull.
     - Are any indentations or fractures evident? This may be seen with trauma such as flying into the wall of the aviary.
     - Is there haemorrhage in the skull bones?
   - Beware of drawing conclusions about cranial haemorrhage based upon bloodstaining in the skull bones. This is often a 'normal' agonal change at time of death or it may be extravasation into bony sinuses post-mortem.
   - Cranial haemorrhage is suspected if there are blood clots or an excessive collection of blood on, in or under the meninges, or if there is rupture of one of the cranial blood vessels visible on the surface of the brain. This author has had the opportunity to examine several birds that died after flying into a hard surface; most did not have any grossly visible changes to the blood vessels of the brain or the cervical structures.

29. The cranial cavity should be opened by dissecting around the margins of the skull with the points of sharp scissors (Figure 14.23); in small birds iris scissors are recommended.
   - The author uses the following principles:
     - Removal of just bone, sparing the underlying brain tissue
     - A transverse cut at the anterior aspect just behind the eyes
     - Each lateral aspect of the skull cut, from just behind the eye on each side down to the foramen magnum
     - If there is remaining bone, cut across the caudal aspect near the foramen magnum, allowing removal of a cap of skull bone to reveal the dorsal surface of the brain.
   - Blood found near the cerebellum may be leakage from venous sinuses, rather than haemorrhage.
   - The meninges may also need to be incised as they are attached to the surrounding structures.
   - Meningitis may be seen as congestion or fibrin over the surface of the brain and/or meninges.
   - Collect swabs from meninges or fibrinous exudate for microbial investigation.

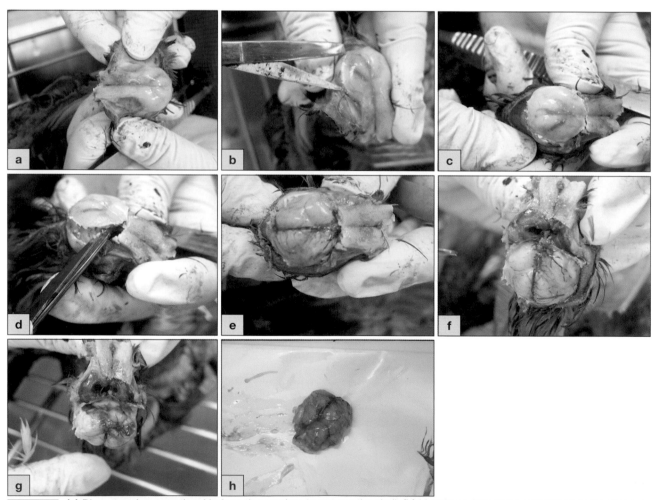

14.23 (a) Dissect and remove the skin from the cranium to expose the skull. (b) Use the points of the scissors to score and cut into the skull around the lateral circumference. (c) The bone of this skull has been scored so it is ready to be removed. (d) Use the points of the scissors to carefully elevate the skull. (e) The brain is revealed. Carefully remove the bone around the cerebellum. (f–g) Hold the head upside down so gravity is pulling the brain out of the cranial cavity to reveal the structures that need to be incised to allow removal of the brain. (h) Continue to carefully incise the nerves at the base of the skull and the brain will fall out.

- To collect the brain, begin dissection at the cranial olfactory lobes and sever the attachments to the base of the skull while holding the skull upside down so gravity pulls the brain downwards.
- Reach in with the tips of the iris scissors and carefully incise the optic chiasma and other cranial nerve attachments, and the brain will be gradually pulled out of the skull by gravity.
- Take care with removing the cerebellum as it often has a fragile bony surround that needs careful, gentle dissection.
- Once the whole brain has been removed, carefully inspect all surfaces for lesions; note that many brain diseases will not have obvious lesions.
- Place the whole brain in 10% buffered formalin to allow fixation for histopathology.
- Harvest the pituitary gland in the bony base of the skull.
  - Pituitary adenomas have been reported in several species but are most common in the Budgerigar and Cockatiel (Harrison and Lightfoot, 2006).

30. The brachial and sciatic plexuses should be examined as they leave the vertebrae (Figure 14.24).
- Examine the spinal cord and vertebrae.
- Look for fractures or deformities of the vertebrae.
- This author does not routinely remove the spinal cord for examination, but if paresis or other neurological deficits associated with the spine or peripheral nerves have been suggested by clinical signs in the history or seen during the external examination, it should be done.
  - Be patient and set aside enough time to complete the task; rushing can lead to poor samples.
  - Use sharp instruments for cutting bone and slowly chip away at the vertebrae. The author tends to use approaches to removing bone similar to a hemilaminectomy in dogs.
  - A fine dental burr can also be a useful tool for removing bone.

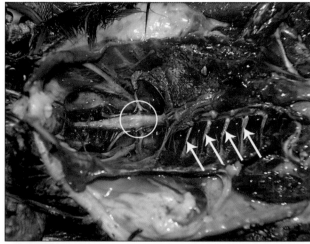

14.24 When the lungs and kidneys are removed, the ribs (arrowed) and the lumbar nerves (sciatic nerves; circled) are revealed.

Toxicology

Birds may be exposed to many different toxins. If organophosphate or organochlorine toxicity is suspected, collect as much fat tissue as possible and freeze for analysis at a later date. For other toxins, collect samples of liver, kidney and feathers as they may be useful for analysis.

For all toxicology submissions, a pathologist at the preferred pathology laboratory should be contacted prior to sending the samples, to ensure:

- Appropriate samples are collected
- Appropriate transportation and packaging of the samples
- A cost estimate is obtained, which is then discussed with the owner prior to committing to testing.

Histopathology

Practitioners must be aware that gross lesions are seldom pathognomonic. Many gross lesions can be misleading. With few exceptions, specimens should be carefully selected for further diagnostic tests, such as bacteriology or histopathology, to aid in a definitive diagnosis. Any sample intended for histopathology needs to be stored in greater than 10 times its own volume of buffered 10% formalin (Figure 14.25). Any tissues for fixation should not be greater than 5 mm thick. If tissues are congested with blood they should

---

Important questions for consideration during dissection

- Have specimens/samples appropriate to the abnormal or suspicious signs in the history and external examination been collected?
- Have specimens/samples of all abnormal or suspicious lesions detected during the post-mortem examination been collected?
- Is the crop full or empty?
  - Has the bird been eating recently?
  - Is there any evidence of anorexia or impaction?
- Is there grit in the ventriculus? Is the size and volume of the grit normal?
- Are internal parasites a problem?
- Is the bird obese?
- Is the bird's reproductive system cycling as it should be?
- Is an infectious or non-infectious primary disease suspected?
- Does the management of remaining birds need to be changed?

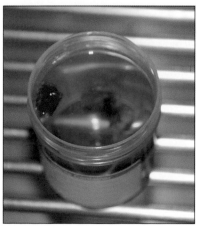

14.25 Place samples in 10 times their own volume of formalin.

be sliced more thinly than normal, as the formalin cannot penetrate as well as into normal tissue. Lungs and the brain are placed into formalin intact. The container should be swirled intermittently during the time prior to dispatch to assist in fixation.

Small birds, including neonates, can be opened in the ventral midline with a scalpel, from beak to cloaca, and then placed in an appropriate volume of buffered 10% formalin, otherwise intact. Further dissection is difficult on such small specimens.

Tissues routinely submitted for histopathology

- Crop lining
- Oesophagus
- Thymus (if present)
- Trachea
- Lung
- Air sac membrane (usually from internal surface of keel bone or any other site that is abnormal)
- Heart (myocardium) and great vessels
- Liver
- Spleen
- Proventriculus, isthmus and ventriculus
- Duodenum/pancreas
- Small intestine (from anterior, middle and posterior segments)
- Caecum (if present)
- Large intestine
- Cloaca/vent (include bursa of Fabricius if present)
- Kidney/gonad/adrenal gland (often removed as one piece and fixed together)
- Other tissues are added as indicated by signs and lesions:
  - Neurological (brain, spine, nerves)
  - Upper respiratory tract (nasal cavity, turbinates, periorbital sinus tissue)
  - Miscellaneous (bone, bone marrow, muscle, thyroid gland, pituitary gland, eyes, skin lesions)

To make the task of the pathologist easier, a full history sheet should accompany any samples sent to an external laboratory for testing.

Clinical pathology techniques used with post-mortem examination

Quite a few useful clinical pathology tests used in a small animal practice can be used equally as well for avian examination. It is advisable to perform as many cytological tests as possible in-house and send out to an external laboratory any for which the diagnosis is uncertain, to assist in learning.

When investigating disease in birds, it is important to appreciate that the inflammatory response is slightly different from that in mammals. The response is usually more frequently fibrinous than suppurative, more frequently forming granulomas than abscesses and involving heterophils rather than neutrophils, but the basic processes in both birds and mammals are similar (Harrigan, 1981).

The most useful cytology tests routinely performed in-house are:

- Impression smears of air sacs or serosal surfaces of organs (e.g. liver, spleen, obvious lesions)
  - Use Gram stain, Macchiavello, modified Ziehl-Neelsen (MZN), Gimenez, Diff-Quik®
- Warm saline smears
  - Intestinal wall scrapings for ova or oocysts (usually select three separate sites along the small intestine)
  - Faecal smears
  - Crop washes/scrapes for trichomonosis
  - These smears can be air-dried and then stained with Gram, Diff-Quik®, etc.
- Faecal flotation.

Samples can also be taken for in-house enzyme-linked immunosorbent assay (ELISA) tests such as those for *Chlamydia* infection.

Most other clinical pathology tests (e.g. bacterial culture and sensitivity testing of swabs from heart blood, tissues, body fluids or intestinal/crop contents, polymerase chain reaction (PCR)) are beyond the resources of a small in-house laboratory.

Summary

Avian practitioners should develop a good working relationship with an experienced avian pathologist. Histopathology, virology, serology, toxicology and exfoliative cytology, as well as more detailed bacteriology, are best handled by a veterinary pathologist. These tests will often give the definitive diagnosis that is not available from an in-house laboratory.

Post-mortem examination is one area of avian medicine that is underserviced and underutilized at present. It needs to be portrayed as a vital part of any aviary management programme. A methodical approach combined with good records will enable a practitioner working in conjunction with an experienced avian veterinary pathologist to offer a high-quality service to clients to eliminate many of the problems that are a direct result of keeping birds in captivity.

References and further reading

Australian Government (2006) Post mortem procedures and protocols for captive and wild birds. In: *Hygiene Protocols for the Prevention and Control of Diseases (Particularly Beak and Feather Disease) in Australian Birds*. Department of the Environment and Heritage. www.environment.gov.au/node/16193

Baraibar MA and Schoning P (1985) Effects of freezing and frozen storage on histological characteristics of canine tissues. *Journal of Forensic Sciences* 30(2), 439–447

Cooper JE and Cooper ME (2008) The exotic side of CSI: Forensics in non-domesticated animals. In: *Proceedings of the North American Veterinary Conference 2008*, pp. 1909–1911. NAVC, Florida

Harrigan KE (1981) Coping with and caring for dead birds. In: *Refresher Course for Veterinarians, Proceedings No. 55, Refresher Course on Aviary and Caged Birds*, ed. TG Hungerford, pp. 397–432. The Post-graduate Committee in Veterinary Science, The University of Sydney, Sydney

Harrison GJ and Lightfoot TL (2006) *Clinical Avian Medicine, Volume 2*. Spix Publishing Inc., Palm Beach

King AS and McLelland J (1984) *Birds: their structure and function*, p. 166. Baillière Tindall, London

Orosz S (2008) The path to histo results. In: *Proceedings of the North American Veterinary Conference 2008*, pp. 1697–1698. NAVC, Florida

St Leger J (2010) It's dead. Now what? Pathology for unusual species. In: *Proceedings of the North American Veterinary Conference 2010*. NAVC, Florida

Basic techniques

Andrés Montesinos

Avian patients pose particular challenges in terms of restraint, sample collection and performing clinical techniques. Some of the techniques discussed in this chapter may be part of the clinical examination or diagnostic investigation, while others may be the primary reason for the bird's presentation (e.g. beak trimming or wing clipping). Although most procedures used in canine and feline medicine are easily adapted to birds, anatomical and physiological differences require practitioners to familiarize themselves with the unique features of their avian patients.

Injection techniques

Intramuscular injection

This is the most common route by which parenteral drugs are given to birds. Intramuscular injections are typically administered into the pectoral musculature along either side of the mid-keel region. Traditionally, especially in raptors, the muscles of the legs have been used for intramuscular injections; however, these muscles are less voluminous than pectoral muscles and more prone to injury if the bird moves suddenly. Additionally, the presence of the renal and portal venous systems make intramuscular injections in the legs risky, and the legs should therefore be used only in cases where it is not possible to use the pectoral muscles (e.g. where the breast area is bandaged or has undergone surgery).

To perform the injection, the feathers are moved away from the featherless tract along the ventral midline of the keel using alcohol (Figure 15.1a). The needle is inserted at a shallow (<30-degree) angle into the muscle (Figure 15.1b). Injection into the cranial portion of the muscle mass should be avoided to prevent inadvertent injection into the pectoral vasculature, which is located in this cranial region. Prior to injecting, the operator should draw back the plunger to ensure that the drug is not being injected into a blood vessel. Further general considerations are detailed below.

- The choice of the needle (size and length) is important. A needle can cause significant tissue damage, especially in the smaller species of birds.

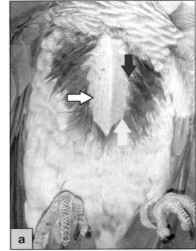

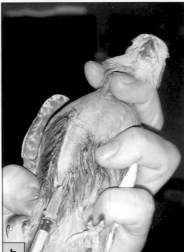

15.1
Intramuscular injection. **(a)** The feathers are wiped away with alcohol, exposing the sternal apterium or featherless tract of the skin (white arrow). Injection into the cranial portion of the muscle (red arrow) should be avoided to prevent inadvertent injection into the pectoral vasculature, located in this region. The correct place for injection is marked with the yellow arrow. **(b)** The smallest available needle size, especially for smaller birds, should be used for intramuscular injection. The needle should be inserted into the muscle at a shallow angle.

In general terms, a needle of as narrow a gauge and as short a length as is consistent with efficient administration of the drug is desirable (25 to 30 G needles are most commonly used). However, too thin a needle may prove unsatisfactory for thick, viscous compounds, and too short a needle may make it impossible to place a depot drug deep into the musculature.

- The volume of the injected medication must be considered. An injection of 0.1 ml into a 500 g bird is equivalent (on a weight:weight basis) to a single injection of 14 ml into a 70 kg human. Care should be taken when injecting large volumes as this may be a source of pain in an already sick bird. As a general guideline, the maximum volumes that can be given per site are as follows:

- Macaws and large cockatoos, 1 ml
- Amazons and Grey Parrots, 0.5 ml
- Cockatiels and small conures, 0.2 ml
- Budgerigars, 0.1 ml
- Canaries or finches, 0.05 ml

■ A volume of up to 1.5 ml can be administered in birds weighing >1.5 kg. If larger volumes are required, these should be administered via several injection sites. Note: multiple injections in the same side of the breast or the use of irritant drugs may result in muscle necrosis or atrophy.

■ Certain drugs (e.g. enrofloxacin, doxycycline hyclate, long-acting oxytetracycline preparations, tylosine and some meloxicam injectable preparations) may be extremely irritant. It is advisable to avoid intramuscular administration of these drugs where possible.

■ The site choice must be made in the context of the bird's individual circumstances. For example, large volumes or irritant drugs will cause muscle degeneration and, likely, some impairment of muscle function around the injection site. Therefore, it is recommended to inject such compounds into muscle mass that is less likely to cause the bird inconvenience or adverse effect. For example, more terrestrial birds that prefer to walk rather than fly (e.g. many companion parrots) should generally have injections into their pectoral muscles, whereas a performance raptor should be injected in the leg muscles (Note: when leg muscles are used, only small volumes are acceptable and the cranial tibial muscle should be used).

Subcutaneous injection

This is a very useful route for administering fluid and large volumes of drugs; however, irritant drugs and very large volumes can result in skin sloughing. Fluids can be administered subcutaneously in the inguinal, interscapular or axillary region, but the preferred site is the large precrural fold (Figure 15.2 and see Subcutaneous injection clip on CD). Volumes as great as 20 ml/kg may be administered in one location. Generally, absorption from subcutaneous sites is rapid and large volumes of fluid may be absorbed within 15 minutes. The rate of absorption depends on the species; whereas raptors and passerines are able to absorb large volumes of fluids, the majority of psittacine birds cannot and often develop oedema. Care should be taken not to enter the body cavity inadvertently while injecting or to damage the blood vessels, which can bleed profusely, especially in small passerines. Fluids administered subcutaneously are poorly absorbed during severe dehydration and hypovolaemic shock.

Intravenous injection and blood collection

Venous blood is the most commonly collected avian haematological sample, but the best peripheral vein site depends partly on the bird's anatomy, the clinician's experience and the volume of blood desired. The right

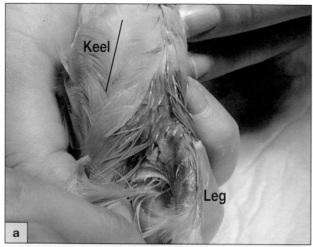

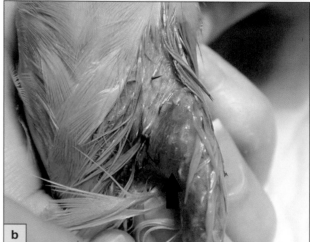

15.2 Subcutaneous injection. **(a)** View of the precrural fold of a lovebird. Note the available 'space' under this fold for large volumes of fluid. **(b)** The precrural fold, after the injection of subcutaneous fluids, is arrowed.

jugular vein is the most frequently used venepuncture site in pet bird species (see **Jugular blood sample** and **Jugular blood sample – anaesthetized** clips on CD). Other common and less commonly used blood collection sites are described in Chapter 12. (See also **Intravenous injection** clip on CD.)

Intravenous catheterization

Intravenous catheterization may be required in some situations, either for continuous or bolus fluid therapy, or where repeated use of intravenous drugs is needed. A small (24–26 G) over-the-needle Teflon®-coated catheter is guided into the vein, butterflied with tape, and secured with acrylic glue or sutures to the skin. The catheter may be placed into the basilic, medial metatarsal (Figure 15.3 and see **Intravenous catheter** clip on CD) or jugular vein. When using the basilic vein, the wing should be wrapped in a figure-of-eight bandage. When using a jugular catheter, the neck should be wrapped lightly in cotton padding and self-adherent bandages. A fluid pump that can administer small fluid volumes, such as a syringe pump, should be used. In the case of birds with powerful beaks, a plastic power-line protector can be used to surround the fluid line; parrots tend to remove the catheter as soon as they start to recover.

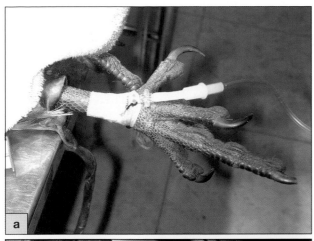

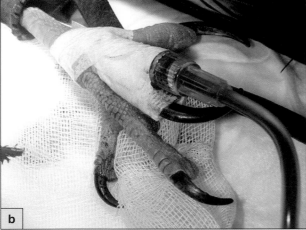

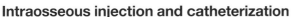

15.3 Intravenous catheterization. **(a)** Intravenous catheter, connected to an infusion pump, in the metatarsal vein of a vulture. **(b)** Intravenous catheter placed in the digital vein of a Harris' Hawk using a 24 G over-the-needle catheter.

Intraosseous injection and catheterization

Intraosseous catheters provide a rapid, stable and accessible route for fluid therapy. Any drug or fluid injectable by the intravenous route, with the exception of extremely caustic drugs (e.g. chemotherapeutic drugs), can be administered by the intraosseous route. Either the tibiotarsus (see **Intraosseous catheter – tibiotarsus** clip on CD) or ulna (see **Intraosseous catheter – ulna** clip on CD) may be used, depending on the patient's clinical condition and the clinician's preference. Only the tibiotarsus and ulna can be used, as avian bones are pneumatized; however, in altricial youngsters the femur is not pneumatized until full growth is reached, and so offers an alternative location for catheterization. As a rule of thumb, if the chick is still covered by down feathers, the femur can be used (Figure 15.4).

Intraosseous catheters are recommended for smaller species and for short procedures such as intra-operative administration of fluids or blood transfusions. The needle used can be a specialized bone needle, a spinal needle of appropriate length or a standard injection needle (18 G, 38 mm for birds >700 g; 21 G, 25 mm for birds between 200 and 700 g; 23 G, 20 mm for birds <200 g). For birds <100 g a 27–30 G standard needle can be used, and the needle hollow can be filled with fluid in order to avoid marrow material getting stuck in the needle.

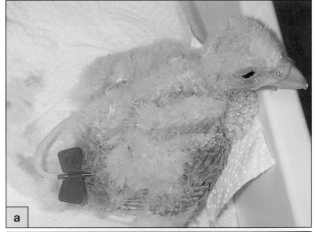

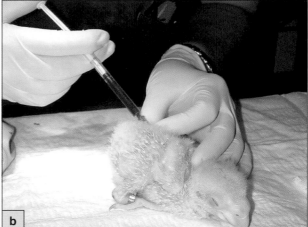

15.4 **(a)** Intraosseous approach to the femur of a falcon chick using a butterfly needle. In young chicks whose bone air sacs are not yet developed, the femur can be used for intraosseous catheterization. **(b)** Blood transfusion in a Jardine's Parrot chick using the femoral intraosseous approach. All the substances that can be injected intravenously can be injected intraosseously, including blood. Note the small syringe used for intraosseous injections.

The tibiotarsal approach is easily performed:

1. The bird should be anaesthetized, unless it is extremely weakened, as intraosseous catheterization is a painful procedure. It is placed in dorsal recumbency with the chosen leg extended and flexed at the stifle.
2. The proximal end of the stifle is prepared for an aseptic procedure. Local anaesthesia can be used over the zone but care must be taken with the dose used (diluting the drug as much as necessary).
3. The tibiotarsus is grasped in one hand, and the thumb and index finger used to determine the position of the tibiotarsus bone.
4. The needle is inserted into the cnemial crest through the insertion of the patellar tendon that is aligned with the diaphysis. Gentle pressure is placed on the needle and it is carefully rotated. The needle is advanced to a point approximately one-third to one-half the length of the bone.
5. A tape 'butterfly' can be placed on the hub of the needle and sutured to the skin of the stifle.

Alternatively, an intraosseous catheter may be placed into the distal ulna.

1. With the bird anaesthetized, the feathers of the dorsal and distal ulna are plucked from the area of the wrist joint. This joint is just proximal to the superficial ulnar artery and superficial digital flexor tendon, which may be seen through the skin (Figure 15.5a).
   The wing is supported in one hand while, with the other hand, an appropriately sized needle is positioned at the distal end of the ulna parallel to the diaphysis and then driven carefully into the medullary canal using firm pressure and a slight twisting motion (Figure 15.5b).
2. When the needle penetrates the cortex, it should pass without resistance once in the narrow cavity. Aspiration of the syringe should produce a small amount of marrow in the hub of the needle. Resistance when driving the needle indicates that the needle is crossing another cortex and the needle must be redirected. A protection cup using a piece of cut syringe can be used (Figure 15.5c).
3. To confirm correct positioning, a small volume of fluid may be injected while watching the basilic vein, where the bolus may be seen, or radiographs may be taken (Figure 15.5d).
4. Once placed, the needle can be flushed with heparinized solution and secured (Figure 15.5e), first with a 'butterfly' of tape sutured to the skin and then with a light figure-of-eight bandage to immobilize the wing.

The most common complication with intraosseous catheterization is osteomyelitis, so it is recommended that the equipment should not be left in place for more than 3 days. In cases of osteoporotic birds, an iatrogenic fracture may result. Placing intraosseous catheters in female birds with increased medullary bone density may be impossible due to the lack of a medullary canal.

As bone is not an elastic structure, high-pressure fluids can cause intense pain. Therefore, small syringes, not bigger than 3 ml, should be used; several 1 ml syringes are preferred to one of 5 ml. The use of small syringes allows for easy fluid delivery and the bird will be comfortable.

Intraosseous drugs can be delivered in boluses or using syringe drivers, the latter of which is especially useful to avoid high pressure during infusions and overloading of fluid in the body of the patient. Raptors tolerate the use of fluid lines connected to the syringe driver well; parrots are likely to interfere with the fluid line using their powerful beaks.

The intraosseous approach can also be used to obtain bone marrow in cases of chronically anaemic birds.

Oral medication

Administration of medications via drinking water is generally not recommended for pet birds. Flocks of birds are often treated with medicated food or water, but therapeutic drug concentrations are seldom achieved in companion and aviary birds. Most of the avian species seen in practice refuse to drink water with an abnormal taste, which can result in dehydration; therefore, most infections in companion birds cannot be adequately treated with medicated water.

It is also difficult to achieve a therapeutic concentration with medicated feeds. Sick birds eat less food. If the medication is placed in food different from the usual diet of the bird, even palatable medicated food may be refused. Crushed tablets, oral suspensions and powders can be mixed with moist food (especially for passerines and raptors); however, the energy content and palatability of the diet will affect the amount consumed and therefore the dose of the medication

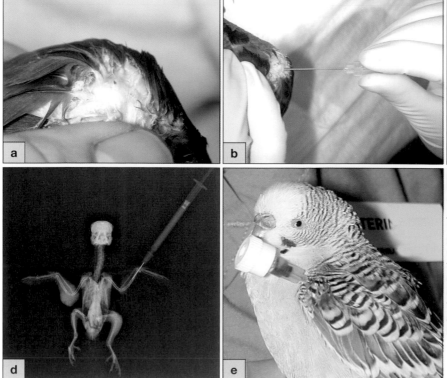

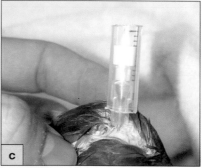

15.5 Intraosseous catheter placement. **(a)** View of the dorsal condyle of the ulna near the wrist joint. **(b)** The catheter is carefully driven into the medullary canal using firm pressure and a slight twisting motion. **(c)** A small protection cup may be fashioned using a cut piece of a syringe. **(d)** Radiographs should be taken if there is doubt about the correct positioning of the catheter. **(e)** Use of a 25 G needle as an intraosseous catheter in a Budgerigar; bandage not yet applied in this image.

ingested. Tetracycline-medicated formulated commercial diets are available in some countries and can be used to treat chlamydiosis. Tetracycline-impregnated millet seed is also available in some countries and is readily accepted by Budgerigars and finches.

Oral medications may be difficult to administer in some avian species, such as parrots. It can be particularly difficult to get parrots to open their mouths, and some birds will refuse to swallow the medications. Medications can be mixed with a palatable liquid such as lactulose syrup or fruit juice to increase acceptance. In the case of tame parrots, clinicians should invest some time in explaining medication training to bird owners; parrots learn very quickly to take medicine from a syringe, and to introduce the syringe as a basic training tool or as a toy may help to medicate the bird when it becomes necessary (see **Oral medication** clip on CD). Capsules that dissolve rapidly can be used in birds of prey. Some raptors will vomit when some medications are given hidden in food or directly administered.

Crop tubing

Fluids and food may be administered orally through a red rubber or stainless steel ball-tipped feeding tube. Metal crop tubes are recommended (Figure 15.6a); however, they should always be used with care, as oesophageal perforation is possible with rigid tubes. Using a tube with a diameter greater than the tracheal diameter reduces the risk of inadvertent tracheal placement.

1. The bird should be firmly restrained in an upright position with the neck as extended as possible. The crop should be palpated before infusion to estimate fluid volume and to avoid overfilling and regurgitation. In larger species, a speculum (such as a nylon dog bone or plastic syringe case) can be used. A speculum should always be used with red rubber tube gavaging to prevent biting, severing and/or swallowing of the tube.
2. The tube should be mildly lubricated (Figure 15.6b), inserted into the left side of the mouth (Figure 15.6c) and guided dorsal and lateral to the glottis, down the oesophagus on the right side of the neck and into the crop.
3. The neck should be palpated for the presence of both the feeding tube and the trachea (Figure 15.6d), and the oral cavity should be inspected during the infusion for the appearance of fluids or food.
4. When the position of the feeding tube has been confirmed as safe, close the oesophagus using two fingers of the hand restraining the neck of the bird (Figure 15.6e).

Crop capacity may be estimated at roughly 30–50 ml/kg bodyweight, although smaller volumes (20 ml/kg) are often used in sick birds to decrease the risk of regurgitation and aspiration.

Fluids and food should not be administered orally (or this should be done only with extreme caution) in birds with regurgitation, gastrointestinal stasis, neurological diseases or orthopaedic problems of the legs,

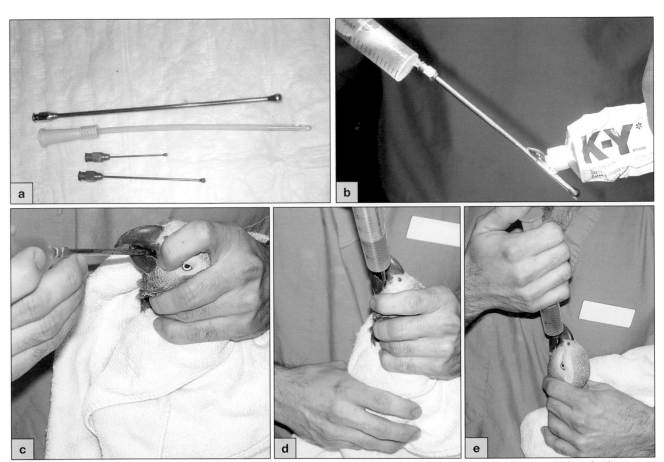

15.6 Crop gavaging. **(a)** Commercial metal crop tubes are recommended, but in raptors and psittacine chicks, plastic or silicone tubes may be used. **(b)** Proper lubrication of the tube is essential. **(c)** The neck is extended and the tube is passed lateral and dorsal to the trachea. **(d)** The tube should be palpated within the crop. **(e)** The oesophagus may be closed around the tube using two fingers.

because of the risk of aspiration. Fluids and food should always be warmed before use, but care must be taken to avoid overheating and burns. Fluids administered by the oral route are poorly absorbed in cases of extreme dehydration or hypovolaemic shock, as a result of peripheral vasoconstriction.

Greater care should always be taken with passerines and owls, as these birds have an underdeveloped or no crop. Therefore, the gavaging tube is placed into the distal oesophagus and a smaller volume of fluid (up to 12 ml/kg) given as a bolus. (Note with this approach, more frequent gavaging may be required.) In the case of sick diurnal raptors, the tube should bypass the crop and introduce food or fluids into the proventriculus.

Crop tubing may also be used for diagnostic sampling or therapeutic crop washing. For sample collection, the tube should be inserted and warmed saline passed into the crop. A small volume is aspirated and submitted for diagnosis (see Chapter 12). For crop washing in birds with impacted contents of the crop, warm saline or water is infused, massaged and aspirated back into the syringe; this procedure can be repeated as many times as it is needed.

Oesophagostomy tube placement

Oesophagostomy tube placement is indicated in cases of severe beak trauma and diseases of the oral cavity or proximal oesophagus, such as abscesses and neoplasia, or when intensive nutritional care is needed. In the experience of the author, it is also very useful in macaws and birds of prey with chronic anorexia or problems in emptying the crop. Oesophagostomy tubes may be directed down the post-crop oesophagus, bypassing the crop in cases of severe crop burn or severe trichomonosis. Silicone or polyurethane catheters are softer and stiffen less with age than red rubber or polyvinylchloride tubes, although all of them can be used for this procedure. The procedure is always done under isoflurane or sevoflurane anaesthesia. The basic technique is as follows:

1. The anaesthetized bird should be placed in left lateral recumbency and the feathers from the mid-cervical region overlying the right neck plucked. The incision site is then aseptically prepared.

2. An appropriate size and type of feeding tube is chosen. The end of the tube is placed at the base of the keel and the level where it reaches the plucked area is marked on the tube.

3. Curved haemostats should be inserted into the oral cavity and passed down the oesophagus to the level of the prepared site. The skin is tented with the curved haemostats through the oesophagus (Figure 15.7a).

4. A stab incision is made through the skin over the tip of the haemostats and into the oesophagus, and the incision is then penetrated with the tips of the haemostats (Figure 15.7b).

5. The tips of the haemostats are spread and the end of the feeding tube is grasped with the tips. The feeding tube is then pulled through the skin and into the oesophagus. The tube is held as the haemostats are removed from the mouth.

6. Once the tube end is out of the mouth, the end held by the haemostats is released and repositioned toward the back of the throat. A small amount of sterile water-based lubricant is placed on the end of the tube.

7. The terminal end of the tube is pushed down the oesophagus, past the incision site, and into the crop. With gentle pressure, the tube should be manipulated past the crop and into the distal oesophagus (Figure 15.7c). This may be time-consuming in macaws but more easily performed in raptors. The tube must not be forced, as excessive force may lacerate the crop.

8. The tube is inserted until the mark created when measuring the tube is at the level of the incision (Figure 15.7d). A purse-string suture is placed through the skin surrounding the tube and secured with a Roman sandal suture or, alternatively, a tape 'butterfly' can be applied to the tube next to the skin and then sutured to the skin to secure the tube in place (Figure 15.7e).

The tube should be capped with a tube adapter and an injection cap. A tube crimp can also be placed for added security. On some occasions, the tube can be cut short so that it is at the level of the bird's neck, or it can be left long enough to secure wrapped over the bird's back. It is extremely important to confirm correct tube placement by radiography (Figure 15.7f).

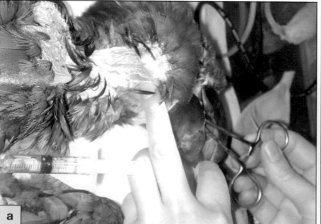
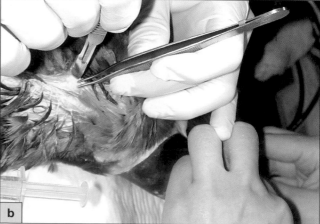

15.7   Placement of an oesophagostomy tube in an anaesthetized Hyacinth Macaw. **(a)** The skin is tented with curved haemostats through the oesophagus. **(b)** A stab incision is made and penetrated with the tips of the haemostats. (continues)

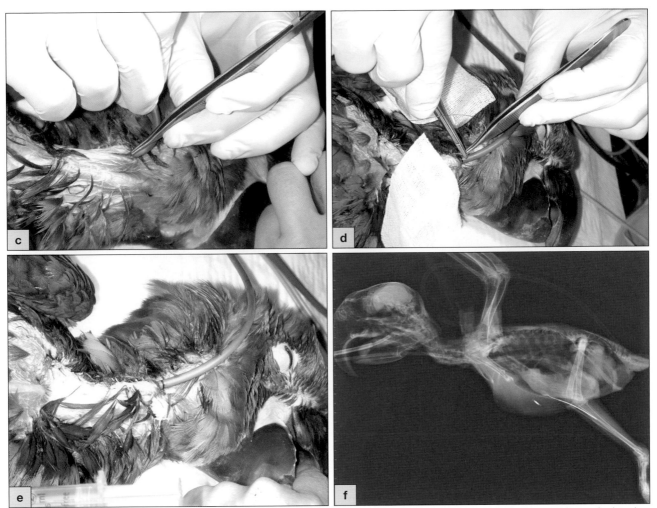

15.7 (continued) Placement of an oesophagostomy tube in an anaesthetized Hyacinth Macaw. **(c)** The tube is manipulated past the crop and into the distal oesophagus. **(d)** The tube is inserted until the mark created when measuring the tube is at the level of the incision. **(e)** The tube is secured in place. **(f)** Radiography confirms correct placement of the tube.

Nasal flush

Nasal flushing can be used diagnostically to collect fluid (and sometimes solid debris) representative of the space between the external nares and choanal cleft. This space represents the ventral aspect of the middle nasal concha, the suborbital chamber and, sometimes, the preorbital diverticulum of the infraorbital sinus. Oral contamination must be considered when interpreting culture results; if the intent of this procedure is to collect microbiological samples, the choanal cleft should be cultured first to help distinguish oral from nasal flush organisms. Aspiration must be avoided.

With the bird adequately restrained and the beak pointed slightly down, a Luer-tip syringe containing 3–10 ml of sterile saline is pressed against one of the nares, forming a seal. Gently flush both nares with equal amounts of saline (see **Nasal flushing** clip on CD), and then collect the resultant sample from the choanal cleft. With obstruction, some fluid may flow out of the lacrimal duct (bubbling or watering in the eye on the same side) or out of the opposite naris, but not into the oral cavity.

Nasal flushing can also be used therapeutically to administer medications locally, break up debris and flush out some foreign bodies. Naris discharge, foreign bodies and undetermined upper beak and rostral head area irritation are all indications for nasal flushing.

Nail trimming

Overgrown claws, nails and talons (Figure 15.8) are frequently found in captive birds from several orders, but in particular those from the Psittaciformes, Passeriformes and Falconiformes. This condition is usually caused by insufficient wear associated with the use of perches too small in diameter and perching surfaces that are too soft. The claws and talons of birds are composed of a hard keratinized casing covering the dorsal and lateral aspects, while the ventral surface is formed of a softer structure.

In small birds (e.g. canaries and finches), nails are trimmed using small nail clippers, such as those commonly used for children. Cat nail clippers or Spencer scissors can also be used. In these small species, nail trimming is easy and fast and anaesthesia is not usually required (Figure 15.9a).

The claws and talons of raptors can be trimmed using nail clippers, a utility knife with a curved blade, a set of small metal files or fine-grain files, as appropriate. To trim the talons of larger birds of prey, a guillotine-type nail clipper, such as that used commonly for dogs, is preferred. Rotary hobby tools can also be used (Figure 15.9b). The overgrown nails are cut and then reshaped using metal files (for larger birds) or fine-grain files (for smaller species). A hand-held modeller grinding tool or a hand drill with grinder attachments can also be

221

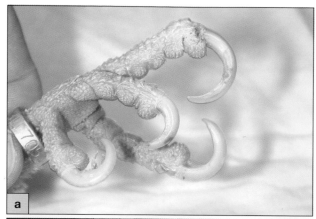

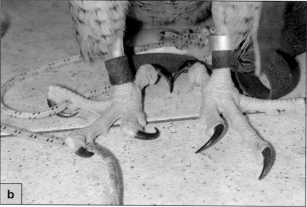

15.8 Overgrown **(a)** nails and **(b)** talons are frequently found in captive birds. This condition is usually caused by insufficient wear associated with small perches.

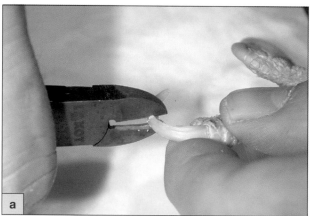

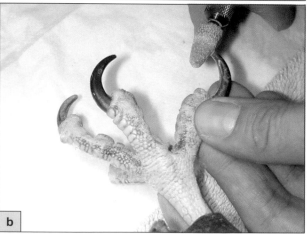

15.9 **(a)** Small nail trimmers or small wire cutters can be used for nail trimming. Note that the nail is being cut side to side. **(b)** A grinding tool being used to reshape the talon of a Harris' Hawk.

used to reshape strong talons (see **Nail trimming** clip on CD). During the trimming process, haemorrhage may occur if the nails or talons are cut too short. Usually it is only necessary to trim the tips by 3 mm in smaller species and up to 8 mm in larger birds. Haemorrhage can be stopped using a silver nitrate pencil, thermocautery or electrocautery.

Parrots possess a zygodactyl foot, meaning that digits I and IV face backward and digits II and III face forward. Parrots are often presented for nail clipping when the nails become intolerably sharp or long enough to become entrapped. The quick of the nail is quite long and easy to see in white-nailed birds. Some Amazon parrot species and Grey Parrots have black nails. There is no set length to achieve when cutting the nails and each case should be evaluated individually. As a rule of thumb, a good limit to cut will be the cross point where an imaginary line projected from the plantar surface of the digit meets the nail, or to clip the nail at the level where it would form a quarter circle (Figure 15.10). Haemorrhage can be treated as described for nail trimming in raptors. Some owners are able to file nails at home with small-grain files.

The author recommends using a rotary hobby tool for performing nail trimming in parrots. A hand-held grinding tool may be used to grind the tips short and blunt, and haemorrhage can usually be stopped by the heat created by the tool. In general, anaesthesia is not required to perform clipping unless the nails are heavily overgrown and haemorrhage will be almost unavoidable in bringing the nails to a normal length.

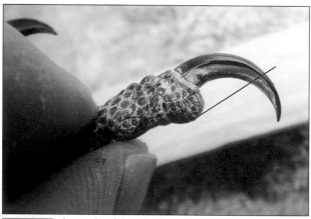

15.10 As a rule of thumb, the nail should be cut to the length where an imaginary tangent line from the ventral surface of the digit transects the nail (red line).

It should be kept in mind that there is always an important underlying cause for overgrown nails.

- Perch width and perch material. Perches should be appropriate to the bird's size; this is particularly important for passerines and small parrots. Overgrown nails can be seen in conjunction with pressure lesions on the feet. Generally, 1 cm diameter perches are recommended for passerines. A concrete perch may be useful for wearing down nails in parrots but, if the bird is not perching properly, the skin can be damaged and pododermatitis can develop.
- Malnutrition or liver disease. Abnormal protein metabolism in conjunction with obesity may result in

an adult bird suddenly developing overgrown nails, associated with hepatic lipidosis. Amazon parrots and Budgerigars are particularly prone.

- Failure to perch properly. Arthritis or a dislocated digit phalanx can preclude friction of the nail with the perch, so it is necessary to keep the nails short.

Nail trimming should be repeated if and when required; there is not an ideal interval and many birds never need a clip. Provision of suitable perches and a good diet is the best advice to avoid regular nail clipping.

A detached or broken claw or talon is another common presentation. A protective cover can be made using multiple layers of cyanoacrylate glue, antibiotic powder and talcum powder. Alternatively, cyanoacrylate glue and fine sodium bicarbonate powder can also be used to the same effect.

Beak trimming

Birds kept in ideal conditions, with well designed cages and provided with appropriate enrichment (e.g. toys, wood or bones to gnaw), can use their beaks more naturally and generally do not require beak shaping. If kept in less than ideal conditions, beak trimming or shaping is usually necessary; cage and aviary birds and birds of prey are prone to beak overgrowth due to lack of wear.

In the majority of the species commonly seen in veterinary practice, the premaxilla is a hollow bone. A very thin layer of vascular tissue covered with an equally thin layer of hard keratin epidermis overlies this bone. The dermis is attached to the periosteum. Within this dermal layer there is a high concentration of sensory nerve organs, causing the tissue to be highly sensitive to pressure and vibration. The keratinized layer grows from the upper germinal bed at the cere down to the tip at a rate of 0.6–1.3 cm a month. The lower mandible consists of two bony projections with a keratinized horn growing in a sweeping arc up and outward. The central portion, which grows upward, is thick, hard and often ground to a very sharp edge. It meets the inside of the upper beak at the occlusal shelf. The sides of both the upper and lower beak are much thinner and almost brittle in comparison to the leading edges.

The tip of the beak functions primarily to pick up and manipulate food items. The majority of mastication occurs at the occlusal shelf with the lower mandible. The majority of wear on the beak also happens at this surface. Many birds, especially parrots, may often be heard grinding their beaks while roosting at night. The beak is kept in shape by:

- The wear of upper against lower beak
- Grinding the beak against itself
- Grinding the beak against the perch or another object.

A beak that is out of alignment will rarely regain proper alignment without assistance. Continued wear only continues to reinforce the malalignment regardless of any toys or objects the bird chews on. In addition to problems with husbandry, there are diseases that can also cause the beak to wear improperly and become overgrown, often necessitating frequent trims:

- Congenital malformation in young birds
- Rickets or malnutrition in young birds
- Beak trauma
- Parasites (e.g. cnemidocoptic mites in Budgerigars)
- Sinusitis or rhinitis affecting the upper germinal bed at the cere (common in canaries)
- Neoplasia
- Abnormal protein metabolism; maxillary beak elongation and hyperkeratosis may be associated with liver disease and warrant clinical investigation
- Iatrogenic causes; bruising of the rictal phalanges or bruising caused by feeding syringes in hand-fed birds is a common cause of 'scissor beak' as the pain from this causes the bird to use its beak differently.

The aim of beak shaping is to return the beak to the normal shape for that species rather than simply making the beak shorter. Basic anatomy and shape should be known before starting the procedure; for psittacine birds the basic design is the same but there is some species variation. In the case of raptors, the normal or abnormal presence of the tomial tooth must also be known.

The tomium and outer keratin layers of the beak should be filed down with a rotary hobby tool fitted with a stone or sandpaper tip (Figures 15.11 and 15.12 and see **Beak trimming** clip on CD); only for very small birds, such as Budgerigars or small passerines, can nail files or nail trimmers be used. Beak layers should be taken back carefully and slowly. The sandpaper tips are disposable, reducing the risk of disease transmission between birds.

If the beak is trimmed too short, the highly vascular deeper tissues can bleed significantly. Haemorrhage can be controlled by direct pressure or application of a styptic gel, silver nitrate and sometimes using cyanoacrylate glue or a bipolar electric scalpel. A single injection of meloxicam or other analgesic must be given to any bird that bleeds during beak trimming.

It is also recommended that the procedure is carried out under general anaesthesia, as careful reshaping is almost impossible in the conscious bird (especially when dealing with the larger species of

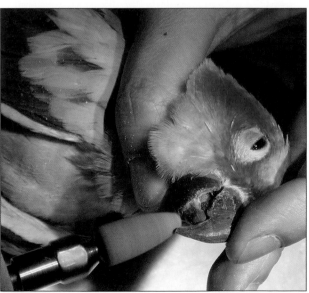

15.11 A modeller's grinding tool being used to reshape the overgrown beak of a Sun Conure.

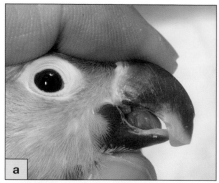 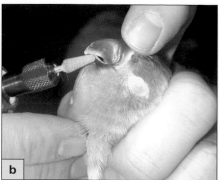 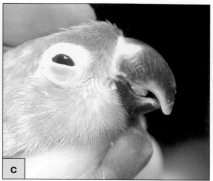

15.12   **(a)** Deformed beak of a 4-year-old lovebird after repeated traumatic cage bar chewing. **(b)** Use of the grinding tool with a small sandstone for reshaping the beak. **(c)** Final result after beak reshaping.

parrots) without damaging the tongue, the beak or the handler. Anaesthesia or heavy sedation also minimizes stress caused to the bird.

If for any reason the procedure has to be done without anaesthesia or sedation, the maxillary beak can be reshaped by forcing it against the lower beak. Then, the mandible is trimmed straight across to even out the surface. To facilitate this, it is possible to manipulate the upper beak tip to sit inside the lower.

Feather techniques

Wing clipping
Trimming of the remiges (or flight feathers) is designed to curtail flight capabilities of birds; it is particularly used for parrots and some other pet species. This is a very simple procedure to perform but it is complicated by ethical considerations.

Benefits include prevention of injury from flying into solid objects such as walls or windows and prevention of accidental escape. It also has use as an aid to training and taming. However, birds with clipped wings tend to lack confidence and empowerment, their musculoskeletal system and eye/body/wing coordination may fail to develop normally, and improper trimming can result in irritation and cause some birds to preen excessively or begin feather destruction behaviour. Clipped birds may still fly, escape and be vulnerable to predators. Excessive trims may result in laceration of the skin and muscle of the keel, fracture of the wings or legs, or chipping of the tip of the beak due to crash landing.

Wing trimming has an important role in avian practice. Although it can be booked in as a quick procedure, wing trimming should be seen as an opportunity to introduce training and management procedures to the owner. The author books two types of appointments for avian patients: a longer one to thoroughly explain the relative advantages and disadvantages of wing trimming and management, and another short one to perform the trim if it is still required. Most owners are happy with these procedures and the majority prefer to bring their birds to the practice to allow the clinician to perform the wing trimming.

Practitioners should encourage owners to get their birds clipped only at a veterinary practice. The following points should be discussed with the owner.

- No wing clip is 100% effective. When a wing trim is properly performed, the bird should not be able to

fly or gain lift, but can still gently glide to the ground over the distance of a few metres. Birds should not be taken outside with the assumption that a wing trim will keep them from flying. Owners should be warned that the bird may still be able to fly, especially in wind. In addition, moulting a few feathers can markedly improve the bird's ability to fly.
- Young birds (especially those that have been hand-reared) should learn to fly and develop landing skills before their first trim. This allows them to develop balance, grace and agility.
- The house and the surroundings are still not safe from parrots' destructive behaviours; many birds feel very comfortable walking on the floor and all are capable of climbing.
- Basic training should include step-up/step-down and returning on command (see Chapter 5).

It is probably correct to state that there is no single clipping technique that is best for every bird in every situation (Figure 15.13). Much has been written about which is the most appropriate method, but a consensus has been established by the Association of Avian Veterinarians. To summarize, the bilateral trimming technique is the primary recommended method, and there are some variations depending on the species treated:

- Long-tailed, slim-bodied birds (e.g. macaws, conures and parakeets): clip primaries 5–10
- Short-tailed, heavy-bodied birds (e.g. Amazon parrots, Grey Parrots): clip primaries 6–10 (Figure 15.14).

A variation of this clipping is used by many practitioners, including the author. A cosmetic clip can be performed leaving the outermost one or two primaries (9 and 10) unclipped for aesthetic purposes and, theoretically, protecting the distal soft tissues and wing bone from injury (Figure 15.15). Some practitioners believe that this kind of clip allows the bird to gain height, but it also causes the bird to lose manoeuvrability, increasing the risk of injury during flight attempts. In the experience of the author, immature birds (particularly Grey Parrots and Cockatiels) are clumsy and tend to fall hard and frequently, resulting in injuries at the wing tip. Leaving the outer two feathers will protect the bird against these accidents and also support new blood feathers. In the case of Grey Parrots, two feathers are left and the next eight primaries cut. In the case of Cockatiels, only one feather is left and the next nine are clipped.

Technique	Advantages	Disadvantages
One-winged (unilateral)	The most effective method to avoid flight in a bird	May cause the bird to spiral during flight attempts and fall, increasing the risk of injury
Two-winged (bilateral)	Better balance so the bird is better able to land without injury	Some birds can still fly by increasing the flapping frequency Light broad-winged birds, such as Cockatiels, cope best with this method
Removing outer primary feathers (6–10)	Fewer feathers need to be removed Result in reduction in lift with less effect on landing, enabling safer descending glide	Less cosmetic as outer feathers are removed; it is obvious that bird is clipped New feathers tend to come through unprotected and be more prone to damage More likely that the bird will chew feathers
Removing inner primary feathers (1–5)	More cosmetic appearance More considerate of moulting sequences Outer feathers will protect the new growing feathers	The bird will not be able to glide to descend Some lightweight birds can fly short distances
Removing all the primary feathers except the two outermost	Cosmetic appearance Outer feathers will protect the new growing feathers Best way to avoid keel injuries in heavy-bodied birds; juvenile Grey Parrots and Cockatiels are clumsy and tend to fall hard and frequently, resulting in injuries at the wing tip. Leaving the outer two feathers will protect the bird against these accidents and also support the new blood feathers	Flight capabilities may remain intact in light birds Some birds can have lift capabilities This method is the least protective against escape

15.13 The advantages and disadvantages of different wing clipping techniques.

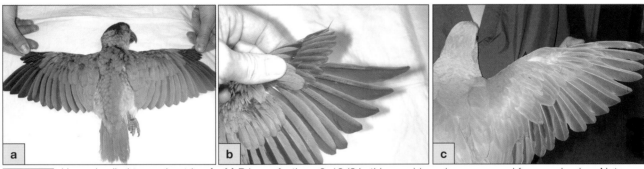

15.14 Heavy-bodied type wing trim. **(a–b)** Primary feathers 6–10 (6 in this case) have been removed from each wing. Note that no cut ends protrude beyond the covert feathers. Compare with **(c)** a normal wing.

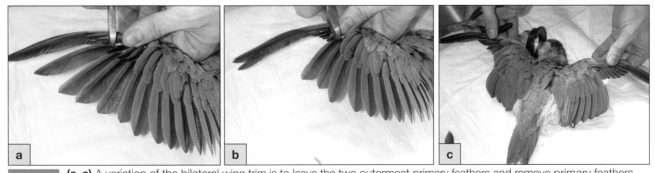

15.15 **(a–c)** A variation of the bilateral wing trim is to leave the two outermost primary feathers and remove primary feathers 3–10.

Unilateral wing clipping is likely to reduce flight more effectively than a bilateral clip, but it may cause the bird to spiral during flight attempts and fall, increasing the risk of injury. The unilateral wing clip should be elected only in special cases or in cases of birds with a high risk of escape.

The bird should be tested indoors to check whether enough feathers have been removed. The bird can be held on a perch or arm and quickly dropped downward, causing it to flap its wings and jump off the perch. If the bird can gain lift, more primary feathers need to be clipped. Clip conservatively and remove additional feathers as needed to prevent the bird from gaining lift. A simple rule of thumb is to remove another primary feather if the bird is able to fly further than 7.5 m.

Whichever method is chosen, the procedure has some essential points.

- To perform a wing trim, the wing is extended while the bird is restrained. The wing is held gently and firmly, supporting the humerus to avoid fracturing the wing. Visualize the shaft of the feathers and cut the elected feathers on both wings, beginning at the tip of the wing.
- Cat claw clippers, wire clippers or sharp scissors can be used (Figure 15.16 and see **Wing trimming**

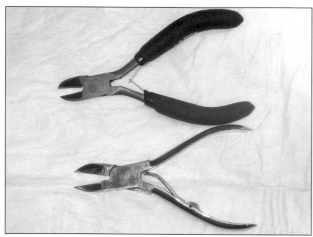

| **15.16** | Wire cutters or small pliers should be used for wing trimming in order to cut the calamus sharply, to avoid splitting the feather. |

clip on CD). This reduces the chance of damage to the wing tip and the feathers are cut in a sharp way and not left splintered.

- Each feather is identified and visualized before clipping across the rachis proximal to the first vane (cut along the shaft of the feather proximal to the loose barbules at the base of the feather), below the level of the covert feathers (see Figure 15.15a).
- Feathers should not be cut flush with the skin; a small length of calamus should be left to provide some protection for adjacent growing feathers. The remaining cut end of the feathers should not protrude beyond the intact covert feathers as this may stimulate feather chewing behaviour.
- Avoid trimming blood feathers (growing feathers with a vascular shaft) because these will haemorrhage if cut. If a blood feather is found during the trimming, leave it in place, remove the next one and test the bird's flight ability.

Bleeding blood feathers

Birds are often presented with damaged and bleeding blood feathers. During the growth phase of a primary feather, which can take 3–4 weeks or longer, the feather is vulnerable to trauma. A cracked blood feather can bleed copiously and should be the first differential diagnosis in a bird presented with profuse bleeding. A damaged blood feather may ooze blood, requiring extraction.

Haemorrhage can be life-threatening and the bleeding should be controlled in the correct manner. The use of clotting powders or other haemostatic compounds is not advised; these agents may be effective in the short term, but bleeding will recur and there is a risk of infection. Bleeding blood feathers should be extracted, although some distal feather bleeds can be stopped using cotton as a short-term solution. To extract the feather, the bird is restrained and the wing held and braced securely to protect it from trauma. Straight haemostats or needle-nosed pliers are used to grasp the calamus of the bleeding feather. Firm and steady traction is applied to the feather while being slightly twisted as it is pulled from the follicle in its natural direction. When the feather is broken or sheared within the follicle, sterile haemostats may be guided between the feather and the follicle to grasp it. Pressure is applied to the empty follicle for a few seconds to a

minute or so, to stem any bleeding. As blood feathers are often broken within the follicle, and there is some risk for injury to the wing because of the significant attachment of the flight feathers to the periosteum, owners are typically not advised to attempt blood feather extraction at home due to the risk of iatrogenic damage.

Imping

Feather repair or 'imping' is the art of repairing bent or fractured feathers. The integrity of the primary feathers (remiges) and tail feathers (rectrices) is vital for flight performance in species destined for release back into the wild, for birds of prey used in the sport of falconry or for birds used in flying shows. Feather repair is also very important to help some pet birds to stop feather chewing behaviour, because imping restores the full length of the feather and the capability of flight, providing mental stimulation for the bird. Relatively frequently, the feathers of captive birds tend to suffer bends or fractures, especially in rescue or rehabilitation centres and also due to crash landing or fighting with prey during training or hunting (falconry birds).

For a total or partial feather replacement or splinting, it is best to use a feather that is from the same species and position (e.g. wing feather), and of the same size and colour. It is preferable to use one of the bird's own feathers, and owners should be advised to keep moulted remiges for potential future use in imping. If it is not possible to use the bird's own feathers, feathers from other birds can be used, but there is a risk of infectious disease spread. Avian practitioners should try to maintain a small collection of feathers from different species, but feathers should be stored only from birds that are negative for psittacine beak and feather disease (PBFD, avian circovirus), polyomavirus, proventricular dilatation disease (PDD, avian bornavirus) and paramyxovirus (PMV). If a suitable feather from another bird is available, the feather can be sterilized using ethylene oxide or frozen prior to use in order to reduce the risk of contamination. As a last resort, feathers from other species can be used (e.g. between different falcon species or different macaw species).

Imping is an easy and simple procedure; falconers and rescue centres involved in raptor medicine usually maintain a collection of moulted feathers and feathers obtained from carcasses, and have developed their own techniques. However, it is recommended that imping is performed under general inhalant anaesthesia at the veterinary practice, for efficiency and more complete feather examination (Lierz, 2000).

Bent feather repair

The treatment for bent feathers depends on the severity of the damage. In mild cases, the bent feather may be straightened up by applying steam for a couple of minutes (e.g. from an iron or from a boiling kettle). In more severe cases, hot water may be applied directly to the bent area and the feather straightened up by digital manipulation or using small pliers. The bent feather should be isolated from the other feathers and from the skin using towels or surgical drapes, in order to avoid accidental burns.

For the more severe cases, the following technique has been developed (Samour, 2008). The technique aims to straighten the bent feather on its axis using a small pair of fine-tipped curved electrician's pliers.

1. Make a longitudinal incision (using a scalpel with a No. 15 blade) over the fracture site, extending about 1 cm in both directions. The incision should include only the upper layer of the feather shaft.
2. An elongated wad of cotton wool is inserted snugly into the feather shaft using the blunt side of the blade.
3. A couple of drops of methacrylate glue are placed directly on the incision, impregnating the wad of cotton wool.
4. Pressure is then applied laterally over the incision using the pliers until the glue sets. When dried, the glue-impregnated cotton wool provides a strong inner reinforcement to the damaged feather shaft.
5. The surface of the feather shaft around the incision is roughened using a fine nail file.
6. A thin layer of methacrylate glue is applied over the area.
7. A small amount of sodium bicarbonate powder is sprinkled directly over the glued surface. The powder binds with the glue, creating a strong cement-like layer over the bend.
8. The upper surface of the newly created layer is filed using the fine nail file.
9. This procedure can be repeated 2 or 3 times in order to create a thicker layer, should this prove necessary. The external splint is translucent, so colouring is unnecessary.

Feather replacement

This procedure is indicated if the fracture has occurred at the mid-shaft or at the distal end of the feather. A similar fragment must be procured or if the lost fragment is still available, this may be reattached. The basic technique is as follows (Figure 15.17).

1. The stump of the damaged feather is trimmed with fine-pointed scissors and a nail file so that the exposed end is smooth.
2. The replacement feather is trimmed to 'fit' on to the end of the old calamus, creating a new feather of the same length as the original. For this reason the equivalent feather should be used if possible (e.g. right primary 1 to right primary 1, right primary 2 to right primary 2).
3. An imping needle of suitable length and diameter is trimmed and/or whittled so that it fits snugly into the base of the feather at one end and the calamus of the new feather at the other. Imping needles may be adapted from small-diameter plastic knitting needles, kebab skewers or bamboo pegs.
4. Cyanoacrylate (tissue) glue is applied to each end of the needle and it is inserted into the new and old feather calami. It is extremely important that the apposition of the old and new feathers is exact and that the replacement feather is oriented correctly.
5. Pressure should be applied over the imping site with fine-tipped electrician's pliers for approximately 30 seconds to allow the glue to set.
6. The dorsal and ventral aspects of the fracture line are then filed with a nail file. Additional layers of cyanoacrylate glue and sodium bicarbonate powder can be used in order to produce a stronger bond to support the new feather.

This imping technique may be used to replace almost the whole feather, as is more commonly required in psittacine birds that chew their feathers. In these cases, when the calamus is bigger than the shaft at the medium length of the feather, fast-setting epoxy glue may be used instead of cyanoacrylate glue because

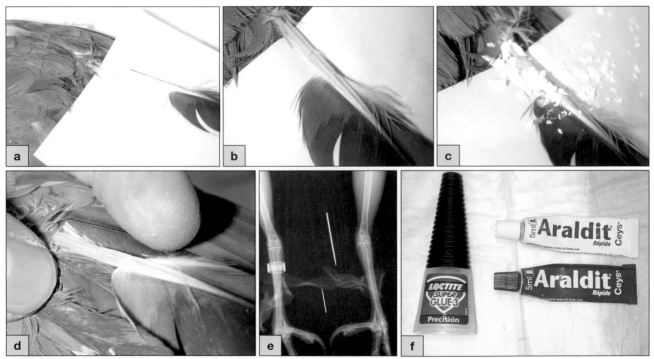

15.17 Imping technique. **(a)** A rod (in this case a 0.6 mm steel pin) is glued into the replacement feather. The ends of the feathers have been trimmed and smoothed to fit together closely. **(b)** A small amount of epoxy resin is placed into the remnant calamus, and then the replacement feather with the rod attached is advanced into the calamus. A piece of paper is used to protect the other feathers from inadvertent glue leakage. **(c)** Sodium bicarbonate powder is sprinkled over the imping to absorb the rest of the glue. **(d)** A small nail file may be used to smooth the surface of the repaired feather. **(e)** Radiograph of a Goshawk showing the needles used for imping feathers. **(f)** The most common glues used for imping feathers: rapid cyanoacrylate and rapid epoxy resin.

epoxy resins are able to fill the hollow space found in the base shaft of the feathers. In general, these grafted feathers can be surprisingly strong and are quite capable of allowing flight, and birds tolerate them very well. The main disadvantage with this method is that the feather is vulnerable to breaking near the tip of the rigid imping needle when subjected to stress.

Ring removal

A huge variety of identification rings are available (see Chapter 3). In the UK, it is a legal requirement for all captive raptors to be identified with a numbered, closed ring. Marking parrots or passerines in this way is, at present, voluntary for captive birds. However, both open and closed rings can pose a health risk to birds and may require removal.

Potential problems associated with rings include entrapment of the leg in enclosure accessories and the accumulation of a constrictive ring of keratin debris (usually associated with malnutrition or *Cnemidocoptes* mites) between the band and the leg that can lead to impaired circulation and necrosis (Figure 15.18). Flat bands that are too wide to comfortably ride on the tarsal bone can lead to traumatic exosteal bone formation. When a ring of an inappropriate size has been placed, an underlying pressure necrosis of the skin may result; this is also found in macaws, as they walk with the entire ventral surface of the metatarsus. Some parrots, particularly macaws, have a tendency to chew steel rings, flattening them and entrapping the leg.

In some cases an owner may request ring removal in order to prevent problems occurring. Any details of the leg ring should be recorded in the bird's records prior to removal. The client's consent should always be obtained before the ring is removed, and the ring should be returned to the client. A microchip should be encouraged as an alternative method of identification, and implanted as soon as possible.

Rings and bands are easiest to remove before they begin to constrict the tissues. It is generally recommended that the bird is anaesthetized with inhalant anaesthesia to prevent it from suddenly moving during the ring removal process, which can result in lacerations or even fractures of the leg. When removing any ring or band, it is important that the force is applied to the ring and not the leg (Figure 15.19).

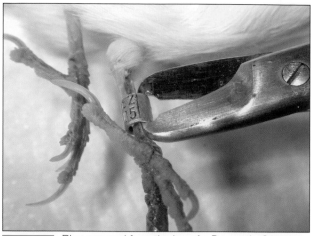

15.19 Ring removal from the leg of a Domestic Canary using specially designed ring removal scissors.

Small closed rings made of plastic or aluminium, as used for the majority of passerines, can be easily transected with Heath stitch scissors. Two diagonally opposing cuts are made and the ring falls off in two parts.

Steel rings are not easy to remove. Routine equipment found in clinics may not be appropriate, as many types of clippers, cutters and saws will damage the underlying tissues directly or through twisting of the ring when cutting, the most common cause of iatrogenic fractures during ring and band removal.

Practices dealing with avian patients should invest in specialist ring cutters, ring removal scissors and a modeller grinding tool (or dental drill) with cutting burrs for removing the biggest rings (Figure 15.20).

Steel or metallic rings can be removed using a rotating tool with a diamond disc making a diagonal cut. Keep in mind that there will be a great production of heat during the procedure and it is important to protect the underlying leg with wet swabs and regularly check for overheating, adding more cold water if necessary during the procedure (Figure 15.21). When removing small steel rings, make two small bites over opposite vertical borders of the ring, then use a ring cutter to cut through the two marks. This method avoids twisting of the ring because the cut is completely vertical. Two pairs of ring removal scissors (or two pairs of small pliers) are then used to apply opposing forces at the site of the cut to separate the cut ends (see **Ring removal** clip on CD).

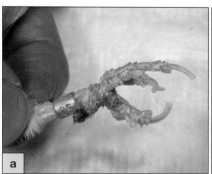 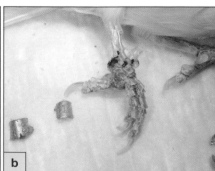 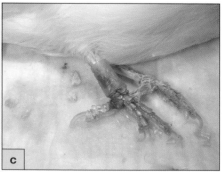

15.18 **(a)** Constricting ring associated with hyperkeratosis in a Domestic Canary. **(b)** Following ring removal. The debris released should be examined under a microscope in order to confirm *Cnemidocoptes* infestation. **(c)** After ring removal, the bone is often left exposed. In this case a hydrocolloid dressing is used over the wound. Bandages are also very useful to promote healing.

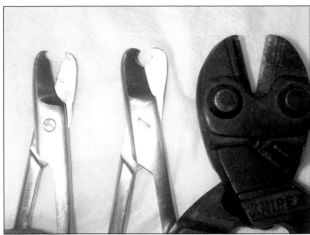

15.20 Specialist ring removal tools are a recommended investment for avian practices.

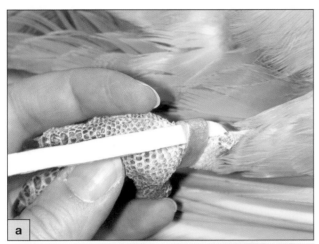

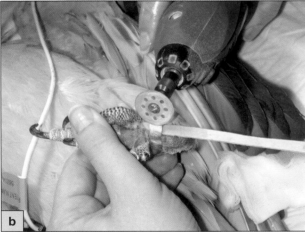

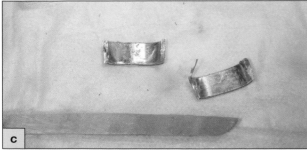

15.21 Removing a steel ring. **(a)** A tongue depressor is used to protect the underlying tissues from the tool and the heat produced. **(b)** A grinding tool equipped with a diamond disc cuts through the steel ring. **(c)** Two cuts in the resistant ring are required to remove it without risking damage to the leg.

Rings that are associated with constrictive accumulations of keratin are best removed using a variable-speed hobby tool and fine-tipped ring removal scissors. Anaesthesia is always advised but more necessary in these cases. The leg should be held by the operator using the hobby tool to prevent slipping of the tool or leg, which can result in severe laceration. Aluminium foil can be used to protect the leg in very small birds with little space between the leg and the ring. Some clinicians prefer to use a fine-tipped cutting bit attached to the tool; others use a diamond disc and perform the cut in the diagonal. The constrictive rings of accumulated keratinized debris should be removed by moistening them with lubricant gel or saline and gently peeling them away. A bandage or light splint may be necessary to support the bone if it has been weakened by the constricting material or if the skin surrounding the bone is lost after ring removal (see Figure 15.18).

Microchip placement

Microchips are small electronic devices that are injected into the musculature or subcutaneously to provide permanent identification. Microchipping is an effective means of identifying an individual bird as it is very difficult for the bird or a person to damage or modify the microchip. The microchips are coded and the code can be read using an appropriate reader. Not all readers are able to read all microchips, so radiography of the whole bird should be performed in order to prove conclusively that there is no microchip present. If a microchip fails or is unreadable by commonly used readers, it may be necessary to implant another.

Prior to microchip insertion, the bird should be scanned completely. There is not a standardized place for microchip implantation and there are different guidelines depending on the different authorities, countries and species of bird. As a result, microchips can be found in the pectoral muscles, subcutaneously in the neck region, in the precrural fold or in the thigh.

The British Veterinary Zoological Society recommends that the microchip should be inserted into the left pectoral muscle mass. This may be done with the bird conscious or anaesthetized; the author recommends that all birds weighing less than 200 g should be anaesthetized for this procedure and, in any bird, some kind of analgesia is always recommended.

It should be noted that microchip implantation may be inappropriate for very small passerine birds, as damage to the very small muscle mass cannot be avoided. Subcutaneous placement may cause less damage (although skin closure with glue or sutures will be required); however, it is very easy to find and remove microchips placed subcutaneously. Whatever the species of bird, the smallest microchip should always be used. Within the EU there are two kinds of veterinary microchips marketed, with two different sizes, and for birds, the smaller one should always be used.

After checking that the bird does not have an existing working microchip, the technique for microchip implantation is as follows:

1. The feathers of the pectoral region are parted and the skin is prepared aseptically (Figure 15.22a).

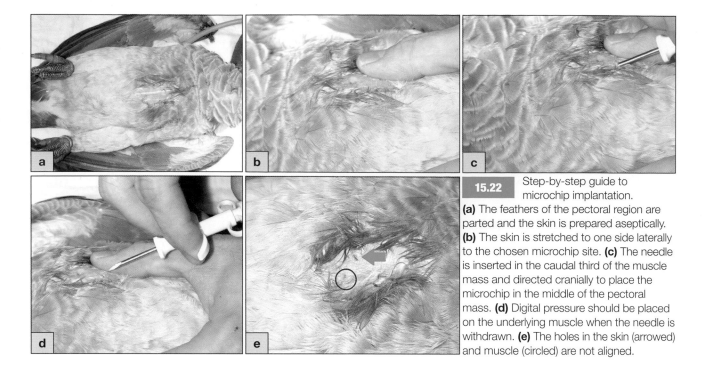

15.22 Step-by-step guide to microchip implantation. **(a)** The feathers of the pectoral region are parted and the skin is prepared aseptically. **(b)** The skin is stretched to one side laterally to the chosen microchip site. **(c)** The needle is inserted in the caudal third of the muscle mass and directed cranially to place the microchip in the middle of the pectoral mass. **(d)** Digital pressure should be placed on the underlying muscle when the needle is withdrawn. **(e)** The holes in the skin (arrowed) and muscle (circled) are not aligned.

2. The skin is stretched to one side laterally to the microchip insertion site elected (Figure 15.22b).
3. The needle is inserted in the caudal third of the muscle mass (as described in the 'Intramuscular injections' section) and directed cranially so that the microchip is placed in the approximate middle of the muscle mass between the superficial and deep pectoral muscles. It is extremely important not to place the device too far cranially, to avoid the large plexus of nerves and blood vessels in this region (Figure 15.22c).
4. Digital pressure should be placed on the underlying muscle when the needle is withdrawn, to reduce the chance of the microchip being withdrawn with the needle (Figure 15.22d).
5. The skin is released so that the holes in the skin and muscles are not aligned (Figure 15.22e).

6. The implantation site should be checked for haemorrhage and pressure applied until it has ceased.

See **Microchipping** and **Microchipping – anaesthetized** clips on CD.

Euthanasia

For more information about euthanasia, see QRG 15.1.

References and further reading

Lierz M (2000) Imping feathers in birds of prey. *Exotic DVM* **1(6)**, 13–15
Samour J (2008) Feather repair. In: *Avian Medicine, 2nd edn*, ed. J Samour, pp 185–191. Mosby Elsevier, Philadelphia

CD extras

- **Beak trimming**
- **Intraosseous catheter – tibiotarsus**
- **Intraosseous catheter – ulna**
- **Intravenous catheter**
- **Intravenous injection**
- **Jugular blood sample**
- **Jugular blood sample – anaesthetized**

- **Microchipping**
- **Microchipping – anaesthetized**
- **Nail trimming**
- **Nasal flushing**
- **Oral medication**
- **Ring removal**
- **Subcutaneous injection**
- **Wing trimming**

QRG 15.1: Euthanasia of birds

John Chitty and Deborah Monks

Important considerations

- Decision-making with the owner:
  - Clinical/welfare need
  - Costs
  - Inability to keep/rehome
- Does the owner wish to be present?
  - Is this appropriate (e.g. intraoperative, delay causing welfare compromise)?
- What does the owner wish to do with the body (i.e. take for burial or practice to arrange cremation)?

Technique

If owner **not** present:

1 If anaesthesia is indicated, mask induce with isoflurane.

2 Select vein; ideally use the right jugular vein. If the right jugular vein is inappropriate (e.g. in pigeons; has already been used for sampling), use the basilic (ulna) vein or medial metatarsal vein.

3 Part the feathers to expose the vein and moisten the skin with surgical spirit.

4 Insert a catheter or directly inject pentobarbital intravenously to effect.

If owner is present:

1 In a private area, explain the euthanasia process to the owner.

2 Sedate the bird using intranasal midazolam (2 mg/kg) plus butorphanol (2 mg/kg).

3 Wait 10–15 minutes.

4 Select vein; ideally use the basilic (ulna) vein. If this is not appropriate (e.g. in pigeons; has already been used for sampling), use the right jugular vein or medial metatarsal vein.

5 Part the feathers to expose the vein and moisten the skin with surgical spirit.

6 Insert a catheter or directly inject pentobarbital intravenously to effect.

7 Determine death, then give the owners time alone with the bird if desired.

Basic anaesthesia

16

Brian L. Speer

Anaesthesia is utilized for a variety of reasons in avian species. Overall, there are comparatively fewer routine or elective anaesthetic procedures in avian practice compared with feline and canine practice. The decision-making process regarding when or when not to employ the use of anaesthesia is not a simple one. Some veterinary surgeons (veterinarians) may tend to overuse anaesthesia on occasions; it is not always needed for some procedures, such as when performing routine examinations and venepuncture. Clinicians can develop the skills to use low-stress handling techniques, careful patient observation and assessment, and conscious sedation to avoid unnecessary anaesthesia.

On the other hand, some veterinary surgeons may avoid anaesthesia due to an awareness of the potential risks, even when it may be indicated in order to benefit the patient. The comparatively smaller average size of pet birds requires experience and enhanced anaesthesia and surgical skill-sets, and this is probably responsible for a large portion of the general perception of increased anaesthetic and surgical risk in birds. The relative risk of anaesthesia in birds is multifactorial, and there is currently comparatively little data regarding mortality risks. Yaakov *et al.* (2007) cited an anaesthetic death percentage of 3.7% in one retrospective study of 310 pet birds and 564 anaesthetic procedures. In that study, anaesthetic death was defined as any unexplained death during the anaesthetic episode or within 2 hours of the anaesthetic procedure. Birds euthanased on the table due to surgical findings, or birds that died due to surgical complications including haemorrhage, were not considered anaesthetic deaths. Anaesthetic episodes in birds weighing <100 g were found to have a higher risk of death (8.5% for birds <100 g *versus* 2.6% for birds >100 g, respectively, $p = 0.04$). In another study, Brodbelt *et al.* (2008) cited an anaesthetic mortality rate of 16% in the Budgerigar, 4% in parrots and 2% in other birds, with anaesthetic death defined as death within 48 hours of a gas anaesthetic procedure. McKeown *et al.* (2012) described an overall anaesthetic procedural mortality of 7.38% in 732 anaesthetic procedures. Deaths due to anaesthetic mortality were not distinguished from those including surgical complications, but birds euthanased intraoperatively were excluded. There was no apparent correlation with procedural time and risk of death, and there was no correlation with patient size and risk of death as was seen in earlier studies. In this study, it was presumed that mortality was less linked to anaesthetic risk, but was more associated with the severity of the disease process being anaesthetically and surgically addressed (e.g. advanced coelomic neoplastic disease, multiple intracoelomic adhesions and emergency tracheal obstruction) and the decision-making processes for anaesthesia that were involved.

Preparation

Informed consent

When discussing with an owner the indications for the use of anaesthesia for a patient, good communication skills are key. Although there will always be some degree of inherent risk, it is important for the attending veterinary surgeon to relay the true need for anaesthesia, the other potential options that may be applicable (if any) and the anticipated outcome of the procedure. Informed consent from owners requires that they have been provided with enough information with which to decide and authorize the proposed course(s) of action. In evaluating whether clients have been provided with enough information about the proposed procedure, practitioners should ask themselves: 'Have we discussed this to the point that a reasonable client would be able to make an informed decision?' Veterinary surgeons should explain at least the following:

- The contemplated procedure in **non-technical language**
- The medical and surgical **alternatives** to the proposed procedure, regardless of whether clients may or may not be able to afford the alternatives
- The availability of **specialists** and second opinions
- The **expected results** of the proposed procedure, including whether the client's bird will be cured or predictions of increased longevity and comfort
- The foreseeable minor and major **complications**
- The type, extent and cost of **follow-up care** and who will be responsible for it
- An **estimate** of the cost of the veterinary services.

BSAVA Manual of Avian Practice: A Foundation Manual. Edited by John Chitty and Deborah Monks. ©BSAVA 2018

The surgical suite

Prior to inducing anaesthesia, the surgical suite should be fully prepared. A pre-surgical conference, where all potentially involved parties of the veterinary medical team discuss the anaesthetic and procedural plan, can have great value. For more complicated (and, therefore, potentially higher risk) procedures, surgeons should consider whether the procedure is necessary, within their current capability and/or if specialist consultation would be beneficial.

When anaesthetizing most companion bird species, the surgery room itself is best maintained at a warmer temperature than usual, in order to help minimize heat loss by the patient. The room should be arranged to facilitate the anaesthetist's focus on the patient and minimize any potential distractions (Figure 16.1). An anaesthetist's assistant is helpful. Supportive and monitoring equipment should be functional, in position, and all associated staff should be familiar with it.

Emergency drugs should be pre-calculated, drawn up and readily available. Atropine, doxapram, adrenaline (epinephrine) and colloid fluids (hetastarch, oxyglobin, whole blood) are examples that can be prepared, depending on anticipated need. Whole blood, if needed, is ideally obtained from a homologous species donor, although heterologous species transfusions may have merit in some settings. All surgical equipment that may be needed, suture materials, bandaging materials and other supplies should be anticipated, and made easily available.

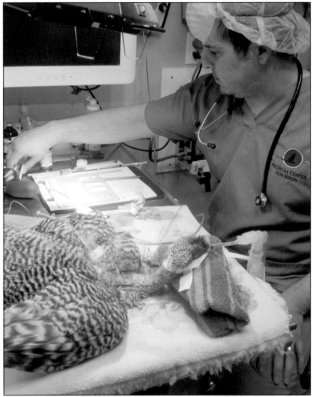

16.1 The primary anaesthetist should be seated comfortably in a position with easy patient access and control; they should not be required to vacate this position during the procedure. Note the patient anaesthetic chart and anaesthesia controls to the right, emergency drugs are pre-drawn and there is easy access to the rebreathing bag for manual intermittent ventilation.

Planning for an anaesthetic procedure: preoperative conference considerations

Operating room and personnel preparation

- What is the planned anaesthetic/surgical procedure and outcome expectations?
- What problems are anticipated?
- Can the room temperature be adjusted and controlled as desired?
- Are the surgeon's and anaesthetist's locations designated?
- Are chair and table heights adjusted and appropriate?
- Are the surgical instruments to be used or potentially used made available?
- Is the monitoring equipment to be used functional and ready?
- Is an operating microscope or magnification tool to be used? Is this adjusted for the surgeon's needs?
- What manner of thermal support will be used?
- Who will be the support person for the anaesthetist?
- Will this person need to be continually present or at specific times only?
- What tasks will be designated to that person?

Patient preparation

- Has food been withheld for the appropriate time that is needed?
- What is the preoperative analgesia plan and timing prior to induction?
- Will there be a local block?
- Will preoperative antibiosis be utilized?
- Are there any specific handling or restraint-associated needs that should be implemented?
- Will there be a pre-oxygenation need prior to induction?
- What is the planned method for induction and maintenance?
- What will the patient positioning be?
- What will be the intraosseous or intravenous fluid access route and location?
- Will there be a need to have whole blood available for transfusion?
- What is the anticipated duration of this procedure?

Patient recovery

- Is there a heated recovery cage or brooder designated and prepared?
- What enrichments (e.g. toys) are to be used postoperatively and when?

Pre- and perioperative patient considerations

Before performing a procedure that requires anaesthesia, the foundational tenets of good veterinary medicine must be employed. In all cases, patient history, physical examination findings, a working diagnosis or problem list, and laboratory or other diagnostic evaluation findings all factor into the decision of whether to use anaesthesia, when to do so, and to guide planning for the procedure. Diagnostic tests, including haematology, serum biochemistry and imaging, may be used to assist in the planning of the anaesthetic or surgical procedure, although they are not necessary in all patients.

Unless an emergency procedure is required, patients should be fasted and adequately stabilized prior to anaesthesia (Echols, 2004). As a general rule of thumb, the bird should be fasted and the crop should be emptied prior to surgery to minimize the risks of regurgitation and aspiration. Depending on the species and the planned procedure, fasting periods as short as 1 hour (small bird species) and up to 8 hours or more (larger bird species) may be employed. Longer periods of fasting are more often used for planned gastrointestinal surgery, including endoscopy. With the exception of some critically ill birds, the overall risk of hypoglycaemia is generally viewed to be minimal with a reasonable pre-anaesthetic fasting period.

If coelomic distension is present and it is determined to contain fluid, coelomocentesis can provide rapid relief from its associated pressure on the air sacs and ventilatory capacity of the patient. Coelomocentesis may be guided using a transilluminating light (to identify clear pockets to target) or ultrasonography. Blind coelomocentesis carries an increased risk of inadvertent penetration of the coelomic organs and, although it may be effective, should be avoided where possible. Pre-oxygenation, combined with the use of conscious sedation (midazolam with butorphanol) and the provision of flow-by oxygen during the procedure, may help facilitate and reduce the procedural risk of coelomocentesis. In the vast majority of circumstances, it is best to remove as much of the fluid as possible to relieve respiratory compromise, allow the patient to stabilize, and then proceed with the anaesthetic and surgical plan. If frank blood is seen during coelomocentesis, the procedure should be stopped immediately, as this may indicate inadvertent penetration of a vascular structure.

Analgesia

Analgesia is an important component of pre-induction, the planned anaesthetic/surgical procedure itself and the postoperative patient management plan. Even in current times, analgesia remains less frequently used as a component of anaesthesia and patient care in avian medicine than it should be. Concurrently, there is a requisite of careful attention to the comfort and degree of fear experienced by the bird. Evidence of pain, increases in escape/avoidance behaviours, aggression and apathy all require consideration in order to help shape treatment methods.

Recognizing the presence of pain in birds is challenging (Paul-Murphy, 2006; Hawkins and Paul-Murphy, 2011). Clinical signs of pain are not necessarily universal, are often species-dependent and are individually variable between birds. Although heart rate, respiratory rate and blood pressure can increase during pain, these parameters can also be influenced by perceived fear, light and temperature. As a result, these parameters alone may not be reliable as quantifiable measurements of pain in a patient. Many of these clinical signs are vague and, as a result, they can be challenging to confidently correlate with pain in many individual patients; therefore, it is generally recommended that clinicians err on the side of caution and overestimate of the presence of pain, assuming that conditions that would be painful to humans are equally painful to birds (Paul-Murphy, 2006; Hawkins and Paul-Murphy, 2011). Generally, observed behavioural criteria are the primary traditional 'tools' utilized to help assess pain in birds and other animals, as there typically will be a change or absence of one or more normal behaviours for that animal.

Acute pain is often more easily recognizable compared with chronic pain. Acute pain should be more readily recognizable through demonstrated rapid withdrawal reflexes or aggression when a painful body part is stimulated or touched. Although these behaviours correspond to the conscious perception of the stimulus, their interpretation requires that the bird be fully cognizant of its environment and physically capable of reacting. There is also a requirement that the hospital personnel take the time to observe and carefully interpret what they see in regard to the pain and comfort of the patient.

Chronic pain in many bird species can be manifested by a reduction in social grooming behaviours, decreased activity, agitation or removal of oneself from the flock. There is little scientific data on the behaviour of raptors, passerines and parrots experiencing pain. Among other species, chickens experiencing arthritic pain most predictably demonstrated an absence of dust-bathing behaviours. Progressive removal of feathers from chickens caused marked changes in behaviour, ranging from an initial alert and agitated response to periods of crouching immobility following successive removal (Gentle and Hunter, 1991). Pigeons, after orthopaedic surgery, showed trembling of the wings and body as the behaviour that correlated most frequently with pain. A reduction in the frequency or duration of comfort and self-maintenance behaviours, sometimes mimicking these other species examples, can certainly be seen in companion parrots as well. Aggression can be seen in some birds with pain, either in an effort to remove a painful stimulus from the environment or non-specifically manifested in some individual cases. Feather-grooming behaviours may either be increased or decreased in frequency for an individual bird that is experiencing pain. In circumstances where there is general withdrawal from daily activities due to pain, a decrease in preening behaviour can be seen. Some birds may show feather-damaging behaviours, either non-specifically or regionally directed to a painful location of their body. Appetite and feeding behaviours can be decreased, resulting in weight loss or a potential failure to gain weight. Birds may display similar tonic immobility postures postoperatively and with chronically painful conditions. Tonic immobility (cataplexy) is an innate fear response that is characterized by a profound and reversible state of motor inhibition.

As a simple guide, it is important for the attending nursing and veterinary staff to envision what their behaviour may be if they, for example, had a migraine headache or a localized pain in their body. With a migraine, most humans will close their eyes, speak less with others (decreased social interaction), separate themselves from others (social isolation), eat less (hyporexia, anorexia) and move less (decreased motor activities). Clinicians should anticipate and look for similar signs of acute and chronic pain in birds, qualified by the normal behaviours of the individual.

Due to the inherent variability of drug kinetics and dynamics in the multiple bird species that the avian clinician treats, the routine use of bimodal analgesia has even greater merit than in domestic mammal species. Opioids combined with non-steroidal anti-inflammatory drugs (NSAIDs) are common components of bimodal analgesia strategies for companion bird species.

Local anaesthetics

Local anaesthetics are used to produce regional anaesthesia and analgesia by blocking the transmission of noxious impulses. When used preoperatively, local anaesthetics block the site of tissue manipulation, which helps prevent central nervous system sensitization. Both lidocaine and bupivacaine act by blocking sodium channels in the nerve axon, interfering with the conduction of action potentials along the nerve. These anaesthetics are applied through regional infiltration, local line blocks or 'splash' block methods (Paul-Murphy, 2006; Hawkins and Paul-Murphy, 2011). The sites for local anaesthetic injection are typically the areas of injury or planned incision, as in mammals. In general, the total dose of lidocaine administered should not exceed 4 mg/kg, and a maximum dose of 1 mg/kg of bupivacaine has been suggested. It is recommended that when using the common dosage range for lidocaine of 1–4 mg/kg, the commercially available concentration should be diluted at least 1:10. An overdose of lidocaine has been reported to cause seizures and death in small birds. In mammals, analgesia from bupivacaine (4–10 hours) lasts much longer than lidocaine (1–3 hours), but the duration of analgesia from these drugs in avian species is not known. Intra-articular administration of bupivacaine (3 mg in 0.3 ml saline) was shown to be effective for treating musculoskeletal pain in chickens. Toxic side effects of these drugs can include fine tremors, ataxia, recumbency, seizures, stupor, cardiovascular effects and death.

Opioids

Drugs in this family bind reversibly to specific receptors (mu, kappa and delta) in the central and peripheral nervous systems. Of these drugs, butorphanol (mixed agonist-antagonist) is the best studied opioid analgesic, with primarily kappa agonist actions. In Grey Parrots, butorphanol, administered intramuscularly, to a plasma concentration of 2 mg/kg has a mean residence time of less than 2 hours, with suggestive analgesia for approximately 4 hours. Butorphanol (1–3 mg/kg) is currently the primary recommended opioid for analgesia in common companion bird species, and it can be given as a preoperative and postoperative analgesic (Paul-Murphy, 2006; Hawkins and Paul-Murphy, 2011). It is also recommended for acute, severe pain that often accompanies trauma. Tramadol has been shown to have a dynamic analgesic effect in

Hispanolian Amazon Parrots when administered at 30 mg/kg orally q8–12h. There is currently minimal evidence to support that buprenorphine has analgesic merit in its studied dosages in companion parrot species. Common analgesics used in the author's primarily companion bird practice include butorphanol, tramadol, carprofen and meloxicam.

Non-steroidal anti-inflammatory drugs

NSAIDs interfere with eicosanoid synthesis by inhibiting the cyclooxygenase (COX) enzymes. These enzymes are involved in reactions that result in polyunsaturated acids being converted to eicosanoids such as prostaglandins and thromboxanes, which are released at sites of tissue injury and cause inflammation and sensitization of nerve endings. A reduction of prostaglandins and thromboxanes results in a decrease of inflammation at the site of injury and has some modulating effect within the central nervous system. NSAIDs can be used for many forms of acute and chronic pain in birds, and are often used in combination with other analgesics (opioids and/or local anaesthetics) to produce a synergistic analgesic effect (Paul-Murphy, 2006; Hawkins and Paul-Murphy, 2011). Common NSAIDs used in avian practice include ketoprofen, meloxicam, carprofen, celecoxib and piroxicam. With the use of these drugs pre- or postoperatively, there remains minimal evidence of direct potential for harm in a well hydrated patient that has acceptable gastrointestinal health. Regardless, many veterinary surgeons, the author included, often add in NSAIDs parenterally to the treatment plan at recovery from an anaesthetic procedure. Ketoprofen exhibits actions similar to those of other NSAIDs, in that it possesses antipyretic, analgesic and anti-inflammatory activity. Its purported mechanism of action is the inhibition of COX catalysis of arachadonic acid to prostaglandin precursors (endoperoxides), thereby inhibiting the synthesis of prostaglandins in tissues. As an anti-inflammatory analgesic, ketoprofen is administered at 2 mg/kg i.m. q8–24h. Meloxicam is also an oxicam NSAID; it has greater activity against COX-2, which suggests it may have a wider safety margin in mammalian species. Current recommended dosages for meloxicam are 1.6 mg/kg orally q12–24h, or 1 mg/kg i.m. q12–24h (Molter et al., 2013). Analgesic effects of meloxicam at 1 mg/kg i.m. q12h have been described in Hispaniolan Amazons with experimentally induced arthritic pain. Carprofen may be a specific COX-2 inhibitor, and is available in oral and injectable forms. Its primary effect is on inflammation while potentially sparing physiological prostaglandins. Pharmacokinetic studies with broiler chickens indicated that peak plasma levels of carprofen were reached between 1 and 2 hours after a subcutaneous dose, and pain thresholds were raised for at least 90 minutes after chickens received 1 mg/kg subcutaneously. Carprofen at this same dose and route of administration has been shown to increase the walking ability and speed of lame broiler chickens. Piroxicam is a NSAID approved for use in humans and is used in mammals to treat chronic inflammatory conditions, such as arthritis. It has been administered to treat pain associated with chronic degenerative joint diseases in birds and appears to provide mild to moderate improvement.

The option of using sedation in place of general anaesthesia

Although general anaesthesia is used on occasion to facilitate minor procedures, conscious sedation may in many situations be a safe and effective alternative. Pre-anaesthetic doses of midazolam (0.25–1 mg/kg i.m.) and butorphanol (0.5–3 mg/kg i.v. or i.m.) are often more than adequate to facilitate laboratory sample collection, radiographic positioning and imaging, and minor procedures in birds (Lennox, 2011). Rapid reversal can be accomplished with flumazenil at 0.05 mg/kg i.m. Intranasal sedation with midazolam at 2 mg/kg was effective at facilitating a 15-minute manual restraint experience in Hispaniolan Amazons within 3 minutes of administration, and was effectively reversed with flumazenil administered intramuscularly within 10 minutes (Mans *et al.*, 2012).

When anaesthesia is necessary, conscious sedation or premedication might reduce the required dosage of the anaesthetic drug itself, resulting in fewer side effects (Korbel, 2012). There are other options outside the use of midazolam with butorphanol. Ketamine alone (10 mg/kg i.m.) and a ketamine/diazepam combination (10 mg/kg + 0.5 mg/kg i.m.) produced appreciable sedation and decreased the minimum anaesthetic dose of sevoflurane in Blue-fronted Amazon Parrots (Veras Paula *et al.*, 2013). However, midazolam and butorphanol remain the most popular sedation options, with the recognized side effects. Oxygen supplementation should be given as indicated.

Induction and intubation

Pre-oxygenation prior to anaesthetic induction offers value for many avian patients. A few minutes in an oxygen-rich cage environment prior to induction, or oxygen delivered by a facemask (Figure 16.2) if the bird is calm enough to enable such a direct procedure, may be beneficial.

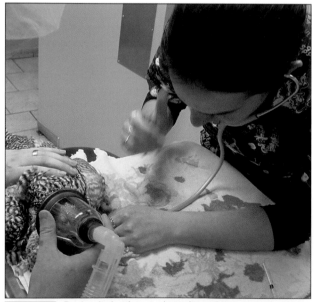

16.2 During induction, a clear view of the patient can be aided by the use of clear facemasks. Good communication between the primary anaesthetist, on the left, and the designated helper, on the right, will function to improve patient safety and shorten the time between induction and the start of the planned procedure.

Anaesthetic induction

Breathing circuits (Figure 16.3) used for avian species are typically non-rebreathing (Bain or Norman elbow) circuits, with oxygen flows from two to three times over minute volume (200 ml/kg/min). Oxygen flow rates of 0.5–1.5 l/kg/min are commonly used during induction of common companion bird species. The smallest available bag should be selected for most common companion bird species (<2 kg bodyweight). Anaesthetic induction is most commonly accomplished by use of a mask with isoflurane, sevoflurane or desflurane. Sevoflurane and desflurane may offer faster induction and recovery in studied patients, as compared with isoflurane. Isoflurane can cause significant respiratory depression in birds. Halothane is no longer considered safe and reliable for avian anaesthesia (Echols, 2004). Clear plastic facemasks facilitate patient monitoring during the induction period. Chamber induction, for the most part, is very uncommonly used, as there is minimal ability to control the bird through its excitatory phase of induction; there are safer methods that can be utilized in most settings. Most birds will be induced with isoflurane at a 5% vaporizer setting, although some may be induced at a lower concentration, with isoflurane maintenance at the 1–3% setting depending on procedure and patient variables.

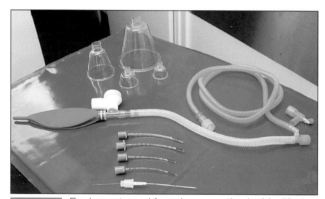

16.3 Equipment used for avian anaesthesia. Modified T-piece breathing system, non-cuffed tubes and a selection of masks.

Intubation

Endotracheal intubation is recommended for most procedures in patients weighing over approximately 100 g, and can be utilized in smaller birds in specific settings and procedures. Birds have complete tracheal rings, and their trachea is typically 2.7 times longer and 1.3 times wider than that of a similar-sized mammal. The laryngeal mound (Figure 16.4) at the base of the tongue houses the visible glottis and is connected distally to the distant syrinx (voice box) by a variably elongated trachea. The syrinx divides into two primary bronchi that enter and pass through the lungs (King and McLelland, 1984). A properly fitted facemask can be used on smaller birds to control respiration and anaesthetic delivery (Echols, 2004). Avian patients rarely develop tracheal obstructive plugs when maintained with a mask but are susceptible to aspiration when not intubated while under anaesthesia (Echols, 2004). With the tongue extended, the glottis can be easily visualized, and an appropriate-sized endotracheal tube passed into the proximal trachea. The bird should be intubated with a small uncuffed or cuffed (non-inflated) endotracheal

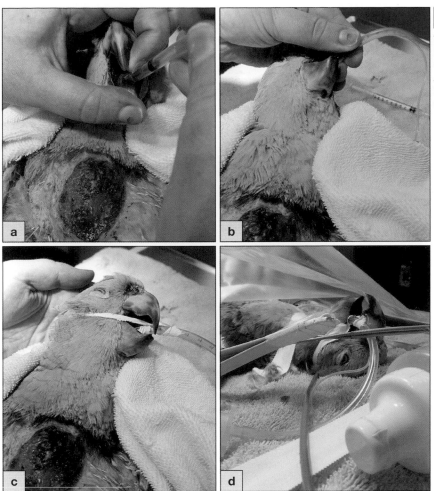

16.4 (a–d) When intubating, extend the tongue (beneath the left thumb) to enable best exposure of the laryngeal mound for placement of the endotracheal tube. This Yellow-naped Amazon is being anaesthetized for surgical biopsy of the lesion shown, which was diagnosed as a squamous cell carcinoma.

tube once anaesthetized. Complete tracheal rings make the tracheal lumen less distensible and more prone to damage from an overinflated endotracheal tube cuff (King and McLelland, 1984). For this reason, uncuffed endotracheal tubes are preferred, and taking care to keep the patient's neck extended and not bent against the end of the endotracheal tube is advised. The endotracheal tube is then taped and secured in position and the patient positioned for the planned procedure. Endotracheal tube-associated trauma can result in the formation of tracheal strictures (Figure 16.5), which are typically seen 1–3 weeks post-procedure.

For those patients where there may be surgery of the trachea planned, or where there is a suspected upper airway obstruction, cannulation of the abdominal or caudal thoracic air sac may be needed to maintain anaesthesia (Echols, 2004) (see Chapter 17). With direct air flow and volatile anaesthetic delivery into the abdominal or thoracic air sacs, oxygen exchange can still occur whilst inspiratory obstruction problems are avoided (King and McLelland, 1984). The air sacs of birds do not participate in gas exchange but function in conjunction with sternal, rib and abdominal movement like bellows, providing tidal air flow through the lungs during ventilation (King and McLelland, 1984). Birds have a two-breath cycle that allows a continuous flow of air to exchange at surfaces, whereas gas exchange for mammals only occurs at the end of inspiration (Degernes, 2008) (see also Chapter 2). Birds tend to breathe more slowly and deeply than mammals, have lower minute ventilation, and have a greater demand for oxygen (Hawkins and Pascoe, 2007).

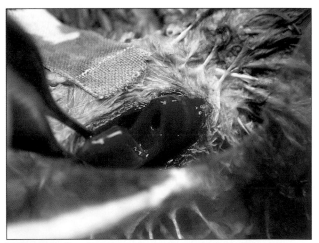

16.5 Surgical view of a tracheal stricture. This stricture was due to a plant foreign body and then granulation tissue, but intubation also carries a risk of tracheal stricture, usually seen 1–3 weeks after the procedure. Avoidance of inflating endotracheal tube cuffs, and careful attention to keep the patient's neck straight during the procedure, should help reduce the risk of this complication, as well as avoiding chemical residues on the endotracheal tubes. (Courtesy of B Doneley)

Monitoring and support

Stability of an anaesthetized patient can change rapidly and unpredictably. Good communication between the surgeon and anaesthetist during the procedure is important to allow optimal coordination between the surgical procedure and anaesthetic support. Once anaesthetized, several patient factors should be evaluated to help determine the depth of anaesthesia (Echols, 2004). Patient respiration is very important to monitor. Reflexes including pedal (foot withdrawal to pinch), palpebral (eyelid closure induced by ocular medial canthus or cere stimulation) and corneal (third eyelid movement in response to corneal manipulation) can all be monitored in birds. At 39–42°C, the normal core body temperature of avian species is higher than that of mammals, and there is increased vulnerability to hypothermia and, less commonly, hyperthermia (Longley, 2008). Most birds have a high surface area to body volume ratio, which increases the risk of heat loss during anaesthesia. Heat loss is directly proportional to the size of the patient: the smaller the bird, the faster the heat loss (Echols, 2004). Heat can be lost from exposed bare skin and this can be augmented by moisture on these exposed surfaces, through the respiratory tract, and from open incisions. Heat loss can also be increased by the delivery of non-humidified, cool anaesthetic gases. A common sign of hypothermia is decreased respiration, which can result in decreased oxygen exchange, leading to patient hypoxia. Providing radiant warmth (in the form of an overhead heat lamp) is an effective means of maintaining body temperature in anaesthetized birds (Echols, 2004), and appears to be superior to underlying heating pads. The heat lamp should be adjusted so that the temperature on the bird is approximately 37.8°C. Although more costly and somewhat awkward, heated air units (e.g. Bair Hugger®) are the most effective at maintaining core body temperature in anaesthetized birds (Rembert et al., 2001). Circulating warm water pads can offer some degree of thermal support, but are inferior to circulating air or radiant heat sources. The body position of anaesthetized birds has an effect on their respiratory system, with mean lung volume and partial air sac volumes in Red-tailed Hawks shown to be greatest in sternal recumbency, followed by right lateral and dorsal recumbency (Malka et al., 2009). This means that patient position can influence the ventilation of the patient, and that probably the most common position used, dorsal recumbency, should be accompanied by the use of intermittent positive pressure ventilation (IPPV). The heavier the pectoral musculature of an anaesthetized bird in dorsal recumbency, the greater the need to artificially ventilate.

Fluid support for anaesthetized birds can be delivered by intraosseous (Figure 16.6), subcutaneous and/or intravenous routes (see Chapter 15). Fluids should be warmed to approximately 39°C, and should be considered in all anaesthetized or debilitated patients (Echols, 2004). Even a low level of supplemental fluids may be beneficial in healthy avian patients undergoing non-invasive anaesthetic procedures. Fluids can be given at 30–60 ml/kg/h safely in most birds; however, balanced electrolyte solutions are more commonly given at 5–10 ml/kg/h i.v. or i.o. to birds under anaesthesia (Echols, 2004). Although frequently discussed as a concern, anaesthetized birds probably rarely become hypoglycaemic. When given intravenously, 5% dextrose may cause significant electrolyte imbalances and is generally discouraged. Balanced electrolyte solutions, such as lactated Ringer's solution and Normosol®, are more commonly used and recommended crystalloid fluids for use during anaesthetic

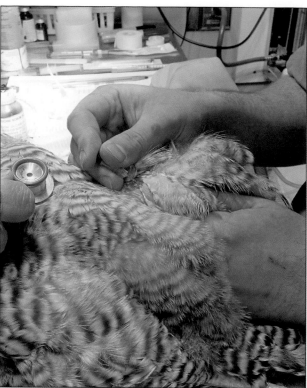

16.6 Intraosseous catheters are relatively easy and quick to place, and offer direct venous access in anaesthetized patients. This chicken has a 22 G spinal needle being placed in the left proximal tibiotarsus during the immediate post-induction period, in preparation for a surgical coeliotomy.

procedures. Hetastarch at 10 mg/kg or smaller volumes can be important to have available for those patients where total serum solids or protein levels may be subnormal prior to surgery, or where there has been a precipitous drop in indirect blood pressure noted during an anaesthetic procedure. Oxyglobin may be an additional colloid choice, should hetastarch not be available.

IPPV or continuous ventilation should be used throughout avian anaesthesia to help counteract decreased respiration, tidal volume and ultimately patient oxygenation. Most commonly, IPPV is applied manually during the procedure. Anaesthetic depth is best monitored by physical observation by the anaesthetist; respiratory rate and character must also be closely observed. Subtle changes in character can be very significant in the anaesthetized avian patient.

All monitoring devices should be placed quickly just prior to, or during, surgical preparation. Respiratory monitors are available that monitor rate, and can have value as an aid in patient monitoring; however, regardless of what monitoring equipment is used, it is always important that the anaesthetist stays completely focused on the actual patient, and no monitor should be used to function as a sole substitute for constant expert observation. Many of the monitoring devices that are used for monitoring mammals may not be as reliable in birds and there is often a lack of normal values in many of the species being anaesthetized. Their potential for providing trends, however, is where many of their benefits can be found.

The heart is monitored for rate and rhythm. An oesophageal stethoscope can aid the anaesthetist in monitoring the patient, but does not offer a 'hands-free' means of monitoring. An 8 MHz Doppler pulse monitor (Figure 16.7) is an important tool that is very helpful for monitoring heart rate and also for the purpose of monitoring indirect blood pressure (Figure 16.8). Although indirect Doppler blood pressure readings are likely not comparable to true arterial pressure, the trends that are observed throughout an anaesthetic procedure can have great value. These units offer a 'hands-free' means of monitoring, but are also vulnerable to being dislodged during the procedure. Doppler probes are best placed over one of the visible vessels, such as the cutaneous ulnar/wing vein and ulnar artery, crossing over the ventral aspect of the elbow region of the metatarsal vessels of the pelvic limbs, and provide an audible sound with each pulse.

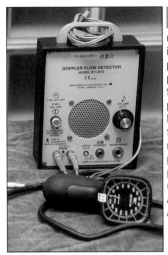

16.7 The use of a Doppler ultrasound pulse monitor is invaluable when monitoring patients under anaesthesia. It provides continual 'hands-free' audible monitoring of the pulse of the patient. The Doppler monitor also facilitates the intraoperative monitoring of indirect blood pressure, further augmenting patient monitoring acuity. (Reproduced from *BSAVA Manual of Canine and Feline Nephrology and Urology*)

Small blood pressure cuffs can be placed around the proximal humerus or femur/proximal tibiotarsus and used in conjunction with a distally placed Doppler probe to provide indirect blood pressure readings. As a simple rule of thumb, if blood pressure drops below 90 mmHg, give hetastarch at 5 ml/kg i.v. or i.o. until blood pressure is greater than 90 mmHg (Echols, 2004). Usually only one or two boluses of hetastarch are required.

Pulse oximeters are not calibrated for use in birds, and their accuracy unknown, but they can on occasion be used to acquire trend data for monitoring some anaesthetized patients and their relative degree of blood oxygenation. Electrocardiography (ECG) can also be used to record heart rates that are too rapid to count manually and may alert the anaesthetist to arrhythmias. Not all ECG equipment is capable of providing accurate readings on the relatively rapid heart rates of some birds, and if there is a plan to use such equipment, prior awareness of exactly how to use it and its limitations is important. The electrodes are placed at the propatagium and inguinal skin web locations with either flattened alligator clips or with small hypodermic needles passed through the skin and attached to the clips (Degernes, 2008).

Mechanical ventilators can be beneficial during longer anaesthetic procedures. Capnography can provide information on how well the patient is being ventilated. It is important to anticipate that during a surgical procedure, painful stimuli can affect the level of anaesthesia of birds, as it does with other species. Birds may require deeper or more shallow planes of anaesthesia, depending on current or anticipated events. As a general rule, pain from the skin and bone tends to be more of an aversive stimulus in birds than manipulation of coelomic organ structures.

Recovery

With most of the more common companion bird species, 'hands-on' postoperative recovery is preferred. During this period, careful observation of the respiratory rate, auscultation of the heart and physical stimulation of the patient all combine to assist in bringing these patients back to consciousness safely. An increasing respiratory rate and deepening character should indicate that the anaesthesia is becoming lighter and the bird is recovering. Sternal excursions should be monitored for increases in depth and frequency. Heart rate and quality should also be monitored. Decreases or changes in heart rate are often mirrored and preceded by changes in respiration. During patient recovery, the anaesthetist should smell the endotracheal tube for volatile anaesthetic fumes; as full recovery is approaching, this odour should diminish. Minimize human exposure to these fumes before, during and after anaesthesia. Mechanical stimulation of the bird's legs, wings and scratching the pectorals help to increase the rate and depth of respiration, speeding up recovery.

As the importance in monitoring the recovering patient decreases, all anaesthesia monitoring and supportive devices should be progressively removed. These include the Doppler pulse monitor, blood pressure cuff, ECG leads, endotracheal tube, supplemental oxygen, other monitors that have been used and, ultimately, the catheter (unless this is needed postoperatively for continued fluid support or venous

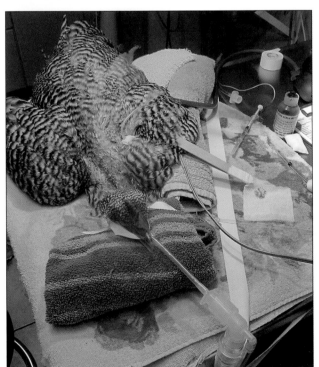

16.8 Indirect blood pressure can be a helpful trend to monitor during anaesthetic procedures. This hen has a Doppler probe placed over the ventral carpus and held in place with light pressure provided by two taped tongue depressors. The pressure cuff is placed about the mid-humeral region of the same wing, and a sphygmomanometer is attached to that.

access). Most often, in the author's practice, intra-osseous or intravenous catheters are removed within 5–30 minutes of recovery from anaesthesia. Immed-iately before or after extubation, examine the patient's oral cavity and glottis and the endotracheal tube itself for any regurgitated food, blood or mucus that may be present, and clean as needed.

Most companion birds are wrapped or held lightly in a towel during recovery to help control any delirious flap-ping or struggling, but it is very important to continue to pay close attention to respiratory rate and character. Most birds experience some degree of delirium during recovery and following anaesthesia (Echols, 2004). This post-anaesthesia excitement phase usually occurs shortly after discontinuing anaesthetic gas delivery, and can result in vigorous wing flapping, vocalization and chewing or biting behaviours. These same behav-iours can also be seen when the recovering patient is experiencing considerable uncontrolled pain at recovery. There is a risk of injury to the anaesthesia and surgical staff as well as the patient during this period of recovery if the patient is not adequately restrained and recovered; it is possible for large birds to fracture their wings at this time. The duration of this excitable phase is typically quite short, measured in a few seconds to minutes. Injectable anaesthetics such as ketamine, if used, may produce more severe post-anaesthetic delirium. The patient should be directly monitored until it is fully awake.

Once an apparent full anaesthetic recovery has been achieved and the bird is stable enough to stand, it should be returned to a warm environment, and moni-toring can be progressively relaxed. Most, but not all, birds should have auxiliary heat provided in the peri-operative period until such time as they are homeo-thermic. Most postoperative birds generally benefit from a warm (29.4–32.2°C), quiet environment with easily accessible food and water. Obese birds, or those with some forms of respiratory disease, may need to be maintained at a slightly lower temperature (23.9°C). With time and observation, as recovering birds become capable of homeothermia, the environmental temper-ature is progressively lowered to room temperature. This is ideally accomplished prior to discharge from the hospital. Generally, food may be offered within 30 minutes to 1 hour for most birds, possibly sooner for some smaller species. Food and/or water are more often provided later and in modified forms for gastro-intestinal surgical patients. Air sac breathing tubes that have been placed and that are to be maintained in the patient should be evaluated for patient comfort and patency. Patency of these tubes can be verified by holding a small contour or down feather to their open-ing and, as the patient breathes, watching for exhaled air to move the feather. Pharyngostomy tubes that have been placed during the surgical procedure should be evaluated for patency as well as patient comfort.

Postoperative patient support

Although they are somewhat of a common practice in canine and feline practice, the 'routine' use of Eliza-bethan or other types of collars is probably much less indicated in common companion avian species. In the author's experience, it is very uncommon for most birds to damage their post-surgical incisions, as long as their analgesia and stress levels are attended to optimally.

Large-sized sutures that are rigid in the skin (e.g. PDS®, Prolene®) may be much more irritating than a smaller suture size of the same material or a softer choice (e.g. Vicryl®). Tissue handling technique during surgery that was more traumatic than desired may result in more inflammation, pain and the potential for chewing at an incision site. Bandages that are excessively heavy, uncomfortable or constricting can also result in increased attention and chewing. With many bandaging techniques, considering the effective-ness combined with patient comfort, less may be best. If the patient's postoperative general and regional analgesia is less than optimal, the suture material used is irritating, the bandaging techniques are cumbersome or uncomfortable to the bird, or the surgeon's tissue handling skills have resulted in increased amounts of tissue trauma and inflammation, a bird may show more focus at its surgery site and there is potential for bandage or incision trauma. In these situations, a collar or the use of sedatives may be recommended or applied, although this may not necessarily be the most appropriate or balanced decision in many cases (Brown, 2006).

It is not uncommon for a bird that chews at the wound site to be labelled as a 'mutilator', thereby justi-fying the need for applying collars and/or other restraint devices; however, wound mutilation may be a clinical sign of discomfort, rather than a behavioural diagnosis. Ideally, a restraint device is only used when absolutely needed, and the use of collars or other restraint devices is probably accepted as a necessity more often than it may really be. Collars can also mechanically impede the bird's ability to eat normally, forage, interacting and per-form many self-comforting behaviours. A bird that has become apathetic to the presence of a collar and 'toler-ates' its presence should not necessarily be viewed as a good thing (Molter et al., 2013). In essence, the use of collars postoperatively or therapeutically should be eval-uated ethically along the lines of best practice (least intrusive, most effective), considering the short- and long-term benefits and risks to the patient.

Behavioural aspects of supportive care are also an important component of the clinical management of pain. Reducing fear and augmenting patient comfort are invaluable both pre- and postoperatively. A warm, calm and soothing hospital environment that has no noxious or anxiety-generating stimuli (e.g. noise, pred-ators) is very important. Companion birds that are accli-mated to human interactions should benefit from caring and positive human interaction, over the course of their hospital stay as part of their daily treatment regimes. On the other hand, those birds that are fearful of human interaction or unaccustomed to it, may benefit best from antecedent arrangement strategies through environmental modification, with a de-emphasis on providing human social interaction.

References and further reading

Brodbelt DC, Blissitt KJ, Hammond RA et al. (2008) The risk of death: the confidential enquiry into perioperative small animal fatalities. *Veterinary Anaesthesia and Analgesia* **35**, 365–373

Brown C (2006) Restraint collars. Part II: specific issues with restraint collars. *Laboratory Animals (NY)* **35(3)**, 25–27

Degernes LA (2008) Anesthesia for companion birds. *Compendium on Continuing Education for the Practicing Veterinarian* **30(10)**, E1–E11

Echols MS (2004) Avian anesthesia. *Proceedings of the Western Veterinary Conference*, Las Vegas 2004

Elliott J and Grauer G (2007) *BSAVA Manual of Canine and Feline Nephrology and Urology, 2nd edn*. BSAVA Publications, Gloucester

Friedman SG, Elding T and Cheney CD (2006) Concepts in behavior: Section I. (The natural science of behavior) In: *Clinical Avian Medicine*, ed. G Harrison and T Lightfoot, pp. 46–59. Spix Publishing, Palm Beach

Gentle MJ and Hunter LN (1991) Physiological and behavioural responses associated with feather removal in *Gallus gallus* var. *domesticus*. *Research in Veterinary Science* **50(1)**, 96–101

Hawkins MG and Pascoe PJ (2007) Cagebirds. In: *Zoo Animal and Wildlife: Immobilization and Anesthesia*, ed. G West, D Heard and N Caulkett, pp. 269–297. Blackwell, Ames

Hawkins MG and Paul-Murphy J (2011) Avian analgesia. *Veterinary Clinics of North America: Exotic Animal Practice* **14(1)**, 61–80

King AS and McLelland J (1984) *Birds: their structure and function*. Bailliere Tindall, Philadelphia

Korbel R (2012) Avian anaesthesia and critical care. *WSAVA/FECAVA/BSAVA World Congress 2012 Proceedings*, Birmingham

Lennox AM (2011) Sedation as an alternative to general anesthesia in pet birds. *Proceedings of the Association of Avian Veterinarians*, pp. 289–292, Madrid 2011

Longley L (2008) *Anaesthesia of Exotic Pets*. Elsevier Saunders, London

Malka S, Hawkins MG, Jones JH *et al.* (2009) Effect of body position on respiratory system volumes in anesthetized red-tailed hawks (*Buteo jamaicensis*) as measured via computed tomography. *American Journal of Veterinary Research* **70(9)**, 1155–1160

Mans C, Guzman DS, Lahner LL, Paul-Murphy J and Sladky KK (2012) Sedation and physiologic response to manual restraint after intranasal administration of midazolam in Hispaniolan Amazon parrots (*Amazona ventralis*). *Journal of Avian Medicine and Surgery* **26(3)**, 130–139

McKeown B, Speer B, Olsen G and Hawkins S (2012) Retrospective review of avian anesthetic procedures and mortalities. *Proceedings of the Association of Avian Veterinarians*, pp. 263–264, Louisville

Molter CM, Court MH, Cole GA *et al.* (2013) Pharmacokinetics of meloxicam after intravenous, intramuscular, and oral administration of a single dose to Hispaniolan Amazon parrots (*Amazona ventralis*). *American Journal of Veterinary Research* **74(3)**, 375–380

Paul-Murphy J (2006) Pain Management. In: *Clinical Avian Medicine*, ed. G Harrison and T Lightfoot, pp. 233–239. Spix Publishing, Palm Beach

Rembert MS, Smith JA, Hosgood G, Marks SL and Tully Jr. TN (2001) Comparison of traditional thermal support devices with the forced-air warmer system in anesthetized Hispaniolan Amazon parrots, *Amazona ventralis*. *Journal of Avian Medicine and Surgery* **15(3)**, 187–193

Veras Paula V, Otsuki DA, Auler JOC *et al.* (2013) The effect of premedication with ketamine, alone or with diazepam, on anaesthesia with sevoflurane in parrots (*Amazona aestiva*). *BMC Veterinary Research* **9**, 142

Yaakov DR, Rosenthal KL, Golder FJ and Shofer FS (2007) What is the mortality rate of anesthetized birds? *American College of Veterinary Anesthesiologists Annual Meeting*, September 2007

QRG 16.1 Avian intubation

Equipment

- Endotracheal (ET) tube
- Atraumatic forceps
- Tie
- Plastic wrap
- Facemask
- Towel

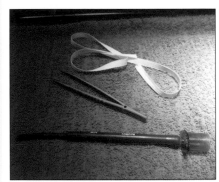

(© Deborah Monks)

Technique

1 Masks are covered in plastic wrap, to allow for a tighter seal around the bird's head.

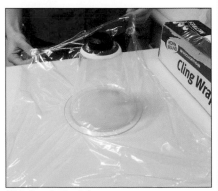

(© Deborah Monks)

2 The bird is adequately restrained in a towel (to prevent wing trauma) and the head is gently pushed into the mask through a small hole.

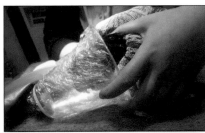

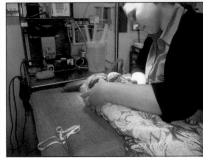

(© Deborah Monks)

3 The rhinotheca is held by an assistant, who also supports the back of the head.

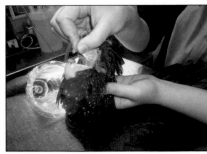

(© Deborah Monks)

4 The glottis is visualized, and the ET tube inserted.

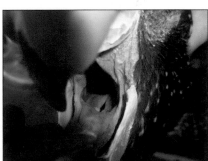

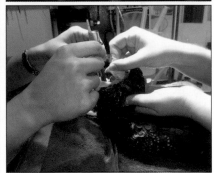

(© Deborah Monks)

5 The ET tube is secured with a tie.

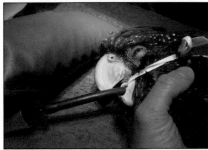

(© Deborah Monks)

Basic surgery

M. Scott Echols

Surgery is an integral part of day-to-day veterinary practice and this applies to avian patients as well as the more traditionally kept species such as cats and dogs. The popularity of pet birds means that more requests than ever are being made for advanced veterinary care. Veterinary surgeons (veterinarians) treating pet birds should at least be aware that surgical options for a large variety of disorders are available. While not exhaustive, this chapter provides clinicians information on selected soft tissue surgical procedures that may be encountered in pet avian practice. Orthopaedic disorders are also commonly encountered in birds and are covered in the *BSAVA Manual of Psittacine Birds* and *BSAVA Manual of Raptors, Pigeons and Passerine Birds*.

Principles of avian surgery

A basic understanding of general surgical principles is required prior to performing avian surgery. While basic surgical techniques are very similar, there are many anatomical and physiological differences between birds and mammals. Due to the small patient size and anatomical differences (e.g. avian air sacs), microsurgical instrumentation with magnification and focused light are recommended for efficient bird surgery. For larger birds, such as some birds of prey, standard surgical instruments are often used. Due to their variable physiology and anatomy, anaesthetic and analgesic management practices in avian species are very different and are discussed elsewhere (see Chapter 16) (see also the *BSAVA Manual of Psittacine Birds* and *BSAVA Manual of Raptors, Pigeons and Passerine Birds*).

Over 100 years ago, Dr William Halsted devised a list of surgical principles to maximize surgical success, and these still hold very true today:

- Gentle handling of tissue
- Meticulous haemostasis
- Preservation of blood supply
- Strict aseptic technique
- Minimal tension on tissues
- Accurate tissue apposition
- Obliteration of dead space.

These principles are simple but crucial to understand and practise during all avian surgical procedures.

Other key aspects of surgery that must be considered are:

- Pre-surgical patient evaluation
- Anaesthetic techniques
- Perioperative support (including fluid therapy, antimicrobials and pain control as needed)
- Longer term pain management.

The reader is encouraged to pursue education related to these topics prior to performing bird surgery.

Fluid therapy

Fluid therapy may be delivered subcutaneously, intravenously (Figure 17.1) or intraosseously for most surgery cases. Ideally, an intravenous or intraosseous catheter should be placed prior to surgery (see Chapter 15), such that the veterinary team has access to the bird's vascular system. The author commonly uses Plasma-Lyte®, Normosol®-R or 0.9% sodium chloride (normal saline) for avian surgeries. Intravenous and intraosseous fluids are generally given at a rate of 10 ml/kg/h during surgery. Perioperative subcutaneous fluids are usually given at 5% of bodyweight once or twice a day.

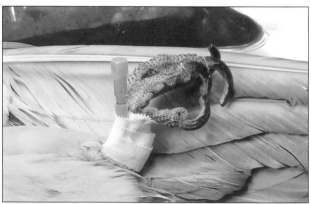

17.1 The pre-surgical avian patient should be carefully evaluated and prepared for surgery. This includes an assessment of appropriate anaesthesia and the requirement for perioperative fluid support, which may be intravenous (such as in this Blue and Gold Macaw), subcutaneous or intraosseous, antimicrobials and pain management.

Antibiotics

Perioperative antibiotics should be considered with contaminated or infected wounds, gastrointestinal exposure, prolonged procedures or if sterile technique was breached during surgery. The author prefers perioperative ceftazidime (100 mg/kg i.m. or i.v. q8–12h) or piperacillin (200 mg/kg i.m. or i.v. q8–12h) because these achieve relatively good tissue distribution and penetration, and cause relatively few reactions at injection sites. If available, culture and sensitivity results of infected tissues may dictate the use of different antimicrobials.

Analgesia

The study of avian analgesia is rapidly expanding, with updated drugs, dosing, frequency and routes. Currently, the author commonly gives butorphanol tartrate (2 mg/kg i.m. q2–4h), tramadol (5–30 mg/kg orally q8–12h) (note: significant species dose variation has been described) and/or meloxicam (1–2 mg/kg i.m. or orally q12–24h) perioperatively for pain control. Butorphanol tartrate serves as both a short-term analgesic and a pre-anaesthetic medication, often reducing the need for delivered isoflurane and possibly sevoflurane and other inhalational anaesthetics. The reader is encouraged to keep current on avian analgesia practice (Carpenter, 2013; Meredith, 2015).

Education

The author also encourages those interested in avian surgery to actively pursue continuing education. One of the best continuing education experiences is performing post-mortem examinations (necropsies) at one's own hospital. With the owners' permission, perform as many post-mortem examinations on birds as possible to gain experience and exposure to avian anatomy, tissue handling and instrument use (see also Chapter 14). Numerous continuing education courses that teach avian medicine and surgery are also available. Journals that focus on avian topics provide numerous well referenced papers on surgical techniques, in addition to medical topics (see 'References and further reading').

Surgical tools

Clinicians should become familiar with the range of surgical 'tools' available (Figure 17.2). These 'tools' include radiosurgery, microsurgical instruments, endoscopes, high-magnification microsurgical loupes with light, operating microscopes, laser units and other items that have become commonplace in avian surgery. Advanced diagnostics including digital radiography, ultrasonography and high-resolution computed tomography (CT) and magnetic resonance imaging (MRI) may be used to help better define the scope of the disease being addressed and better guide the surgeon.

Referral

While it is common practice to refer a challenging soft tissue or orthopaedic cat or dog case to a specialist small animal surgeon, general practitioners may not be aware that such avian specialists capable of complex bird procedures exist. In fact, board certification (or equivalent specialist qualification) for avian practice is available in Europe, Australia and North America. An avian species specialist may be board-certified as a Diplomate of the American Board of Veterinary Practitioners or certified in avian medicine and surgery by the Australian and New Zealand College of Veterinary Scientists or by the European College of Zoological Medicine. Individual countries may also have their own qualifications indicating specialization or increased knowledge/experience in dealing with these species (e.g. the Royal College of Veterinary Surgeons in the UK) (see 'Useful contacts').

If the veterinary surgeon is unsure about the complexity of the case or the procedure is expected to be above their medical or surgical skill level, referral is an excellent option. By contacting one or more of the above board certification groups, a regional specialist can be located. While not all clients will choose referral, this option should be considered for challenging cases.

Suture material and patterns

Suture material has been poorly studied in living avian species. However, limited research suggests that polydioxanone (e.g. PDS®) is at least acceptable, in terms of

Tool	Relative cost	Frequency of use	Space requirements	Special notes
Radiosurgery	££	1–2	+	Can cause more lateral tissue damage than standard and microsurgery instruments. Most commonly used on skin and to ligate small vessels
Microsurgical instruments	£	3–4	+	Reduce tissue damage but can lengthen surgery time and take time to learn proper use
Endoscopy	£££	1–2	++–+++	Most useful for pre-surgical scouting, biopsies and retrieving foreign bodies (respiratory and gastrointestinal systems)
Magnification loupes with focused light	£	4	+	Extremely beneficial with surgical and non-surgical procedures
Operating microscope	££	1	++	Most beneficial for peripheral surgeries (eyes, legs, wings)
Laser	££–£££	1–2	++	Can cause more lateral tissue damage than radiosurgery
Computed tomography	££££	1	++++	Usually only found at referral centres. Requires specialized training to operate and interpret images
Magnetic resonance imaging	££££	1	++++	Usually only found at referral centres. Requires specialized training to operate and interpret images

17.2 Tools commonly used in avian surgery. A scale of £ (least) to ££££ (most) (relative cost), 1 (least) to 4 (most) (frequency of use) and + (least) to ++++ (most) (space requirements) is used to rate each item. All tools take experience to master and proper use is assumed.

minimal tissue reaction, slow absorption and suture strength, for most avian surgeries (Bennett *et al.*, 1997; Pollock *et al.*, 2006). The author primarily uses PDS® and Monomend® MT (mid-term synthetic absorbable monofilament suture made of glyconate) sutures (generally 1–2 metric, 5/0–3/0 USP) for most avian surgeries. Monomend® MT tends to be more pliable and easier to tie than PDS®. Based on clinical experience and limited studies, PDS® or Monomend® MT are commonly used as the primary monofilament absorbable suture material in bird surgeries, and are implied throughout this chapter when no specific details are given. Of course, other suture materials may be used with bird surgeries and their use is often dictated by the tissue being sutured and, ultimately, surgeon preference.

Suture patterns used in birds are similar to those in other animals. For example, gastrointestinal incisions are often closed with a simple interrupted pattern followed by a continuous inverting pattern. Bird skin is quite forgiving and tends to heal well with minimum scarring by completing closure with adequate apposition and minimum tension. As a result, just about any suture pattern works well on avian skin. The author commonly closes avian skin with horizontal mattress (everting) or simple continuous patterns. Doing so decreases closure time compared with placing simple interrupted sutures (which are more commonly performed on small animal skin).

Wound management

The general principles of wound management in birds are similar to those used in cats and dogs. Anatomical and physiological differences do exist that may impact some wound treatment strategies.

All wounded avian patients require a complete history to be taken and a physical examination prior to devising a treatment plan. Antibiotics should be considered with bite wounds, necrotic and infected tissue, and whenever infection is a concern. When possible, culture and sensitivity testing should direct antibiotic choice, otherwise safe broad-spectrum antibiotics are recommended. Birds must be stabilized as much as possible prior to anaesthetic events and provided with cardiorespiratory, dietary and fluid support, pain management and haemorrhage control, as needed.

Open wounds can be protected with bandages, surgical closure and/or semi-occlusive bandages. Necrotic wounds must be debrided prior to closure. Consider primary closure for clean wounds less than 24 hours old (Riggs *et al.*, 2004). Burn wounds should be given 3–7 days post-injury in order to better delineate normal and dead tissue prior to surgical wound closure. Avian skin is very thin and is rapidly revascularized, therefore free skin grafts work better in birds than most other animals (Riggs and Tully, 2004). When cleaning the injured site, create a 2–3 cm circumferential featherless zone around the wound (Riggs and Tully, 2004; Ritzman, 2004).

The function of the bird and how the injury will affect the avian patient should be considered. With some exceptions, injured wild birds should be managed with the intent to release the patient back to the wild. Many wounds may not be initially life-threatening; however, they may result in long-term injuries that preclude normal flying, hunting or escape. Some of these birds may need to be humanely euthanased.

Addressing each type of possible avian wound goes beyond the scope of this chapter. General principles will be provided.

Avian skin

Birds have epidermal, dermal and subcutaneous layers, but the epidermis is extremely thin with typically only 3–5 cell layers (except over the thicker non-feathered areas such as the feet, beak, legs and face) (Riggs and Tully, 2004; Ritzman, 2004). With the exception of the uropygial gland, avian skin typically lacks glands and is dry and inelastic over much of the body. However, individual keratinocytes act as holocrine glands and can produce oils.

Avian wound healing has been described in three chronological phases: the inflammatory phase, the collagen phase and the maturation phase (Ritzman, 2004). Wound healing in birds begins with a clot and inflammatory response much as with mammals (Riggs and Tully, 2004). Heterophils and monocytes, later followed by lymphocytes, infiltrate the avian wound during the inflammatory phase. Fibroblasts and then capillaries proliferate in the following collagen phase. Finally, collagen fibres organize and ultimately orient in relation to the tension placed on the edges of the wound in the maturation phase. In this last phase, the wound contracts, attempting to bring epithelial margins back together, closing the wound; this phase can take weeks or months to complete (Riggs and Tully, 2004; Ritzman, 2004) (Figure 17.3).

Normal bruising results in a greenish discoloration in the bird (Ritzman, 2004). After haemoglobin is broken down, biliverdin pigment accumulates, giving the greenish colour within 2 to 3 days post-injury (Ritzman, 2004).

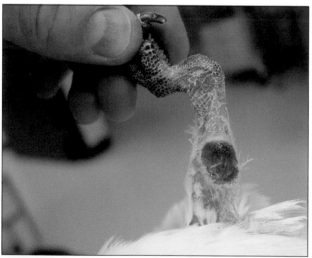

17.3 A self-induced mutilation wound on the medial crus of a Goffin's Cockatoo. The wound is beginning to contract at the edges, suggesting the lesion is changing from the collagen to maturation phase.

Skin protective devices

Except for instances of self-mutilation, most birds will not continue to traumatize their wounds. When sutures are properly placed with minimal tension, birds rarely pull at them after surgery. If birds do self-mutilate their wounds, this suggests pain, and the cause should be investigated and dealt with as needed (e.g. analgesics, evaluation of the surgery site). Birds that have primary wounds from self-mutilation require a full medical and behavioural work-up. Bandages can be useful when birds self-traumatize their wounds or when open wound management is needed (see 'Bandaging').

As a general rule, adherent bandages are used during the initial inflammatory stage of healing while non-adherent bandages are reserved for the proliferative and remodelling phases (Ritzman, 2004).

Non-stick (e.g. Tegaderm™) or minimally adhesive bandaging material can be used to protect a tissue bed and prevent serum leakage from a wound (Riggs and Tully, 2004). Semi-occlusive dressings may be poorly adhesive but can be laid over a cleaned wound and then covered with a bandage. Cyanoacrylic products or tissue glue (e.g. Nexaband®) can be used to repair minor incisions or lacerations.

Wet to dry bandages are beneficial in large wounds that are not amenable to primary closure (Riggs and Tully, 2004) (Figure 17.4). The wound should be cleaned and debrided before gauze bandages soaked with an antiseptic or sterile isotonic fluid are applied. A thick layer of dry gauze sponges on top of the wet sponges and a bandage to hold everything together should then be applied. Bandages need to be changed frequently as removal debrides and cleans the wound and helps stimulate granulation tissue. Once a healthy granulation tissue bed is present, non-adherent bandages can be used. If the wound does not completely contract and eventually close, surgical assistance may be required (Riggs and Tully, 2004) (Figure 17.5).

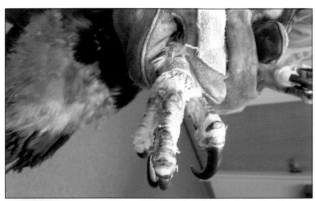

17.4 The foot of a young Golden Eagle damaged in a wildfire. A week after the initial injury, the foot was still in the healing process but did well with wet to dry bandages soaked in chlorhexidine solution and topical 1% silver sulfadiazine cream.

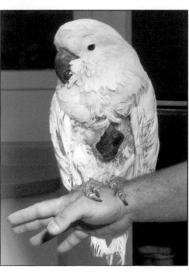

17.5 Large open wounds, as seen in this Moluccan Cockatoo, may require surgically assisted closure.

The simplest distracting device is to place a tape tag over a bandage that the bird can otherwise reach and damage. Butterfly the central portion of a tape strip leaving two sticky ends. The sticky ends are then applied to the bird's bandage leaving a tape tag sticking out. The bird may chew on the tag until it gets used to the bandage.

Neck collars should be reserved for birds that insist on self-traumatizing their wounds. The cause of the self-mutilation should be identified and corrected if possible. Neck collars should be temporary. There are a variety of neck collars available, from homemade (e.g. plastic and radiographic film 'E-collars', foam pipe insulation) and manufactured (e.g. plastic clam shell, plastic circular discs) models. The author primarily uses foam pipe insulation because it is inexpensive, effective, easily placed and, because it is soft, it tends to not cause pressure wounds (Figure 17.6). Some clinicians and owners have also successfully created 'T-shirts' and other devices that limit the bird from self-mutilation but do not impair respiration or wound healing.

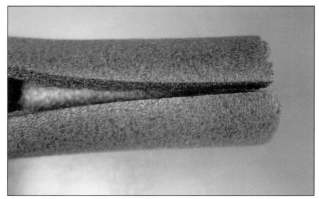

17.6 Foam pipe insulation material can be used to make a temporary neck collar. Primarily reserved for parrots, the pipe insulation material is placed on the bird's neck and cut to the appropriate length to prevent the patient from self-mutilating. When properly placed, the patient can eat, drink and ambulate with no difficulties. These types of collars should be rarely used and only for short periods of time. Every effort to understand the underlying cause of mutilation should be determined and treatment instituted as soon as possible.

Skin disinfectants

Most skin wounds are cleaned prior to surgical closure or bandaging. While sterile saline and other isotonic solutions can safely be used to clean and irrigate superficial wounds, chemical disinfectants are often needed with contaminated wounds. Povidone–iodine (1%) and chlorhexidine diacetate (0.05%) have both been found to be equally effective at cleaning skin (in mammals). However, povidone–iodine has been associated with skin reactions in some dogs (Bowles et al., 2006). Povidone–iodine has also been shown to be toxic to fibroblasts in concentrations as low as 1–5% (Ritzman, 2004). Chlorhexidine (0.05%) is considered very effective and safe as a wound irrigating solution (Ritzman, 2004). Hydrogen peroxide (3%) is minimally effective against most bacterial organisms but is sporicidal and can be useful to clean wounds that may be contaminated with clostridial organisms (Riggs and Tully, 2004). Hydrogen peroxide is also toxic to fibroblasts and other tissues and is best used as a single lavage treatment (Ritzman, 2004).

In birds, water-miscible ointments are optimal and can be applied to skin wounds (Ritzman, 2004). Avoid or sparingly use oil-based ointments because these inhibit normal thermoregulatory function of the feathers. A 1% silver sulfadiazine cream (e.g. Silvadene) is effective against most bacteria and fungi, promotes epithelialization and penetrates necrotic and eschar tissue (good for burn wounds) but can damage fibroblasts and impede wound contraction (Ritzman, 2004). It is best to avoid all topical steroid products as these compounds may be absorbed systemically from the skin in birds and cause life-threatening side effects.

Bandaging

Bandaging techniques are useful for stabilizing fractures, traumatic injuries, intravenous and intraosseous catheters and feeding tubes. Bandages are rarely used to limit self-trauma in pet birds. Most bandages are used for pre- and post-surgical fracture stabilization. Tape splints and figure-of-eight wing bandages are commonly used as the primary treatment of fractured bones in small birds (Chavez and Echols, 2007).

Bandages offer a lower-cost means to stabilize fractures than surgery. Properly applied bandages can be just as effective as (and lower risk than) surgery in some cases. Closed and minimally displaced fractures and those 'splinted' by surrounding intact bones (such as the ulna or radius, and major or minor metacarpal) often heal well with proper bandaging. Another important consideration is patient temperament; well adjusted and non-fractious patients tend to not continually traumatize bandaged appendages and have a better chance at healing conservatively set fractures than do fractious patients.

Most bandages are best placed with the patient sedated or anaesthetized. However, some bandages can be adequately placed in calm or subdued patients. When placing bandages, stabilizing the joint above and below the fracture site is ideal but is not always possible with all avian fractures. If both joints on either side of the fractured bone(s) cannot be stabilized, at least one joint is properly immobilized and the bird's environment should be arranged to limit activity and stress to give the bone(s) the best opportunity to heal.

A properly placed bandage is comfortable. When birds pick at or chew at their bandage, it is an indication that something needs to be modified. If the bird continually picks at its bandage, consider the following as potential causes: improper placement causing pain or unstable fracture(s); uncontrolled infection; and boredom. Bandages may need to be periodically removed, inspected and then replaced to ensure proper bone healing, joint mobility and infection control. Analgesics may need to be added or adjusted. The bird's environment may also need to be arranged to reduce boredom and create a situation where productive and safe behaviours can be performed (such as foraging).

Tape splint

Tibiotarsal and tarsometatarsal fractures are easily diagnosed by palpation and can be supported with the use of a tape splint in birds weighing less than 300 g. Radiographs are useful to better characterize the fracture(s) (Figure 17.7). For larger birds, a Schroeder–Thomas splint, a bandage incorporating support

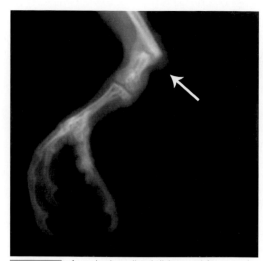

17.7 A malunion distal tibiotarsal fracture (arrowed) in a Timneh Grey Parrot resulted from a poorly placed leg bandage. As a result, the leg had to be refractured, surgically reduced and set with an external fixator.

material (e.g. a modified Robert Jones bandage) or surgical fixation is recommended. If the fracture is chronic or open and infected, surgical fixation and antibiotics are usually indicated.

For either tibiotarsal or tarsometatarsal fractures, place a 0.5–1 cm wide strip of flexible minimally adherent bandage material (e.g. Vetrap®) around the affected leg from the foot up to the stifle. The bandage material should be loosely applied and overlap by about 50% with each pass. Next, butterfly white medical tape strips (0.5–2 cm depending on the size of the bird) are applied over the bandage material up and down the wrapped leg. The butterfly tapes should be evenly placed over the leg, overlapping such that the tibiotarsal–tarsometatarsal joint is in the normal resting position and a relatively solid 'cast' is created. Both ends of the butterfly tape are crimped using a haemostat and the excess tape is cut and removed. If the toes become discoloured (dark), loosen the tape to improve distal circulation. This technique is illustrated in Figure 17.8.

During the healing period, keep the bird in a smooth-sided container such as a large fish tank or plastic storage box. The idea is to keep the bird from climbing and reinjuring the leg until it is healed. Food, water, low perches and safe toys must be placed on the bottom of the container. The tape splint should be carefully removed after 3–5 weeks. Activity is further restricted to the same container for another 2 weeks. If the leg is palpably stable after 2 weeks, the bird can be returned to its normal environment.

Schroeder–Thomas splint

The use of a Schroeder–Thomas splint is limited to fractures of the tarsometatarsus and distal one-third of the tibiotarsus (Degernes, 1994; Roush, 1996). These splints are used for tarsometatarsal fractures in small parrots (which are too small for surgical repair) and fractures close to the hock. This bandage should not be used with femoral or proximal (two-thirds) tibiotarsal fractures. The wire material used in the splint should be made with two right-angled bends next to a ring at the top so that the splint is parallel to the long axis of the leg (Figure 17.9). Position the leg so that there is some flexion at the hock joint. A light bandage is

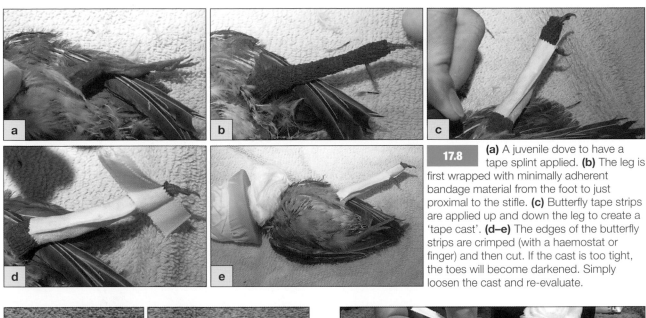

17.8 **(a)** A juvenile dove to have a tape splint applied. **(b)** The leg is first wrapped with minimally adherent bandage material from the foot to just proximal to the stifle. **(c)** Butterfly tape strips are applied up and down the leg to create a 'tape cast'. **(d–e)** The edges of the butterfly strips are crimped (with a haemostat or finger) and then cut. If the cast is too tight, the toes will become darkened. Simply loosen the cast and re-evaluate.

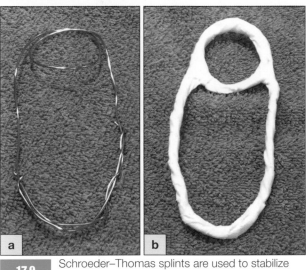

17.9 Schroeder–Thomas splints are used to stabilize distal tibiotarsal and tarsometatarsal fractures. **(a)** Each splint is custom made to match the leg dimensions of the bird with a ring that encircles the femur and two sides that run parallel to the length of the leg. **(b)** The wire frame splint is padded by covering it with tape.

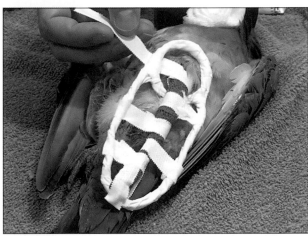

17.10 A Schroeder–Thomas splint is used to stabilize a distal tibiotarsal fracture in a dove (*Zenaida* sp).

applied to the leg with gauze and tape. The leg is suspended within the splint by alternating strips of tape placed cranially and caudally, with the toes extended to the end of the splint (Figure 17.10). The splint is covered with bandage material. Fracture healing should occur over 3–5 weeks, and the bandage should be changed every other week.

In most cases, a tape splint is more simple to place and as equally effective as a Schroeder–Thomas splint. However, the latter effectively immobilizes the entire leg and can be more beneficial with fractious or active birds and less stable fractures, resulting in better healing than that achieved with a tape splint.

Spica bandage

Spica splints can be used for simple aligned fractures of the femur in birds that weigh less than 300 g. A splint can be moulded from light- or heat-activated dental and human orthopaedic products such as Orthoplast® or Hexcelite® or padded aluminium finger splints. At room temperature, Orthoplast® and Hexcelite® are firm but, after placing in hot water, they can be made to

conform to the shape of a bird's limb. This splint is a modified Robert Jones bandage, except that the padded moulded splint extends from the tibiotarsus proximally and over the bird's synsacrum in an inverted U-shape to immobilize the femur against the body of the bird. As with most fractures of avian long bones, 3–5 weeks of fracture stabilization followed by 2 weeks of rest is needed for proper healing.

Modified Robert Jones bandage

The modified Robert Jones bandage should be limited to tibiotarsal fractures or soft tissue injuries of the hock joint and distal to the hock joint, and can be used in birds weighing up to 500 g (Degernes, 1994; Roush, 1996). Start by cutting light- or heat-activated dental and human orthopaedic products in an L-shape (with an approximately 60-degree angle). The size of the arms of the 'L' needs to be adjusted for the size of the patient's tibiotarsus (long arm) and tarsometatarsus (short arm) and angled to match the normal resting position of the tibiotarsal–tarsometatarsal (hock) joint. Next, place a layer of padding material around the leg from the foot up to just above the stifle. Follow the cast padding with a layer of cling or cotton gauze, tightening gently while wrapping. Heat or light activate the splint until it becomes malleable. Position and shape the splint along the lateral aspect of the leg and wrap the final layer of flexible minimally adherent bandage material around the splint before it hardens. The splint is left on for 3–5 weeks for fractures and generally shorter times for soft tissue injuries.

Note: loosely placed modified Robert Jones bandages can result in distal slipping. This can weight the distal limb, placing more strain on the fracture site, leading to non-union fractures and healing failure.

Ehmer type bandage

As with dogs and cats, the Ehmer bandage, or sling, can be used for a dislocated hip or for temporary stabilization of fractures involving the leg in birds. Without overflexing the hock, the tarsometatarsus is folded against the tibiotarsus and gauze is wrapped around both. If necessary, the tarsometatarsus and tibiotarsus can be bound to the body by extending the wrap over the synsacrum and across the ventral coelom back to the leg. Anatomical differences between birds and mammals mean it is difficult to achieve the same forces that direct a dislocated head of the femur back into normal position. The sling will likely need to be adjusted to best position the hip, and this will depend on the species of bird. However, the Ehmer sling is a reasonable bandage to use with acute hip dislocations. Radiographs are used to confirm reduction of the hip after bandage placement. The bandage and hip position may need to be checked every 2–4 days to ensure continued reduction until the joint is fully reduced and stable (which may take 2–3 weeks). Unstable hip dislocations usually require surgical reduction. As this bandage effectively hobbles the patient, the bird's environment needs to be adjusted to prevent further injury.

Figure-of-eight wing bandage

Patients with wing fractures commonly present with a dropped wing. Some fractures heal well after treatment with external coaptation, with return to full function. However, surgical reduction and fixation is generally considered the best treatment for most wing fractures, especially in performance flying birds, such as many birds of prey. Wing bandages may also be used to support soft tissue injuries and protect medical equipment such as intravenous and intraosseous catheters. Bandages can be used to treat most wing fractures in birds not required to return to full flight (aviary and cage birds). Due to the lack of significant soft tissue coverage, wing fractures are commonly open. Many acute open fractures can be adequately stabilized and can heal with bandaging, the wounds should be thoroughly cleaned, skin wounds closed (if needed) and the patient placed on systemic antibiotics, such as ceftazidime or piperacillin. Open humeral fractures should be carefully and minimally lavaged as the humeral lumen is directly connected to the respiratory system in birds. The wing is especially amenable to splinting because it can be placed in normal anatomical resting position.

A figure-of-eight bandage provides adequate stabilization for fractures of the radius and ulna. As the name implies, this bandage makes a figure-of-eight pattern. Small birds (<750 g) generally only need one layer of flexible minimally adherent bandage material, while larger birds often benefit from a first layer of roll gauze followed by a layer of flexible minimally adherent bandage material. Rarely, an additional protective layer

made of duct or similar tape may be needed for some parrots. Parrots may also benefit from distraction tabs (butterflied white tape) placed on the outside of the bandage without using the 'protective layer' (Figure 17.11). A protective layer or distraction tabs are not substitutes for poorly placed bandages. As discussed above, if a bird persistently chews at the bandage this may indicate uncontrolled pain or an improperly placed wing bandage.

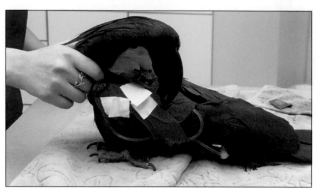

17.11 Distraction tabs made of butterflied white tape are placed on the outer layer of this figure-of-eight wing bandage in a Palm Cockatoo. The bandage was placed simply to protect the intravenous catheter and line, while the distraction tabs give the patient something to groom or chew on without destroying the bandage. Distraction tabs are not a substitute for a poorly placed uncomfortable bandage. If the patient is chewing at the actual bandage, re-bandage the wing and consider analgesics to help manage pain.

The goal of the figure-of-eight bandage is to provide as much support as possible with minimal bulk, whilst allowing the wing joints to remain at natural angles. The bandage should allow the wing to lie normally against the body, resulting in minimal discomfort to the patient. The bandage should be easily removed and replaced to allow for physical therapy and evaluation of the injury until the fractures are adequately healed. The bandage removal, physical therapy and bandage reapplication process should be completed every 2–4 days to prevent joint fibrosis and contracture.

The figure-of-eight bandage is one of the most commonly utilized bandages in avian medicine and is arguably one of the most challenging to properly place for novices. However, with a little practice, the figure-of-eight bandage can be easily placed and provide good support for wing injuries.

Whether using one or two layers, the bandage material used is positioned in a similar fashion, starting on the medial aspect of the wing (as high in the axilla as possible), to keep it away from the elbow and reduce tension on the propatagial tendon. Bandage material laid close to or covering the elbow may impinge upon the propatagial tendon, which over time damages the tendon and reduces flight capabilities. The wrap should be continued on the dorsal surface of the wing up to the carpus (Figure 17.12a) and then circle the carpus from a lateral (dorsal) to medial direction, ending on the ventral portion of the carpus (Figure 17.12b). The final stage is to pass the bandage along the wing surface from the carpus and back to the axillary region (Figure 17.12c); the whole cycle should be repeated until the wing is held lightly but securely in a flexed position (Figure 17.12de). If needed, a second layer of wrap can be placed (Figure 17.12f).

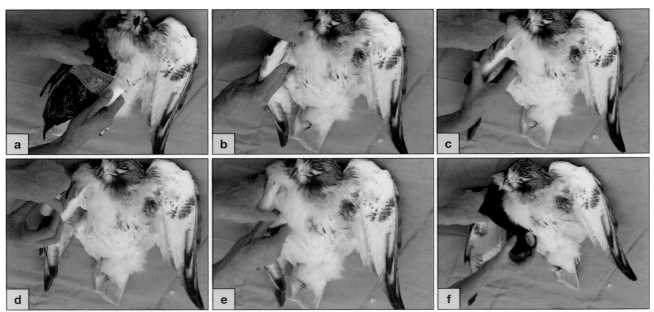

17.12 A figure-of-eight wing bandage demonstrated on a deceased Red-tailed Hawk. **(a)** The bandage (in this case a first layer of roll gauze) is started high in the axilla and carried over the dorsal aspect of the wing to the leading edge of the carpus. **(b)** Next, the bandage material is wrapped around the carpus from lateral (dorsal wing) to medial, **(c)** circling the carpus to the medial side of the wing and ultimately being pulled high in the axilla to **(d–e)** be brought around the dorsal side of the wing for a second pass. **(f)** A second layer of flexible minimally adherent bandage material is placed following the same pattern as the first.

Body wrap wing bandage

In order to protect injuries to the humerus and pectoral girdle, a body wrap can be used (Degernes, 1994; Roush, 1996). Adherent but non-feather-destructive tape (such as Durapore™) should be used to hold the wrapped wing next to the body in a natural position. The body wrap can also be used in conjunction with a figure-of-eight bandage to stabilize multiple wing injuries.

Start by placing the tape over the breast at the middle part of the keel and wrap around the body, keeping relatively high in the axilla (Figure 17.13a).

Pass the tape once or twice around the body. Next, bring the tape around the dorsal aspect of the wing and back over the previously laid tape on the breast (ventrally). The wing should be laid in a normal resting position (Figure 17.13b). Make one or two passes incorporating the wing to the body bandage. The overall bandage should be light and not contribute to any discomfort to the bird. Pass one or two fingers under the tape bandage where the wing is folded up against the body (Figure 17.13c). If properly placed, the wing will be stabilized and the tape will not interfere with respiration or leg movements.

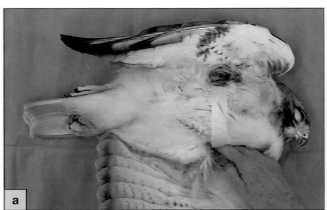

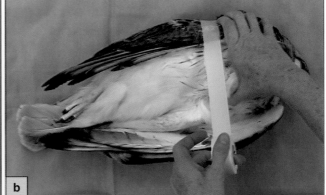

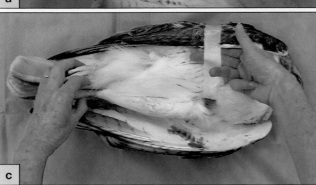

17.13 A body wrap is demonstrated on a deceased Red-tailed Hawk. **(a)** Start by placing tape over the central portion of the keel and wrap it around the body, keeping the tape relatively high in the axilla. 3M™ Durapore™ is used here because it is adherent but minimally damages the feathers when removed. **(b)** Next, bring the tape around the dorsal side of the injured wing over the middle portions of the humerus, radius, ulna and phalanges, such that the wing lies in a normal resting position. **(c)** After making one or two passes stabilizing the wing against the body, insert one or two fingers under the tape to ensure the bandage is not too tight.

Simple foot bandage

For simple foot and toe injuries, including mild bumblefoot (Figure 17.14), a flexible minimally adherent bandage can be used. Usually only one layer is required. With the foot and toes in natural positions, start by wrapping the bandage around the distal tarsometatarsus. After one or two passes, carry the bandage material under the plantar surface of the foot, then the dorsal surface of the foot and back to the distal tarsometatarsus (Figure 17.15a). Next, go between each digit, making sure that normal position is achieved (Figure 17.15b). Cut the bandage material to make it as narrow as needed for the size of the bird. If necessary, the bandage can be extended to cover a digit.

Ball bandage

The ball bandage is used to immobilize the toes and is most commonly used with birds of prey. The bandage is used to aid healing of more serious foot and toe injuries and also during procedures (e.g. radiography, surgeries) to prevent birds of prey from unexpectedly impaling their talons in handlers. A large ball of soft (roll or square) gauze is placed within the centre of the foot and the bird is allowed to grasp down on the

padding (Figure 17.16a). A layer of roll gauze is started around the distal tarsometatarsus and carried over and around the foot (Figure 17.16bc). Next, flexible minimally adherent bandage material is wrapped around the foot and gauze, safely securing the toes in a semi-perching position (Figure 17.16de). If only one foot is bandaged, the awake patient should be able to bear weight on the wrapped foot.

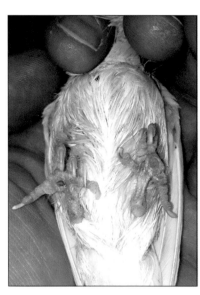

17.14 A Budgerigar with bumblefoot lesions on both feet. Such lesions can benefit from perch management, addressing underlying illness (especially arthritis and obesity), topical medications and a simple foot bandage.

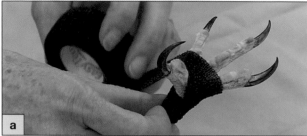
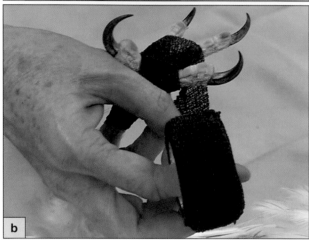

17.15 A simple foot bandage demonstrated on a deceased Red-tailed Hawk. **(a)** Start by wrapping the distal tarsometatarsus with minimally adherent bandage material. Carry the bandage under the plantar surface of the foot, then over the dorsal foot, and back to and around the distal tarsometatarsus. **(b)** Next, pass the bandage material between each toe, going from plantar to dorsal, until all interdigital spaces are covered. The bandage can be extended to one or more toes as needed. An excessively tight bandage may result in tissue necrosis and should be monitored.

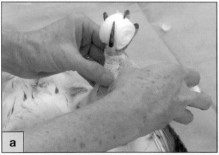
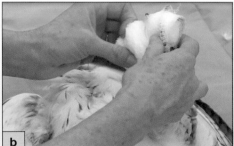
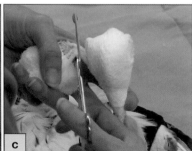
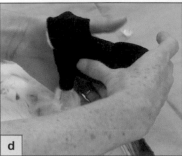
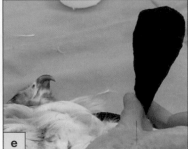

17.16 A ball bandage demonstrated on a deceased Red-tailed Hawk. Ball bandages are reserved for more serious foot injuries and also used as needed to prevent birds of prey from impaling handlers during procedures. **(a)** Roll gauze or square gauze pads are placed into the central plantar surface of the foot and the bird is allowed to grab the material. **(b–c)** Next, a layer of roll gauze is started at the distal tarsometatarsus and carried over and around the foot with the toes kept in a semi-perching position. **(d–e)** This is followed by a layer of minimally adherent bandage material laid in the same fashion.

Surgical procedures

The procedures discussed within this chapter will be rated on a 1 to 3 scale of difficulty.

- **Level 1: Basic procedures.** These procedures include primarily topical surgeries of the skin or others that require minimal expertise and equipment. Complications are generally minimal if performed correctly.
- **Level 2: Intermediate procedures.** These are surgeries that require at least some familiarity with avian anatomy and tissue handling and, often, penetration into a body cavity. Complications are generally limited to the region of interest but can be significant.
- **Level 3: Advanced procedures**. These are surgeries that require advanced knowledge of avian anatomy and tissue handling, result in penetration into a body cavity and come with a relatively high risk of variation (in terms of findings and adjustments that may be needed) and patient risk (e.g. excessive bleeding, prolonged anaesthesia time).

The upper respiratory tract

Diseases of the sinus, especially related to infections, trauma and cancer, are occasionally noted in pet birds, some of which require surgical intervention. The classic and non-specific signs of sinus disease include swelling of various diverticula of infraorbital sinuses, ocular and naris discharge, naris distortion and head shaking. Solid masses, such as tumours and walled-off granulomas, may present with infraorbital sinus swelling only (Figure 17.17; see also Chapter 20).

Due to the cavernous anatomy of the infraorbital sinus and its many diverticuli and chambers, fluid, soft tissue and inflammatory debris can build up unnoticed. Once the debris fills one portion of the infraorbital sinus, it either spills over into an adjacent chamber or diverticulum (which may continue to go unnoticed) or reaches a point where a swelling is evident externally. Oculonasal discharge, conjunctivitis and/or head shaking may or may not be present before a physical swelling is noticed by the owner or attending veterinary surgeon. By the time a bird is identified as having a sinus mass or supportive clinical signs, it may have advanced disease that affects many regions of the infraorbital sinus(es).

Diagnostics such as skull radiography (Figure 17.18), choanal or nares inspection via magnified light or endoscopy, CT, MRI, infectious disease testing (e.g. polymerase chain reaction (PCR), culture and sensitivity), sinus aspiration (with or without flushing small amounts of sterile saline) and cytology can be used to better characterize the cause and distribution of the swelling (see also Chapter 20). While early cases of infectious sinusitis (before the debris becomes caseated) may respond to appropriate antibiotic therapy, advanced cases often require surgical attention.

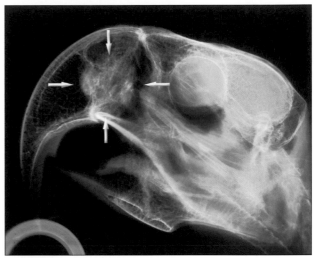

17.18 Advanced diagnostics such as radiography, computed tomography and magnetic resonance imaging are often needed to better characterize sinus disease in birds. In this case, a large soft tissue dense mass is identified in the rostral diverticulum of the infraorbital sinus (in the base of the upper mandible, outlined by arrows) in a Blue and Gold Macaw.

Unless guided differently by advanced diagnostics, incisions are best made directly over swollen sinus tissue and away from the eye (Figure 17.19a). Skin overlying inflamed sinus tissue is often very vascular and haemostasis is generally needed. Conversely, once inside the sinus the tissue is generally poorly vascular unless a mass is attached to the sinus wall or surrounding bone and muscle, as sometimes occurs with tumours. The beak may be opened to increase potential sinus space to improve visualization.

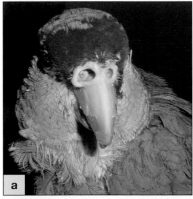 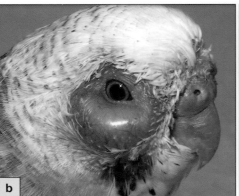 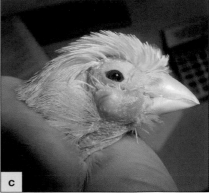

17.17 **(a)** As a result of chronic upper respiratory disease and accumulation of caseous debris, the right naris of this Green-cheeked Amazon is severely distorted. **(b)** A Budgerigar with a swollen infraorbital sinus and discharge from the nares. This is more typical of the classic presentation of advanced sinusitis. **(c)** Some sinus masses are solid and may manifest as a visible swelling only with no discharge, as in this Canary.

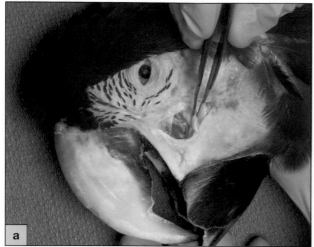

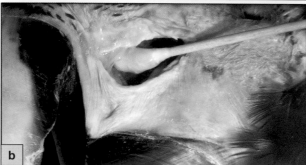

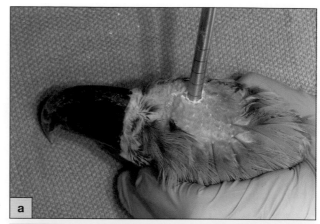

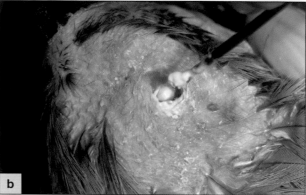

17.19 **(a)** When performing an infraorbital sinusotomy, incise directly over the swollen area but away from the eye, as shown with this Green-winged Macaw (cadaver). By opening the beak, the potential space within the infraorbital sinus can be increased, thereby increasing exposure and working room. **(b)** A cotton-tipped applicator is used to remove mucoid discharge. Microsurgical and miniaturized instruments, such as loop ear curettes, can all be used to help retrieve infectious and foreign material from the sinus.

17.20 Trephination is sometimes required, especially when sinus masses are hidden behind bony structures. **(a)** A trephine is drilled into the frontal sinus of a Blue and Gold Macaw with caseous sinusitis. **(b)** After trephination, caseous debris is scooped out with an ear curette.

Magnification with light is often required to adequately inspect the infraorbital sinus. Common tools such as cotton-tipped applicators can be used to retrieve debris (Figure 17.19b), but microsurgical and miniaturized instruments are also beneficial when retrieving debris from deep recesses within the sinus. The normal sinus space should be clear with no visible debris or discharge. Any discharge, foreign bodies or debris are removed. Submit collected tissue for cytology, culture and sensitivity testing, other infectious disease testing and/or histopathological evaluation if not done so previously.

The sinus space can hold a surprising amount of material and every attempt to remove all debris should be made. Invasive material may extend into the beak diverticuli and the opposite side of the head. Occasionally, multiple surgical entries are required to reach visible debris. Trephination (Figure 17.20) into the beak or skull is rarely needed for addressing sinus disease; however, it may be considered if necessary. Referral to an experienced avian surgeon should be considered for trephination (Speer, 2012).

Once the bulk of the fluid, debris and abnormal tissue is removed, the surgical site can be left open to drain (if infectious disease is suspected) or closed, if the sinus was clean (e.g. with an excised encapsulated mass). Postoperative care may include flushing the open wound once or twice daily with an appropriate antiseptic solution (such as dilute chlorhexidine) until

the wound closes. Use caution with any flush solution that is highly tissue reactive, such as hydrogen peroxide, as this may cause more inflammation and inflammatory fluid and debris accumulation. Also, aggressive flushing may result in excess fluid entering the respiratory system and subsequent patient respiratory distress and, rarely, death. Open sinusotomy wounds generally heal rapidly and make flushing difficult within 3–5 days. If appropriate, sinusotomy closure is standard and any sutures placed can generally be removed in 10–14 days. Systemic antibiotics and analgesics are given as needed.

> **Procedure difficulty level: 1–2**

The beak

The craniofacial and beak anatomy is highly complex and variable between bird species (see Chapter 2). Injuries to the beak can involve multiple muscles and bones of the craniofacial apparatus in addition to the obvious injuries to the upper or lower mandibles (Figure 17.21). Overgrown, twisted or otherwise misaligned beaks may be associated with underlying disease and often require thorough patient evaluation in addition to precise beak trimming (Figure 17.22). Improperly performed beak trims can result in further damage to the beak–craniofacial apparatus and negative behavioural consequences for the patient. Due to the complexities of beak anatomy and function, the reader is encouraged to review the literature or refer to a veterinary surgeon experienced with beak injuries, especially

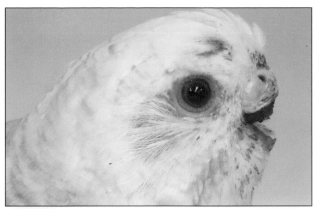

17.21 The upper mandible was bitten off this Budgerigar by a larger parrot. Such severe beak injuries require supportive care until the bird can learn to eat on its own.

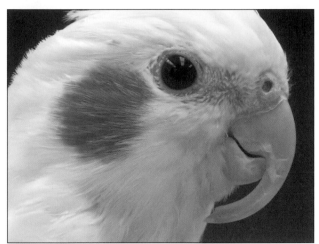

17.22 The upper mandible of this Cockatiel is severely overgrown and related to an underlying liver disease. Simply trimming the beak without treating the underlying disease will not address the cause of the beak abnormality.

serious injuries, such as avulsions, fractures, dislocations and significant crush damage.

However, minor injuries that include simple chips and cuts in the rhinotheca (covering of the upper mandible) or gnathotheca (covering the of lower mandible) can be easily protected to allow for adequate healing (Figure 17.23). The wound is cleaned and any depressed segments of keratin are gently replaced without disrupting the blood supply. Use sterile saline or dilute chlorhexidine to gently flush the wound. For more chronic wounds, debride necrotic tissue and consider antibiotics. Once the keratin and/or dermal sections are replaced in as normal an anatomical position as possible, apply common ethyl-2-cyanoacrylate ('super glue') on and around the fractured tissue. Immediately following, sprinkle sodium bicarbonate (baking soda) on the glue. This results in a near instantaneous hard resin (Redig, 2006). Roughen the beak keratin with a grinding tool as needed to improve adherence of the super glue–baking soda compound. Apply more glue and baking soda layers as needed to create a stable and protective cap over the wound. If needed, the cap can be shaped with a grinding tool and painted to match the surrounding beak. The protective cap can simply be allowed to fall off as the beak grows out or gradually ground down as needed.

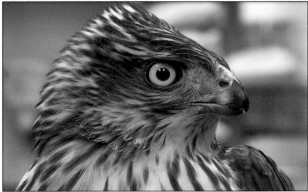

17.23 A minor injury such as this beak tip damage in a Cooper's Hawk can be patched with cyanoacrylate adhesive (super glue) and baking soda, providing temporary protection until the beak adequately heals. The bird will likely benefit from analgesia.

Procedure difficulty level: 1

The coelom

The specific surgical approach to the coelom (coeliotomy) is determined by the access needed, surgeon preference and individual bird anatomy and physical condition. Each entry point has distinct advantages and disadvantages. The approaches generally require the bird to be in dorsal or lateral recumbency. If ascites or significant organomegaly is present, elevating the proximal half of the body may help reduce pressure on the heart, lungs and more cranial air sacs, improving ventilation.

Left lateral coeliotomy

A left lateral coeliotomy provides good exposure to the proventriculus, ventriculus, spleen, colon and left male and female reproductive tracts, hepatic lobe, lung, heart apex, kidney and ureter (Dennis and Bennett, 1999). The anaesthetized patient should be placed in right lateral recumbency with the wings pulled dorsally, right leg caudally and left leg cranially (Figure 17.24ab); the left leg is pulled caudally when a more cranial approach to the lateral coelom is required. The extremities are taped in place and a longitudinal incision from cranial to caudal made in the left paralumbar fossa (Figure 17.24c). The incision may extend from the cranial extent of the pubis to the uncinate process of the last rib. The incision can be further extended cranially by incising through the last rib(s) at the costochondral junction(s) if needed. Use radiosurgery, laser, sutures or simple haemostasis to control haemorrhage.

Once through the skin, bluntly dissect through the lateral coelomic muscles, including the external oblique, internal oblique and transversus abdominis muscles. The muscles should be dissected in the direction of their fibres to reduce excessive tearing. At this point the abdominal air sac should be visible dorsally. The air sac is commonly punctured to approach more dorsal structures but should be preserved if possible. Palpebral or similar retractors are very useful to better expose the underlying structures. Individual muscles, if clearly defined, can be closed via a simple interrupted pattern. Skin may be closed via multiple patterns and the

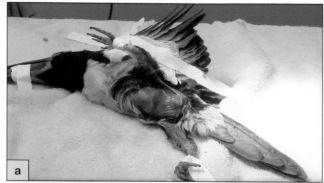

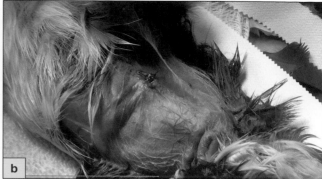

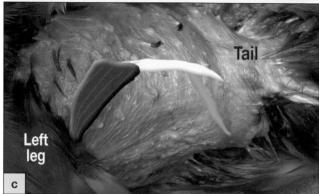

17.24 **(a)** A left lateral approach is used with this aracari. With the patient in right lateral recumbency, the wings are taped dorsally, the right leg is taped caudally and the left leg is taped cranially (for a more cranial approach to the coelom and in this case an endoscopic renal biopsy). **(b)** The closed endoscopic entry site. **(c)** With the bird in right lateral recumbency, the paralumbar fossa is bound cranially by the caudal thigh muscles (pink), dorsally by the synsacrum (white) and caudally by the pubis (green).

choice of which to use is based on surgeon preference. Monitor for subcutaneous emphysema and air leakage through the skin incision and re-suture as needed.

Right lateral coeliotomy

A right lateral coeliotomy is used to expose the duodenum and pancreas, lung, heart apex, kidney, ureter, hepatic lobe and right male or female reproductive tracts. This approach is far less commonly performed compared with a left lateral or ventral coeliotomy. The approach is otherwise reversed from a left lateral coeliotomy and closure is routine.

Ventral coeliotomy

A ventral midline, transverse or combination coeliotomy is used to expose the middle and/or both sides of the coelomic cavity, gaining access to the liver, intestines, pancreas, kidneys, ureters, cloaca and the oviduct. The testes and ovaries can also be accessed via a ventral approach but this requires manipulating surrounding tissues to improve exposure. Make an incision on the ventral midline from just caudal to the sternum extending caudally to the interpubic space. The supraduodenal loop (ileum) lies relatively ventral along the midline of the caudal coelom and can be easily transected if care is not taken. Additionally, the ileum may be adhered to the ventral body wall as is sometimes seen with coelomitis, cancer and other disorders of the coelom. As a result, the midline incision should be made as cranial as possible unless the caudal ventral coelom must be explored, as with some cloacal surgeries (Figure 17.25). After the skin incision is made, the linea alba is tented upward and carefully transected, being careful not to damage underlying organs (Figures 17.26 and 17.27). The air sacs are normally preserved using ventral approaches.

The transverse and combination ventral coeliotomy can be used to increase exposure. A transverse incision is made just caudal to the sternum. If needed,

a ventral midline incision is used in conjunction with the transverse incision ('T' incision) to increase exposure. Alternatively, a transverse incision can be made on the left or right half of the midline, combined with a ventral midline incision, creating an inverted 'L' incision. The 'T' or 'L' incision is only made if increased exposure is needed. As discussed above, underlying structures should be carefully avoided when incising through the underlying coelomic wall.

The linea alba and other transected muscles are closed in a simple interrupted pattern (Figure 17.26c). In some overweight birds, the subcutaneous tissue may need to be closed (commonly in a simple continuous pattern). Skin closure is routine (Figure 17.26d).

Procedure difficulty level: 2–3

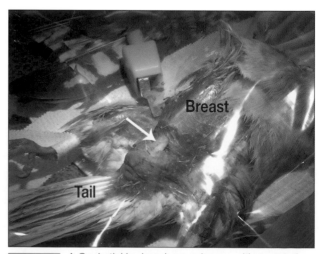

17.25 A Cockatiel in dorsal recumbency with a ventral midline incision (arrowed). Note the cranial extent of the incision just caudal to the sternum.

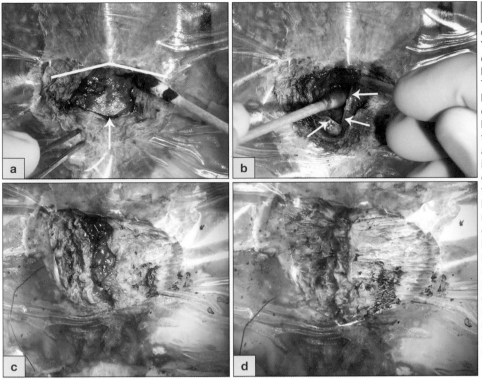

17.26 Ventral coeliotomy. **(a)** A ventral midline coelomic incision is made on a Yellow-naped Amazon. The caudal extent of the sternum is highlighted by the white lines. The skin only has been incised, leaving the underlying ventral coelomic muscles visible, and the linea alba is barely visible along the midline (as indicated by the arrow). **(b)** The linea has been incised and its margins are outlined by the arrows. Cotton-tipped applicators are used for blunt dissection. **(c)** The ventral midline coelomic incision is closed in two or three layers. The linea alba has been closed with monofilament absorbable suture material in a simple interrupted pattern. **(d)** The skin has been closed with a horizontal mattress pattern using monofilament absorbable suture material. Obese birds may require a middle subcutaneous layer closure.

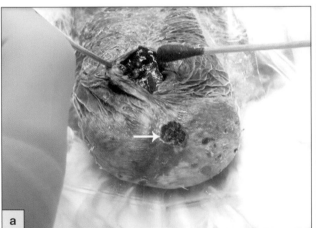

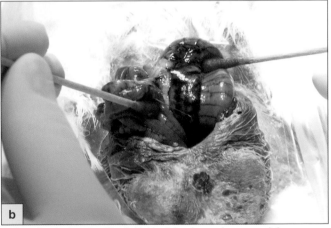

17.27 **(a)** An Umbrella Cockatoo presented with a large ventral coelomic hernia. The initial incision is made as cranial as possible. The pendulous ventral coelom has an ulcer (arrowed) from contact with the ground. **(b)** Inflamed intestines are carefully exteriorized through the incision.

The gastrointestinal tract

The gastrointestinal tract, from oral cavity to vent, may require surgical corrective procedures in pet birds. The beak, while technically the starting point of the gastrointestinal tract, is highly specialized and variable between species and was briefly discussed previously in this chapter.

Due to the potential for leakage of food or intestinal contents and dehiscence, careful attention should be paid to aseptic technique and meticulous closure. Antibiotics may be required for many gastrointestinal surgeries and should be considered on a case-by-case basis.

Crop surgery

Ingluviotomy may be indicated for identification of crop masses (such as neoplasia, food impaction and foreign bodies), to screen for proventriculuar dilatation disease (PDD), to repair damaged tissue (e.g. thermal burns) and to gain access to the thoracic oesophagus, proventriculus and ventriculus via intraluminal endoscopy.

Incise the skin over the bird's right side or the middle of the crop near the thoracic inlet (Figure 17.28a). Bluntly separate the skin and crop until the crop can be pulled partly out of the incision (Figure 17.28b). Incise the crop wall. Remove abnormal tissue, masses, impacted food or foreign bodies if present. If screening for PDD, remove a large (1–2 cm) section of crop including the visible blood vessels (Figure 17.28cd). A two-layer closure works best with crop incisions. The first layer is closed with an inverting suture pattern (Figure 17.28e). One reference notes that the skin and crop should not be closed together as a single layer as this may increase the risk of dehiscence (Bowles *et al.*, 2006); however, the author closes the skin and crop together as the second layer and has not noted problems in multiple clinical cases (Figure 17.28f).

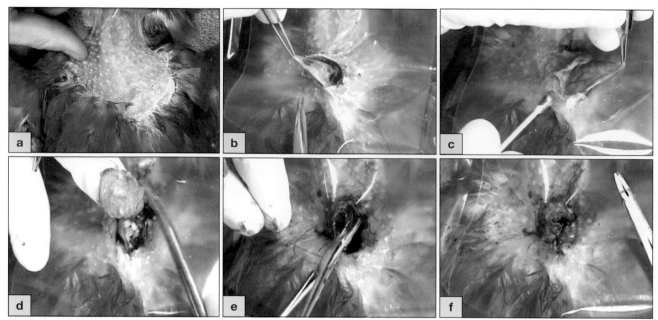

17.28 **(a)** In preparation for an ingluviotomy, the skin over the ventral caudal neck (proximal to the thoracic inlet) is prepared. **(b)** Bluntly separate the overlying skin from the crop, which is held in the forceps here. **(c)** Excise any abnormal tissue for biopsy. When screening for proventricular dilatation disease, select a highly vascular area of the crop to collect neurovascular tissue. **(d)** A large sample of crop tissue has been collected for proventricular dilatation disease screening. Note the seeds still in the now exposed crop lumen. **(e)** Upon completion of the ingluviotomy, close the crop with a continuous inverting pattern using monofilament absorbable suture material. An initial simple interrupted layer may be placed first. **(f)** The final skin closure for the ingluviotomy site can include the underlying crop wall or this may be closed separately.

Crop repair is most often indicated following trauma, especially thermal burns in hand-fed chicks. Prior to surgery, wait until the margins of the necrotic tissue are clearly visible (usually 4–7 days after the incident). Remove all necrotic tissue and close as described above. The crop has an incredible ability to stretch and even large crop resections seem to be well tolerated by most birds. Subsequent feedings will obviously need to be reduced depending on the postoperative size of the crop. Occasionally, a proventricular feeding tube may be required if crop resection is extensive and this area needs to be bypassed during the healing process (see also Chapter 15).

Procedure difficulty level: 2

Proventricular and ventricular surgery

The 'stomach' of birds consists of the proventriculus, isthmus and ventriculus (gizzard). In general, the proventriculus and isthmus are soft muscular organs and the ventriculus is composed of strong contractile muscles with a tough inner lining (koilin layer) designed to crush food, sometimes with the aid of ingested grit. The proventriculus secretes digestive enzymes that help prepare the food for mechanical digestion in the ventriculus. The isthmus is the short region between the proventriculus and the ventriculus.

Birds that eat a coarse diet, such as granivores (most parrots and passerines), have well developed paired thick and thin muscles with a thick koilin layer on the mucosal surface (Degernes *et al.*, 2012). Birds that consume a soft diet, such as planktivores, piscivores and carnivores, have a relatively thin-walled ventriculus and koilin layer (Degernes *et al.*, 2012). Variation can also be found within groups. For example,

lories feed on a diet primarily of nectar, flower buds and some insects and are quite different from other more granivorous parrots. As a result, lories have a thin-walled ventriculus. Depending on the type of bird and its diet, the ventriculus may range from poorly to well developed.

Proventriculotomy and ventriculotomy are reserved primarily for the removal of foreign bodies not eliminated via conservative therapy or non-retrievable using endoscopy or other less invasive techniques. Gastrointestinal impactions related to foreign bodies are reported in multiple species including ratites, kiwis, Umbrella Cockatoos, Micronesian kingfishers, Sarus cranes and bustards (Honnas *et al.*, 1991; Honnas *et al.*, 1993; Speer, 1998; Bailey *et al.*, 2001; Kinsel *et al.*, 2004). The author has also noted gastrointestinal foreign bodies in numerous species of passerines, parrots and raptors (Figure 17.29). Gastrointestinal foreign bodies should be considered possible in all bird species, as evidenced in the literature and anecdotally.

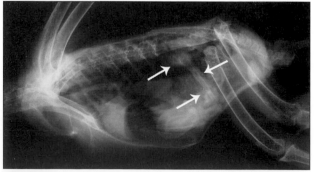

17.29 Penetrating ventricular foreign bodies, such as this bone outlined by arrows in a Harris' Hawk, represent an emergency. Rare circumstances such as the one presented here require aggressive medical therapy and exploratory coeliotomy.

The same approaches to the proventriculus and ventriculus are also used to obtain biopsy samples (e.g. for neoplasia and PDD diagnosis), to address perforating ulcers and diverticula and to explore the serosal surface of the proventriculus, isthmus and ventriculus (Figures 17.30). Note: the crop is a preferential site for PDD screening as there is significantly less danger from perforation compared with a proventricular or ventricular biopsy. Prior to surgery, conservative therapy using bulking agents, fluid therapy and basic support should be attempted.

The ventriculus consists of two opposing muscle pairs: the cranial and caudal thin muscles and the lateral and medial thick muscles (Hall and Duke, 2000). The alternating contractions of the thin muscles, duodenum, thick muscles and proventriculus make up the gastroduodenal motility sequence in poultry (Degernes et al., 2012).

The myenteric nerves cover the entire surface of the thin ventricular muscles and isthmus. These nerves should ideally remain intact to preserve gastroduodenal motility (Chaplin and Duke, 1990; Hall and Duke, 2000). A traumatic and precise surgery is needed when incising and handling the isthmus.

For adult birds undergoing proventriculotomy or ventriculotomy, fast the patient for at least 12 hours to help 'clean' the gastrointestinal tract. Juvenile birds should be fasted for shorter periods of time (1–4 hours), depending on the animal's age, size and health status. If possible, use hand-feeding formula 1–2 days prior to surgery as these easily digestible foods tend to leave little residue in the ventriculus. Discontinue feeding formula food 6–12 hours prior to surgery. Pre- and postoperative antibiotics (such as parenteral ceftazidime or piperacillin) and analgesics (parenteral butorphanol and/or tramadol) should be considered as with other animals undergoing enterotomies.

A left lateral or ventral midline combined with transverse coeliotomy may be used to approach the ventriculus (Figure 17.31a–c). If the ventriculus is displaced medially (as supported by contrast study radiographs), the ventral midline approach is more appropriate. Some surgeons prefer a ventral midline approach to enter the ventriculus through the caudoventral sac (see below). However, the proventriculus and isthmus are approached via a left lateral coeliotomy.

With either approach, place stay sutures in the white tendinous portion of the ventriculus to help retract the organ(s) out of the coelomic cavity and improve exposure (Bennett, 1994). Due to its location, the proventriculus cannot be exteriorized, but visualization is improved by retracting the ventriculus (Figure 17.31d). Pack moist sponges around the retracted organs to help prevent coelomic contamination. Via a left lateral coeliotomy, incise into the relatively avascular isthmus and extend the incision orad into the proventriculus or aborad to the ventriculus as needed (Figure 17.31e).

Both the proventriculus and ventriculus can be explored (Figure 17.32a). Due to the massive mobile muscular tunic and high tensile strain on the tendinous centres, the body of the ventriculus does not have a good site for incisional entry (Ferrell et al., 2003). Additionally, an endoscope may be introduced to improve visualization and help retrieve foreign bodies. The caudal thoracic (cranial coelomic) oesophagus can be partially evaluated via this approach (Figure 17.32b). Irrigation and suction are often needed – be careful not to contaminate the coelomic cavity or flood the respiratory system. The author commonly instils gastroprotective agents, such as sucralfate, into the incision prior to closure (Figure 17.33a). This intra-surgical application ensures direct protectant application on the surgically damaged mucosal tissue. Use fine monofilament absorbable suture material in a simple continuous pattern to close the wound. If possible, oversew with a continuous inverting pattern. Use meticulous closure to help prevent dehiscence (Figure 17.33b). Reappose any transected ribs. Close the muscle and skin in standard fashion (Figure 17.33c–e).

Through the ventral midline coeliotomy, the ventriculus may also be approached via the caudoventral sac (Bennett, 1994). The ventriculus has two blind sacs (craniodorsal and caudoventral) covered with relatively thin muscles. Slightly rotate the ventriculus clockwise to help expose the caudoventral sac. Incise through the muscle fibres to enter the ventricular lumen. Again, use meticulous closure. This tissue does not invert, so use interrupted sutures placed close together. In studied Japanese quail undergoing caudoventral sac ventriculotomy, ventricular mucosal healing was not complete until 21 days post-surgery (Ferrell et al., 2003).

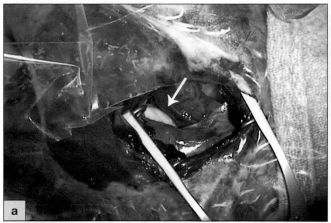
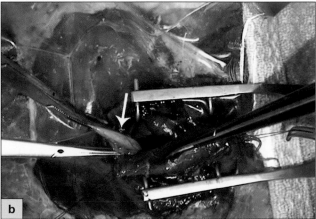

17.30 When performing a proventriculotomy to ventriculotomy, look for other abnormalities that may be present, such as masses and diverticula. **(a)** During removal of a ventricular foreign body, a large cystic mass (arrowed) was found on the dorsal surface of the proventriculus of a Yellow-naped Amazon. The cyst was aspirated to remove its fluid contents and collect samples for culture and sensitivity testing. **(b)** The cyst was exteriorized, ultimately removed and submitted for histopathological analysis.

While collagen and endogenous fat patches have been suggested in mammals to help intestinal wounds heal, they may be detrimental to birds. Compared with non-grafted controls, porcine submucosal collagen and endogenous coelomic fat patches placed over the serosal surface of the ventricular suture line in Japanese quail that underwent ventriculotomies, resulted in a statistically significant increase in gross or microscopic perforations and serosal inflammation, respectively (Ferrell *et al.*, 2003; Simova-Curd *et al.*, 2013).

> **Procedure difficulty level: 3**

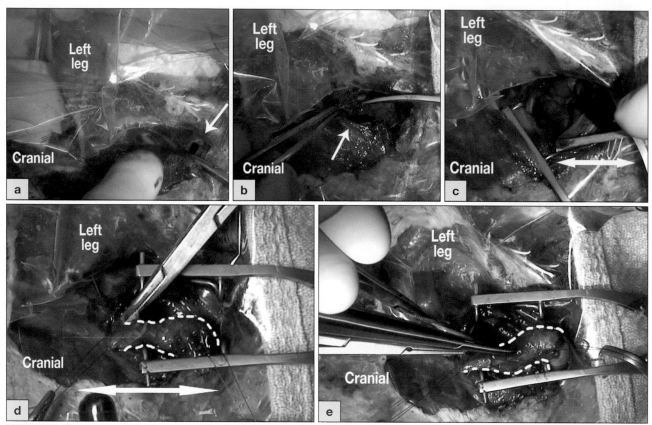

17.31 The approach to the proventriculus, isthmus and ventriculus demonstrated on a Yellow-naped Amazon. **(a)** The left leg is pulled cranially and is abducted from the body. The inguinal skin has been incised and forceps have been used to puncture through the lateral coelomic muscles (arrowed) just caudal to the ribs. **(b)** The last two ribs have been cut (arrowed) to increase exposure. **(c)** Thumb screw retractors (double-headed arrow) are used to expand the surgical entry into the left lateral coelom. **(d)** The proventriculus (cranial dashed lines) and ventriculus (caudal dashed lines) are exteriorized with the aid of stay sutures (double-headed arrow). Ideally, two stay sutures should be placed in the tendinous portion of the ventriculus. If placing sutures in the proventriculus, as shown here, minimal tension should be applied. Most, if not all, of the tension should be on the ventricular stay sutures. Due to an unusual proventricular cyst in this parrot, a single stay suture was placed in the proventriculus to better examine the cyst. **(e)** Using precise technique, incise into the isthmus (narrowed junction between the proventriculus and ventriculus, both outlined by dashed lines), being careful to cause as little damage as possible.

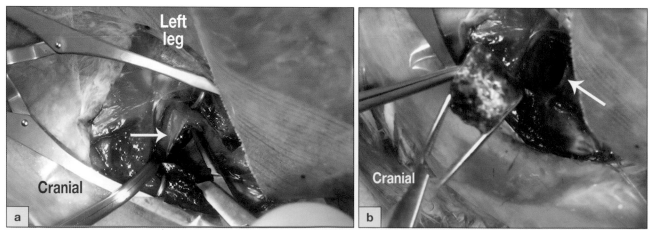

17.32 **(a)** Carefully probe orad (into the proventriculus) and aborad (into the ventriculus) for foreign material. Microfine mosquito haemostats are used to probe the proventricular lumen through the isthmus incision in this Red-fronted Macaw. **(b)** This bird had a large foreign body (shown within the jaws of a microfine mosquito haemostats) obstructing the distal oesophagus. The arrow points to the large isthmus incision.

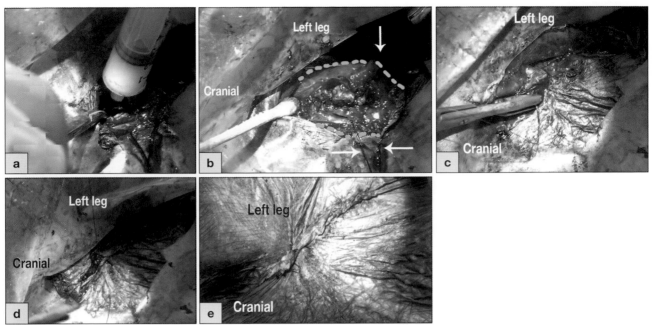

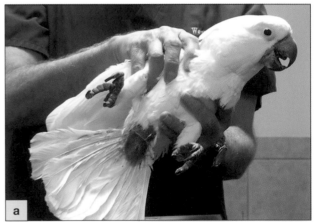

17.33 **(a)** Sucralfate is instilled into the proventricular–ventricular lumen via the isthmus incision after successful removal of a metal screw in this hornbill. By directly instilling the sucralfate, delivery to the affected area is ensured (incised proventricular, isthmus and/or ventricular mucosal surface). Sucralfate reacts with hydrochloric acid in the 'stomach' to form a cross-linking, viscous material capable of acting as an acid buffer and ultimately protecting ulcers or, in this case, a surgical incision. **(b)** The isthmus incision is closed in a simple interrupted appositional pattern using fine monofilament absorbable suture material. The orad proventriculus, isthmus and aborad ventriculus are outlined by a green dotted line with the closed incision roughly in the centre. Due to the relatively large size of this bird, a continuous inverting suture pattern was sewn over the isthmus incision. Ventricular stay sutures are denoted by the arrows. **(c)** The left lateral body wall is closed, taking care to re-appose ribs (if needed). The underlying muscle layer is closed such that no air leaks during positive pressure ventilation. **(d)** The overlying skin can be closed separately or by incorporating the underlying muscle and subcutaneous (if identifiable) layer(s) as needed to prevent a potential space. **(e)** The finished closure.

Ventplasty

Ventplasty is reserved for chronic cloacal prolapse (Figure 17.34). In the author's experience, chronic cloacal prolapses are most commonly associated with prolonged egg laying and, especially in male cockatoos, masturbation behaviours (Figure 17.35). However, other causes of cloacal prolapse are possible and should be determined and resolved prior to considering surgery. If the prolapse is chronic, the cloacal muscles and supporting structures may be permanently stretched and non-functional. The goal of ventplasty is to reduce the vent size such that cloacal prolapse does not recur. It should be understood that ventplasty will likely fail if the underlying causes of the prolapse are not resolved and the bird continues to strain postoperatively.

The extent of the dilated vent will determine how much tissue to resect. For mild to moderate dilatation, usually one section of the vent is resected. For more

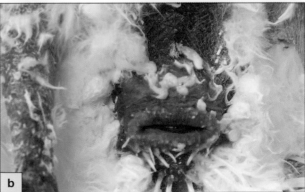

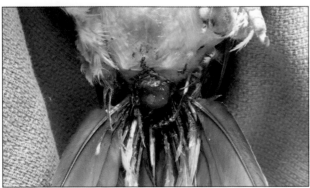

17.34 Ventplasty is not recommended for acute cloacal prolapses, as seen with this Black-capped Caique.

17.35 **(a)** A male Umbrella Cockatoo with a chronic (>10 years) cloacal prolapse. **(b)** A male Umbrella Cockatoo's significantly dilated vent associated with chronic cloacal prolapse (the prolapsed tissue was easily replaced prior to photographing this patient).

severe dilatation, two areas of vent resection may be required. The basic incision is the same; however, the choice of one *versus* two resections is based on surgeon determination in relation to the animal's needs. Consider pre- and postoperative antibiotics based on culture and sensitivity results of a cloacal swab or cloacal tissue culture.

Prior to performing surgery, estimate how much tissue needs to be resected in order to make a normal vent diameter (Figure 17.36a). Triangular incisions work best with the 'base' of the triangle on the leading edge of the vent and the 'point' away from the vent. A single incision works best over the cranial ventral side of the vent, while two opposing incisions can be performed at the right and left lateral sides.

After determining the resection site(s), excise the desired triangular area(s), taking epidermis and dermis. Save excised tissue for biopsy and culture and sensitivity testing if needed. Spare the sphincter and transverse cloacal muscles if visible. The dermis can usually be bluntly resected from the underlying muscular and submucosal tissue layers. When apposed, the new epidermal edges should form the desired vent diameter. Remove more epidermal/dermal tissue as needed.

With the 'new' vent margins, close the surgery site. First close the submucosa (Figure 17.36b). Place simple interrupted absorbable sutures medial (which represents the new vent wall) to lateral for all tissue layers. Next, close the dermis in the same fashion (Figure 17.36c). Finally, close the overlying epidermis. The distal cloacal mucosa should extend distally to the vent epithelial margins. If not, simply suture the mucosa in place as needed. The end result should be one suture line extending cranially (single vent resection) or one suture line extending laterally on the left and right sides of the vent (double vent resection). The new vent diameter should be just large enough to easily allow passage of droppings. Use lubricated cotton-tipped applicators to test the patency of the vent. Sutures are absorbable but can be removed in 2 weeks if needed.

If the patient is female, egg laying must be controlled either via a salpingohysterectomy, behaviourally or chemically, otherwise dystocia or rupture of the ventplasty sutures may result.

Procedure difficulty level: 2

The liver

At this time, liver surgery is generally limited to partial hepatectomy to remove solitary masses, and liver biopsy. Numerous non-invasive diagnostics, such as serum biochemistry, radiography, ultrasonography, high detail CT and MRI, are described elsewhere to help determine if liver surgery is necessary.

Liver biopsy is a fairly common procedure and is useful in determining hepatic pathology. Liver biopsy is obviously indicated when hepatic disease is suspected and is also used to evaluate environmental toxins and in determining response to therapy. A thrombocyte estimate and capillary clot time (normal is less than 5 minutes) can be performed prior to surgery (Jaensch, 2000). With that stated, avian platelets can only be estimated as they tend to clump in birds. If a coagulopathy is suspected, give vitamin K_1 (0.2–2.5 mg/kg i.m.) 24–48 hours preoperatively (Zebisch *et al.*, 2004). If ascites is present, as much fluid as possible should be drained via coelomocentesis prior to surgery.

Minimally invasive endoscopic, ultrasound-guided and blind percutaneous biopsies can be considered (Taylor, 1994; Jaensch, 2000; Nordberg *et al.*, 2000). However, ultrasound-guided liver biopsy may result in inadequate biopsy samples and unnecessary risk to the patient (Zebisch *et al.*, 2004). The author cautions against relying on endoscopic liver biopsy as the samples harvested often represent capsular, and not parenchymal, tissue. The end result is that endoscopically obtained liver biopsy specimens contain smaller samples, compared with the larger wedge specimens, and are at greater risk of being non-diagnostic.

A cranial ventral midline coelomic (just caudal to the sternum) approach works well for most hepatic surgeries (Figure 17.37). With hepatomegaly, the liver is readily visible and the right lobe is usually larger. With microhepatica, the liver is tucked under the sternum. Use cup-end biopsy forceps or curved haemostats to collect as large a piece of liver as possible without undue risk of haemorrhage. As an example, 0.5 g and 1.2 g (6% and 18% hepatectomies, respectively) liver biopsy samples were safely collected from a total of 16 Galahs in one study (Jaensch *et al.*, 2000). In general, the author attempts to collect a liver sample measuring at least 5 x 3 mm in birds weighing less than 100 g. Much larger samples can be collected in bigger birds, determined by the liver size and surgeon experience.

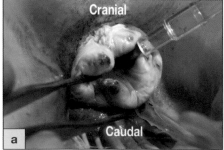
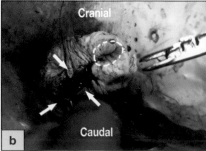
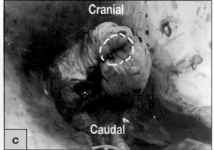

17.36   **(a)** A grossly dilated and disfigured vent in an Umbrella Cockatoo due to chronic cloacal prolapse and multiple local surgeries. The goal of ventplasty is to reduce the vent opening to a normal size and thereby prevent further prolapse of cloacal or other tissue. This particular bird required intensive behaviour modification and lifestyle changes prior to surgery. **(b)** Ventplasty in a male Umbrella Cockatoo. A triangular wedge has been resected from the left and right sides of the vent. The bird's left side ventplasty has already been performed, leaving the right to finish. The 'new' vent diameter is outlined with dashed lines. The submucosal layer has been closed (area outlined by arrows) with monofilament absorbable suture material. **(c)** The ventplasty procedure is continued and the dermis has been sutured closed. At this point only the overlying skin needs to be closed and the vent diameter (dashed lines) should be normal for the species and easily allow for waste material to pass.

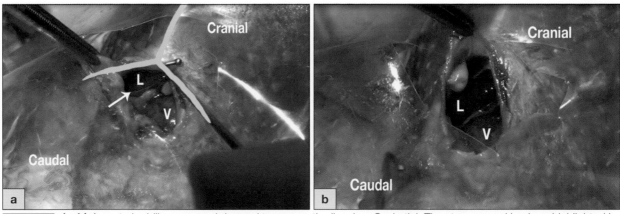

17.37 **(a–b)** A ventral midline approach is used to access the liver in a Cockatiel. The sternum and keel are highlighted in green. Note the cranial extent of the ventral midline incision. The right liver lobe (L) is located behind a coelomic membrane (arrowed) and lateral to the ventriculus (V). The liver is enlarged with a rounded edge.

Typically, the edge of the liver is biopsied using either instrument, while the cup-end forceps are more appropriate for selecting specific lesions and with microhepatica. When biopsying the edge of the liver, bleeding is often minimal and sutures are rarely required (Figure 17.38). If haemorrhage is persistent, use haemostats to clamp the bleeding area until haemostasis is established. Absorbable haemostatic agents may also be placed along the cut edge of the liver to further reduce bleeding. If possible, collect extra tissue for culture and electron microscopy. Close the muscle and skin layers as with other coelomic surgeries.

Although complications such as uncontrolled haemorrhage, perforation of intestines and other underlying organs, and introduction of ascitic fluid into the air sacs are reported, these problems are fairly uncommon with the coelomic approach discussed above (Jaensch, 2000). If ascites is present, perform coelomocentesis prior to surgery and/or collect fluid (often using a butterfly catheter) intraoperatively. Selected laboratory values will likely change following a liver biopsy. In pigeons and quails undergoing ultrasound-guided Tru-cut liver biopsies, aspartate aminotransferase (AST), creatinine kinase (CK), lactate dehydrogenase

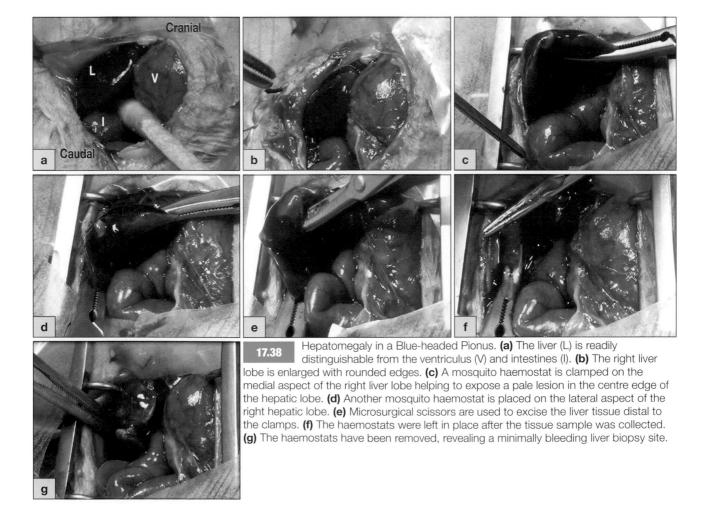

17.38 Hepatomegaly in a Blue-headed Pionus. **(a)** The liver (L) is readily distinguishable from the ventriculus (V) and intestines (I). **(b)** The right liver lobe is enlarged with rounded edges. **(c)** A mosquito haemostat is clamped on the medial aspect of the right liver lobe helping to expose a pale lesion in the centre edge of the hepatic lobe. **(d)** Another mosquito haemostat is placed on the lateral aspect of the right hepatic lobe. **(e)** Microsurgical scissors are used to excise the liver tissue distal to the clamps. **(f)** The haemostats were left in place after the tissue sample was collected. **(g)** The haemostats have been removed, revealing a minimally bleeding liver biopsy site.

(LDH), alkaline phosphatase (ALP), total protein (TP) and albumin were measured before and 1 week after surgery. In pigeons, AST and albumin both significantly increased post-surgically, while only AST increased in the quails (Zebisch *et al.*, 2004). In a study of mixed wild raptors, 'liver and kidney values' increased within 5 days of liver biopsy (Lierz *et al.*, 1998). With the exception of mildly elevated alanine aminotransferase (ALT) immediately following biopsy (18% liver weight), Galahs that underwent 6% and 18% hepatectomies had normal serum bile acids and elevated AST, CK and ALP values that were statistically no different from sham-operated birds immediately following and 4 and 7 days post-surgery. This last report suggests that these 'liver enzymes' were elevated as a result of coeliotomy and not liver trauma.

With a little experience, surgical liver biopsies can be easily and safely performed in birds.

> **Procedure difficulty level: 2**

The pancreas

The avian pancreas seems to tolerate surgery well. Based on the author's experience and published studies, pancreatic biopsies and partial debulking are well tolerated in birds.

Pancreatic biopsy

Pancreatic biopsy is indicated when pancreatic disease, such as pancreatitis and neoplasia, is suspected and accurate diagnosis is needed for individual case management. A cranial ventral midline approach is used. The dorsal and ventral pancreatic lobes rest between the ascending and descending duodenal loop (Figure 17.39). The duodenum is located to the right of the midline and is often covered by a thin coelomic

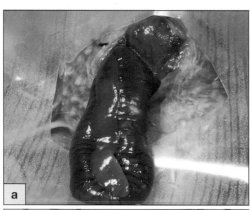

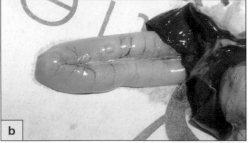

17.39 **(a)** The ventral (pictured) and dorsal pancreatic lobes rest in between the ascending and descending duodenal loop, as in this Blue-headed Pionus. **(b)** An atrophied pancreas is noted in this Monk Parakeet at post-mortem examination. Notice the lack of recognizable tissue in between the duodenal loop.

membrane. Incise through the thin membrane and gently retract the duodenal loop. After examining the pancreas and duodenum for gross abnormalities, select the distal (free) end of the dorsal pancreatic lobe (unless another site is clearly abnormal). Using haemostats, clamp the pancreas just distal to its distal-most vessel coming off the duodenum. Remove the distal pancreatic fragment and submit for histopathological evaluation (Figure 17.40). Commonly, a 3–8 mm section of pancreas is harvested. Remove the haemostats. Reapply if bleeding occurs. Sutures to control haemostasis are rarely indicated. Coelomic closure is routine.

> **Procedure difficulty level: 2**

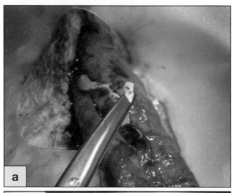

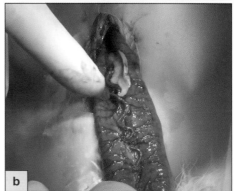

17.40 **(a)** A small section of the distal aspect of the ventral pancreatic lobe is simply cut off in a curassow. **(b)** No haemostasis was required here; however, sutures, haemostatic agents or just direct pressure can all be used as needed to control bleeding.

The urinary tract

Renal surgery

Due to the dorsal coelomic location within the renal fossae, complex vascular anatomy and close association with the lumbar and sacral plexuses, kidney surgery is often limited to focal procedures, such as biopsy and superficial mass removal.

Most cases of avian renal disease can be managed conservatively. However, the only means to definitively diagnose avian renal disease and specific pathological patterns is with a kidney biopsy and histopathological evaluation. A renal biopsy is most frequently performed during endoscopic examination of the coelomic cavity and, specifically, kidneys (Figure 17.41). However, a renal biopsy can be performed using 5-French cup biopsy forceps during exploratory coeliotomy.

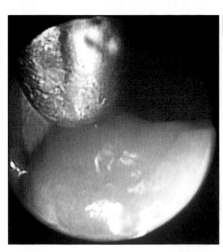

17.41

A kidney biopsy (endoscopic view) is the only means to accurately characterize renal pathology.

Using a left lateral paralumbar fossa (most common with endoscopy) or ventral midline approach (coeliotomy), the kidney is identified dorsal to the abdominal air sac. A right lateral approach may be used if disease is suspected to be limited to that side. The kidney is visualized and examined as much as possible. A small incision is made through the abdominal air sac and any other overlying membranes to expose the serosal surface of the kidney. Generally, one to three 5-French cup biopsy samples are collected from the cranial renal division in an effort to avoid the large vessels coursing through and around the kidneys. The middle renal division may also be biopsied. Once the tissue is collected, the site is monitored for excessive bleeding. Direct pressure using a cotton-tipped applicator or haemostatic agent may be used if needed. Kidney biopsy samples are immediately placed in formalin and body wall closure is standard.

In a study of 89 free-living birds of prey, 126 endoscopic renal biopsy samples (two biopsy samples from 37 birds) using 1.8 mm biopsy cup forceps were taken (Müller *et al.*, 2004). Post-biopsy haemorrhage averaged 67 seconds (10–172 seconds). The average biopsy sample taken was 2.2 mm long, 1.3 mm wide and 1 mm deep. All samples contained proximal and distal tubuli and 1–89 glomeruli, with most having 25–29 glomeruli per histological slide. Of 126 samples, 113 could be evaluated well or very well; 66 samples revealed lesions including subcapsular bleeding (19/66), inflammation (16/66), cell casts (12/66), periodic acid–Schiff positive reactions (8/66) and protein casts (6/66). Correlation between endoscopically visible change and histological disease was 76.1% (96/126). The cranial division was considered the best site to collect biopsy samples. The authors noted it was possible to obtain specimens from the middle and caudal renal divisions in larger birds (Müller *et al.*, 2004).

Many different diseases cause similar kidney changes. As such, renal histological lesions are rarely pathognomonic for a specific disease process. The author encourages veterinary surgeons to work with a pathologist familiar with avian histology. Often, it is the pathologist's interpretation of a renal biopsy specimen combined with the attending veterinary surgeon's case familiarity that enables both parties to make a definitive diagnosis or build a reasonable differential diagnoses list compatible with the kidney lesions identified.

Procedure difficulty level: 2–3

The female reproductive tract

Reproductive tract disease is very common in captive female birds. Often, domesticated birds have been selectively bred over decades and have a high reproductive drive. This translates into prolonged egg-laying seasons and complications resulting from this physically and energetically demanding process. The physiological changes associated with egg laying (such as weight gain and medullary hyperostosis) can result in unwanted consequences (e.g. fatty liver disease, fractures) when the process becomes more continuous with shortened rest periods.

Emergency surgery of the avian reproductive tract is rarely indicated. Pre-surgical preparation is recommended for all stable birds with reproductive tract diseases to improve the chance of a positive surgical outcome. Basic husbandry such as diet and behaviour modification should be improved prior to surgery. Pre-surgical conditioning may require several weeks to months and depends on the problem(s) and health status of the bird.

The drive to produce eggs is very strong in some pet birds. Behavioural management, gonadotropin-releasing hormone (GnRH) agonists and other means may be used to help reduce it. The reader is encouraged to review these options, discussed in this manual and elsewhere (see Chapter 4).

Environmental, dietary and behavioural modifications are often needed for long-term successful management of reproductive tract diseases in hens, before and after surgery. Occasionally, short- and long-term GnRH agonist use is required, especially if the owners are non-compliant with other recommended modifications or if used as a form of chemotherapy for some types of reproductive tract neoplasia. Even if the oviduct and most of the ovary are surgically removed, the reproductive drive remains high in some captive birds. Continued stimulation can result in internal ovulation and other problems. These issues should be discussed with owners prior to considering surgery.

Diseases of the oviduct

Oviductal disorders may be incidental findings or clinically relevant and are surgically addressed as needed. Birds with oviductal disease may present with non-specific clinical signs. The most commonly recognized abnormalities with oviductal disease are related to a space-occupying coelomic mass, including compression of surrounding organs, coelomic distension, coelomitis and ascites. Abnormal oviductal tissue is removed at the time of exploratory surgery.

Cystic, neoplastic, hyperplastic, torn, torsed, infected and prolapsed oviductal tissue (Figure 17.42) commonly requires removal (salpingohysterectomy) (Figure 17.43). Viable prolapsed oviductal tissue should be manually replaced in an attempt to spare the reproductive tract. However, if the prolapsed tissue is devitalized or significantly infected, salpingohysterectomy is often the recommended procedure. Persistent right oviducts are often removed if cystic or large. Free eggs in the coelom and inflammatory debris (egg yolk coelomitis) are removed during surgery. Free cysts and any other abnormal tissue should be carefully removed and/or biopsied. If septic coelomitis or salpingitis are suspected, collect samples for culture and sensitivity testing.

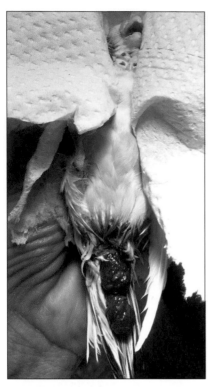

17.42

A Budgerigar with a prolapsed oviduct. This represents a true reproductive tract emergency.

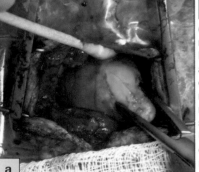

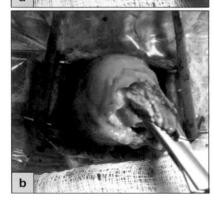

17.43

(a–b) A Yellow-naped Amazon Parrot with salpingitis and an impacted oviduct having a necrotic egg removed via salpingotomy. Ultimately the entire oviduct was removed.

causes and is commonly associated with functional (malformed eggs, cloacal masses and obesity), metabolic (calcium imbalance and nutritional deficiencies), environmental (temperature changes, lack of exercise and other stressors) and hereditary diseases.

Most cases of egg binding and dystocia are managed medically and are discussed elsewhere (see Chapter 25). Surgical intervention (primarily exploratory coeliotomy) is rarely required (Figure 17.44).

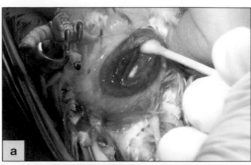

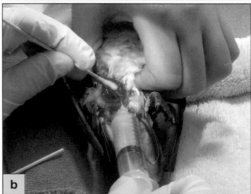

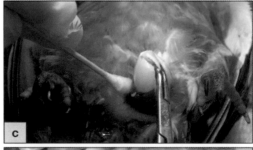

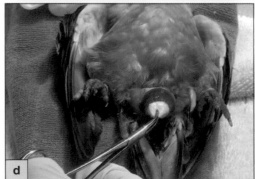

17.44   Dystocia in a Sun Conure. This conure presented depressed and anorexic for 2 days with a swollen ventral coelom and a palpable egg. **(a)** The white colour of the egg is visible through the vent, supporting the hypothesis that it is located in the distal oviduct. **(b)** The egg is aspirated by directing the needle through the shell without penetrating any other tissue. **(c)** The egg is then manually collapsed by using two fingers on the outside body wall and pressing on the now empty egg. The cloaca is swabbed with sterile lubricant jelly and the shell is grasped with haemostats. **(d)** The collapsed egg shell is carefully removed.

Egg binding and dystocia

Egg binding and dystocia are commonly described problems in pet bird medicine. Oviposition is the expulsion of the egg from the oviduct and is conducted by vigorous contraction of the oviductal muscles and peristalsis of the vagina. Egg binding is simply defined as prolonged oviposition (the egg is arrested in the oviduct longer than normal for the given species), while dystocia implies the developing egg is within the distal oviduct either obstructing the cloaca or prolapsed through the oviduct–cloacal opening. Dystocia is often more advanced than egg binding alone, has many potential

Salpingohysterectomy

Salpingohysterectomy is the surgical removal of the oviduct and infundibulum to the uterus, and is indicated for chronic egg laying and any oviductal disease that cannot be medically managed. Every attempt should be made to understand the bird's overall health status prior to surgery, and the patient should ideally be stable. While rare compared with sterile inflammation, birds with septic yolk coelomitis generally carry a poor prognosis. Underlying health problems such as various lung, liver and kidney diseases can also complicate surgery; however, healthy salpingohysterectomy candidates typically do well with the procedure.

Oviductal hypertrophy occurs secondary to elevated oestrogen levels during sexual activity and can take up most of the left side of the intestinal–peritoneal portion of the coelomic cavity. This oviductal hypertrophy includes increased vascularity and so there is an increased risk of bleeding during surgery (Orosz, 1997) (Figure 17.45a). If the patient is stable, time permits and increased reproductive tract vascularity is suspected, the author prepares the bird prior to surgery as described previously in this chapter. The goals are to improve the overall physical health of the bird and decrease reproductive tract vascularity.

In the author's experience, a left lateral approach offers the most direct access to the left female avian reproductive tract. However, a ventral midline approach is better for exploratory coeliotomy, especially when normal anatomy is significantly distorted and the degree of coelomic disease is unknown.

Perform a left lateral coeliotomy (Figure 17.45b–d). After incising through the left abdominal air sac, the ovary and oviduct are readily visible (Figure 17.45e). Gently retract the cranial oviduct (infundibulum area) via the incision and haemoclip or cauterize suspensory ligament vessels as needed (Figure 17.46). The closer the bird is to laying, the larger the vessels present will be. Depending on the size, the cranial, middle and/or

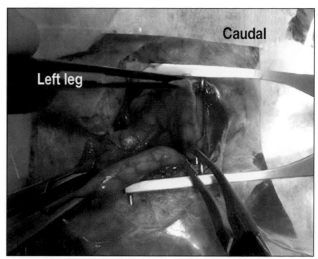

17.46 A left lateral coeliotomy in an Eclectus Parrot with the left leg pulled cranially. As more of the oviduct is exteriorized, large vessels should be occluded with haemoclips as needed to limit haemorrhage.

caudal oviductal artery may need to be haemoclipped or cauterized. Once visualized, haemoclip the base of the oviduct just proximal to its junction with the cloaca. Be certain to not incorporate the distal ureter in the haemoclip. Excise the oviduct.

When performing a ventral midline coeliotomy, the air sacs do not need to be breached (Figure 17.47). A careful evaluation of the caudal coelom is made and the right oviductal tissue, in addition to the more normal left, is identified and removed as described above. When present, right oviductal tissue is often cystic. With a little more difficulty, right oviductal tissue can also be accessed from a left lateral approach.

Well developed pre-ovulatory follicles (F1 and F2 ± F3 and F4) may pose a risk for intracoelomic ovulation and can usually be easily removed (Figure 17.48). Use cotton-tipped applicators to rotate the follicle in one

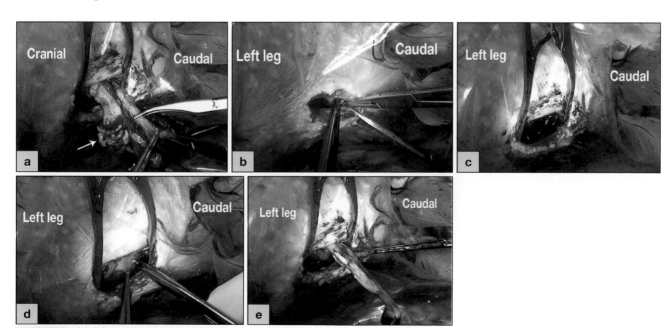

17.45 A left lateral coeliotomy in a hybrid macaw. **(a)** This hen was reproductively active at the time of surgery, as supported by the presence of a highly vascular oviduct (arrowed) exteriorized through the incision. **(b)** The initial incision is made in the paralumbar fossa. **(c)** The underlying lateral coelomic muscles are cut in the direction of the fibres. **(d)** Thumb screw retractors are used to improve access to the left oviduct. **(e)** The abdominal air sac is often incised to directly visualize the oviduct and ovary. The air sac is variable between species and does not always need to be transected. The proximal portion of the oviduct (infundibulum) is retracted out of the incision if possible.

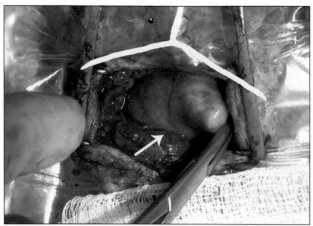

17.47 A ventral midline coeliotomy is used to approach an impacted oviduct (arrowed) in this Yellow-naped Amazon. The margins of the keel and sternum are outlined in white.

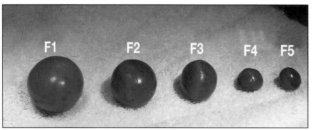

17.48 F1–F5 follicles removed from a domestic duck. The F1 follicle is fully developed and ready to be released by the ovary and caught by the oviductal infundibulum. Leaving such large follicles after salpingohysterectomy increases the risk of egg yolk coelomitis.

direction continuously until it separates from its pedicle (Figure 17.49). This may require 20–40 full rotations until the follicle is free. Once free, simply remove the follicle. If concerned about a well developed vascular pedicle, use haemoclips and then excise the follicle.

Cystic follicles should either be aspirated (drained) or, ideally, be removed. If a follicle is accidentally incised, yolk will leak into the coelom. Excess yolk and other fluid, if present, should be 'mopped up'; use a dry cotton-tipped applicator to remove large amounts of free yolk and fluid. Use sterile fluid-moistened cotton-tipped applicators to carefully remove yolk material

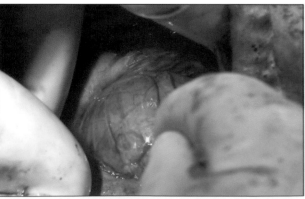

17.49 A large F1 follicle is being 'twirled' such that it can be easily removed. Use a cotton-tipped applicator to rotate the follicle 20–40 times until the blood vessels are no longer visible. At that point, the follicle should simply come loose as its vascular supply is cut off and the pedicle literally twists off.

more adherent to surrounding tissues. If done too aggressively, local tissues may bleed. Remove as much of the visible yolk material as possible without causing damage to surrounding tissues. Collect samples for culture and histopathological evaluation as needed.

> **Procedure difficulty level: 3**

Caesarean section and reproductive tract sparing

Caesarean section is indicated when the bird's reproductive capabilities need to be spared and is typically limited to cases of egg binding with an otherwise normal, or minimally diseased, oviduct. Depending on the location of the egg, a caudal left lateral or ventral midline approach is used. The oviduct should be incised directly over the bound egg and away from prominent blood vessels. After removing the egg, inspect the oviduct for other abnormalities and collect biopsy and culture samples as needed. Close the oviduct in a single simple interrupted or continuous layer using fine (1.5 metric, 4/0 USP or smaller) absorbable suture material. Coelomic closure is standard. Rest the hen from reproductive stimuli for at least 2 to 4 weeks as dictated by culture and/or histopathological results.

> **Procedure difficulty level: 3**

Lower respiratory tract

Air sac breathing tube

An air sac tube can be used if the oral cavity or trachea is occluded preventing proper induction or maintenance of anaesthesia, an endotracheal tube cannot be used (e.g. during head surgery) or the air sacs need to be medicated (Jenkins, 1997; Curro, 1998; Ludders, 1998; Brown and Pilny, 2006). Patients with oral masses, tracheal obstructions, etc. should be mask- (if possible) or box-induced. Anaesthesia delivered via air sac breathing tubes has been successfully used in patients as small as Zebra Finches (Brown and Pilny, 2006).

Once anaesthetized, place the patient in lateral recumbency and, quickly, surgically prepare the paralumbar fossa (just behind the last rib) (Figure 17.50a). Generally, the left side is used, however, a right approach is also possible. A small skin incision is made over the paralumbar fossa (same site as for surgical sexing), exposing a relatively thin layer of lateral abdominal wall muscles (Figure 17.50b). Use right-angled forceps to 'punch' through the muscle layer and into the underlying air sac (Figure 17.50c). Place a sterilized endotracheal, red rubber feeding or other tube into the air sac (either caudal thoracic or abdominal air sac, depending on the bird species and placement) and suture (the tube) to the skin (Figure 17.50d–h). Butterflied tape affixed to the tube, Roman sandal suture pattern or even directly suturing the tube to the surrounding skin can all be used to anchor the breathing tube. The tube diameter should approximate the bird's tracheal size.

The tube may exit just dorsally above the wing feathers or be directed caudally and lie along the bird's back. Whichever position is used, the tube should be relatively comfortable such that the bird does not pick or pull at the tube. Reposition as needed. Analgesics are used as indicated.

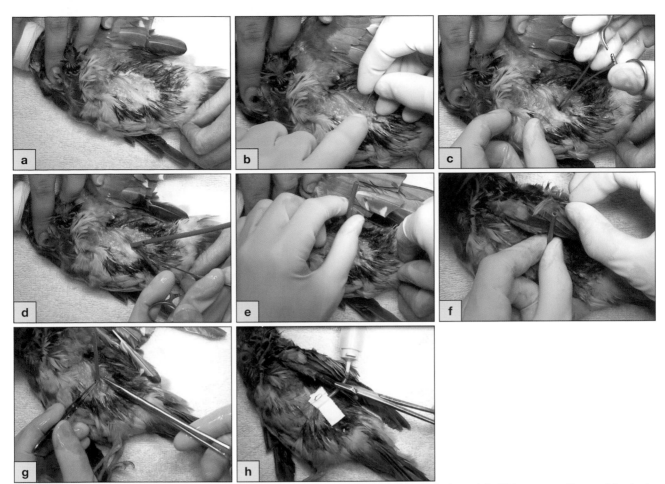

17.50 An Eastern Rosella is placed in right lateral recumbency with the left leg pulled caudally. This exposes the cranial extent of the paralumbar fossa, which is the palpable depression just cranial to the thigh muscles. **(a)** The area is plucked and surgically prepared for an air sac tube placement. **(b)** A nick incision using a No. 15 blade is made over the cranial extent of the paralumbar fossa just enough to cut through the skin. **(c)** A straight, curved or right-angled mosquito haemostat is used to 'punch' through the lateral body wall muscles and into the immediately underlying air sac (either caudal thoracic or abdominal depending on the exact position and species). **(d)** Next, a red rubber feeding, endotracheal or similar sterile tube is guided by open haemostats into the air sac space. **(e)** The internal diameter of the tube should approximate the patient's tracheal lumen size. Do not place the tube too deep as vital structures can be speared and damaged. Next, the tube is trimmed to make its size more manageable and decrease the dead space. **(f)** Prior to securing the tube, test the patency by placing a small feather over the opening and force ventilate the patient. If air is not adequately moving the test feather, reposition the air sac tube. Once the tube patency is determined, attach it to the body wall. This can be accomplished by **(g)** directly suturing the tube to the body wall, **(h)** via butterflied tape or a Roman sandal suture.

When properly placed, one can hold a down feather over the tube opening to watch for air movement, or place a slide and watch for condensation (Brown and Pilny, 2006). Due to progressive microorganism infection and air sacculitis, air sac breathing tubes should not be left in avian patients for more than 5 days (Mitchell *et al.*, 1999). In addition to infection, air sac breathing tubes can result in coelomic organ damage, life-threatening blood loss (from vessel laceration/trauma), air sac damage and subcutaneous emphysema (which is usually self-limiting) (Brown and Pilny, 2006).

The tube and bird are frequently monitored as obstruction with fluid, debris or even tissue may occur. Gentle suction or cleaning with a sterile cotton-tipped applicator or microbiology swab may be needed periodically. Occasionally, the tube may need to be replaced if completely occluded.

In studied Sulphur-crested Cockatoos, delivering isoflurane and oxygen via caudal thoracic air sac intubation provided a reliable method of maintaining anaesthesia and resulted in minimal alteration in respiratory function, similar to endotracheal tube administration. In the same study, clavicular air sac intubation did not provide adequate ventilation or maintenance of anaesthesia (Jaensch *et al.*, 2001).

> **Procedure difficulty level: 2**

References and further reading

Bailey TA, Kinne J, Naldo J *et al.* (2001) Two cases of ventricular foreign bodies in the kori bustard (*Ardeotis kori*). *Veterinary Record* **149**, 187–188

Bennett RA (1994) Techniques in avian thoracoabdominal surgery. In: *Association of Avian Veterinarians Core Seminar Proceedings*, Nevada, 45–57

Bennett RA, Yaeger MJ, Trapp A and Cambre RC (1997) Histologic evaluation of the tissue reaction to five suture materials in the body wall of rock doves (*Columba livia*). *Journal of Avian Medicine and Surgery* **11**, 175–182

Bowles HL, Odberg E, Harrison GJ and Kottwitz JJ (2006) Surgical resolution of soft tissue disorders. In: *Clinical Avian Medicine Volume II*, ed. GJ Harrison and TL Lightfoot, pp. 775–829 Spix Publishing, Palm Beach

Brown C and Pilny A (2006) Air sac cannula placement in birds. *Lab Animal* **35**, 23–24

Carpenter JW (2013) *Exotic Animal Formulary, 4th edn*. WB Saunders Company, Pennsylvania

Chaplin SB and Duke GE (1990) Effect of denervation of the myenteric plexus on gastroduodenal motility in turkeys. *American Journal of Physiology* **259**, G481–489

Chavez W and Echols MS (2007) Bandaging, endoscopy and surgery in the emergency avian patient. *Veterinary Clinics of North America: Exotic Animal Practice* **10**, 419–436

Chitty J and Lierz M (2008) *BSAVA Manual of Raptors, Pigeons and Passerine Birds*. BSAVA Publications, Gloucester

Curro TG (1998) Anesthesia of pet birds. *Seminars in Avian and Exotic Pet Medicine* **7**, 10–21

Degernes LA (1994) Trauma medicine. In: *Avian Medicine: Principles and Application*, ed. BW Ritchie, GJ Harrison and LR Harrison, pp. 418–433. Wingers Publishing, Lake Worth

Degernes LA, Wolf KN, Zombeck DJ *et al.* (2012) Ventricular diverticula formation in captive parakeet auklets (*Aethia psittacula*) secondary to foreign body ingestion. *Journal of Zoo and Wildlife Medicine* **43**, 889–897

Dennis PM and Bennett RA (1999) Ureterolithiasis in a double-yellowheaded Amazon parrot (*Amazona ochracephala*). In: *Association of Avian Veterinarians Annual Conference*, Louisiana, pp. 161–162

Doolen M (1997) Avian soft tissue surgery. In: *Association of Avian Veterinarians Annual Conference*, Nevada, pp. 499–506

Ferrell S, Werner J, Kyles A *et al.* (2003) Evaluation of a collage patch as a method of enhancing ventriculotomy healing in Japanese quail (*Coturnix coturnix japonica*). *Veterinary Surgery* **32**, 103–112

Hall AJ and Duke GE (2000) Effect of selective gastric intrinsic denervation on gastric motility in turkeys. *Poultry Science* **79**, 240–244

Harcourt-Brown N and Chitty J (2005) *BSAVA Manual of Psittacine Birds, 2nd edn*. BSAVA Publications, Gloucester

Hawkins MG, Barron HW, Speer BL *et al.* (2013) Birds. In: *Exotic Animal Formulary*, ed. JW Carpenter , and CJ Marion, pp. 183–437. Elsevier, St Louis

Honnas CM, Blue-McLendon A, Zamos DT *et al.* (1993) Proventriculotomy in ostriches: 18 cases (1990–1992). *Journal of the American Veterinary Medical Association* **202**, 1989–1992

Honnas CM, Jensen J, Cornick JL, *et al.* (1991) Proventriculotomy to relieve foreign body impaction in ostriches. *Journal of the American Veterinary Medical Association* **199**, 461–465

Jaensch S (2000) Diagnosis of avian hepatic disorders. *Seminars in Avian and Exotic Pet Medicine* **9**, 126–135

Jaensch SM, Cullen L and Raidal SR (2000) Assessment of liver function in galahs (*Eolophus roseicapillus*) after partial hepatectomy: A comparison of plasma enzyme concentrations, serum bile acid levels and galactose clearance tests. *Journal of Avian Medicine and Surgery* **14**, 14–171

Jaensch SM, Cullen L and Raidal SR (2001) Comparison of endotracheal, caudal thoracic air sac, and clavicular air sac administration of isoflourane in sulphur-crested cockatoos (*Cacatua galerita*). *Journal of Avian Medicine and Surgery* **15**, 170–177

Jenkins JR (1997) Hospital techniques and supportive care. In: *Avian Medicine and Surgery*, ed. RB Altman, SL Clubb, GM Dorrestein *et al.*, pp. 232–252. WB Saunders, Philadelphia

Kinsel MJ, Briggs MB, Cranq RF and Murnane RD (2004) Ventricular phytobezoar impaction in three micronesian kingfishers (*Halcyon cinnamomina cinnamomina*). *Journal of Zoo and Wildlife Medicine* **35**, 525–529

Lierz M, Ewringmann A and Göbel T (1998) Blood chemistry values in wild raptors and their changes after liver biopsy. *Berliner und Münchener Tierärztliche Wochenschrift* **111**, 295–301

Ludders JW (1998) Respiratory physiology of birds: considerations for anesthetic management. *Seminars in Avian and Exotic Pet Medicine* **7**, 3–9

Meredith, A (2015) *BSAVA Small Animal Formulary, 9th edn – Part B: Exotic Pets*. BSAVA Publications, Gloucester

Mitchell J, Bennett RA and Spalding M (1999) Air sacculitis associated with the placement of an air breathing tube. In: *Association of Avian Veterinarian Annual Conference*, Louisiana, pp. 145–146

Müller K, Göbel T, Müller S *et al.* (2004) Use of endoscopy and renal biopsy for the diagnosis of kidney disease in free-living birds of prey and owls. *Veterinary Record* **155**, 326–329

Nordberg C, O'Brien RT, Paul-Murphy J and Hawley B (2000) Ultrasound examination and guided fine-needle aspiration of the liver in Amazon parrots (*Amazona* species). *Journal of Avian Medicine and Surgery* **14**, 180–184

Orosz S (1997) Anatomy of the urogenital system. In: *Avian Medicine and Surgery*, ed. RB Altman, SL Clubb, GM Dorrestein and K Quesenberry, pp. 614–622. WB Saunders, Philadelphia

Pollock C, Wolf K, Wight-Carter M and Nietfeld J (2006) Comparison of suture material for cloacopexy. In: *Association of Avian Veterinarians Annual Conference*, Texas, pp. 31–32

Redig PT (2006) Raptors: practical information every avian practitioner can use. *Conference of the Association of Avian Veterinarians*, Texas, pp. 203–212

Riggs SM and Tully TN Jr (2004) Wound management in nonpsittacine birds. *Veterinary Clinics of North America: Exotic Animal Practice* **7**,19–36

Ritzman TK (2004) Wound healing and management in psittacine birds. *Veterinary Clinics of North America: Exotic Animal Practice* **7**, 87–104

Roush JC (1996) Avian orthopedics. In: *Current Veterinary Therapy XII Small Animal*, ed. RW Kirck, pp. 662–673. WB Saunders, Philadelphia

Simova-Curd S, Foldenauer U, Guerrero T *et al.* (2013) Comparison of ventriculotomy closure with and without coelomic fat patch in Japanese quail (*Coturnix coturnix japonica*). *Journal of Avian Medicine and Surgery* **27**, 7–13

Speer BL (1998) Chronic partial proventricular obstruction caused by multiple gastrointestinal foreign bodies in a juvenile umbrella cockatoo (*Cacatua alba*). *Journal of Avian Medicine and Surgery* **12**, 271–275

Speer B (2012) Surgical procedures of the psittacine skull. In: *Conference of the Association of Avian Veterinarians*, Kentucky, pp. 181–191

Taylor M (1994) Endoscopic examination and biopsy techniques. In: *Avian Medicine: Principles and Applications*, ed. BW Ritchie, GJ Harrison and LR Harrison, pp. 327–354. Wingers Publishing, Lake Worth

Zebisch K, Krautwald-Junghanns ME and Willuhn J (2004) Ultrasound-guided liver biopsy in birds. *Veterinary Radiology and Ultrasound* **45**, 241–246

Useful contacts

American Board of Veterinary Practitioners (ABVP): www.abvp.com

Australian and New Zealand College of Veterinary Scientists (ANZCVS): www.anzcvs.org.au

European College of Zoological Medicine (ECZM): www.eczm.eu

Royal College of Veterinary Surgeons (RCVS): www.rcvs.org.uk

Basic radiography

Lorenzo Crosta, Alessandro Melillo and Petra Schnitzer

Radiography is one of the most commonly used, non-invasive and direct diagnostic tools in veterinary medicine. Radiographs are easy to interpret and most clients appreciate their usefulness. Furthermore, most small animal practices already have an X-ray machine, and usually this works well for birds.

Although digital radiography, which eliminates technical problems related to screens and films, is becoming more common, many veterinary practices still have conventional X-ray machines.

Whether using digital or conventional X-ray machines, the practitioner has to decide, on a case-by-case basis, whether it is better to anaesthetize the patient or not (see Chapter 16). Furthermore, even experienced avian practitioners require a good-quality X-ray machine. As radiograph interpretation skills increase with daily usage of the X-ray machine, radiography becomes a valuable tool.

Equipment

Radiography machines

It is a mistake to presume that the reduced body size of birds implies the use of low-capacity radiography units; high-capacity machines are still required to allow for accurate study. Birds have a high respiratory rate, which may cause a loss of sharpness in radiographs; therefore, a very short exposure time (0.015–0.05 seconds or less) is recommended. Another technical problem is that whilst the avian skeleton is easy to visualize, differentiation of the soft tissues is difficult.

Radiographic exposure factors are more critical in birds than in mammals. Small variations in X-ray output are very noticeable on avian radiographs, especially those made with lower peak kilovoltage (kVp) techniques; therefore, the X-ray generator must be in excellent condition (Silverman and Tell, 2010). These difficulties indicate the need for a high-frequency X-ray machine.

The X-ray generator should be able to produce at least 300 milliamps (mA); settings should have a range of 40–90 kVp, and be adjustable in 2 kVp increments. High-frequency X-ray generators are recommended because they produce a uniform X-ray output.

Portable X-ray machines

Portable X-ray equipment is commonly used by equine or zoo veterinary surgeons (veterinarians), whose patients are difficult, if not impossible, to be moved. However, nowadays the avian veterinary surgeon can also utilize portable X-ray machines designed for dentistry. Although these machines look like a normal digital camera, they do not directly display an image; they emit X-rays and the image is recorded on to a substrate (a standard X-ray film or a digital cassette). Portable X-ray machines are ideal for field work. Small details are more easily radiographed (Figure 18.1a), as well as total body images of larger parrots and cockatoos (Figure 18.1b).

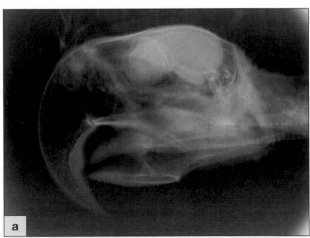

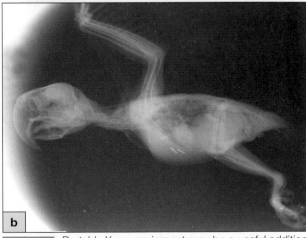

18.1 Portable X-ray equipment may be a useful addition to the avian clinician's toolkit. Radiograph of **(a)** the head and **(b)** the whole body of a Green-winged Macaw taken with portable X-ray equipment.

Preparation

Use of anaesthesia

The question of whether to anaesthetize a bird for taking a radiograph or not is still a debatable issue, with strong arguments on both sides. Proponents argue that radiographs performed under anaesthesia are more efficient and of higher quality, as the birds can be positioned with less physical restraint, with an associated reduction in the potential for iatrogenic fractures (Silverman and Tell, 2010). Harcourt-Brown (1996) advises that anaesthesia of the bird allows the clinician to work within the requirements of the Health and Safety at Work Act whilst achieving better positioning; inhalant anaesthesia (isoflurane or sevoflurane) is recommended (Helmer, 2006).

However, Krautwald-Junghanns and Trinkaus (2000) advise that sedation for radiography must be considered on a case-by-case basis, and that it is often not necessary in routine practice. The process of preparing for parenteral anaesthesia if inhalation apparatus is not available (including weighing and post-anaesthetic supervision) can increase the time, and therefore associated risk, of the procedure (see also Chapter 16).

In the routine practice of the authors, most birds to be radiographed will be anaesthetized. Generally, for a simple diagnostic radiograph, quick inhalation anaesthesia with isoflurane is adequate, but there are cases (e.g. before or after an orthopaedic surgery) when deeper anaesthesia or pre-anaesthesia are required. There may also be cases when a mild sedation (midazolam at 2 mg/kg intranasally) is enough for taking radiographs.

The health status of the individual bird must always be considered. It is **always** advised to anaesthetize the following birds:

- Very excited/not tame birds, which may struggle excessively and be hurt (e.g. iatrogenic traumas or fractures)
- Potentially dangerous patients (such as large eagles), as they may inflict serious wounds to the operators.

On the other hand, anaesthesia could be avoided in the following cases:

- Tame birds that can be easily handled and restrained by a Plexiglas® or acrylic positioning device
- Very weak patients in a critical condition, for which the anaesthesia maybe dangerous (e.g. egg-bound females)
- Very young birds, especially if hand-fed, as the semi-liquid formula may easily be regurgitated and suffocate the patient.

Patient positioning

The interpretation of avian radiographs is complicated by several factors:

- Viscera are very compact in the coelomic cavity; this may lower the ability to distinguish between different organs
- Due to the absence of a diaphragm, there is a lack of separation between abdominal and thoracic organs; this makes the differentiation even more difficult

- Compared with mammals, birds have a reduced amount of perivisceral fat, which normally helps in telling the different organs apart
- Avian fat has a radiopacity that is very similar to that of the soft tissues, and this limits the interpretation even further.

For these reasons, in order to avoid misinterpretation of the radiographs, it is imperative that the patient is positioned in a perfectly symmetrical way and that the practitioner has a very good knowledge of the normal radiological avian anatomy in each given species or, at least, group.

Whether or not the patient is anaesthetized, positioning can be assisted by:

- Special Plexiglas® traps/boards (Figure 18.2). The positioning boards have been designed for this specific purpose, are easy to use and patients are quickly released from the board. On the other hand, some clinicians believe they are very stressful for the non-anaesthetized patient

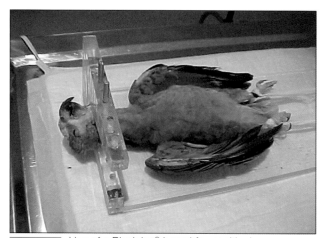

18.2 Use of a Plexiglas® board for positioning a medium-sized parrot.

- Some relatively heavy objects, such as sand bags or radioprotective lead gloves (Figure 18.3). These can be adjusted according to the specific needs of the case and the patient
- Tape or other adhesive strips (Figure 18.4). Tape is mostly used for the smaller species, since positioning boards may be too large and bags and gloves too heavy.

A good ventrodorsal (VD) view requires the bird to be:

- Lying on its back
- Head and neck extended cranially
- The keel bone (sternum) must be perfectly aligned (superimposed) over the spinal column
- The wings can be extended laterally or not, but they must be perfectly symmetrical
- The legs will be pulled caudally and parallel.

In the experience of the authors, the required alignment is more easily achieved standing at the feet of the patient and trying to position the bird by manipulating its wings and legs; working this way will give the operator a very good perspective of the bird's position.

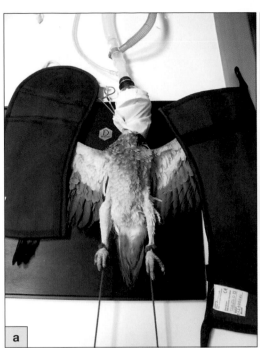
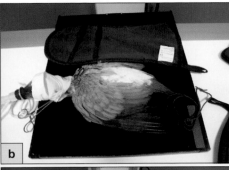
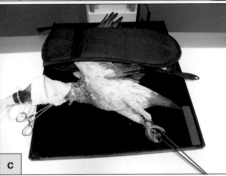

18.3 **(a)** Positioning of an African Grey Parrot for a ventrodorsal radiograph. Radiology gloves and foot straps are utilized. **(b)** To achieve good positioning for the laterolateral view, it is best to put something of the right thickness between the wings; this will prevent rotation of the body. **(c)** Final positioning for the laterolateral radiograph.

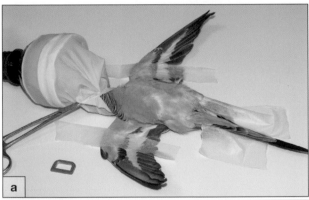
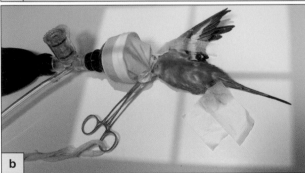

18.4 **(a)** For the smallest species, such as Budgerigars, it is better to use tape, instead of a heavy object to aid positioning. Excessive tension on the wings can cause impediment to lateral excursions of the body wall, compromising respiration. **(b)** Budgerigar placed in a laterolateral position using tape.

When the bird is positioned for the laterolateral (LL) view, it will be:

- Lying on its right side (right lateral recumbency). This is the standard position, unless specific needs require the patient to be on its left side
- The head and neck will be extended
- The shoulders will be superimposed
- The wings will be extended dorsally and superimposed (in most species it is important to put a thick pad between the wings, in order to avoid

rotation of the body when the upper (left) wing is stretched out). Note: excessive tension on the wings can cause impediment to lateral excursions of the body wall, compromising respiration
- The legs will be stretched ventrocaudally. Unless there is a specific need, the authors prefer the hips and legs to be superimposed and parallel.

When radiographs of the hips are needed, the bird is positioned on one side and the upper leg is stretched outwards; this will allow a good visualization of the contralateral hip. Once this is done, the same process is carried out on the other side.

Avian radiology

It is important for avian practitioners to be familiar with the normal radiographic appearance of parrots (Figures 18.5 and 18.6) and raptors (Figures 18.7 and 18.8). For further details on avian anatomy, see Chapter 2.

Skull

As with many other species, the standard procedure for radiographing the avian head includes at least two images: a VD (Figure 18.9a) and LL (Figure 18.9b) view.

All birds have a chain of scleral bones in the eye, and these bones are easily spotted during radiography. Another common feature of avian skulls are the sinuses; these vary between species and are often very complex. Striking anatomical differences exist between different species groups; for example, in some taxonomic groups (e.g. Psittaciformes) the upper bill–frontal bone joint is movable.

Positioning is a key point when viewing the avian skull, and several different techniques can be used to maximize the final outcome. For a good VD view of the head, the bird is better positioned on its back, although some authors prefer the dorsoventral (DV) view. If the body is kept in the right position, then the head can be extended with different tools, such as a small string or wire loop (Figure 18.10). The same technique can be used for the lateral view.

271

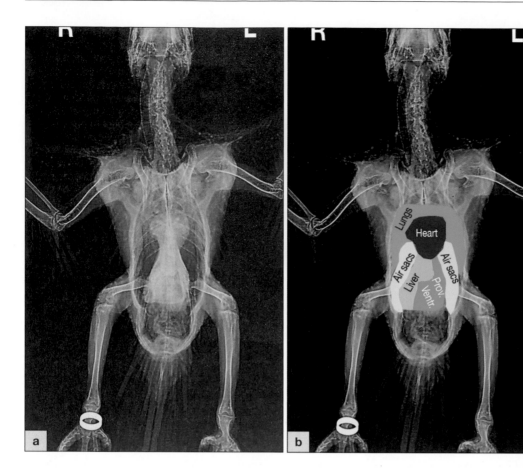

18.5

Blue and Gold Macaw.
(a) Ventrodorsal view
and **(b)** with organs
highlighted.
Prov. = proventriculus;
Ventr. = ventriculus.

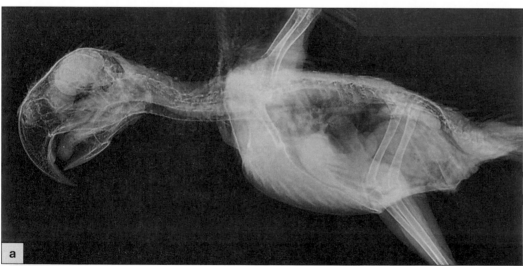

18.6

Blue and Gold Macaw.
(a) Laterolateral view of
a bird with spleno-
megaly. **(b)** View with
organs highlighted.
Note the enlarged
spleen.
Prov. = proventriculus;
Ventr. = ventriculus.

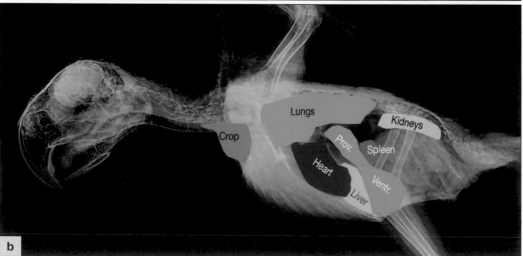

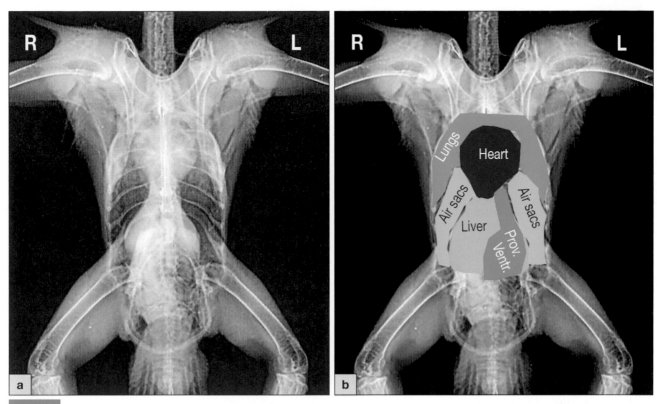

18.7 Saker Falcon. **(a)** Ventrodorsal view and **(b)** with organs highlighted. Prov. = proventriculus; Ventr. = ventriculus.

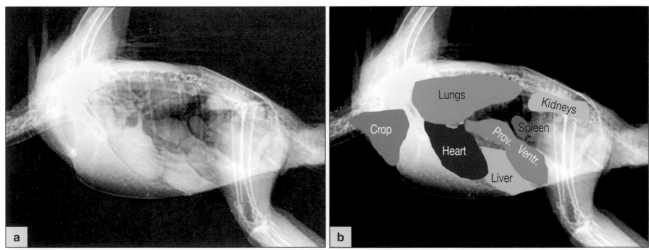

18.8 Saker Falcon. **(a)** Laterolateral view of a bird with splenomegaly. **(b)** View with organs highlighted. Note the enlarged spleen. Prov. = proventriculus; Ventr. = ventriculus.

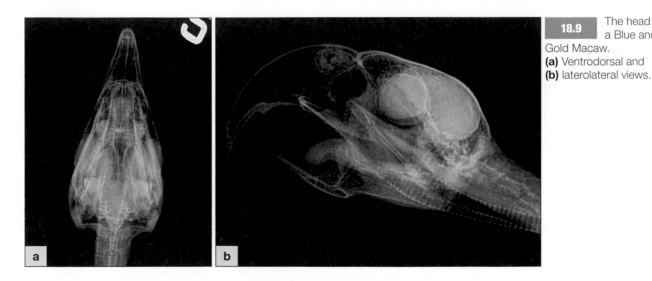

18.9 The head of a Blue and Gold Macaw. **(a)** Ventrodorsal and **(b)** laterolateral views.

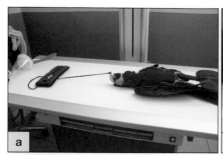
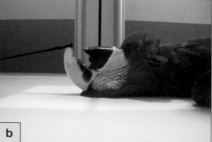
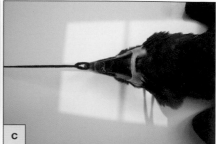

18.10 **(a)** An anaesthetized Green-winged Macaw positioned for a ventrodorsal radiograph of the head. **(b–c)** A small strap can be tied to the upper beak, in order to extend it.

Several types of lesions may be observed in the avian skull, in the bones (Figure 18.11) and in the soft tissues (Figure 18.12). It is imperative to know the anatomical differences between different avian species, as there are some striking variations.

Spinal column

The number of vertebrae may vary between different species and taxonomic groups; however, the subdivisions of the spinal column are the same as in mammals.

- **Cervical column:** in birds the number of cervical vertebrae varies between 10 and 25, depending on species. As a general rule, parrots have 12 cervical vertebrae.

- **Thoracic:** like the fuselage of an aircraft, the avian thorax must support the action of flying. To do this, it has to be stiff and not foldable. For this reason, the thoracic vertebrae of most adult birds are fused in a long os dorsale or notarium.
- **Synsacrum:** also called *os lumbosacrale*, or *os pelvicum*, the synsacrum is a rigid unit, consisting of ankylosed vertebrae in adult birds. The synsacrum includes one or more thoracic vertebrae, the lumbar vertebrae and some of the caudal vertebrae.
- **Free caudal vertebrae:** these can also be spotted in the typical avian radiograph.
- **Pygostyle:** also known as the pygostilus, urostylus or coccyx, this is a compound bone, formed by the ankylosis of the last three to six free caudal vertebrae.

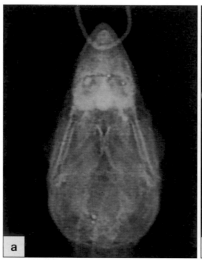
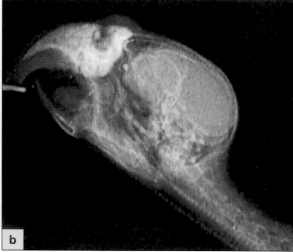

18.11 A lovebird with an inflammatory process of the maxillary bones. **(a)** Ventrodorsal and **(b)** laterolateral views. The owner refused further investigation and the aetiology remains unknown.

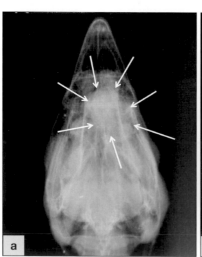
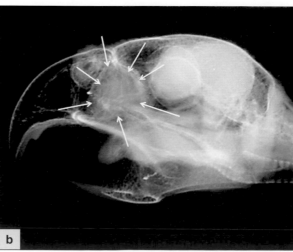

18.12 Blue and Gold Macaw with a radiodense mass in the sinuses (arrowed). **(a)** Ventrodorsal and **(b)** laterolateral views. Compare with Figure 18.9, which shows a healthy head of a Blue and Gold Macaw.

Radiographically, the avian spinal column is best visualized on the LL view (Figure 18.13), even if some lateral deviations can be better diagnosed on the VD view.

Sternum and pectoral girdle

The avian pectoral (or shoulder) girdle (Figure 18.14) is formed by three bones. The clavicle and the scapula are homologous to the bones of the shoulder of most mammals but the coracoid does not exist in therian mammals.

- The two clavicles are fused together distally, to form the furcula ('wishbone').
- The coracoid is a strong bone that connects the sternum to the shoulder and the humerus. Although coracoids can be visualized on a LL radiograph, they are best studied on the VD view.

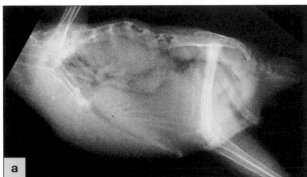

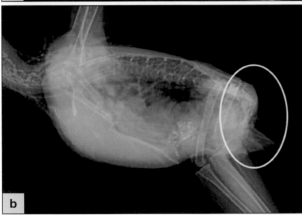

18.13 (a) Dusky-headed Conure with severe scoliosis. (b) Yellow-naped Amazon with severe ventral deviation of the last portion of the spinal column (circled). These lesions often have a traumatic origin.

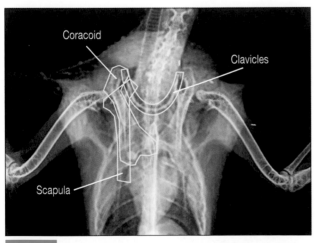

18.14 The pectoral girdle of a Yellow-fronted Amazon.

- The avian scapula is long and thin compared with its mammalian counterpart. This tiny bone is not easily spotted, and it is best seen on the VD view.

The sternum of parrots, raptors and passerines has a keel that serves to anchor the powerful pectoral muscles. For good VD positioning, it is important that the keel of the sternum is perfectly superimposed over the spine.

Wings

The skeleton of the proximal and mid-wing includes basically the same bones that form the forelimbs of mammals (Figure 18.15). The bones become different in the distal part, from the wrist down. However, in a proximal–distal sequence:

- **Humerus:** a large bone that supports the power of the pectoral muscles and wing together
- **Radius:** the smaller bone in the bird's forearm; on the VD view the radius is seen over the ulna
- **Ulna:** the secondary remiges (flight feathers) are intimately connected to the periosteum of the caudal ulna, so this bone supports most of the power produced by the wing during flight. This explains why the ulna is the largest bone in the avian forearm (Figure 18.16)

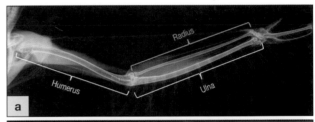

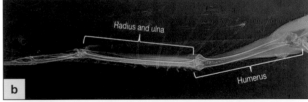

18.15 The normal wing of a Brown Wood Owl. **(a)** Mediolateral and **(b)** caudocranial views.

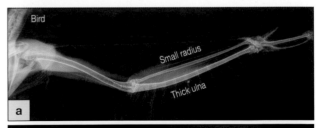

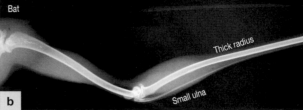

18.16 Comparison between the **(a)** avian and **(b)** bat wing; an example of convergent evolution. While birds developed a strong ulna to support the power of the secondary remiges that are intimately connected to the ulnar periosteum, bats have a thicker radius, needed to support the large propatagium.

- **Carpal bones:** these are two tiny bones that form the carpal joint.
- **Carpometacarpus:** this is fused out of the distal carpal bones and the metacarpal bones to a single two-strutted bone
- **Hand:** this includes the bones of the alula, metacarpus and phalanges.

When a thorough study of the wing is required, it must be evaluated mediolaterally and caudocranially. It is also recommended that the contralateral wing is radiographed for comparison (Figure 18.17), and a good understanding of the development of avian long bones is important when dealing with young patients (Figure 18.18).

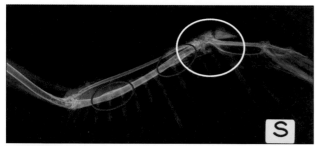

18.17 Mediolateral view of a Brown Wood Owl with old lesions of the ulna and carpal bones (circled). Although these lesions apparently are not severe, the most distal (white circle) can limit the ability to fly.

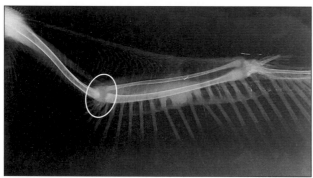

18.18 The wing of a young Eurasian Eagle Owl, in which ossification is not yet complete (circled). Note this is normal for the stage of development.

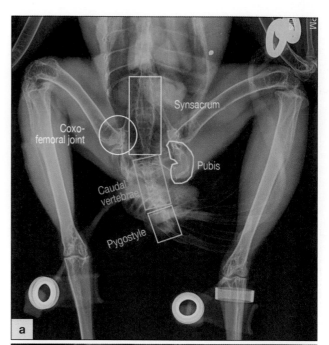

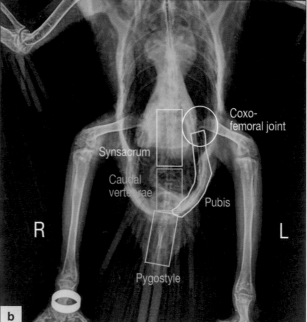

18.19 Pelvic girdle of **(a)** a Harris' Hawk and **(b)** a Blue and Gold Macaw.

Pelvic girdle

The avian pelvic girdle includes the:

- **Synsacrum:** although the synsacrum is a subdivision of the spine, and has already been explained above, it also forms part of the pelvic girdle
- **Ilium and ischium:** these are fused together in birds
- **Pubis:** this is not fused.

Generally, the avian pelvic girdle is better evaluated on the VD view and perfect symmetry of the bones is a prerequisite for good interpretation (Figure 18.19).

With some experience, lesions can be spotted on the hips and pelvis but in most cases birds are not really symptomatic, even when they have impressive skeletal lesions.

Lower limbs

Although some of the bones in the avian leg are the result of fusion of several bones found in other types of animals (e.g. tibiotarsus, tarsometatarsus), the skeleton of the avian leg includes bones that are, more or less, the same as in mammals:

- Femur
- Patella
- Tibiotarsus
- Fibula
- Tarsometatarsus
- Phalanges (usually four).

To obtain a good VD view, the legs must be extended caudally and be parallel (Figure 18.20).

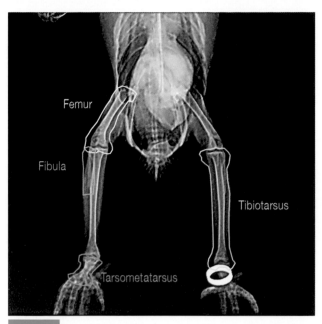

18.20   The lower limb bones of a Yellow-fronted Amazon.

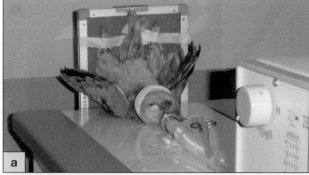

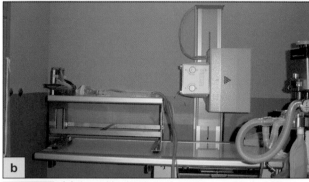

18.22   (a) A positioning board can be used to hold the patient in a more physiological position, in this case for obtaining a radiograph of the feet of a Blue-fronted Amazon. **(b)** The board accommodates the X-ray cassette vertically and the X-ray beam is directed horizontally.

When an evaluation of the hips has to be undertaken, then at least three views are needed:

- A standard VD view of the lower body that includes both legs; legs well extended and parallel
- A left LL view, with the left leg lying on the table and extended ventrocaudally, while the right leg is pulled outwards as much as possible, allowing a good view of the left hip
- A right LL view; this will mirror the left LL described above.

Special positioning may be required when good radiographs of the feet are needed. In these cases either the feet can be taped to the X-ray table (Figure 18.21), or the X-ray beam can be directed horizontally, to allow for more physiological positioning of the avian patient (Figure 18.22).

Besides the more obvious leg lesions, such as fractures and luxations, more subtle abnormalities can be detected via radiography (Figures 18.23 and 18.24).

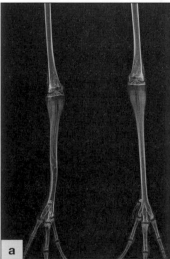

18.23

(a) Ventrodorsal view of a Crowned Crane with a curved right tibiotarsus. **(b)** Laterolateral view. Juvenile osteomyelitis was found to be the cause of limited bone growth.

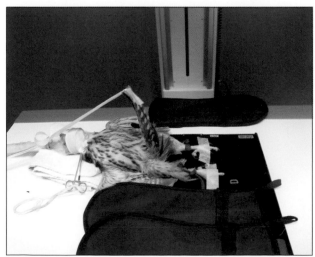

18.21   In order to obtain a clear view of the feet, the tail of this Saker Falcon has been taped away from the field of view.

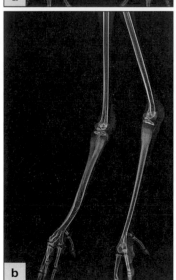

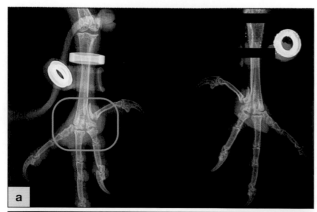

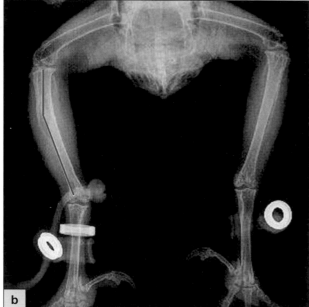

18.24 (a) Saker Falcon with mild ulcerative pododermatitis (bumblefoot); swelling of the footpad is evident (circled). (b) Proximal view of the legs. The deviation of the right tibiotarsus (red line) does not allow for normal perching. This deviation requires surgical correction.

Respiratory system

The respiratory system possibly represents one of the most striking differences between birds and mammals; from a physiological and radiological point of view. It includes several parts and all of them can be evaluated with radiography.

Trachea

The trachea is easily identified on radiographs, especially because it is formed of closed cartilaginous rings, which are easily recognizable. However, it is still better evaluated on the lateral view. In some species the trachea has an unusual shape; for example, in toucans and mynahs, just before entering the thorax, the trachea forms an angle with a ventral apex (Figure 18.25).

Lungs

The lungs should be evaluated on both LL and VD views, in order to fully examine any pulmonary lesions or abnormalities and reach a suspect diagnosis.

Due to the structure of the distal portion of the parabronchi, on the LL view the avian lungs show a distinct honeycomb pattern.

Any respiratory disease may alter the radiodensity of the image, making it darker, or even clearer (Figure 18.26).

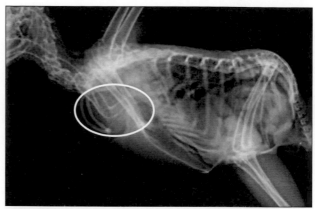

18.25 It is important to be aware of species variations such as curved tracheas. This Hill Mynah has a typical curved trachea (circled), but also has severe kyphosis.

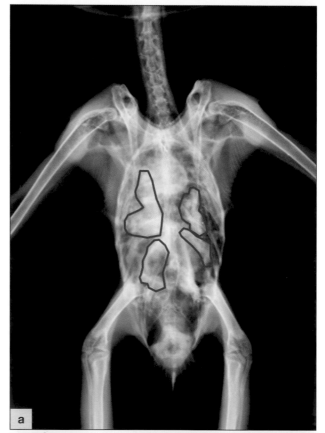

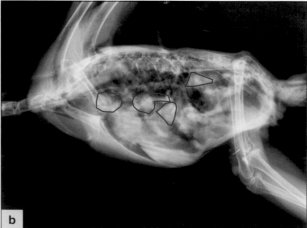

18.26 Snowy Owl with respiratory granulomas (highlighted). (a) Ventrodorsal and (b) laterolateral views. These lesions are indicative of aspergillosis.

Air sacs

The air sacs are not involved in gaseous exchange; their function is to support the air flow/ventilation within the respiratory system. The majority of the avian species that are commonly seen in practice have nine air sacs, which appear as dark (air-filled) areas within the body cavity.

When radiographing the air sacs, the following must be taken into consideration:

- Being virtually empty spaces, air sacs are basically identified by their borders with other organs
- Normally they are of the same grey tone as the air outside the body (but consider that the soft tissues in between will alter the shade of grey a little)
- In cases of air sacculitis, the radiological appearance of the air sacs may change, both in shape and shade of grey, as well as with the presence of focal lesions (Figure 18.27).

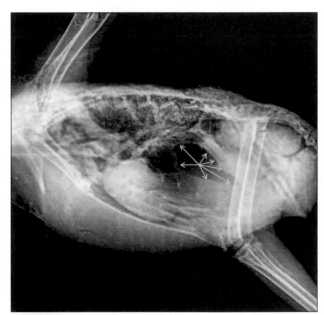

18.27 African Grey Parrot with air sacculitis. The deposits of fibrin over the air sac wall (arrowed) have resulted in an increase in radiodensity.

It is important to remember that for a good diagnosis of air sac lesions, both a VD and a LL view must be obtained; this is because some lesions may be shown on only one view, and also because the triangulation achieved by comparing the two views helps in locating the exact sites of the focal lesions.

Circulatory system

As in mammals, only the heart and the large vessels of birds can be studied by radiography without the use of specific contrast media. Angiography has been performed in birds, but it remains a very rare procedure. The most common radiographic procedures performed on the avian circulatory system are probably the measurement of the heart where cardiomyopathy is suspected, and the evaluation of the large cardiac vessels.

In most species, the heart is located between the second and sixth rib. In captive parrots, the width of the heart base is between 51 and 61% of the maximum width of the coelomic cavity, but this measurement may change dramatically in birds that actively fly.

In a VD view the heart forms an hourglass figure with the liver; the shape may change with different

diseases. Heart problems that can be spotted via radiography include:

- Cardiomegaly (Figure 18.28)
- Reduced size of the heart (very rare)
- Arteriosclerosis with mineralization of the great heart vessels.

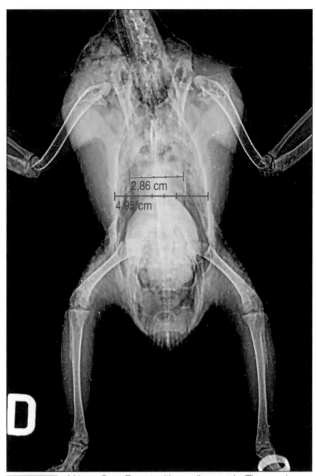

18.28 African Grey Parrot with cardiomegaly. The maximum width of the heart should not be more than 61% of the maximum width of the coelomic cavity at this level.

Digestive system

Birds have a relatively short digestive system compared with mammals. Although the anatomical subdivisions of the avian gastrointestinal (GI) tract are similar to those of mammals, the distal portion is very difficult to identify via radiography. The avian GI tract is divided into:

- Cervical oesophagus
- Crop
- Thoracic oesophagus
- Proventriculus
- Ventriculus
- Intestine
- Cloaca.

See 'Contrast media' for more information on imaging of the GI tract.

Cervical oesophagus and crop

Most avian species have a crop (owls are a notable exception). On the VD view, the cervical oesophagus and the crop will lie on the right side, but some extension to the left is normal. However, if the crop is shown only on the left side, it is very likely pathological.

Proventriculus and ventriculus

The appearance of the avian stomach varies significantly between the various species, mostly dependent on diet; however, there are some patterns that are common to the majority of avian groups.

- Proventriculus:
  - On the VD view, it is slightly on the left side
  - On the LL view, it lies dorsally to the liver.
- Ventriculus:
  - Is easily identified (often contains some grit)
  - On the VD view, it is slightly on the left side of the coelomic cavity
  - On the LL view, it is located caudoventrally to the proventriculus.

The best way to evaluate the digestive system, for a general diagnosis, is a contrast study with barium (Figure 18.29) or some other radiopaque substance (see 'Contrast media'). The displacement of portions of the GI tract, as seen with contrast studies, is also used indirectly to evaluate enlargement or displacement of different surrounding organs.

Obviously, there are cases when a simple radiograph is enough for a diagnosis; for example, in the case of radiopaque foreign bodies (Figure 18.30), or when the proventriculus is dilated (Figures 18.31 and 18.32).

Spleen

In parrots the spleen is a rounded organ, visible at the junction of the proventriculus and ventriculus. Radiography is not usually a good diagnostic tool for spleen pathology as it cannot always be identified; the only view in which it may be possible to find the spleen is the LL view (Figure 18.33).

Liver

In most avian species the liver is better evaluated on a LL view. In several bird species, particularly parrots, the hepatic and the cardiac silhouettes together form an hourglass shape (Figure 18.34). Most alterations of the shape of the cardiohepatic silhouette depend on heart or liver problems, but a pathological enlargement of the proventriculus could also be the cause.

In the case of parrots, a general idea of liver size can be assessed in the following ways:

- On a VD view, the liver borders should not pass an imaginary line that goes from the shoulder joint to the acetabulum
- On a LL view, the liver should not pass the sternum.

Kidneys

The avian kidneys are typically divided into three lobes (cranial, medial and caudal). Like the mammalian kidneys, the kidneys of birds are extraperitoneal organs and give rise to the ureters, but since birds do not have a urinary bladder (another point to remember when interpreting the radiographs of birds), the ureters open directly into the urodeum (the middle portion of the cloaca).

Healthy avian kidneys are not easy to spot on the VD view, since there are several other structures superimposed in the image; however, they are easily spotted on the LL view, where their silhouette is evident in the dorsal part of the coelomic cavity, almost as if the kidneys are 'hanging' from the synsacrum.

Typical renal alterations that can be diagnosed via radiography are swelling (Figure 18.35) and mineralization (Figure 18.36).

Gonads and reproductive apparatus

The gonads of birds can be seen on the LL view, where they appear as slightly radiodense organs, located cranioventrally to the cranial lobe of the kidney. However, the quality of a radiographic image is not good enough to assess the gender of a bird.

Two exceptions to this rule are ovulating and laying females; in the first case, a developing egg (ovum) can be seen. In the experience of the authors, it is very rare to be able to identify this stage. On the other hand, a shelled egg is unmistakable (Figure 18.37).

There are cases, often when a bird is suspected to be egg bound, where the patient is so stressed and dyspnoeic that physical or chemical restraint can be dangerous. In these cases, the patient can be radiographed on a wooden perch (tame and well

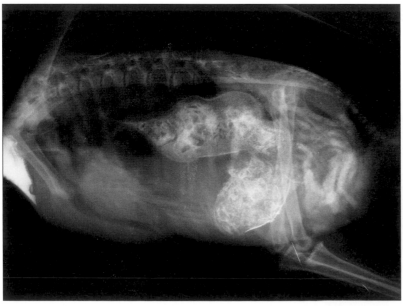

18.29 Contrast medium evaluation of the gastrointestinal tract of an Eclectus Parrot. Most of the contrast medium was still in the proventriculus and ventriculus after 24 hours. This bird died from polyomavirus disease.

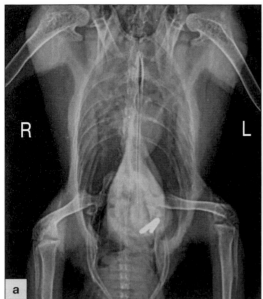

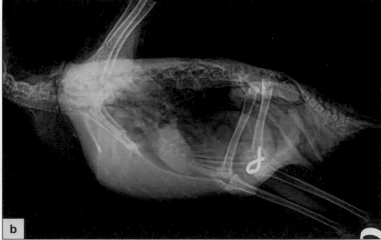

18.30 Blue and Gold Macaw with a metal foreign body in the ventriculus. **(a)** Ventrodorsal and **(b)** laterolateral views. Metallic foreign bodies of this size will not pass the gastric compartment and it is always better to retrieve them with an endoscope, or even via a surgical approach.

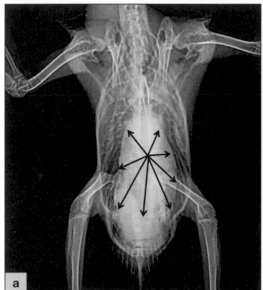

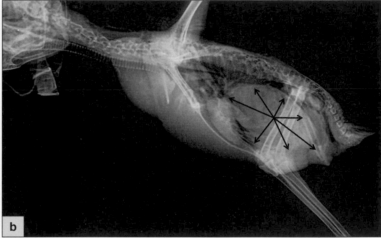

18.31 Red-fronted Macaw with suspected proventricular dilatation disease (PDD). **(a)** Ventrodorsal and **(b)** laterolateral views. The arrows denote the dilated gastric compartment. This patient tested positive for avian bornavirus.

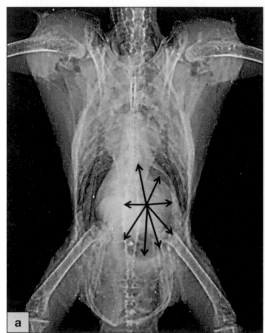

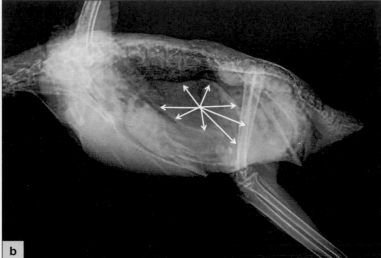

18.32 Umbrella Cockatoo with a dilated proventriculus (arrowed). **(a)** Ventrodorsal and **(b)** laterolateral views. This bird was negative for bornavirus (polymerase chain reaction and serology), which may have been due to it being a very recent infection, poor sample collection or a laboratory error; however, not all dilated stomachs are the result of bornaviral infection.

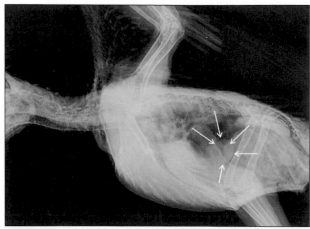

18.33 The spleen may be identified on laterolateral views (arrowed), as shown in this Blue and Gold Macaw.

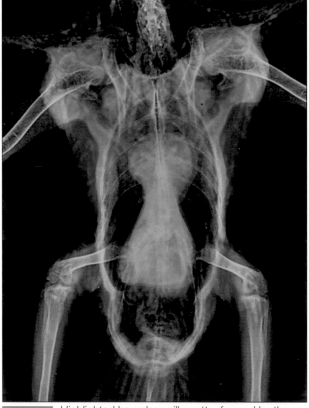

18.34 Highlighted hourglass silhouette, formed by the heart and the liver, in a Blue and Gold Macaw.

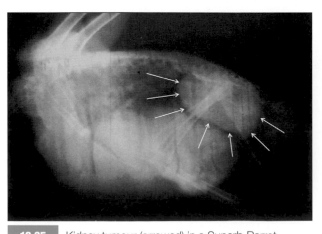

18.35 Kidney tumour (arrowed) in a Superb Parrot.

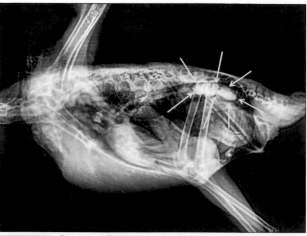

18.36 Blue and Gold Macaw with renal mineralization (arrowed). These lesions must also be evaluated with other diagnostic tools, such as a kidney biopsy.

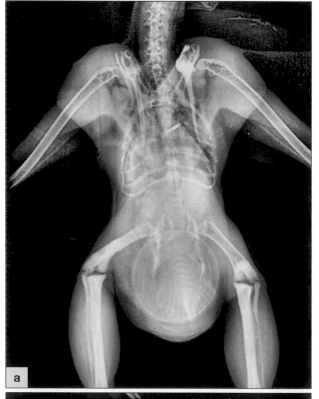

a

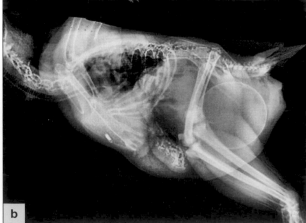

b

18.37 Egg-bound Spectacled Owl. **(a)** Ventrodorsal view. This was a mild case that resolved with calcium, fluid therapy and a warm cage. **(b)** Laterolateral view. In cases of egg binding, it is always important to take both ventrodorsal and laterolateral views.

trained birds) (Figure 18.38), or radiography can be performed with the bird in a cardboard box (Figure 18.39). In both cases, the main purpose is to ascertain the presence of an egg, and this can be achieved without specific positioning. If there is an egg, then a decision must be made regarding the best diagnostic and therapeutic approach, but this is a step further.

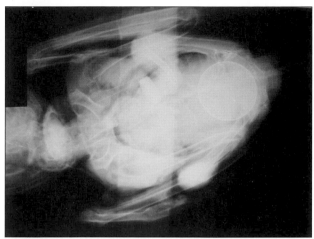

18.38 A tame and trained egg-bound bird, such as this Blue and Gold Macaw, can be easily radiographed on a wooden perch. The presence of a calcified egg is unmistakable.

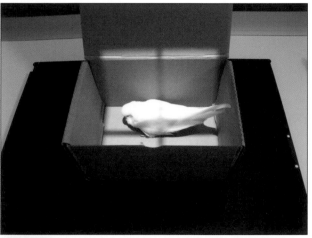

18.39 In order to avoid any unnecessary stress to egg-bound birds, with small patients the first radiograph can be taken with the bird in a cardboard box.

Contrast media

In avian radiology, contrast media are mostly used for studying the digestive system. Not only can the different parts of the GI tract be identified and studied, but their position and/or dislocation within the coelomic cavity can also be determined, which serves as a tool to diagnose other masses/organs/systems that are not easily visualized with normal radiography. For example, when the ventriculus is displaced ventrally and on the right side this may be due to enlargement of the oviduct, whereas when the ventriculus is displaced dorsally it may be due to enlargement of the liver. This can be a very good indication to start the diagnostic work-up.

A contrast study is generally started with a standard 'empty' set of radiographs. As a general rule, birds are fasted for 2–3 hours before the contrast study, but this varies between different species. It is important not to prolong the recommended fasting time, as this may alter the transit time in the GI tract, which is one of the indications for diagnosis.

Barium sulphate is still considered the standard contrast medium for birds because it is easy to use and relatively safe. For birds, the commercial preparation should be diluted to obtain a 25–45% barium solution, and this is administered at a dose of 20 ml/kg. Barium sulphate should not be used if an intestinal rupture is suspected.

A good alternative to barium sulphate is iohexol; 10 ml/kg of a 250 mg/ml solution should be administered by gavage. It is important to note that the GI transit time of iohexol is double that of barium sulphate (Krautwald et al. 2011).

After the first empty radiographs have been taken, the contrast medium is administered by crop gavage to the patient. Subsequent sets of radiographs are taken at 0, 30 (Figure 18.40), 60 and 120 (Figure 18.41) minutes, but this may vary with the different species (Krautwald et al., 1992; Krautwald-Junghanns et al., 2011). Patients are woken up between each exposure.

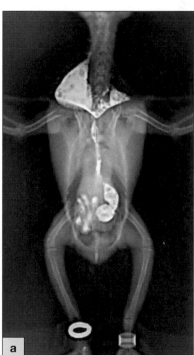

18.40 Contrast study of a Peach-faced Lovebird, 30 minutes after barium gavage. **(a)** Ventrodorsal and **(b)** laterolateral views.

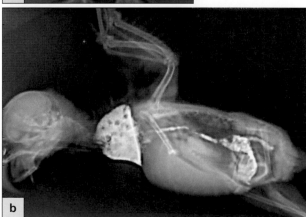

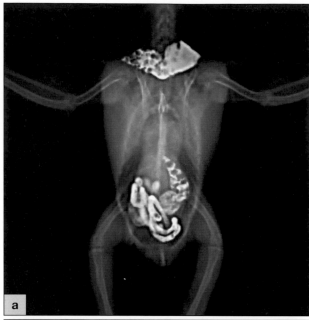

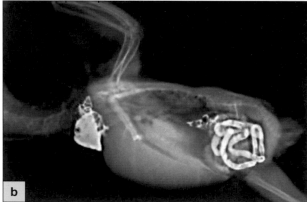

18.41 Contrast study of a Peach-faced Lovebird, 120 minutes after barium gavage. **(a)** Ventrodorsal and **(b)** laterolateral views.

Historically, birds were not anaesthetized for radiographic contrast studies. This was done to avoid alterations of GI transit time. A joint study, presented by Dr Angela Lennox (USA) and the veterinary staff of the Loro Parque (Spain) in 2002, showed that isoflurane anaesthesia does not significantly alter GI transit time; therefore, birds can safely be anaesthetized for contrast studies, although the risk of regurgitation/aspiration of the contrast medium must be taken into consideration. It is recommended that the bird is intubated instead of having a simple facemask placed, as is often done for quick procedures, at least until the contrast medium is no longer in the crop.

Contrast urography

Contrast urography is seldom performed in avian patients; this is mostly due to the fact that birds do not have a urinary bladder, renal pelvis or urethra, thus urography is only used to visualize the ureters and this is not a common need in avian diagnostics. However, if contrast urography has to be performed, iodine compounds can be used. Published doses vary between 700 and 800 mg/kg iodine. The iodine compound should be administered intravenously immediately before taking the image, as it will be cleared by the kidneys very quickly.

- The bird should be deeply anaesthetized and monitored on the X-ray table. An intravenous catheter connected to a drip system should be in place.
- All the required drugs must be ready before starting the procedure.
- The patient is positioned exactly as needed as indicated by the specific circumstances and fixed in place.
- The X-ray machine should be already on and the cassette in place (in the case of conventional or indirect digital radiography).
- One operator should be ready to take the radiograph whilst another delivers the iodine compound intravenously.
- Immediately after the drug has been administered, and when the operator is no longer in the X-ray field, the first image is taken.
- Within 5 minutes (preferably within 2–3 minutes), another image is taken.

Contrast angiography

- To perform angiography, the bird must be anaesthetized.
- A solution containing 380 mg iodine/ml (e.g. iopamidol) is slowly injected intravenously via a catheter. The total delivered iodine dose is about 2–4 mg/kg (Krautwald-Junghanns *et al.*, 2011).
- Alternatively, an iohexol solution containing 240 mg/ml can be injected as a bolus at 2 ml/kg (Beaufrère *et al.*, 2010).

Contrast rhinosinography

Although the best technique for evaluating the nasal sinuses is computed tomography (CT), most general practitioners do not have access to such equipment and/or the procedure is too expensive for most clients. Contrast rhinosinography is an alternative diagnostic tool.

- Depending on the size of the bird, 0.1–1 ml of a solution containing 200–250 mg/ml of iodine is injected directly into the paranasal sinus (Krautwald *et al.*, 2011).
- The needle is directed toward a point midway between the eye and external nares, keeping parallel with the side of the head. The needle passes under the zygomatic bone, which lies between the lower corner of the rhinotheca (upper beak) and the ear (Campbell, 1994).
- After the required X-ray images have been taken, the contrast media must be flushed away with warm saline solution.

Contrast cloacography

Another positive-contrast study technique is positive-contrast cloacography, although it is seldom used in birds. This technique is the final stage of contrast urography. The cloaca will be highlighted between 2 and 5 minutes after the iodine compound is injected. However, an easier technique to evaluate the cloaca is a double-contrast study, using air and barium sulphate as contrast media: 10 ml/kg of a 25% barium sulphate suspension is given orally or intracloacally. Immediately after administration of the barium sulphate, the bird is given air via the same route. The volume of air given should be roughly twice the volume of barium sulphate.

Use of contrast media in other imaging techniques

Magnetic resonance imaging (MRI) is considered the gold standard diagnostic technique for the nervous system; however, avian MRI faces several problems, including:

- Most birds have a metal leg ring
- The procedure is fairly long

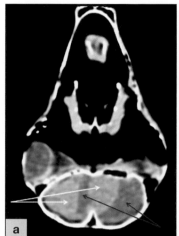

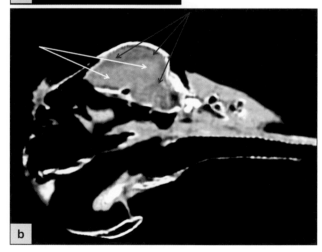

18.42 Computed tomography images of the head of a Moluccan Cockatoo performed using contrast medium. White arrows show brain areas with contrast medium; red arrows show areas without contrast medium. **(a)** Ventrodorsal and **(b)** laterolateral views.

- The anaesthetic machine cannot be located inside the MRI room and stays outside; this implies a huge dead space in the anaesthetic circuit, and subsequent problems with monitoring the anaesthetized bird for a fairly long time.

For these reasons, contrast media have been used for CT scanning of the central nervous system in birds (Figure 18.42). This technique offers undoubted advantages:

- It is a shorter procedure
- There are no limitations where metal objects are concerned
- The patient can be easily monitored during anaesthesia
- The anaesthetic machine can stay near the bird.

References and further reading

Baumel JJ, King AS, Breazile JE, Evans EE and Vanden Berge JC (1993) *Handbook of Avian Anatomy: Nomina Anatomica Avium, 2nd edn*. Nuttall Ornithological Club, Cambridge

Beaufrères H, Pariaut R, Rodriguez D and Tully TN (2010) Avian vascular imaging: A review. *Journal of Avian Medicine and Surgery* **24(3)**, 174–184

Campbell T (1994) Cytology. In: *Avian Medicine, Principles and Applications*, ed. BW Ritchie, GJ Harrison and LR Harrison. Wingers, Lake Worth

Harcourt-Brown NH (1996) Radiology. In: *BSAVA Manual of Raptors, Pigeons and Waterfowl*, ed. PH Beynon, NA Forbes and NH Harcourt-Brown, p. 92. BSAVA Publications, Gloucester

Helmer P (2006) Advances in diagnostic imaging. In: *Clinical Avian Medicine*, ed. GJ Harrison and T Lightfoot, pp. 251–257. Spix Publishing, Palm Beach

Krautwald ME, Tellhelm B, Hummel G, Kostka G and Kaleta EF (1992) *Atlas of Radiographic Anatomy and Diagnosis of Cage Birds*. Paul Parey Scientific Publishers, New York

Krautwald-Junghanns ME and Trinkaus K (2000) Imaging techniques. In: *Handbook of Avian Medicine*, ed. TN Tully, MPC Lawton and GM Dorrestein, p. 53. Saunders Elsevier, St Louis

Krautwald-Junghanns ME, Pees M, Reese S and Tully T (2011) *Diagnostic Imaging of Exotic Pets*. Schlütersche, Hannover

Lennox AM, Crosta L and Buerkle M (2002) The effects of isoflurane anesthesia on gastrointestinal transit time. *Proceedings of the 23rd AAV Annual Conference*, California, pp. 53–55

Samour JH and Naldo JL (2007) *Anatomical and Clinical Radiology of Birds of Prey*. Saunders Elsevier, St Louis

Silverman S and Tell LA (2010) Radiology equipment and positioning techniques. In: *Radiology of Birds*, ed. S Silverman and LA Tell, pp. 1–16. Saunders, St Louis

Infectious diseases

Petra Zsivanovits

Biosecurity in the veterinary practice

When considering disease control, veterinary surgeons (veterinarians) need to reflect on three fundamental aspects: individual patient care; disease control within the facility; and avoiding the spread of disease from the facility to birds/patients in the outside world. Veterinary practices can be described as a source of infectious disease, due to the grouping of a large number of birds with potentially unknown history. The birds are often kept in a limited space with the potential for direct or indirect contact with each other. These are ideal conditions for the accumulation of pathogens and the transfer of infection between individuals. Furthermore, birds presented to veterinary surgeons are often young, old, debilitated or the victims of trauma, factors that add to the stress level of a bird, making it more prone to shedding pathogens. Chronic stress also abets immune suppression, rendering the birds more likely to develop disease after exposure to pathogens.

The transmission cycle can be interrupted by cleaning (removing particles) and disinfecting (destroying surface receptors on pathogens that allow binding to somatic cells, or destroying their nucleic acid) the environment, by quarantine of potentially diseased birds and by controlling modes of transfer (e.g. fomites, aerosol control, faecal–oral contact).

Disinfection is a fundamental element of disease control management, but it does not replace thorough hygiene protocols in preventing the spread of infectious disease. It is important to note that organic matter (soil, food, faeces, blood or mucus) can increase the survival time of pathogens by serving as a protective matrix. Therefore, thorough cleaning prior to any disinfection is absolutely crucial (Figure 19.1). The use of high-temperature programmes in dishwashers and washing machines is valuable as they combine washing with hot water and heat drying.

Disinfectants need to be in direct contact with the microorganism for a suitable period of time to be effective, but often in veterinary practices the contact time is only seconds (e.g. wiping tables). Pathogen-specific appropriate contact times need to be considered, and the surface needs to be soaked for the specified

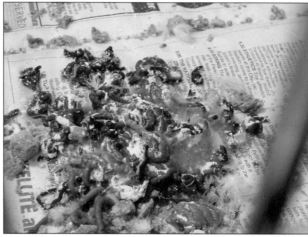

19.1 Dirty cages contaminated with leftover food, faeces, damp bedding and even fungal growth provide a great environment for pathogens, resulting in a high risk of infection. Thorough cleaning and removal of all organic matter is vital before considering disinfection.

period. Certain disinfectants can be corrosive and damage surfaces such as metals or plastic. Concentration of the disinfectant is also important, as some organisms require more concentrated exposure for effective inactivation. The variation in composition of the same active pharmaceutical ingredient in different brands can also alter its efficacy in killing pathogens.

Most failures of disinfectants are related to improper use (Ritchie, 1995; Kroker, 1997). Repeated exposure to inadequate disinfection can result in the development of resistance; therefore, the manufacturer's recommendations should always be followed carefully. Any disinfectant (including its fumes) that destroys microorganisms can present a potential health hazard to staff or birds via frequent exposure. Figures 19.2 and 19.3 show an overview of commonly used disinfectants.

Spread of disease can occur by multiple methods, such as direct contact (bird to bird, human to bird), mechanical vectors/fomites and aerosol (feather or faecal dust being transported by air). Direct contact with the potential transfer of mucus, nasal or ocular discharge, blood or faeces is an obvious way of transferring disease. Frequently washing one's hands with a soap containing a detergent followed by using a hand

Infectious agent	Specific pathogen	Disinfectants
Bacteria	Including *Chlamydia* and *Mycoplasma* spp.	■ Alcohol/ethanol 70% ■ Aldehyde/glutaraldehyde/formaldehyde ■ Phenol/cresol derivatives ■ Detergents (synthetic) ■ Halogens (iodine, chlorine) ■ Chlorinated compounds (bleach) ■ Quaternary ammonium derivatives ■ Guanidine derivatives (chlorhexidine) ■ Peracetic acid
	Mycobacterium spp.	■ Aldehyde/glutaraldehyde/formaldehyde ■ Phenol/cresol derivatives
Enveloped viruses	Herpesviridae, Coronaviridae, Flaviviridae, Orthomyxoviridae, Poxviridae, Paramyxoviridae, Togaviridae, Rhabdoviridae	■ Alcohol/ethanol 70% ■ Aldehyde/glutaraldehyde/formaldehyde ■ Phenol/cresol derivatives ■ Halogens (iodine, chlorine) ■ Chlorinated compounds (bleach) ■ Quaternary ammonium derivatives; ■ Guanidine derivatives (chlorhexidine) ■ Peracetic acid
Non-enveloped viruses	Adenoviridae, Birnaviridae, Circoviridae, Papovaviridae, Picornaviridae, Reoviridae	■ Aldehyde/glutaraldehyde/formaldehyde ■ Phenol/cresol derivatives ■ Quaternary ammonium derivatives ■ Peracetic acid
Fungi/yeasts	*Macrorhabdus ornithogaster*, *Aspergillus* spp., *Candida* spp.	■ Aldehyde/glutaraldehyde/formaldehyde ■ Peracetic acid ■ Detergents (synthetic) ■ Halogens (iodine, chlorine) ■ Chlorinated compounds (bleach) ■ Guanidine derivatives (chlorhexidine)
Parasites	Protozoa, nematodes, cestodes, trematodes, coccidia	■ Phenol/cresol derivatives ■ Alcohol ■ Perchloroethylene carbon disulphide

19.2 A list of disinfectants that can be used for different infectious agents (DVG (German Veterinary Medicine Society) list of disinfectants; Kroker, 1997). Concentration as well as contact time alter the efficacy of the disinfectant to inactivate different pathogens, therefore the directions for use provided for each product need to be followed.

Disinfectant	Mode of action	Indication	Notes
Alcohol/ethanol 70%	Protein denaturation	Skin, hands, instrumentation, surfaces	Can dissolve rubber or plastic; fumes can be irritating to eyes/mucous membranes
Aldehyde/glutaraldehyde/ formaldehyde	Reaction with free amino groups of proteins	Surfaces, rooms, instrumentation	Irritation to eyes, respiratory tract and skin; some are corrosive to metal
Phenol/cresol derivatives	Protein denaturation, damage to cell membrane	Skin, rooms, surfaces, instrumentation, faeces	Can be irritating to skin, eyes and respiratory tract; need sufficient ventilation and rinsing/drying
Detergents/soap (synthetic)	Reduces attraction of dirt or grease to an object, damage to cell membrane	Skin, hands, equipment (bowls, perches etc.)	Can be irritating to eyes
Halogens (iodine, chlorine)	Inhibition of enzymes, oxidization	Faeces, water (chlorine), skin (iodine)	Iodine can cause irritation to skin; allergic reactions
Chlorinated compounds (bleach)	Oxidization	Surfaces (1:32 dilution)	Solution and fumes are irritating to tissue/mucous membranes; corrosive to metals; need thorough ventilation and rinsing/drying
Guanidine derivatives (chlorhexidine 0.1–0.2%)	Damage to cell membrane	Skin, preoperative	Relatively non-toxic and non-corrosive
Quaternary ammonium derivatives	Damage to cell membrane	Surfaces, rooms	Need ventilation and rinsing/drying; can be toxic when ingested
Peracetic acid (1%)	Oxidization	Surfaces, instrumentation	Irritating to eyes, skin, mucous membranes; at higher concentrations or temperatures can be explosive

19.3 Indications and modes of action for commonly used disinfectants (DVG (German Veterinary Medicine Society) list of disinfectants; Kroker, 1997).

disinfectant is the best way to reduce mechanical vector transfer by veterinary staff (Figure 19.4). At minimum, a water-free hand sanitizer should be used. Again, all contact matter must be removed if disinfection is to be effective. It is crucial to clean and disinfect hands between each patient, and working 'from less infectious patients to more infectious patients' is useful.

Non-medical fomites present another very important mode of transfer of pathogens. Any items travelling between birds can serve as fomites; therefore, cages and any equipment used (bowls, towels, nets, toys, perches, containers, weighing scales, feeding dishes and medical instrumentation) must be thoroughly cleaned and disinfected. Cages and food and water containers need to be cleaned at least daily. Using towels, paper or newspaper on the bottom of the cage allows easy, hygienic and inexpensive removal of faeces and seed husks. Wrapping perches with disposable bandage material will pad them as well as facilitate the removal of organic material (faeces, vomit) that is stuck to the bandages, instead of the perch itself. The level of cleaning must be balanced against the level of disturbance that it creates. Often, it is advantageous to work in a two-person system, with one handling the patient while the other is cleaning and disinfecting the cage and environment. It is important to use individual towels for handling each bird, as well as individual cleaning and feeding tools (sponges, dishes, crop tubes, etc.) for each patient. Disposable paper towels should be used for drying hands as well as for wiping working surfaces when cleaning and disinfecting.

Separation of individuals functions adequately in respect of ecto- and endoparasite management, but it cannot control airborne diseases. Pathogens can travel via air either with dust particles or incorporated in minuscule droplets of liquid from sneezes or coughs. Everyone in a veterinary practice must be aware that by having multiple birds with questionable health status in one facility, there is a risk of disease transfer. An

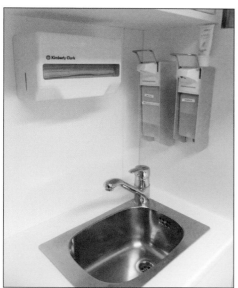

19.4 Spreading disease by handling different patients is an obvious risk, particularly in a veterinary practice. This threat can be minimized by using a detergent soap as well as a hand disinfectant to wash hands between patients. Hands-free dispensers as well as disposable paper towels are recommended next to every sink, not only those in the operating theatre.

isolation ward, with minimal traffic to or from the main hospital, is essential in any avian practice. Providing overalls, scrubs and overshoes that remain within the isolation ward should be considered. Isolation for infectious birds as the first line of defence is a fundamental and vital concept in disease control. Birds from different owners must not be mixed in one enclosure or, for example, be allowed to play on a free-standing playground together. Infectious birds must be kept in isolation.

A veterinary practice must only offer boarding of birds if the boarding unit is completely separated from the hospital unit and/or the clients are well educated about the potential exposure to infectious diseases. Owners can carry infectious agents on their skin, hair or clothing. If allowed to visit inpatients or enter particularly hazardous areas, such as the operating theatre, these agents can be spread around. If visitation is favoured, then a separate visitation room, that can be easily cleaned and disinfected, should be provided.

An avian veterinary surgeon should not consult different flocks of birds on the same day, unless showering and a change of clothes or use of protective clothing is ensured. Within a practice environment, most clinicians will change their clothes after handling a suspected infectious bird.

There is a smaller risk of a disease outbreak in a clean and not overcrowded environment. This starts in the waiting room area of each clinic; avoid having lots of patients with unknown history waiting together by having an organized appointment system (see Chapter 7).

Controlling the transmission of pathogens is important not only to avoid spreading disease from one bird to another, but also to avoid transmission of disease to humans. Those working with birds must be educated about potential zoonotic diseases. Treating and handling infectious birds represents a risk, as does food preparation for raptors or the performance of post-mortem examinations. Zoonotic diseases of special interest include chlamydiosis, mycobacteriosis, salmonellosis, campylobacteriosis, cryptosporidiosis and viruses such as paramyxovirus or influenza A virus. Appropriate protective measures, including disinfection and the use of gloves and facemasks, should be taken, especially during post-mortem examinations.

Common pathogens in avian practice

Viruses

Circovirus

This virus, also called psittacine beak and feather disease (PBFD) virus, has numerous variants with no defined host specificity. Circovirus is found worldwide in captivity and also in free-ranging birds. Scattered accidental viral releases have occurred elsewhere. Circovirus strains that differ antigenically from the psittacine circovirus strain have been demonstrated in pigeons and canaries and seem to cause clinical signs in those species.

Clinical signs include feather dysplasia, haemorrhages in the feather, progressive feather loss and/or necrotic lesions to the beak (Figure 19.5). Necrosis of the bursa and thymus and damage to circulating

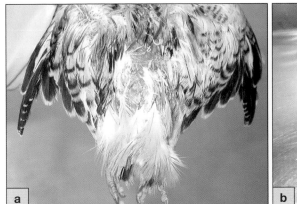
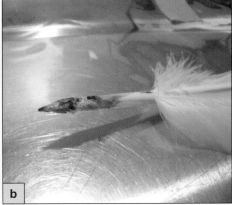
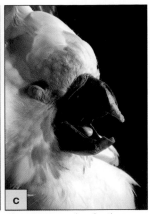

19.5 Birds affected with circovirus present with **(a)** feather dysplasia, **(b)** haemorrhages in the feather, progressive feather loss and/or **(c)** necrotic lesions to the beak. The clinical signs may progress with each moult, potentially resulting in completely featherless individuals. Other individuals, mainly those infected as adults, are able to eliminate the virus after a viraemic period. (b–c, © Deborah Monks)

white blood cells result in immunosuppression. Disease outbreaks are more likely in young birds. Adult birds that mount an antibody response can potentially process the virus without developing clinical disease. Lovebirds and Budgerigars, particularly, can be asymptomatically infected but still shed the virus.

Historically, disease was confirmed by biopsy of feather follicles and the demonstration of intranuclear and intracytoplasmic inclusion bodies. Diagnosis can also be made via polymerase chain reaction (PCR) testing of blood or feathers with cell material (freshly plucked blood feathers or newly grown feathers), ideally using assays that detect the conserved areas of viral genome common to all variants. PCR techniques designed for parrots seem to be unreliable for passerines. Birds that are not showing any clinical signs but are positive on PCR testing may represent transient subclinical infection, or be in the early stages of infection, assuming no sample contamination. These birds may mount an antibody response and become immune. In order to distinguish these birds, the PCR can be repeated after 90 days, or an antibody assay run (only available in certain countries). If the bird is negative on PCR after 90 days, or has a significant antibody response, then it is likely to be clearing the infection. Be aware that the bird may continue to shed the virus from viral feathers for some time after systemic clearance. Particularly in Budgerigars, disease due to circovirus needs to be differentiated from polyomavirus.

Disease transfer occurs directly through feather dust, faeces or crop secretions. The virus is very stable in the environment, therefore transmission via fomites plays an important role.

There is no reliable treatment for this disease. It is recommended that affected birds are separated, as long as quality of life is ensured. Parrots tend to deteriorate within 6–12 months after the onset of clinical signs. Affected Budgerigars or lovebirds can survive for years with this disease, although they are contagious, and quality of life must be monitored.

Circovirus is found in numerous psittacine species, particularly in cockatoos, Eclectus Parrots, Budgerigars, lories, Grey Parrots and lovebirds. Amazon parrots and macaws are rarely infected (Phalen, 2006b). Necrotic beak lesions are most often found in affected cockatoos. Infected juvenile Budgerigars less often have dystrophic feathers; feather loss of the primary and secondary wing feathers or tail feathers is a more common clinical sign in these birds. Juvenile Grey Parrots may show a particular form of disease, presenting with non-specific signs such as weakness, inability to stand, regurgitation, crop stasis and an extremely low white blood cell count. Prognosis in these birds is extremely poor. Circovirus infection is also described in canaries; nestlings show high morbidity and mortality with clinical signs such as a distended abdomen and an enlarged gall bladder.

Avian polyomavirus
Different strains of polyomavirus are thought to show some order specificity; for example, the canary variant is less likely to be infectious to parrots. Disease is typically seen in unweaned nestlings. Budgerigar nestlings have a high mortality rate, abnormal feather development, skin discoloration, abdominal distension and scattered haemorrhages (Figure 19.6). Survivors may show stunted primary and secondary wing feathers and tail feathers, and need to be differentiated from birds suffering from circovirus infection. In other psittacine nestlings, polyomavirus infection results most often in peracute death, although, occasionally, subcutaneous and subserosal haemorrhages and oedema can be found.

In Passeriformes, surviving fledglings might be left with long, tubular, misshapen beaks. Adult birds may process and clear the virus without showing clinical signs, although they are thought to be infectious within this time. If polyomavirus infection causes clinical signs and death in an adult bird, it is very likely that the bird has concurrent circovirus infection (Phalen, 2006b). Polyomavirus seems particularly problematic for Gouldian Finches.

PCR assays (on feathers with cell material, either freshly plucked blood feathers or newly grown feathers, or combined cloacal and choanal swabs) can detect infection and status of shedding. PCR techniques designed for parrots seem to be poorly reliable for passerines. Serology (virus neutralization antibody titres, ELISA) can determine if a bird has been infected in the past by production of a persistent antibody titre within 2 weeks of exposure. Histological examination will demonstrate intranuclear inclusion bodies, although these must be differentiated from adenovirus inclusion bodies.

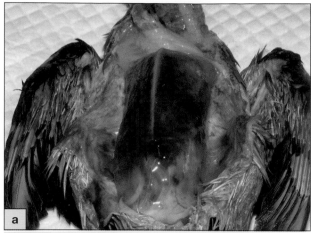

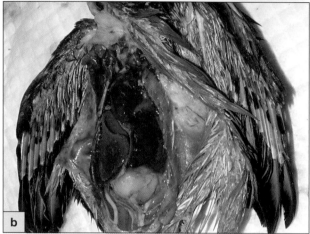

19.6 The clinical picture of polyomavirus differs depending on the species (Budgerigars *versus* non-Budgerigar psittacine birds) and the age (nestlings *versus* adult birds) of the birds affected. In nestlings, **(a)** abdominal distension and **(b)** scattered haemorrhages are the predominant clinical signs. Adult birds might be able to clear the virus without distinct clinical disease. (Courtesy of Robert J. Doneley)

Disease transfer occurs via direct contact via the respiratory route.

There is no reliable treatment for polyomavirus. Outbreaks can be controlled by ceasing breeding for at least 6 months, and removing all adult breeding birds from the facility for this period. Breeders of larger parrots should desist from breeding Budgerigars, Cockatiels and lovebirds as well or make use of a thorough quarantine and screening programme. There is a commercial vaccine for parrots available in the USA, but its protective potential against infection for parrots is controversial, and appears minimal in other groups such as Passeriformes (Sandmeier and Coutteel, 2006).

Polyomavirus is also reported to have been identified in a few buzzards and a falcon (Johne and Müller, 1998).

Paramyxovirus

Within the nine different serogroups of paramyxovirus (PMV) there are numerous strains of differing pathogenicity. PMV-1 occurs in the velogenic viscerotropic form, causing haemorrhagic lesions in the digestive tract, and the velogenic neurotropic form, causing respiratory and neurological signs. PMV-2 has been demonstrated in passerines; clinical signs are mainly mild and the disease is self-limiting. PMV-3 has been demonstrated in various parrots and passerines, particularly African and Australian finches. These birds show neurological signs as well as conjunctivitis, dysphagia, diarrhoea or voluminous starchy faeces consistent with chronic pancreatitis (see Appendix 4).

Diagnosis is made by virus isolation or serology. Histological examination will demonstrate intranuclear and intracytoplasmic inclusion bodies.

Disease transfer occurs through shedding via faeces and respiratory secretions.

The use of vaccines designed for poultry in pet birds is largely debated. There are reports of the successful vaccination of raptors. The best prophylaxis is strict quarantine and screening. In many countries, PMV-1 is notifiable.

Psittacine herpesvirus

Herpesviruses are responsible for two different diseases in parrots: Pacheco's disease and internal papillomatosis (Figure 19.7). These viruses belong to the alpha-herpesviruses and have five different genotypes and, accordingly, serotypes. Disease development depends on the viral serotype and the species of bird infected.

The most common clinical sign of Pacheco's disease is acute death within hours to a few days. Infrequently, there might be lethargy, anorexia, biliverdinuria, regurgitation, haemorrhagic diarrhoea or neurological signs. Survival rate after the development of clinical signs is very low.

Internal papillomatosis is usually noticed because of blood in the bird's faeces or around its cloaca, or the papilloma may be prolapsed. Papillomatous lesions can occur anywhere in the intestinal tract. Cloacal papillomatous lesions are most common, but oral papillomas also occur, particularly in macaws. If the proventriculus or ventriculus is affected, the bird may show regurgitation. Lesions vary from mild with merely a roughening and/or thickening of the mucosa to severe proliferations. The lesions can change in appearance and can even disappear entirely. A moderate number of birds suffering from internal papillomatosis can develop bile duct or pancreatic carcinomas.

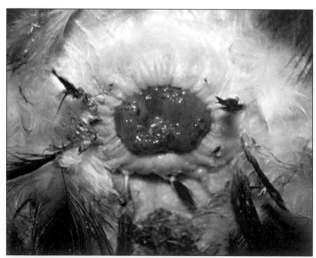

19.7 Internal papillomatosis is caused by psittacine herpesvirus and mainly presents as papillomatous lesions protruding from the cloaca. Oral papillomas may also occur. Approaches to permanently surgically remove these papillomas from the cloacal mucous membranes proved to be of no avail. (Courtesy of Robert J. Doneley)

Herpesvirus can be detected via PCR testing of blood and combined choanal and cloacal swabs. Histological examination will show typical intranuclear inclusion bodies in the liver and spleen of birds with Pacheco's disease. Persistent infection can occur, most often in macaws, Amazons and some conures, particularly the Patagonian Conure. Internal papillomatosis is best diagnosed by biopsy and histological demonstration of typical papillomatous changes.

Disease transfer takes place through direct contact with contaminated oral or conjunctival exudates, vomit or faeces.

The effect of aciclovir in diseased birds is questionable, but prophylactic administration of this drug in the face of an outbreak of Pacheco's disease has proven useful (Phalen, 2006b). Birds affected with internal papillomatosis do not respond to anti-herpesviral therapy. Following principles of biosecurity and disease transfer control is crucial. Several approaches to removing cloacal papillomas have been described, including cryotherapy, electrocautery, chemical cautery, laser surgery and sharp dissection. Often, any remaining parts of the papillomas will regress, but they may also return. The risk of stricture formation with surgery needs to be considered.

Among psittacine birds, macaws, Amazons and conures are particularly susceptible, but other species can also develop Pacheco's disease. Internal papillomatosis has been demonstrated in macaws, Amazons, Hawk-headed Parrots and conures (Phalen, 2006b).

There are three different serotypes of herpesvirus affecting raptors. Diseased birds show a short period of depression, anorexia and biliverdinuria prior to death. There might also be neurological signs such as tremors or seizures. Disease transfer is mostly through the ingestion of infected pigeons. There are reports of successful treatment of this infection in raptors with aciclovir injections but, in general, the prognosis for recovery is poor.

Bornavirus

This virus is regarded as the aetiological agent of proventricular dilatation disease (PDD), which is also thought to be associated with autoimmune reactions. To date, nine genotypes have been identified and infection has been demonstrated in various psittacine species, waterfowl and canaries. There is a gastrointestinal form with wasting, diarrhoea, polyuria or regurgitation and a neurological form with ataxia or tremors, as well as a mixed form. The incubation period can last several years.

There are numerous differential diagnoses for bornavirus, including foreign bodies, neoplasia, parasites, bacterial or fungal gastric infections, heavy metal poisoning and internal papillomatosis. A suggestive diagnosis can be established by demonstration of gastrointestinal dilatation and poor motility (especially of the proventriculus) via radiography, contrast radiography or fluoroscopy (Figure 19.8). Histological demonstration of lymphocytic/plasmacytic infiltrations in the nerves of gastrointestinal organs, adrenal glands or the brain confirms the diagnosis, but the false-negative rate of crop biopsy can be up to 30%, and taking biopsy samples from more sensitive sites (such as the pancreas or ventriculus) has a much higher risk of complications.

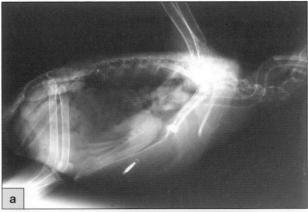
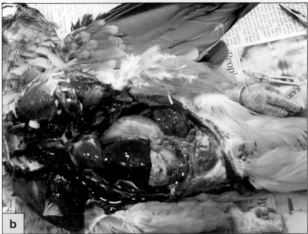

19.8 Proventricular dilatation disease (PDD) has been a concern for many years and is now thought to involve bornavirus as the aetiological agent. Clinical signs vary, including weight loss, regurgitation, polydipsia, polyuria and, in progressed cases, there is often an obviously dilated proventriculus on **(a)** radiography or **(b)** post-mortem examination. The histological proof for this disease is cytoplasmic infiltrations in the nerve plexi of the gastrointestinal tract.

PCR tests, as well as serological immunofluorescent tests, have been developed to identify bornavirus. There is a strong correlation between birds showing clinical signs and being positive on PCR and serology, but some birds with no clinical signs still test positive on serology. Full understanding of the incubation period, pathophysiology and progression to clinical disease is still lacking. Currently there is no reliable treatment for this disease. COX-2 specific inhibitors, such as celecoxib, seem to slow down the clinical process, mainly in the gastrointestinal form. Attempts to treat using antiviral drugs or immunosuppressive drugs, such as ciclosporin, have had varying success. Affected birds should be isolated and their quality of life monitored.

Poxvirus

There are multiple types of poxviruses that show a more or less strict host specificity. There are three clinical pictures.

- The dry or cutaneous form produces raised nodular lesions, mainly in featherless areas around the face or feet. The lesions vary from small and clinically insignificant to extensive neoplasia-like proliferations. They develop from papules to vesicles that burst and form crusts. Often they can ulcerate, and there might be secondary bacterial or fungal infections. This form is mostly self-limiting within several weeks, but it often results in permanent damage to the beak, nostrils or conchal structures, the loss of digital function due to avascular necrosis of digital tendons or the loss of talons due to distal necrosis. Latent infections can occur.

- The wet (mucosal or diphtheroid) form shows diphtheritic lesions in the oral cavity, nasal cavity or trachea. In canaries, there is conjunctivitis, blepharitis and chemosis.
- The systemic or septicaemic form is predominantly seen in canaries and is characterized by chemosis, depression, anorexia or dyspnoea and death within days. Typically there are no respiratory sounds with this form of dyspnoea. Surviving birds can develop cutaneous lesions.

Diagnosis is made using a biopsy sample and histological demonstration of eosinophilic intracytoplasmic inclusion bodies (Bollinger bodies). Disease transfer occurs from direct contact with contaminated exudate or via mosquitoes or red mites as vectors. The virus cannot penetrate intact epithelium, therefore minor trauma, caused by abrasions, picking or parasites, has to be present to facilitate infection.

Treatment consists of supportive care, vitamin A and C supplementation, drying out the lesions with glycerol or iodine–alcohol-based tinctures, and the treatment of secondary infections. There are vaccines available for canaries, poultry and pigeons. Attempts to use these vaccines for other than the designated species have yielded questionable to devastating effects. The use of vaccination in the face of a disease outbreak is controversial, as handling might introduce abrasions to the skin and amplify infection, and there might be the risk of recombination of the vaccine and field virus. Insect vector control is crucial.

Parasites

Parasitic burdens and associated disease are important in avian practice (Figures 19.9, 19.10, 19.11 and 19.12). For further information on treatment refer to appropriate therapeutic formularies (e.g. Meredith, 2015).

Organism	Properties	Host range	Clinical signs	Disease transfer	Diagnosis	Treatment
Lice	Host-specific; spend entire lifecycle on host, short survival time in environment	Occasionally Passeriformes	Often asymptomatic; irritation and feather damage may be seen	Direct contact; wild birds	Clinical examination	Pyrethrin weekly, at least three times
Diptera insects	Blood-sucking; disease vectors	Passeriformes; raptors	Anaemia; dermatitis; irritation	Environmental; direct contact; wild birds	Clinical examination	Pyrethrin; mosquito-proof enclosures; manual removal of larvae
Ticks	Blood-sucking; disease vectors	Raptors; occasionally Passeriformes and Psittaciformes	Anaemia; dermatitis; irritation	Environmental	Clinical examination	Fipronil; disinfection of environment; removal of parasites
Mites						
Red mites (*Dermanyssus gallinae*)	Non-host-specific; blood-sucking; disease vectors; long survival time in environment; on birds during the night	Passeriformes	Feather damage; anaemia; irritation during the night	Environmental; direct contact; wild birds	Clinical examination; white cloth over cage	Pyrethroids/piperonyl butoxide; permethrin; carbaryl powder; fipronil; treatment of environment very important, weekly, at least three times
Feather mites	Host- and site-specific; generally spend entire lifecycle on host	All species	Occasional feather damage; irritation if large numbers, which may also indicate host debility	Direct contact	Clinical examination	Pyrethrin weekly, at least three times; fipronil
Cnemidocoptes mutans, C. pilae (see Figure 19.10)	Long incubation; birds are often asymptomatic carriers	Wide, particularly Budgerigars and Galliformes	Scabs with bore holes to the cere, skin around the eyes or legs; hyperkeratosis	Environmental; direct contact	Clinical examination	Ivermectin/moxidectin weekly, at least three times
Sternostoma tracheacolum	Can be difficult to diagnose and treat	Particularly Passeriformes	Dyspnoea; respiratory tract infection; coughing; gasping; head shaking; loss of voice	Direct contact	Post-mortem examination; transillumination	Ivermectin/doramectin weekly, at least three times; pyrethrin via aerosol
Protozoa						
Trichomonas spp. (see Figure 19.11)	Single-cell organisms; no cyst form	Psittaciformes, particularly Budgerigars; raptors; Passeriformes	Yellow caseous lesions in oropharynx/upper digestive or respiratory tract; dyspnoea; gagging; sinusitis	Direct contact; ingestion of diseased quarry, food or water	Microscopic examination of swab	Dimetridazole; metronidazole; ronidazole; carnidazole; water hygiene

19.9 Parasites commonly found in birds. For further information on treatment refer to appropriate therapeutic formularies. (continues)

Organism	Properties	Host range	Clinical signs	Disease transfer	Diagnosis	Treatment
Protozoa continued						
Giardia spp.	Cyst forms excreted via faeces; survival time outside host 3 weeks	Psittaciformes; Passeriformes; raptors	Diarrhoea; weight loss	Direct contact; contaminated food/faeces	Faecal flotation; intermittent shedding	Dimetridazole; metronidazole; environmental hygiene
Cochlosoma spp.	Asymptomatic in Society Finches	Particularly in young Passeriformes	Diarrhoea; dehydration; death	Direct contact with faeces	Faecal flotation	Ronidazole; dimetridazole; metronidazole
Caryospora, Eimeria spp.	Lifecycle in host (sexual and asexual) and the environment; many intracellular; long survival in environment; some carriers asymptomatic	Particularly in young raptors and Passeriformes	Diarrhoea, often haemorrhagic; inappetence; depression; abdominal distension	Direct contact; contaminated food/water/ faeces	Faecal flotation	Toltrazuril; sulphonamides; environmental hygiene
Atoxoplasma spp.	Asexual lifecycle in liver, lung, spleen or heart	Particularly in young raptors and Passeriformes	Diarrhoea; debilitation; inappetence; hepatomegaly	Direct contact; contaminated food/water/ faeces	Intermittent shedding; post-mortem examination/ impression smear	Toltrazuril; sulphonamides; environmental hygiene
Isospora spp.	Sexual and asexual lifecycle in intestines	Particularly in young canaries	Diarrhoea; weight loss	Direct contact; contaminated food/water/ faeces	Intermittent shedding; post-mortem examination/ impression smear	Toltrazuril; sulphonamides; environmental hygiene
Sarcocystis spp.	Sexual lifecycle in intestines of definitive host (opossum); asexual lifecycle in musculature of intermediate host (birds, cockroaches, rats, flies)	Psittaciformes, Passeriformes	Mostly asymptomatic; sometimes dyspnoea	Digestion of diseased prey; contaminated faeces	Post-mortem examination with cysts in musculature	Trimethoprim; sulphadiazine
Helminths						
Nematodes (roundworms), especially *Ascaridia* spp. (see Figure 19.12)	Worms vary in size and organ systems affected; some require intermediate host. Potential endotoxicosis or intestinal obstruction with treatment, particularly in Budgerigars	Psittaciformes, raptors; less common in Passeriformes	Diarrhoea; debilitation; weight loss; partly asymptomatic	Ingestion of intermediate host; contaminated faeces/water	Faecal flotation	Fenbendazole; ivermectin; moxidectin; levamisole; mebendazole; flubendazole
Capillaria spp.	Earthworm is potential intermediate host	Psittaciformes, raptors; less common in Passeriformes	Affect oesophagus, crop, intestines: diarrhoea, partly yellowish scales in oropharynx; weight loss; regurgitation	Ingestion of intermediate host; contaminated faeces/water	Faecal flotation; microscopic examination of oral/crop swab	Fenbendazole; ivermectin; moxidectin; levamisole; mebendazole; flubendazole
Trichostrongylids	Can cause severe pathology	Psittaciformes, raptors; less common in Passeriformes	Affect oesophagus, crop, intestines: poor condition	Ingestion of intermediate host; contaminated faeces/water	Faecal flotation; post-mortem examination	Fenbendazole; ivermectin; moxidectin; levamisole; mebendazole; flubendazole
Dispharynx, Spiroptera spp.	Can cause severe pathology	Psittaciformes, raptors; less common in Passeriformes	Affect proventriculus: weight loss	Ingestion of intermediate host; contaminated faeces/water	Post-mortem examination	Fenbendazole; ivermectin; moxidectin; levamisole; mebendazole; flubendazole
Syngamus trachea	Lifecycle direct, but earthworm as transport host	Psittaciformes, raptors; less common in Passeriformes	Affect respiratory tract: dyspnoea; coughing; gasping; head shaking	Ingestion of intermediate host; contaminated faeces/water	Faecal flotation; microscopic examination of crop swab; transillumination	Fenbendazole; ivermectin; moxidectin; levamisole; mebendazole; flubendazole

19.9 (continued) Parasites commonly found in birds. For further information on treatment refer to appropriate therapeutic formularies.

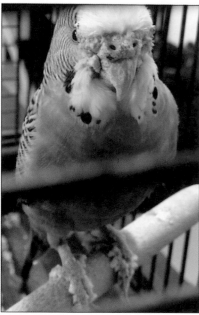

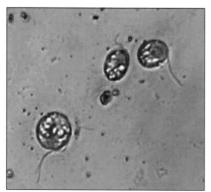

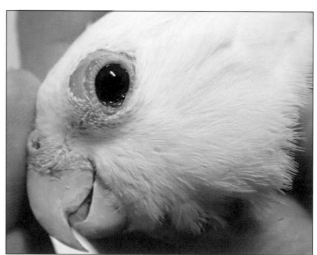

Bacteria

Chlamydia psittaci

Chlamydia psittaci is a bacterial pathogen with an intracellular lifecycle, replicating mainly in white blood cells. Two stages are differentiated: reticulate bodies and elementary bodies, with the former representing the form within cells and the latter the extracellular stage. It is important to appreciate that the reticulate bodies enable infection and active disease, and therefore are susceptible to antibiotics. The non-active, elementary bodies do not respond to antibiotic prophylactic treatment.

Clinical signs of chlamydiosis vary considerably from mild to severe multisystemic disease and include ocular (Figure 19.13), nasal or conjunctival inflammation and discharge, respiratory distress, anorexia, biliverdinuria, diarrhoea, polydipsia and lethargy. Often, clinical signs are associated with hepatomegaly, splenomegaly, leucocytosis, monocytosis and heterophilia. The differential haemogram is consistent with chronic inflammatory diseases, and therefore not pathognomonic for *Chlamydia* infection.

On pathology, organ tissue (liver and spleen) can be stained with Stamp or Macchiavello stain to show the specific elementary bodies in the cytoplasm. There are antibody tests (direct complement fixation, screening

19.10 *Cnemidocoptes* mites are not restricted to poultry and pigeons; they are also found in Passeriformes and parrots, particularly in Budgerigars. The birds develop typical lesions with bore holes over the cere, around the beak or on the feet. As only the larval state can be eliminated by treatment, it is crucial to repeat the applications weekly as long as lesions are visible.

19.11 *Trichomonas* spp. are flagellated single-celled organisms that manifest themselves in the oropharynx and/or crop of birds. This sample is from a crop wash from a budgerigar. There is no species specificity. The organism is diagnosed via wet mount examination of crop smears by identification of their circulating movements. In order to maintain the live organism it is important to perform the examination straight after swabbing the crop and to provide a warm environment (using warm water and warmed slides). (© John Chitty)

19.13 Conjunctivitis is only one clinical sign of psittacosis. Some affected birds show rhinitis, diarrhoea or are simply 'off colour'. This airborne disease needs to be considered when birds from different backgrounds are kept in close proximity. Furthermore, the zoonotic potential of this disease needs to be taken into account. This is a mild conjunctivitis in a Cockatiel, with subtle swelling and erythema and is not pathognomonic of psittacosis.

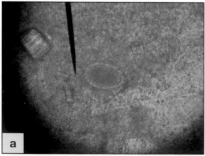
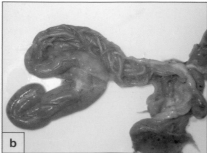
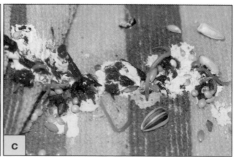

19.12 **(a)** Ascarides are not species-specific and can cause serious disease, particularly in small birds such as passerines or Budgerigars. **(b)** If during treatment too many worms die off at the same time, there is the risk of endotoxicosis or an intestinal ileus. Controlled and carefully dosed treatment allows the bird to excrete the dead worms. **(c)** The need for regular microscopic faecal examinations should be self-evident in open-roofed aviaries.

for IgM; elementary body agglutination, screening for IgG) and antigen tests (ELISA, immunofluorescent antibody test, PCR amplification technology). These tests are carried out on blood, choanal/conjunctival/cloacal swabs or organ tissue. The time from infection to a positive confirmation via testing differs with the test used: 5–15 days with PCR and up to 21 days for serology. A disadvantage of the complement fixation test is that it tends to stay positive for an extended period after treatment. If the birds are treated with an antibiotic such as enrofloxacin, azithromycin or doxycycline, the antigen and PCR testing is prone to giving false-negative results (Phalen, 2006c).

Disease transfer takes place through direct contact, fomites or aerosol. Organisms can be found in nasal discharge, faeces, ocular discharge, crop contents or crop milk. The incubation period is said to be 2 weeks. However, there are many anecdotal reports of more prolonged incubation periods. Any sick parrot that has been in the same air space as another parrot of unknown history within a year should be viewed with caution.

The treatment of choice is doxycycline. Drugs can be given orally on a daily basis or via intramuscular injection on a weekly basis, dependent on the bird's response to handling; off-label weekly depot injections are often required to minimize stress. In Passeriformes, treatment via drinking water, ideally combined with treatment in soft food, has been shown to be effective. The treatment should cover a 45-day period (although there are reports of successful outcomes after 21 days (Tully, 2006)). It is said that after the first 48 hours of treatment the birds stop shedding infectious pathogens. If recognized and treated thoroughly (ensuring that all in-contact birds are treated and that each bird receives its proper dosage for long enough), the disease can be controlled even in bigger collections.

Chlamydia infections affect a range of bird species, including parrots, raptors, finches and pigeons. Cockatiels and Budgerigars can be infected and can spread this bacterium without showing clinical signs of disease. Passeriformes show less specific clinical signs such as apathy, diarrhoea, and nasal and ocular discharge. They seem to be less susceptible than Psittaciformes. Raptors demonstrate nonspecific clinical signs such as 'being off colour', sinusitis, conjunctivitis, biliverdinuria, leucocytosis and sometimes splenomegaly. Clinical disease is rarely recognized in raptors.

The zoonotic potential of this disease needs to be taken into account. If a *Chlamydia* infection in humans remains undiagnosed or inappropriately treated, it can result in very severe health problems or even death.

Other bacteria

Diagnosis of bacterial disease (Figures 19.14, 19.15 and 19.16) is usually made by bacteriological culture of tissue samples or swabs. In most cases, disease transfer takes place through direct contact with nasal/ocular discharge, crop milk or faeces, or by fomites. Treatment is based on antibiotic therapy depending on sensitivity, as well as thorough hygiene protocols. Host ranges are usually wide, including passerines, psittacine birds and raptors.

Yeast

Macrorhabdus ornithogaster

Historically, classification of *Macrorhabdus ornithogaster* (Figure 19.17) was difficult due to the organism's strange staining and growth characteristics. Initially it was thought to be a Gram-positive bacterium, hence the well-known name Megabacterium. However, it has been proven that the organism is in fact a yeast, based on ribosomal DNA sequencing (Tomaszewski et al., 2003).

The clinical picture of *M. ornithogaster* infection can vary considerably. Some birds can be infected but not show any clinical signs. Others develop severe clinical disease with rapid deterioration leading to death. Some birds respond well to treatment, others are refractory. Some birds relapse frequently, others maintain good health after treatment for prolonged periods of time. These different clinical pictures might be the result of a combination of different strains of *M. ornithogaster* with different pathogenicities, different susceptibility of bird species to the organism or further influencing factors such as a compromised immune system of the individual. The clinical signs vary from 'sick bird, fluffed up and off colour' to diarrhoea, with or without melaena, and sometimes with undigested seed, or retching and/or vomiting. Most birds maintain a good appetite but lose weight.

Shedding of the organism can be intermittent, so detection via examination of a faecal wet mount has variable success. Multiple faecal examinations may be necessary, although most clinically diseased birds shed copiously. A more reliable diagnostic tool is a proventricular scraping or flush, but this is not practical in normal clinical practice (Phalen, 2006a).

On post-mortem examination affected birds show a loss of body condition as well as a dilated proventriculus and/or isthmus. There may be evidence of ulceration and inflammation of the gastric mucosa and thick mucus covering these areas. In advanced cases, proventricular and intestinal dilatation is severe enough to be detected radiographically. Undigested seeds and mucus contribute to filling defects on contrast studies.

Disease transfer takes place through direct contact or fomites; the organism is shed in faeces and regurgitated material.

To date, the only effective treatment is amphotericin B orally twice daily for at least 3–4 weeks. Other antifungal drugs are either ineffective or can be toxic to some species (especially Budgerigars). During treatment, extensive cleaning and high hygiene standards are essential. The treatment of infected flocks of birds can be challenging. Ideally, every bird should be treated individually but this is often not practicable. The pharmaceutical form of amphotericin B available in most countries is not water soluble, and in-water treatment for parrots is questionable in general. Numerous additives in food and water (e.g. acidification) have been tried and there are anecdotal reports of successful treatment but no scientific evidence of efficacy thus far.

M. ornithogaster is distributed worldwide and affects a wide host range, including canaries, finches, Budgerigars, Cockatiels, parrotlets and lovebirds and, as well as ostriches, chickens, turkeys, geese and ducks (Phalen, 2006a).

Pathogen	Properties	Host range	Clinical signs	Diagnosis	Disease transfer	Treatment and prevention
Enterobacteriaceae, *Escherichia coli*	Multiple subspecies with differing pathogenicity due to enterotoxins; virulent strains can penetrate intestinal mucosa, non-virulent strains need predisposing lesion; for environmental and/or less virulent strains, it is important to look for underlying causes	Passeriformes	Localized enteritis; rhinitis; polyserositis; salpingoperitonitis; septicaemia – secondary colonization of joints and bone marrow; coligranulomatosis – granulomas in liver, intestinal subserosa, spleen, kidney or skin; to be differentiated from mycobacteriosis	Bacteriological culture of tissue samples/swabs	Poor hygiene, overcrowding, stress factors, nutritional deficiencies, concomitant infections contribute to disease outbreak; environmental contamination often origin of infection	Antibiotic therapy based on sensitivity; hygiene measures
Salmonella spp.	Five subgenera, with subgenus 1 most relevant for birds; production of endotoxins; zoonotic potential	Passeriformes, occasionally Psittaciformes or raptors, some asymptomatic	Acute: lethargy; anorexia; polydipsia. Chronic: central nervous system signs; arthritis; dyspnoea (depending on organ system affected); septicaemia. Grey Parrots: phlegmon; granulomatous dermatitis; arthritis; tendovaginitis. Finches: granulomatous ingluvitis with or without liver and spleen involvement (differentiate from mycobacteria or *Yersinia pseudotuberculosis*)	Serology, but diagnosis is difficult in chronic cases	Aerogenic via faeces, feather dust; vermin as vectors; egg transmission	Antibiotic therapy based on sensitivity; hygiene measures, particularly vermin control and proper food storage
Klebsiella pneumoniae, *K. oxytoca*	Primary or opportunistic with immunosuppression	Psittaciformes; Passeriformes; raptors	Systemic: bacteraemia with renal failure; pulmonary infections. Local infections: sinuses, skin, crop, oral cavity	Bacteriological culture of tissue samples/swabs	Direct contact	Antibiotic therapy based on sensitivity; hygiene measures
Yersinia pseudotuberculosis (see Figure 19.15)	Grows at low temperatures; vermin as vectors; zoonotic potential	Particularly Passeriformes; less so Psittaciformes	Peracute death. Acute: lethargy; diarrhoea; dyspnoea. Chronic: emaciation; flaccid paresis or paralysis	Post-mortem examination: miliary demarcated foci in liver, lungs, spleen, kidneys; in chronic cases progression to granulomas (in combination with Gram-negative coccoid rods on cytology); culture is challenging	Rodents as vectors; free-ranging birds as reservoir	Mostly commonly post-mortem diagnosis. In chronic cases bacteria are encapsulated in granulomas and difficult to treat: enrofloxacin; vermin control; proper food storage. If seen acutely, then treat non-specific signs of severe systemic illness
Pseudomonas aeruginosa, *Aeromonas hydrophila*	Produces extracellular toxins	Occasionally Psittaciformes or raptors	Septicaemia – diarrhoea, dyspnoea, death; oedematous/necrotizing skin lesions; rhinitis, sinusitits, laryngitis; catarrhal to haemorrhagic enteritis. Psittaciformes – upper respiratory tract. Raptors – stomatitis with caseous nodules (sequel to trichomonosis)	Bacteriological culture of tissue samples/swabs	Contaminated water; misting bottles; poorly prepared sprouted seeds	Antibiotic therapy based on sensitivity; hygiene measures; remove waterfowl from affected areas
Campylobacter jejuni	Birds may be symptomatic; often immunocompromised birds; zoonotic potential	Wide	Hepatitis – lethargy, anorexia, diarrhoea, biliverdinuria; catarrhal to haemorrhagic enteritis	Bacteriological culture of tissue samples/swabs; special growth media and microaerophilic environment; Gram stain with comma- to S-shaped Gram-negative rods	Direct contact	Antibiotic therapy based on sensitivity; hygiene measures

19.14 Common bacterial infections. (continues)

Pathogen	Properties	Host range	Clinical signs	Diagnosis	Disease transfer	Treatment and prevention
Pasteurella multocida	Produces endotoxins	Wide	Respiratory tract; septicaemia; arthritis; central nervous system signs; granulomatous dermatitis; with toxins: haemorrhages and coagulation necrosis	Bacteriological culture of tissue samples/swabs	Rodents and free-ranging birds act as reservoirs	Treatment with doxycycline Avoiding vectors; caution with carnivore-related injuries
Staphylococcus aureus	20 subspecies with differing pathogenicity; often epithelium damage, immunosuppression, environmental stressors or prolonged medical treatment required to cause disease	Wide	Septicaemia; thrombi-induced necrosis/ischaemia of digits or adnexa of head or skin; dermatitis; arthritis; synovitis; osteomyelitis	Bacteriological culture of tissue samples/swabs	Direct contact	Antibiotic therapy based on sensitivity; hygiene measures
Streptococcus, Enterococcus spp.	Ubiquitous, need predisposing factors such as immunosuppression or concomitant infections	Particularly Passeriformes	*Streptococcus*: septicaemia; arthritis; respiratory infections; endocarditis. *Enterococcus*: partly autochthonous intestinal flora. *E. faecalis*: pathogenic septicaemia; respiratory disease with tracheitis (respiratory sounds, dyspnoea, voice change)	Bacteriological culture of tissue samples/swabs	Direct contact	Antibiotic therapy based on sensitivity; hygiene measures; poor prognosis for infected Passeriformes
Clostridium spp.	Part of intestinal flora of raptors, Phasianiformes, Galliformes; but *C. perfringens* type A/*speticum*/*novyi* can cause toxin-induced disease; *C. botulinum* produces neurotoxins blocking acetylcholine and damaging vascular endothelium	Vultures and several other raptor species more resistant to infection	Ulcerative enteritis/gastritis; gangrenous dermatitis with feather loss; haemorrhagic skin discoloration; oedema and emphysema. *C. botulinum*: neurotoxins; flaccid paralysis of skeletal musculature. If raptors are affected: peracute to acute depression, regurgitation, haemorrhagic diarrhoea, death	Bacteriological culture of tissue samples/swabs; special growth media and anaerobic environment (*C. botulinum*, mouse animal model)	Direct contact	Antibiotic therapy based on sensitivity; hygiene measures including removal of carcasses, prevention of contact with decaying food and regulation of water levels and temperature
Mycoplasma spp.	Obligate intracellular; no cell wall but three-layered membrane; low survival potential outside host	Particularly Passeriformes, Psittaciformes (e.g. Budgerigars); sometimes in raptors with concomitant infections	Respiratory tract cisease: sinusitis, tracheitis, rhinitis; ocular infections: conjunctivitis, arthritis, synovitis	Bacteriological culture of tissue samples/swabs; special transport/growth media; culture time-consuming and challenging; PCR test; serology if available	Vertical transmission; requires close contact between birds	Enrofloxacin; tetracycline; tylosin; persistent infections occur Reduce population density
Mycobacterium avium-intracellulare, M. genavense (see Figure 19.16)	High survival potential in environment; non-pathogenic/ubiquitous/pathogenic species; long incubation time; asymptomatic but shedding birds have zoonotic potential; mainly environmentally derived infections in humans; risk for immunocompromised humans; increasing concern about multidrug-resistant infections in humans	Passeriformes: atypical picture; raptors more prone to tubercular picture and bone involvement	Atypical picture: enlargement of the liver and spleen. Lepromatous picture: nodular subcutaneous lesions. Tubercular picture: granulomas in the liver/spleen/intestines with no necrotic/calcified centre; weight loss; diarrhoea; polyuria; anaemia; abdominal distension due to hepatomegaly and dilatated intestines; biliverdinuria; lameness; subcutaneous and conjunctival masses; swollen joints; dyspnoea	Cytology: acid-fast stains (Ziehl–Neelsen) only with large numbers of bacteria and no identification; caution with faecal test (cytology or PCR) due to false-negative results and intermittent shedding; culture is challenging and very time-consuming; serology if available. Poultry: intradermal skin tests	Environmental: ponds; estuaries; soil Free-ranging birds can act as reservoirs	Multidrug protocols (to destroy cell wall); long treatment of up to 18 months; client compliance crucial; risk of multidrug-resistant infections in humans to be balanced against urge to treat

19.14 (continued) Common bacterial infections.

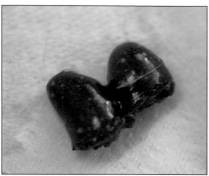

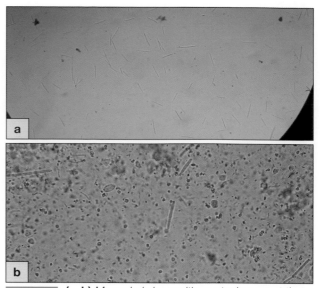

19.15 *Yersinia pseudotuberculosis* causes miliary necrotic lesions in the spleen. This bacterial infection is predominantly seen in Passeriformes and, as it often results in peracute death, diagnosis is mainly made by post-mortem examination. Rodent control is crucial when trying to control the spread of this pathogen. (© John Chitty)

19.17 **(a–b)** *Macrorhabdus ornithogaster* is a yeast that causes haemorrhagic lesions in the mucous membrane of the proventriculus. Multiple species are susceptible, including passeriformes and parrots; Budgerigars are particularly affected. As the disease progresses, the birds lose weight but with continuous appetite. The organism can be identified in the faeces via wet mount. (© Deborah Monks)

References and further reading

DVG (2016) *Desinfektionsmittelliste der Deutschen Veterinärmedizinischen Gesellschaft für die Tierhaltung*. Available at: www.desinfektion-dvg.de

Johne R and Muller H (1998) Avian polyomavirus in wild birds: Genome analysis of isolates from Falconiformes and Psittaciformes. *Archives of Virology* **143**, 1501–1512

Kroker R (1997) Desinfektionsmittel. In: *Pharmakotherapie bei Haus- und Nutztieren*, ed. W Löscher, FR Ungemach and R Kroker, pp. 207–211. Parey Buchverlag, Berlin

Meredith A (2015) *BSAVA Small Animal Formulary – Part B: Exotic Pets, 9th edn*. BSAVA Publications, Gloucester

Phalen DN (2006a) Implications of *Macrorhabdus* in clinical disorders. In: *Clinical Avian Medicine, Vol II*, ed. GJ Harrison and T Lightfoot, pp. 577–582. Spix Publishing, Palm Beach

Phalen DN (2006b) Implications of viruses in clinical disorders. In: *Clinical Avian Medicine Vol II*, ed. GJ Harrison and T Lightfoot, pp. 721–746. Spix Publishing, Palm Beach

Phalen DN (2006c) Preventive medicine and screening. In: *Clinical Avian Medicine Vol II*, ed. G Harrison and T Lightfoot, pp. 705–709. Spix Publishing, Palm Beach

Ritchie BW (1995) An overview of viruses. In: *Avian Viruses: Functional Control, 2nd edn*, ed. BW Ritchie, pp. 7–15. Wingers Publishing, Lake Worth

Sandmeier P and Coutteel P (2006) Management of canaries, finches and mynahs. In: *Clinical Avian Medicine Vol II*, ed. GJ Harrison and T Lightfoot, pp. 879–914. Spix Publishing, Palm Beach

Tomaszewski EK, Logan KS, Snowden KF, Kurtzman CP and Phalen DN (2003) Phylogenetic analysis identifies the 'megabacterium' of birds is a novel anamorphic ascomycetous yeast, *Macrorhabdus ornithogaster*. *International Journal of Systematic and Evolutionary Microbiology* **53**, 1201–1205

Tully NT (2006) Update on *Chlamydophila psittaci*. In: *Clinical Avian Medicine Vol II*, ed. GJ Harrison and T Lightfoot, pp. 679–680. Spix Publishing, Palm Beach

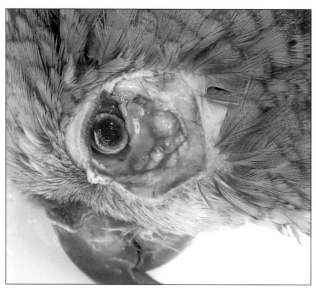

19.16 *Mycobacterium* spp. are still causing disease among companion birds. The atypical form presents with diffuse enlargement of the liver and spleen. The lepromatous form shows nodular to diffuse subcutaneous lesions. In the tubercular form, discrete granulomas develop within and around the liver, spleen and intestines. Sometimes granulomas in the conjunctiva (pictured) might be the only clinical signs. It is crucial to identify such lesions via acid-fast staining methods.

Upper respiratory tract disease

Yvonne van Zeeland

Respiratory tract disease is a common cause of illness in pet birds. Many respiratory diseases quickly develop into life-threatening emergencies, which become overt with the onset of (non-specific) clinical signs such as open-beak breathing, tachypnoea and 'tail bobbing' (an exacerbated vertical motion of the bird's tail whereby the tail is pressed ventrally; this movement can be compared to abdominal breathing in mammals; see **Tail bobbing** clip on CD). Patients can also present with more subtle signs resulting from chronic disease that has been present for several months or even years. Chronic disease will often be more difficult to treat, especially when opportunistic infections develop that further complicate management. Early recognition of clinical signs combined with rapid diagnosis and adequate therapy are therefore important to increase the chances of a successful outcome.

The first and most important step in the work-up of a bird with respiratory disease is to establish whether the respiratory disease originates from the upper (i.e. nares, sinuses, trachea) or lower (i.e. lungs, air sacs) parts of the respiratory system. This will not always be easy, since birds tend to hide their illness and/or predominantly present with non-specific signs. However, some signs can point to the involvement of a specific part of the respiratory tract (see 'Localizing the origin of respiratory disease'). This chapter will deal primarily with the clinical signs, differential diagnosis and step-by-step approach to diseases involving the three parts of the upper respiratory tract. For a discussion on lower respiratory tract disease, see Chapter 22.

Localizing the origin of respiratory disease

There are distinct differences in the diagnostic and therapeutic approach to upper and lower respiratory disease and respiratory disease resulting from non-respiratory causes, therefore the primary goals in any patient with respiratory signs are to:

- Identify whether the disease originates from within or outside of the respiratory tract
- In case of a suspected respiratory cause, determine whether disease is located in the upper or lower respiratory tract.

This distinction can usually be made on the basis of a thorough history and physical examination (Figure 20.1). Once upper respiratory tract involvement has been established, the next step will be to determine which part(s) of the upper respiratory tract is/are involved.

History

A detailed history can provide essential clues with regard to the localization and underlying cause of the disease (Figure 20.1). However, some of these clinical signs (e.g. tail bobbing and open-beak breathing) do not necessarily point towards a specific location but rather reflect the severity of the disease.

When taking the history, attention should be paid to the course and duration of the disease as well as any treatments given to the bird, and their effect. A complete history includes inquiries regarding the patient's general condition (appetite, drinking, behaviour, droppings), housing and nutrition, as this information can help to determine predisposing factors such as inadequate nutrition (particularly hypovitaminosis A), environmental factors and/or recent exposure to other birds (Figure 20.1).

Observation of the patient

As birds often tend to hide their illness and signs are likely to be subtle, a thorough examination of the patient is warranted. However, handling and restraint can significantly alter the bird's respiration. Prior to performing a physical examination, the bird should therefore always be observed from a distance to eliminate the effects of human interference.

Closely observe the bird's respiratory rate and breathing pattern as well as its posture and wing position. In a normal, calm bird, respiration should hardly be noticeable, whereas birds with dyspnoea often show an increased respiratory rate with a characteristic tail bob with every breath (see **Tail bobbing** clip on CD). These signs may be accompanied by open-beak breathing in the case of more severe respiratory problems. Also inspect the eyes, nares and cere for the presence of discharge and other abnormalities, and listen closely for abnormal respiratory sounds as these are an indication of upper respiratory tract disease (URTD) (Figure 20.1). Be aware that some parrots produce noises that are likely to be mistaken

	Signs indicating upper respiratory tract involvement

History	■ Nasal discharge and/or sneezing
	■ Coughing
	■ Change or loss of voice or pitch
	■ Presence of abnormal breath sounds
	■ Head shaking
	■ Frequent scratching and/or rubbing of the head
	■ Rapid and/or laboured breathing
	■ Tail bobbing
	■ Open-beak breathing
	■ Presence of one or more predisposing factors:
	   – Malnutrition, particularly hypovitaminosis A in birds fed an all-seed diet, results in squamous metaplasia of the epithelial cells lining the respiratory tract, formation of hyperkeratotic granulomas and/or increased susceptibility to infectious disease
	   – Environmental factors including low humidity and exposure to environmental toxins and/or irritants (e.g. dust, feather dander, smoke, cooking fumes, aerosols)
	   – Recent acquisition from a breeder or pet store may suggest an underlying infectious cause
	   – Infectious causes are also more likely in multiple-bird households or aviaries, especially when birds have recently been added and/or multiple birds are showing signs of respiratory disease

Observation from a distance	■ Ocular and/or nasal discharge ■ Abnormal facial swellings (particularly in the periorbital region) ■ Increased respiratory rate (tachypnoea) ■ Tail bobbing ■ Open-beak breathing (particularly in more severe cases) ■ Stretching of the neck ■ Wings drooped and/or held away from the body ■ Abnormal respiratory sounds, including sneezing, coughing, stridor ■ Change or loss of voice or pitch
Physical examination	Head and periorbital region: ■ Subcutaneous masses or swellings ■ Inflation of the sinuses concurrent with each breath ■ Exudate expelled from the naris or lacrimal duct upon applying pressure to the infraorbital sinus Nares and cere: ■ (Dried) nasal discharge (with or without obstruction of the naris) ■ Changes in shape and/or size (e.g. erosion, asymmetry, swelling) Oropharynx: ■ Blunting of the choanal papillae ■ Exudate in the choanal slit or glottis ■ Plaques, erosions, swellings or other lesions Neck and trachea: ■ Inflated (overfilled) cervicocephalic air sac ■ Palpable deformities ■ Intraluminal abnormalities seen during transillumination of the trachea, including foreign bodies or tracheal mites (*Sternostoma tracheocolum*); particularly in smaller parakeets and Passeriformes

20.1   Clinical signs indicating upper respiratory tract disease.

for abnormal sounds by the inexperienced owner or veterinary surgeon (veterinarian) unfamiliar with the species (Figure 20.2).

Physical examination

If the bird is well enough to withstand the stress of being handled, a physical examination is performed, during which the bird's overall condition and hydration status, as well as its bodyweight, are assessed and the different parts of the respiratory tracts are more closely examined for abnormalities.

Parrot species	Normal sounds
Amazon parrots (particularly chicks)	'Ak-ak' sound while begging for food
Cockatoos	Hissing
Grey parrots	Growling
Pionus parrots	Sniffling sounds, produced when the bird is excited
All parrots	Mimicking of human sounds (e.g. coughing, sneezing)

20.2   Normal sounds produced by parrots which are sometimes mistaken for abnormal breath sounds.

■ Head, in particular the dorsal and cranial aspects and periorbital region:
   • Inspect for the presence of subcutaneous masses or swellings
   • Observe for rhythmic inflation of the sinuses (simultaneous with each breath)
   • Apply gentle digital pressure to the infraorbital sinus (around and ventromedial to the eye) and check for expulsion of exudate from the naris or lacrimal duct.
■ Nares and cere:
   • Inspect for the presence of (dried) discharge in or around the nares
   • Inspect for the presence of lesions or other deformities
   • Evaluate possible changes in size or shape
   • Note: the nares should normally be bilaterally symmetrical, with a central flap of keratinized tissue (the operculum) present in each naris, which is smooth and dry in appearance.
■ Oropharynx:
   • Inspect the choanal slit and glottis for the presence of discharge or exudate

- Inspect the choanal slit for blunting of the papillae and the presence of plaques or other lesions. Note: the choanal slit is normally lined with slender, tapered papillae, moist and free of discharge
- Inspect the glottis (located just caudally to the tongue) for the presence of swelling and/or lesions
- Note: to enable visualization of the aforementioned structures, it may be necessary to use a mouth gag or speculum (Figure 20.3).
■ Neck and trachea:
  - Inspect the neck for the presence of abnormal swellings (e.g. overfilled cervicocephalic air sac)
  - Palpate for abnormalities
  - Transilluminate the trachea to identify intraluminal abnormalities (e.g. foreign bodies or tracheal mites). Note: this procedure is particularly useful in smaller parakeets and Passeriformes for detection of e.g. tracheal mites (Sternostoma tracheacolum, Figure 20.4)
  - Note: the trachea usually runs along the right side of the neck and is composed of complete cartilaginous rings.

Dependent on the clinical signs noted in the history or physical examination, it may be possible to further specify whether and which part of the upper respiratory tract is affected:

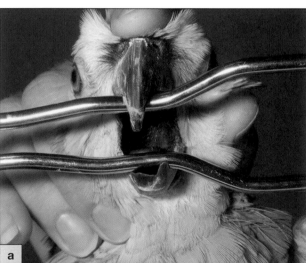

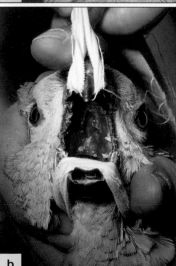

20.3 **(a)** A speculum or **(b)** a mouth gag can be useful to enable better visualization of the structures in the oral cavity. (©Yvonne van Zeeland, Utrecht University)

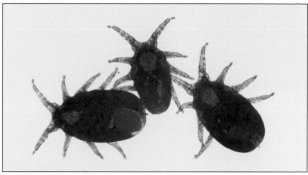

20.4 Tracheal mites (*Sternostoma tracheacolum*) found in the trachea of a Gouldian Finch. (© Yvonne van Zeeland, Utrecht University)

■ Nasal discharge, sneezing and/or staining or dried discharge in the feathers around the nares suggest involvement of the nasal cavity
■ Periorbital swellings or sunken eyes (especially in macaws) point to sinus involvement
■ Coughing, abnormal breathing sounds (stridor) and change in pitch or voice (in psittacine birds) are often noted in birds with tracheal or syringeal disease.

Other signs pointing to the involvement of a specific part of the upper respiratory tract are summarized in Figure 20.5. For each part of the upper respiratory tract, work-up and differential diagnoses are discussed below.

Part of the upper respiratory tract	Clinical signs
Nares and nasal cavity	■ Sneezing ■ Nasal discharge ■ Staining or dried discharge in the feathers surrounding the nares ■ Nasal plugs, occlusion of the nares ■ Abnormally shaped nares ■ Swollen cere ■ Scratching or rubbing of the beak (with or without concurrent feather loss) ■ Head shaking ■ Yawning ■ Discharge or mucus in the choanal slit ■ Open-beak breathing ■ Epiphora, conjunctivitis ■ Longitudinal groove(s) in the beak (chronic rhinitis) ■ Often seen in combination with sinusitis
Sinuses	■ Periorbital swelling (may be soft, firm or fluctuating) ■ Protrusion of the eye (exophthalmos) ■ Sunken eyes (chronic sinusitis, particularly in macaws) ■ Scratching or rubbing of the head ■ Periorbital feather loss ■ Often seen in combination with rhinitis
Trachea and/or syrinx	■ Loss of vocalization ■ Change of pitch or voice ■ Abnormal breathing sounds (stridor), particularly on inspiration ■ Head shaking ■ Coughing ■ Gurgling ■ Dyspnoea, breathing with an open beak ■ Breathing with an extended neck

20.5 Clinical signs associated with disease in specific parts of the upper respiratory tract.

Diseases of the nasal cavity and nares

Patients with URTD located in the nasal cavity often present with sneezing or nasal discharge as the most prominent clinical signs. Occasional sneezing can also be noted in healthy birds. In these birds, the nares should normally remain dry and clean. An increase in frequency, repetitive sneezing and/or the presence of nasal discharge warrants further investigation to identify the initiating cause.

The type and amount of nasal discharge produced by the bird will largely depend on the nature and extent of the disease (see 'History and physical examination'). Dependent on the amount of discharge that is produced, a range of clinical signs can be seen. In birds with limited nasal discharge, a slight staining of the feathers (Figure 20.6) and/or changes in the bird's behaviour (yawning, head shaking, scratching or rubbing of the beak) may be the only clinical signs to indicate a problem in the nasal cavity. If the nasal discharge is copious, it can completely block the nares, thereby resulting in respiratory distress, manifested by the bird breathing with an open beak. Deformed nares or beak deformities are suggestive of chronic nasal disease (Figure 20.7).

Differential diagnosis

Sneezing or nasal discharge often results from disease that is strictly localized to the nasal cavity. Common causes of sneezing and nasal discharge include (bacterial) infections or irritation by draft, dust, smoke or aerosols (Figure 20.8). Due to the close anatomical relationship between the nasal cavity and sinuses, rhinitis and sinusitis are commonly seen in combination and share a similar aetiology. Sneezing or nasal discharge can also manifest as part of lower respiratory or systemic disease (e.g. in birds with chlamydiosis). In these cases, the sneezing and

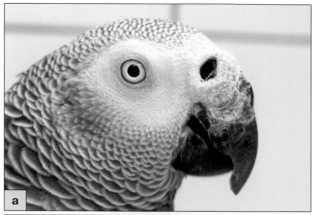

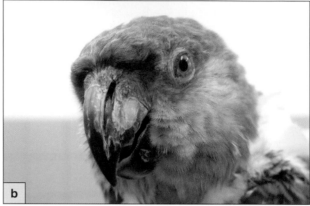

20.7 Deformities of the nares and/or beak, as seen in this **(a)** African Grey Parrot and **(b)** Senegal Parrot, are suggestive of chronic rhinitis.
(© Yvonne van Zeeland, Utrecht University)

nasal discharge will usually be accompanied by other respiratory signs or signs of generalized disease.

Since nasal discharge can result in occlusion of the nares, especially when the amounts produced are copious and/or the exudate dries up, the differential diagnoses for nasal discharge and occluded nares greatly overlap one another. Occlusion of the nares can also occur in the absence of nasal discharge due to morphological changes to the cere or nares. Common causes for these morphological changes include metaplasia and formation of so-called rhinoliths resulting from malnutrition in all psittacine birds (Figure 20.9), and brown cere hypertrophy or parasitic disease in Budgerigars (Figures 20.10 and 20.11). Other differentials for occluded nares can be found in Figure 20.12.

Step-by-step approach to nasal discharge and sneezing

The approach to sneezing and nasal discharge is summarized in Figure 20.13.

History and physical examination

Important points to address in the history and physical examination of a bird with nasal discharge pertain to the characteristics (colour, consistency, amount, unilateral *versus* bilateral) of the discharge that is produced, as these will vary according to the nature of the underlying disease:

- Clear, serous discharge is encountered in birds suffering from allergies, malnutrition or viral, mycoplasmal or chlamydial infections (Figure 20.14)

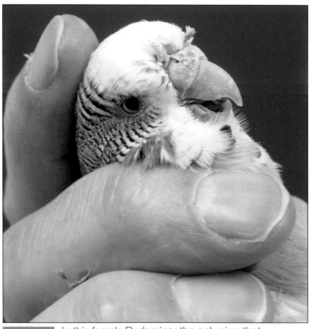

20.6 In this female Budgerigar the only sign that indicated the presence of rhinitis was a slight staining of the feathers.
(© Yvonne van Zeeland, Utrecht University)

Differential diagnosis	Comments
Bacterial infections	
Gram-negative bacteria (e.g. *Escherichia coli*, *Haemophilus*, *Klebsiella*, *Pasteurella*, *Pseudomonas*), Gram-positive bacteria (e.g. *Mycobacterium*, *Streptococcus*, *Staphylococcus*)	Gram-negative infections most common
Spirochaetes	Spirochaetes in Cockatiels 3–10 weeks of age (lockjaw syndrome)
Chlamydia psittaci	All bird species susceptible; consider in all birds that have recently been in contact with other birds; often systemic illness
Mycoplasma spp.	Common in smaller Psittaciformes (Budgerigars, Cockatiels), Passeriformes
Fungal infections	
Aspergillus spp., *Candida albicans*, *Cryptococcus* spp., *Mucor* spp.	Common in birds with malnutrition or stress; formation of granulomas that block the trachea or syrinx; may also affect other parts of the respiratory system
Viral infections	
Avian influenza, herpesvirus, poxvirus, reovirus	Poxvirus common in Passeriformes (canaries), birds of prey
Parasitic infections	
Cryptosporidium spp.	Particularly in birds of prey
Trichomonas gallinae	
Nutritional	
Hypovitaminosis A, resulting in squamous metaplasia and non-infectious granulomas	Particularly in Psittaciformes fed an all-seed diet
Allergic	
Inhalant allergens (e.g. smoke, perfume, feather dander)	Macaws are anecdotally reported to be more susceptible
Toxic	
Cigarette or tobacco smoke, aerosol sprays, ammonia	
Neoplastic	
Lymphoma, fibrosarcoma, (adeno)carcinoma, melanoma, papilloma, etc.	More common in older birds
Environmental	
Low humidity, dust, dander of other birds (particularly cockatoos, Grey Parrots)	Particularly in birds housed under suboptimal conditions
Foreign body	
e.g., millet seed	Can result in secondary rhinitis
Trauma	
Resulting in (subcutaneous) haemorrhage, emphysema and/or fractures	
Coagulopathy	
Bleeding disorders resulting in epistaxis (e.g. conure bleeding syndrome)	Conure bleeding syndrome is specific to conures
Choanal atresia	
Congenital deformity	Young birds (particularly Grey parrots)

20.8 Differential diagnosis for rhinitis and/or sinusitis, as indicated by the presence of, for example, nasal discharge, sneezing, facial and/or periorbital swellings.

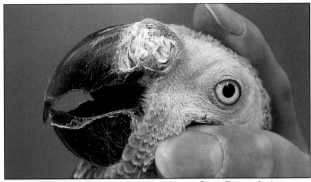

20.9 Rhinolith in an adult African Grey Parrot fed an all-seed diet. These masses usually result from accumulation of sloughed cells, exudate and other debris in the naris. (© Yvonne van Zeeland, Utrecht University)

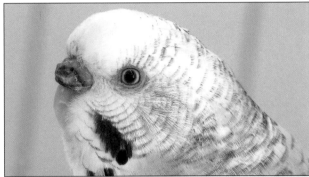

20.10 Brown cere hypertrophy in a female Budgerigar. (© Yvonne van Zeeland, Utrecht University)

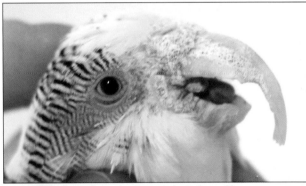

20.11 Scaly face due to an infestation with *Cnemidocoptes pilae* in a Budgerigar. Note the overgrowth of the upper beak resulting from this infection. (© Yvonne van Zeeland, Utrecht University)

Differential diagnosis	Comments
(Dried) nasal discharge or abscess	See Figure 20.8
Cnemidocoptes (scaly mite)	Particularly common in Budgerigars
Brown cere hypertrophy	Hormone-related, female Budgerigars
Rhinolith	Often resulting from nutritional imbalances, particularly hypovitaminosis A, leading to squamous metaplasia of the epithelium
Neoplasia	Lymphoma, melanoma, papilloma, etc.
Trauma	Resulting in stenosis or haemorrhage
Coagulopathy	Bleeding disorders resulting in epistaxis, e.g. conure bleeding syndrome
Foreign body	For example, millet seed

20.12 Differential diagnosis for occluded nares.

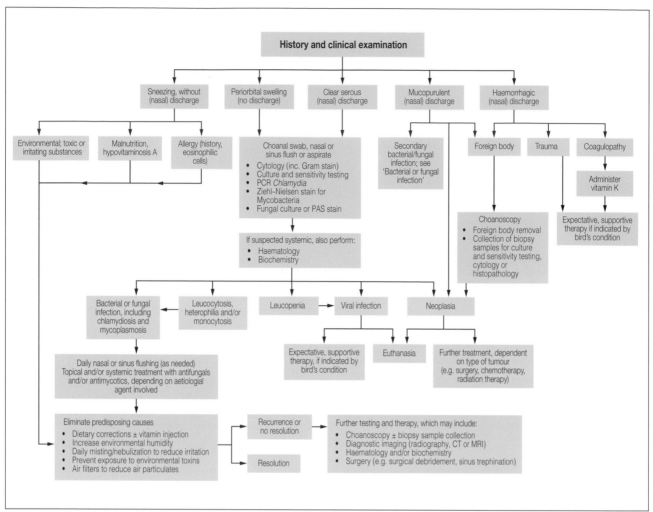

History and clinical examination

- Sneezing, without (nasal) discharge
- Periorbital swelling (no discharge)
- Clear serous (nasal) discharge
- Mucopurulent (nasal) discharge
- Haemorrhagic (nasal) discharge

Sneezing, without (nasal) discharge:
- Environmental; toxic or irritating substances
- Malnutrition, hypovitaminosis A
- Allergy (history, eosinophilic cells)

Clear serous (nasal) discharge:
Choanal swab, nasal or sinus flush or aspirate
- Cytology (inc. Gram stain)
- Culture and sensitivity testing
- PCR *Chlamydia*
- Ziehl–Nielsen stain for Mycobacteria
- Fungal culture or PAS stain

If suspected systemic, also perform:
- Haematology
- Biochemistry

Mucopurulent (nasal) discharge:
- Secondary bacterial/fungal infection; see 'Bacterial or fungal infection'

Haemorrhagic (nasal) discharge:
- Foreign body
- Trauma
- Coagulopathy → Administer vitamin K

Choanoscopy
- Foreign body removal
- Collection of biopsy samples for culture and sensitivity testing, cytology or histopathology

Expectative, supportive therapy if indicated by bird's condition

- Bacterial or fungal infection, including chlamydiosis and mycoplasmosis
- Leucocytosis, heterophilia and/or monocytosis
- Leucopenia → Viral infection
- Neoplasia

Viral infection:
- Expectative, supportive therapy, if indicated by bird's condition
- Euthanasia

Neoplasia:
- Further treatment, dependent on type of tumour (e.g. surgery, chemotherapy, radiation therapy)

Daily nasal or sinus flushing (as needed)
Topical and/or systemic treatment with antifungals and/or antimycotics, depending on aetiologial agent involved

Eliminate predisposing causes
- Dietary corrections ± vitamin injection
- Increase environmental humidity
- Daily misting/nebulization to reduce irritation
- Prevent exposure to environmental toxins
- Air filters to reduce air particulates

Recurrence or no resolution → Further testing and therapy, which may include:
- Choanoscopy ± biopsy sample collection
- Diagnostic imaging (radiography, CT or MRI)
- Haematology and/or biochemistry
- Surgery (e.g. surgical debridement, sinus trephination)

Resolution

20.13 Approach to sneezing, nasal discharge and sinusitis. CT = computed tomography; MRI = magnetic resonance imaging; PAS = periodic acid–Schiff; PCR = polymerase chain reaction.

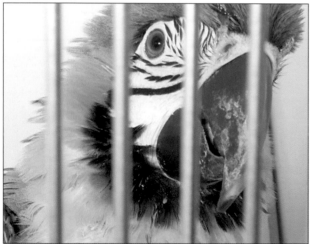

20.14 Clear serous nasal discharge in a Harlequin Macaw. This bird was diagnosed with *Chlamydia psittaci* infection. (© Yvonne van Zeeland, Utrecht University)

- Mucopurulent discharge is encountered in cases of a (secondary) bacterial or fungal infection, neoplasia or foreign body (Figure 20.15)
- Haemorrhagic discharge can be noted in birds with coagulopathies, trauma or foreign bodies
- Unilateral involvement is common in birds that suffer from fungal or bacterial infections, neoplastic conditions, foreign body entrapment or trauma.

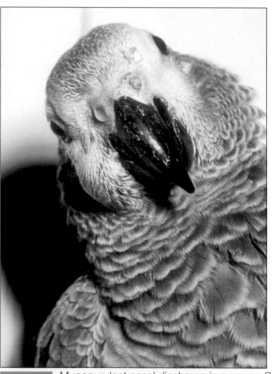

20.15 Mucopurulent nasal discharge in a young Grey Parrot with choanal atresia and secondary bacterial rhinitis/sinusitis. (© Yvonne van Zeeland, Utrecht University)

Other aspects to consider in the history include the presence of other respiratory signs to distinguish localized from generalized disease. Similarly, details regarding the bird's housing, nutrition and exposure to other birds need to be obtained as these will help to identify any predisposing or causative factors such as hypovitaminosis A, low humidity, airborne toxins or preceding trauma.

During the physical examination, the nares should be closely examined for uni- or bilateral involvement as well as their size, symmetry, patency and the nature of nasal discharge, if present. Also check the cere and surrounding feathers for signs of inflammation and dried discharge. An oral examination may reveal signs of blunting or sloughing of the choanal papillae (Figure 20.16), suggestive of hypovitaminosis A, or plaque formation resulting from bacterial (e.g. mycobacteria), fungal (particularly candidiasis) or viral (e.g. poxvirus, herpesvirus) infections, parasitic disease (e.g. trichomonosis, capillariasis), or neoplasia (Figure 20.17). In addition, attention is paid to other parts of the respiratory system (in particular the sinuses) and signs of general illness accompanying the sneezing or nasal discharge, as these can be suggestive of a more generalized respiratory or systemic disease.

Based on the history and findings of the physical examination, specific conditions such as trauma, allergy, toxins and malnutrition can be ruled out or deemed more likely.

Diagnostic work-up

After the history has been obtained and the physical abnormalities have been noted, cytology (including a Gram stain) and culture and sensitivity testing of a choanal swab or nasal flush are often performed as a next step.

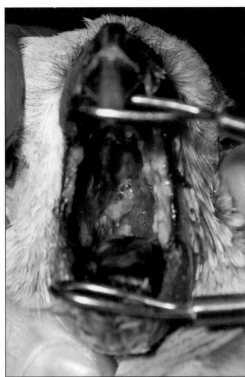

20.17 Plaque formation, as seen in this Amazon parrot, can be seen in birds with bacterial, fungal or viral infections, parasitic disease, or neoplasia. In this bird, mucosal biopsy samples were collected after removal of the plaques. Histopathology revealed a squamous cell carcinoma to underlie the abnormalities. (© Yvonne van Zeeland, Utrecht University)

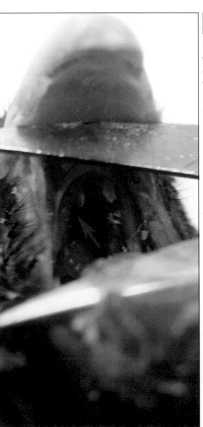

20.16

Blunting of the choanal papillae (arrowed), as seen in this *Rosella* spp., is indicative of chronic malnutrition (hypovitaminosis A). (© Gerry Dorrestein, NOIVBD)

Nasal flush: A nasal flush is easily obtained by applying a syringe filled with sterile, lukewarm saline in one of the nares and tilting the patient upside down, following which the saline is forcefully flushed into the nasal passage while occluding the other naris with a finger (Figure 20.18). Be sure to always perform this procedure with caution and monitor the patient carefully as excessive and/or rapid flushing can cause the patient to aspirate fluids and drown. If performed correctly, the infused saline is forced to leak out via the choana, following which it can be collected and submitted for further testing. In addition, swabs can be collected from the choanal slit to be submitted for e.g. *Chlamydia* testing (Figure 20.19). If fungal disease is suspected, samples can be submitted for periodic acid–Schiff staining or fungal culture, whereas Ziehl–Neelsen stains can be useful in cases of suspected mycobacteriosis. The results should always be interpreted with care since samples collected from the nares or nasal cavity can easily be contaminated with normal flora. (Note: the normal flora of the nasal cavity in birds primarily consists of Gram-positive rods and cocci, and – to a lesser extent – yeasts and/or Gram-negative rods. False-negative results can also occur, especially if *Mycoplasma* spp. are involved, as these are difficult to isolate.)

Haematology and biochemistry: In patients with severe or chronic rhinitis, or patients with systemic signs, a full haematological and biochemical profile (including protein electrophoresis) should be considered. Although results rarely point towards a specific

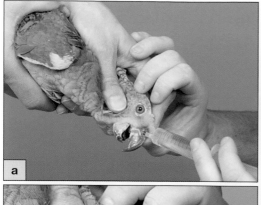

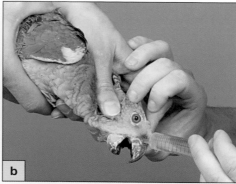

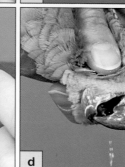

20.18 Nasal flush in a Blue-fronted Amazon Parrot. **(a)** For this procedure, the patient is tilted upside down to prevent water from running into the trachea. **(b)** After applying a syringe filled with sterile, lukewarm saline in one of the nares, **(c)** the saline is forcefully flushed into the nasal passage while the other naris is simultaneously held closed with a finger. **(d)** Often, material leaks out of the choanal slit. This material may be collected for further work-up (e.g. cytology, culture and sensitivity testing). (© Yvonne van Zeeland, Utrecht University)

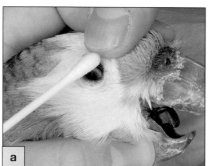

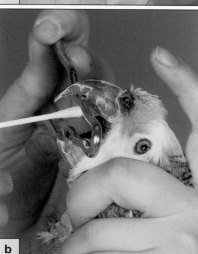

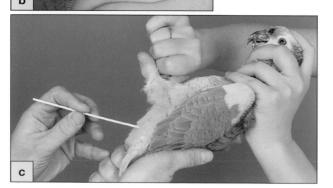

20.19 Collection of **(a)** conjunctival, **(b)** choanal and **(c)** cloacal swabs in an Amazon parrot. After collection, swabs may be submitted for polymerase chain reaction or used to make a smear which can be stained using a Macchiavello's stain for *Chlamydia* testing. (© Yvonne van Zeeland, Utrecht University)

disease, leucocytosis, heterophilia or monocytosis are suggestive of the presence of a (bacterial or fungal) infection or inflammation, whereas leucopenia is more commonly found in patients with an overwhelming viral or bacterial infection.

Diagnostic imaging and endoscopy: Diagnostic imaging modalities and/or choanal endoscopy are warranted in cases of refractory or chronic rhinitis unresponsive to the initiated therapy. In such cases, referral to an avian specialist or veterinary surgeon experienced with birds should be considered.

Therapeutic approach

Management considerations: Most birds with mild rhinitis respond well to environmental and dietary modifications, which help to eliminate any predisposing factors. Advise the owner to convert the bird to a pelleted diet, give parenteral injections with vitamin A (in case of suspected malnutrition) and keep the bird in a well ventilated, dust- and toxin-free environment, preventing exposure to cigarette smoke, strong odours or sprays, or aerosols of any kind. Air filters (e.g. HEPA systems) can help to reduce the number of air particulates, whereas air humidifiers or nebulizers help to increase the humidity in the room. Daily misting or bathing is advised to reduce sneezing caused by excessive dust or dander.

Local and systemic treatment for rhinitis: Dependent on the severity of the rhinitis and presence of other clinical signs, the treatment regimen may consist of local and/or systemic treatment.

Local therapy includes cleaning of the nares, followed by one or more nasal flushes (as needed), and topical medication. If the nasal discharge is tenacious, it may not be possible to flush any fluid through one or both nasal passages. In these cases it can be useful to place one drop of a mucolytic agent (e.g. acetylcysteine) into each naris followed by a new attempt to flush the nares after 5–10 minutes.

Following the flushing and cleaning of the nares, a topical antimicrobial drug can be administered, especially in patients with suspected (secondary) bacterial or fungal infections. Preferably, the choice of drug is based on the results of a culture and sensitivity test, but should these not be available (yet), aminoglycosides (e.g. amikacin, gentamicin or tobramycin), chloramphenicol or fluoroquinolones (e.g. ciprofloxacin, enrofloxacin) will often serve as a good starting point. (Note: according to new regulations concerning antibiotic use in veterinary medicine in the European Union, enrofloxacin and other fluoroquinolones should be used cautiously, preferably being limited to those cases in which culture and sensitivity testing has shown resistance to all other drugs. In exceptional cases (e.g. critical patients with a life-threatening condition that may succumb if not treated promptly) the use of the drug is permitted without availability of the results of the sensitivity test.)

To enable topical administration, the drugs can be dissolved in sterile water, saline or Ringer's solution (dilution of 10–20 mg/100 ml), after which the solution can be used to flush the nares. Suggested volumes are provided in Figure 20.20.

Bird species	Volume[a]
Small-sized birds (e.g. Budgerigar, Cockatiel)	3–5 ml
Medium-sized birds (e.g. Amazon, Grey Parrot)	6–12 ml
Large-sized birds (e.g. large cockatoos, macaws)	12–20 ml

20.20 Guidelines for volumes to be used for nasal flushing. [a]Suggested volume to use for flushing one naris.

Alternatively, ophthalmic solutions can be used, as these are convenient and safe to apply in the proximity of the eye. Solutions containing corticosteroids should be avoided as these are rarely (if at all) indicated and are dangerous to use in birds due to their immunosuppressive effects. Dependent on the severity of the clinical signs and the response to therapy, flushing is performed one to three times daily for several days in a row.

When rhinitis is severe and accompanied by signs of systemic illness or lower respiratory tract infection, parenteral therapy with a broad-spectrum antibiotic or antifungal drug is recommended pending the result of the culture and sensitivity test.

Rhinolith removal: In cases of rhinoliths or obstructed nares, a small curette can be used to remove the excessive debris. If the material is firm, wet cotton swabs or saline flushes can help to moisten the material, thereby facilitating its removal. In most cases, the debris or plug can gently be levered out from the nostril. Be careful not to damage the central operculum (if still present) while performing this procedure.

Once the plug is removed, mucus to mucopurulent material will often appear, which can be flushed out using sterile saline or Ringer's solution and sent for microbial testing. Pending results, local and/or systemic treatment can be initiated, as secondary infections with bacteria (e.g. *Escherichia coli*, *Pseudomonas* spp., *Klebsiella* spp.) or fungi (particularly *Aspergillus* spp.) are common.

Large rhinoliths will often cause permanent distortion of the naris (Figure 20.21) due to progressive destruction of the soft tissues, conchae and bone, thereby predisposing the bird to respiratory infections. Regular cleaning and flushing is advised to minimize the risks of recurrence.

Treatment of choanal or nasal abscesses: Abscesses in the nasal cavity or choana are best approached orally in the anaesthetized bird. Once the bird is sufficiently anaesthetized, a 21 G needle can serve as a stylet to open the abscess, after which a blunt probe can be used to push the inspissated pus out. Treatment for choanal or nasal abscesses may also include flushing and topical and systemic medication, preferably based on the results of culture and sensitivity testing.

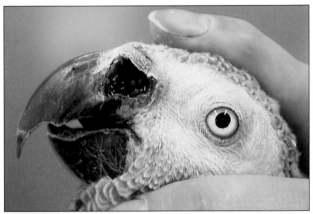

20.21 Grey Parrot from Figure 20.9 after removal of the rhinolith. Large rhinoliths will often cause permanent distortion of the naris.
(© Yvonne van Zeeland, Utrecht University)

Diseases affecting the sinuses

The complex anatomy of the bird's infraorbital sinus, with its numerous diverticula extending into the maxilla and mandible, around the eye and ear canal, predisposes birds to the development of sinusitis. Moreover, the dorsal opening of the sinus into the nasal cavity complicates the course of the disease as secretions are not easily drained, often resulting in chronic disease which does not respond well to medical treatment alone, but also requires surgical intervention.

Disease of the sinuses often manifests as infra- or periorbital swellings (Figures 20.22 and 20.23) or asymmetry of the face associated with the position of the eye globe (i.e. exophthalmos or – in macaws – enophthalmos). Oculonasal discharge can also be noted, resulting in matting or loss of feathers around the eye and cere. Affected birds may also sneeze, shake their head, scratch their face or rub it excessively on perches or other objects in the cage. Hyperinflation of the cervicocephalic air sac, which communicates with the infraorbital sinus, can also be noted (Figure 20.24).

A specific condition, referred to as lockjaw syndrome, occurs in 3- to 10-week-old Cockatiels. An infection with spirochaetes is suspected to be the underlying cause, initially resulting in oculonasal discharge and periorbital swelling, followed by an inability of the birds to open their beak, causing them to die from starvation.

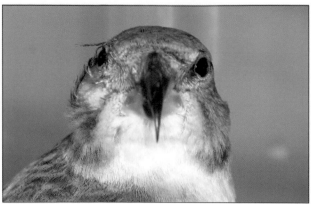

20.22 Crossbill with a marked swelling ventral to the eye. Periorbital swellings or swellings such as noted in this bird are highly indicative of sinusitis. (© Yvonne van Zeeland, Utrecht University)

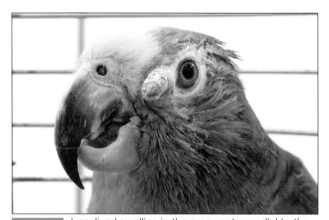

20.23 Localized swelling in the area ventromedial to the eye due to chronic sinusitis in a Yellow-fronted Amazon Parrot.

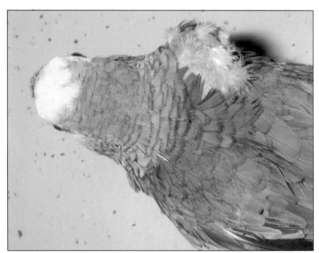

20.24 Hyperinflation of the cervicocephalic air sac in an Amazon parrot. This type of lesion can be observed in birds with (chronic) sinusitis due to obstruction of the connection between the sinuses and cervicocephalic air sacs. (© Yvonne van Zeeland, Utrecht University)

Differential diagnosis

Sinusitis and rhinitis share many of the same features and frequently occur in combination, thereby resulting in a grossly similar differential diagnosis for both conditions (see Figure 20.8).

Step-by-step approach to periorbital swelling
History and physical examination

When taking the history of a bird with suspected sinus disease, specifically ask the owner about the speed of onset (slow *versus* sudden) and duration of the swelling. Other important points that need to be addressed are grossly similar to those discussed for nasal disease (see 'Step-by-step approach to nasal discharge and sneezing' and Figure 20.13) and pertain to the presence of other respiratory signs, recent trauma or exposure to other birds, and details regarding the bird's diet and environment.

Observe the bird for signs of respiratory compromise and specifically pay attention to the structures of the head and neck during the physical examination. Closely examine the eyes and orbital region for abnormalities such as bruising and abrasions, which may indicate preceding trauma or result from repeated rubbing or scratching. When trauma is suspected, the skull and bony orbit should be palpated for possible fractures.

When periorbital swelling is present, note its location and extent (e.g. restricted to the ventral or supraorbital region or completely surrounding the eye) and whether the swelling is uni- or bilateral. Also check the consistency of the swelling, which may be firm, soft or fluctuant, dependent on the nature of the secretions. The rest of the respiratory tract needs to be examined to identify whether disease is limited to the sinuses or also involves other parts of the respiratory tract.

Diagnostic work-up

Cytology and culture of a nasal flush (see Diagnostic work-up) or sinus aspirate are usually helpful to establish the underlying cause of the sinusitis. Other diagnostic testing (i.e. radiographs, computed tomography (CT) or magnetic resonance imaging (MRI), endoscopy, haematology and biochemistry, polymerase chain reaction (PCR) testing for *Chlamydia* infection) follows similar guidelines as previously discussed for rhinitis.

Sinus aspirate: Sinus aspirates can be collected from the ventral and rostral parts of the infraorbital sinus using a 22–25 G needle and syringe. It is preferable to anaesthetize the patient for this procedure, as sudden movement by the patient may lead to puncture of the eye or other vital structures.

The rostral area can be approached by inserting the needle at the commissure of the beak and directing it perpendicular to the skin below the zygomatic bone to a point between the eye and naris (Figure 20.25).

The ventral area can be approached from either of two directions (Figure 20.26):

- Introduction of the needle at a point ventral to the zygomatic bone and just ventral to the eye, while holding it perpendicular to the skin
- Introduction of the needle just caudal to the commissure of the beak while directing it toward the point ventral to the eye and zygomatic arch.

If aspiration fails to produce any material, sterile fluid can be infused into the sinus using one of the abovementioned locations and collected at the choanal slit for further microbial and cytological analysis. Should a surgical approach be indicated (see 'Therapeutic approach'), biopsy samples from the sinus epithelium may be collected for histopathology and/or culture.

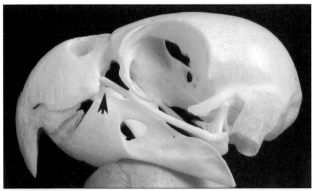

20.25 Location to perform a sinus aspirate of the rostral area (arrowed) indicated on a lovebird skull. (© Yvonne van Zeeland, Utrecht University)

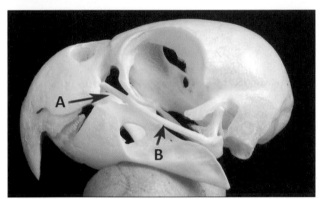

20.26 Locations to perform a sinus aspirate of the ventral area using a rostral (A) or ventral (B) approach (arrowed), indicated on a lovebird skull. (© Yvonne van Zeeland, Utrecht University)

Therapeutic approach
Management of sinusitis includes the identification and correction of any predisposing factors or underlying disease. This often includes dietary corrections (including parenteral administration of vitamin A) as well as environmental modifications, similar to those described in the previous section.

Nasal and sinus flushing: If the nidus of an infection is not identified and removed, sinusitis is likely to recur. It is important to remove all exudate and debris from the sinuses. For this purpose, nasal flushing using physiological saline or diluted acetylcysteine can be attempted. However, the complex anatomy of the sinuses will hinder the successful flushing of these structures. Infraorbital aspiration and flushing, using similar approaches as described for diagnostic sampling, are likely to provide better results.

Surgical debridement: If the material is firm and caseous, aggressive therapy using surgical debridement will often be needed. In birds, this is essentially a form of abscess treatment since the sinuses are not surrounded by bone. Once the sinus is opened, sterile cotton swabs or a curette can be used to clean out the pocket (Figure 20.27; and see also Chapter 17). During this procedure, samples may be collected from the sinus lining for histology, cytology and/or culture. Next, the sinus can be flushed with sterile saline, while carefully monitoring that no fluid is aspirated when it exits the nares or choana. Following the debridement, the sinus is generally left open and flushed 2–4 times per day until the wound granulates.

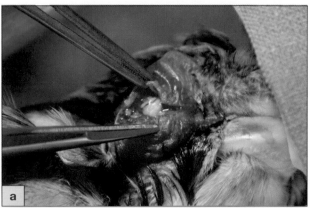
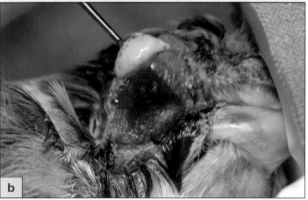

20.27 (a) Opening of the sinus and (b) removal of caseous exudate from the sinus in the Crossbill from Figure 20.22. Culture and sensitivity testing did not reveal a causative agent. (© Yvonne van Zeeland, Utrecht University)

Sinus trephination: In birds with localized lesions in the sinus cavities underneath the cancellous bone, drainage via trephination (using a technique similar to that described in dogs and cats) is often warranted. Commonly used trephination sites include the frontal sinus and nasal diverticulum (Figure 20.28). A proper knowledge of the anatomy and surgical technique is needed prior to performing this procedure, to prevent damage to the underlying structures (eye, nerves). Referral to an avian specialist or veterinary surgeon who sees birds on a regular basis is therefore recommended.

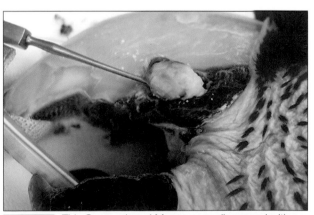

20.28 This Green-winged Macaw was diagnosed with a sinusitis of the nasal diverticulum due to *Aspergillus* infection. After drilling a hole through the cortical bone, the caseous material could be removed. A Penrose drain was subsequently sutured in place to allow for daily flushings with clotrimazole. After several weeks of treatment, the sinusitis resolved and months later, the hole in the beak was completely closed. (© Yvonne van Zeeland, Utrecht University)

Dependent on the results of the culture and sensitivity test, oral and/or parenteral antimicrobial therapy may be initiated. Topical treatment, by nebulization, application of ophthalmic drops into the nares and/or flushes with antibiotic or antifungal solutions, can also be considered.

Overfilled cervicocephalic air sac: An overfilled cervicocephalic air sac can incidentally be seen in birds as a complication of chronic sinusitis, air sacculitis, or trauma. In these patients, the distended air sac can be deflated by lancing it with a scalpel or bevelled edge of a needle repeatedly until the underlying disease has been sufficiently treated. In refractory cases, placement of a stent has been reported, but this measure often only results in temporary resolution of the clinical signs (Figure 20.29).

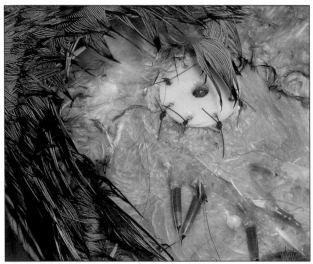

20.29 Stents can be used to deflate the cervicocephalic air sac in chronic refractory cases such as the one shown in Figure 20.24.
(© Yvonne van Zeeland, Utrecht University)

Tracheal disease

Tracheal disease is often accompanied by signs of respiratory distress including breathing with an open beak, tail bobbing and stretching of the neck, particularly if a (partial) obstruction (e.g. due to a foreign body, gran loma, parasites) is present. Wheezing sounds will also be noticeable in these patients (see **Tracheal obstruction** clip on CD). Irritation of the tracheal mucosa can result in coughing, although this is rare in birds (coughing can be observed in parrots mimicking human sounds). A change in pitch or voice, or loss of vocalization, is common, particularly if the syrinx is involved in the disease process.

Differential diagnosis

The differential diagnoses for tracheal obstruction are presented in Figure 20.30. Common causes include:

- Diphtheritic plaques and granulomas due to bacterial (e.g. *Pseudomonas* spp.) or fungal infections (particularly *Aspergillus* spp. in birds with malnutrition or suffering from stress)
- Parasites such as tracheal mites (*Sternostoma tracheacolum*) in smaller passerines, flagellates (*Trichomonas gallinae*) in passerines and small psittacines, or *Cryptosporidium* spp. or gapeworms (*Syngamus trachea*, *Cyathostoma* spp.) in larger passerines
- Foreign bodies (particularly common in Cockatiels due to inhalation of millet seed)
- Tracheal stenosis due to iatrogenic trauma (particularly in macaws, due to intubation with cuffed tubes resulting in pressure necrosis and inflammation)
- Extramural masses or compression due to:
  - Thyroid disease (goitre) (particularly in Budgerigars suffering from iodine deficiency)
  - Fractures of the coracoid
  - Other (e.g. neoplasia).

Differential diagnosis	Comments
Bacterial infections	
Gram-negative (e.g. *Pseudomonas*)	Common in cockatoos; resulting in diphtheritic plaques and granulomas
Chlamydia psittaci	All bird species susceptible; consider in all birds that have recently been in contact with other birds; often systemic illness
Fungal infections	
Aspergillus spp.	Common in birds with malnutrition or stress; formation of granulomas that block the trachea or syrinx; may also affect other parts of the respiratory system
Viral infections	
Adenovirus, avian influenza virus, cytomegalovirus, herpesvirus (e.g. Amazon tracheitis), poxvirus, paramyxovirus	Species commonly affected: Cytomegalovirus: finches Herpesvirus: Amazon parrots – rare Poxvirus: Passeriformes (canaries), birds of prey Paramyxovirus: birds of prey
Parasitic infections	
Cryptosporidium spp. Gapeworms: *Syngamus trachea*, *Cyathostoma* spp. Tracheal mites: *Sternostoma tracheacolum*, *Cytodites* spp. *Trichomonas gallinae*	Species commonly affected: Cryptosporidiosis: birds of prey Gapeworms: larger Passeriformes (e.g. crows, starlings) Tracheal mites: smaller Passeriformes (e.g. canaries, finches) Trichomoniasis: Passeriformes, birds of prey, smaller Psittaciformes

20.30 Differential diagnosis for tracheal disease (voice change, stridor, coughing). (continues) ▶

Differential diagnosis	Comments
Nutritional	
Hypovitaminosis A, resulting in squamous metaplasia and non-infectious granulomas	Particularly in Psittaciformes fed an all-seed diet
Allergic	
Inhalant allergens (e.g. smoke, perfume)	Macaws are anecdotally reported to be more susceptible
Toxic	
Cigarette or tobacco smoke, perfume, aerosol sprays	A thorough history including questions about these potential toxins is required
Environmental	
Dust, dander of other birds	Most likely birds housed under suboptimal conditions. Particularly cockatoos, Grey parrots
Neoplastic	
Carcinoma, adenocarcinoma, papilloma, squamous cell carcinoma, etc	More common in older birds
Foreign body	
e.g. millet seed	Common in Cockatiels
Trauma	
Following intubation with cuffed tubes, resulting in tracheitis and stenosis	Macaws are suggested to be predisposed
Iatrogenic	
Aspiration of food, medication	Can result in acute asphyxia and death
Extramural masses or compression	
Goitre; granulomas; neoplasia Fractures of the coracoid bone (excessive callus formation)	Goitre common in Budgerigars as a result of all-seed diet resulting in iodine deficiency

20.30 (continued) Differential diagnosis for tracheal disease (voice change, stridor, coughing).

Step-by-step approach to suspected tracheal disease

The approach to tracheal disease is summarized in Figure 20.31.

History and physical examination

In any patient with suspected tracheal disease, a full history and physical and faecal examinations need to be performed. The owner should be asked about the speed of onset, duration and course of the disease, as well as the type of respiratory signs that are noted and conditions under which these are seen. If acute dyspnoea and coughing started while the bird was eating, a foreign body inhalation is deemed likely. Inquiries about the bird's diet, environment and exposure to other birds may reveal malnutrition, exposure to respiratory irritants or contagious pathogens. Recent intubation may indicate the presence of tracheal stenosis.

Oral inspection may reveal blunting of the papillae, indicative of vitamin A deficiency, or the presence of plaques (e.g. in poxvirus infections). Closely inspect the glottis and tracheal opening for signs of swelling or inflammation, and check for the presence of mucus, which may indicate tracheitis.

Faecal flotation or direct wet mounts may reveal gapeworm or mite eggs in gallinaceous birds and passerines.

Diagnostic work-up

Tracheoscopy: Tracheoscopy using a rigid endoscope is considered the most useful technique in larger-sized birds, as this allows for visualization of the tracheal lumen and mucosa, which may reveal the presence of foreign bodies, parasites, granulomas or stenosis (Figure 20.32 and **Tracheoscopy** clip on CD). For this procedure, the bird is anaesthetized briefly with isoflurane. When a sufficient depth of anaesthesia is reached, the bird is held in an upright position with its neck stretched, beak open and tongue pulled out to visualize the glottis (Figure 20.33). A rigid endoscope of appropriate size (Figure 20.34) is passed into the glottis and trachea to visualize any abnormalities within the tracheal wall and/or lumen. Care must be taken to ensure the endoscope is passed through the centre of the trachea to avoid damage to the tracheal wall. If abnormalities are visualized, grasping or biopsy forceps, or suction, can be used to collect samples for diagnostic purposes such as cytology, culture and sensitivity, PCR and histopathology.

In smaller birds, transillumination using a bright light may be helpful (Figure 20.35).

> **Editors' note**
> Throughout this volume the emphasis has been on providing care for these species without recourse to specialized equipment. However, tracheoscopy is mandatory when examining and stabilizing the severely dyspnoeic bird. If tracheoscopy is not available then the bird should be referred to the nearest avian veterinary facility as soon as possible and ideally be sent directly to this facility for stabilization. Basic rigid endoscopy equipment (2.7 mm rigid telescope and portable cold light source) can be purchased online for minimal outlay.

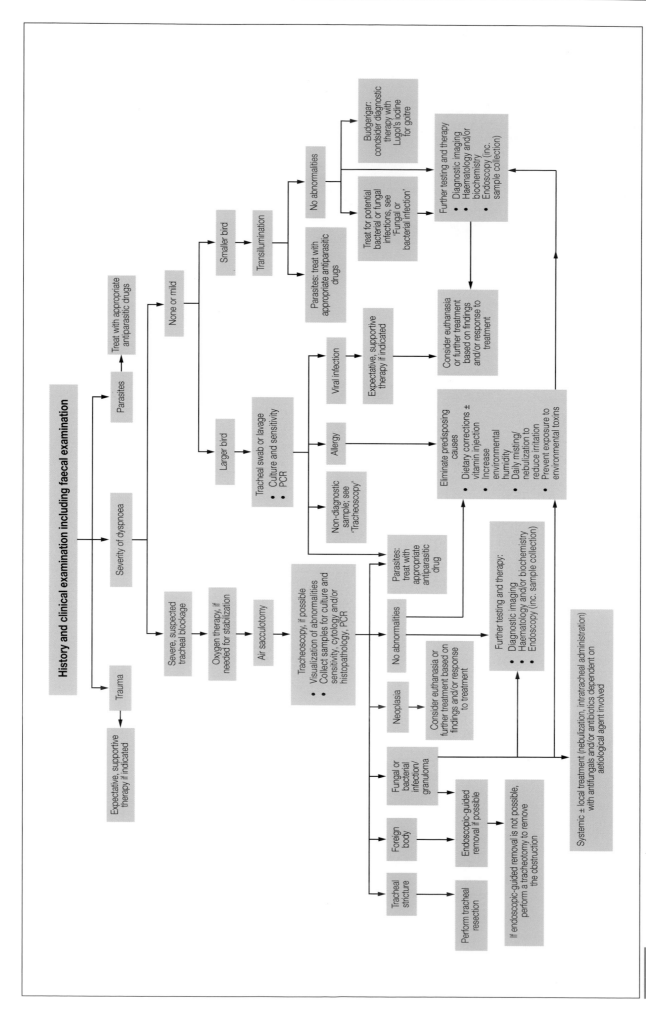

20.31   Approach to tracheal disease (coughing, stridor). PCR = polymerase chain reaction.

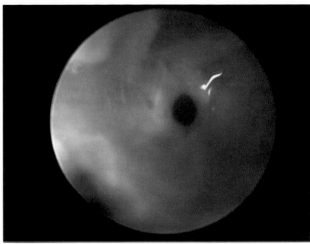

20.32 Upon performing tracheoscopy, a variety of different abnormalities may be encountered, such as parasites, foreign bodies, granulomas and/or strictures. This image, obtained during tracheal endoscopy in a macaw, revealed the presence of a (post-intubation) stricture. (© Yvonne van Zeeland, Utrecht University)

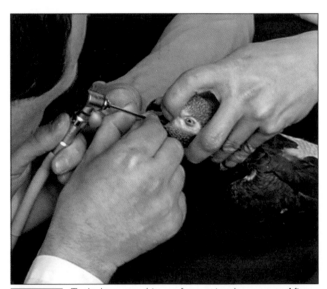

20.33 Technique used to perform a tracheoscopy. After anaesthestizing the bird with isoflurane, an assistant presents the bird with its neck stretched out and beak opened to enable the rigid endoscope to pass into the trachea. (© Yvonne van Zeeland, Utrecht University)

Diameter of the endoscope[a]	Bird species
1.1 mm	Birds <150 g (e.g. Cockatiel, lovebirds)
1.9 mm	Birds >150 g (e.g. corellas, Lesser Sulphur-crested Cockatoo, Timneh Grey Parrot)
2.7 mm	Birds >300 g (e.g. Amazon parrots, Eclectus Parrot, Grey Parrot, Umbrella Cockatoo)
4 mm	Birds >800 g (e.g. Moluccan Cockatoo, macaws)

20.34 General guidelines for endoscope sizes to be used for tracheoscopy in birds. [a]Rigid endoscopes with a 0-degree angle are preferred over those with a 30-degree angle as the former allows for easier manoeuvring in the narrow and straight tracheal lumen.

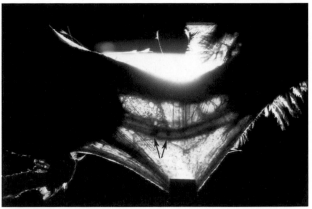

20.35 Transillumination in a small bird, such as this Gouldian Finch, may be useful to detect tracheal mites (arrowed). (© Gerry Dorrestein, NOIVBD)

Diagnostic imaging: Diagnostic imaging may be helpful in some cases, particularly to identify involvement of the lower respiratory tract. On occasion, radiography may reveal intra- or extraluminal obstructions (e.g. foreign bodies, neoplasia, granulomas, callus formation after coracoid fractures). If available, CT imaging is preferred, as this technique provides superior images for diagnosis of tracheal narrowing, obstruction or compression compared with conventional radiographs.

Tracheal swabs or lavage: For cases of tracheitis, tracheal swabs or lavage can be used to collect material for cytology or microbial culture. Tracheal lavage is preferably performed under general anaesthesia, using a soft, sterile tube to infuse sterile saline (0.5–10 ml/kg) into the trachea, which is subsequently aspirated using a sterile syringe that is attached to the tube. Alternatively, 18–22 G Teflon® catheters may be inserted through the skin into the trachea.

Other testing (e.g. haematology and biochemistry, PCR testing for *Chlamydia* infection) follows similar guidelines as previously discussed for rhinitis and sinusitis.

Therapeutic approach

Birds with tracheal obstructions often present as emergency patients, thereby warranting immediate therapeutic intervention. This includes supplementing the patient with oxygen and placement of an air sac cannula to provide a secure airway (see Chapters 16 and 17).

Once the patient is stabilized, endoscopic retrieval or debridement of the obstruction may be attempted using grasping forceps or suction (see **Removal of tracheal obstruction** clip on CD). Throughout this process, materials may be collected for further diagnostic testing. If attempts to remove the obstruction are unsuccessful or if stenosis is present, a tracheotomy and/or tracheal resection can be considered as a next step.

When aspergillomas are present, intratracheal administration of amphotericin B can be helpful, in the author's experience. This treatment may be given as a stand-alone therapy or in combination with nebulization or parenteral administration of antimycotic drugs such as itraconazole, voriconazole and terbinafine. Dependent on the cause, other types of therapy may be initiated. An overview of these is provided in Figure 20.36.

Disease condition	Therapy
Rhinolith	Curettage, treat (secondary) bacterial or fungal infections, dietary correction
Goitre	Lugol's iodine through the drinking water
Bacterial infection	Topical and/or systemic treatment with antibiotics, preferably based on results of a culture and sensitivity test, combined with sinus or nasal flush (in case of rhinitis-sinusitis); treat or eliminate underlying cause
Chlamydia psittaci	Parenteral doxycycline, fluoroquinolones (enrofloxacin) or azithromycin, supportive therapy (if needed). Keep bird in quarantine and notify government as disease is notifiable in many countries. Maintain proper hygiene (zoonotic potential)
Fungal infection	Topical (intratracheal or intranasal, nebulization) and/or systemic treatment with antimycotic drugs such as itraconazole[a], voriconazole, terbinafine. Surgical debridement, endoscopic removal and/or trephination can be considered in case of granulomas. Treat or eliminate underlying cause
Mycoplasma spp.	Tetracyclines, tylosin, fluoroquinolones
Poxvirus	Supportive therapy, administration of vitamin A ointment may be beneficial; treat secondary infections. Canaries can be preventively vaccinated in June-July; also consider insect control (mosquitoes are a vector)
Trichomonas gallinae	Nitroimidazoles (ronidazole, metronidazole)
Cryptosporidium spp.	Paromomycin, azithromycin
Sternostoma tracheacolum	Parenteral or topical ivermectin[b], selamectin; also consider treatment of the environment
Syngamus or *Cyathostoma* spp.	Fenbendazole, levamisole, ivermectin
Hypovitaminosis A	Parenteral vitamin A injection, conversion to a balanced diet
Allergy and/or environmental pollutants	Create a dust-free environment using air filters. Also consider proper ventilation and humidification of the living environment of the bird. Prevent smoking or use of sprays or aerosols in the vicinity of the bird
Neoplasia	Surgical debridement or excision, adjunctive chemotherapy or radiation therapy, dependent on the tumour type
Foreign body	Removal (endoscopic-guided or via tracheotomy)
Tracheal stenosis/stricture	Resection of the section of the trachea containing the stricture; stent placement can also be considered
Choanal atresia	Surgery

20.36 Therapeutic considerations for selected upper respiratory diseases in birds. [a]Itraconazole may be toxic to Grey Parrots and is therefore not recommended for this species. [b]Parenteral ivermectin may be toxic to finches and Budgerigars.

References and further reading

Bailey T (2008) Raptors: respiratory problems. In: *BSAVA Manual of Raptors, Pigeons and Passerine Birds*, ed. J Chitty and M Lierz, pp. 223–234. BSAVA Publications, Gloucester

Brown C and Pilny AA (2005) Air sac cannula placement in birds. *Lab Animal* **35**, 23–24

Doneley B (2008) Pigeons: respiratory problems. In: *BSAVA Manual of Raptors, Pigeons and Passerine Birds*, ed. J Chitty and M Lierz, pp. 320–327. BSAVA Publications, Gloucester

Girling SJ (2005) Respiratory disease. In: *BSAVA Manual of Psittacine Birds, 2nd edn*, ed. N Harcourt-Brown and J Chitty, pp. 170–179. BSAVA Publications, Gloucester

Graham JE (2004) Approach to the dyspneic avian patient. *Seminars in Avian and Exotic Pet Medicine* **13**, 154–159

Hillyer EV, Orosz S and Dorrestein GM (1997) Respiratory system. In: *Avian Medicine and Surgery*, ed. RB Altman, SL Clubb, GM Dorrestein and KE Quesenberry, pp. 387–411. Saunders, Philadelphia

Jenkins JR (1997) Hospital techniques and supportive care. In: *Avian Medicine and Surgery*, ed. RB Altman, SL Clubb, GM Dorrestein and KE Quesenberry, pp. 232–252. Saunders, Philadelphia

Lawton M (1999) Management of respiratory disease in psittacine birds. *In Practice* **21**, 76–88

Morrisey JK (1997) Diseases of the upper respiratory tract of companion birds. *Seminars in Avian and Exotic Pet Medicine* **6**, 195–200

Orosz SE and Lichtenberger M (2011) Avian respiratory distress: etiology, diagnosis and treatment. *Veterinary Clinics of North America: Exotic Animal Practice* **14**, 241–255

Pye GW (2000) Surgery of the avian respiratory system. *Veterinary Clinics of North America: Exotic Animal Practice* **3**, 693–713

Rupley AE (1997) Respiratory signs. In: *Manual of Avian Practice*, pp. 55–90. Saunders, Philadelphia

Tully TN (1994) Pneumonology. In: *Avian Medicine: Principles and Application*, ed. BW Ritchie, GJ Harrison and LR Harrison, pp. 556–581. Wingers Publications, Lake Worth

Tully TN (1995) Avian respiratory disease: clinical overview. *Journal of Avian Medicine and Surgery* **9**, 162–174

CD extras

Removal of tracheal obstruction
Tail bobbing
Tracheal obstruction
Tracheoscopy

Case example 1: Canary with obstructed naris

Presentation and history

A 10-year-old male Atlantic Canary was presented with a unilateral obstruction of the right naris of 3 weeks' duration. The obstruction was due to the presence of a mass that appeared to be increasing in size. The bird showed no other signs of illness and was found to be bright, alert and active. No nasal discharge had been noted by the owner. The bird had no prior history of illness, and was eating and drinking well. The bird was housed solitarily in a large cage in the house and was fed a bird seed diet, supplemented with some fruits and vegetables.

Clinical examination

Upon physical examination, a whitish discoloration of the beak was noted, which was found to be irregular in shape. The right naris was severely disrupted, with a rhinolith present.

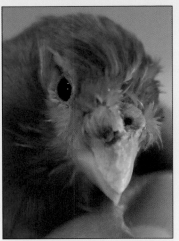

(© Yvonne van Zeeland, Utrecht University)

Sampling

The rhinolith was removed using a small curette, and samples were submitted for culture and sensitivity testing, which yielded no presence of pathogens.

Therapy

The bird was given a multivitamin injection. To prevent future problems, the owner was advised to either convert the bird to a pelleted diet or supplement its current diet with egg food in a 1:1 ratio.

Outcome

Although the naris remained permanently distorted, the bird lived for several years in good health.

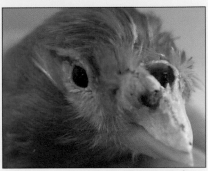

(© Yvonne van Zeeland, Utrecht University)

Case example 2: Cockatiel with swelling below the eye

Presentation and history

A 3-year-old male Cockatiel was presented with a 6-month history of sneezing, inflation of the cervicocephalic air sacs, mild dyspnoea and progressive swelling of the ventral eyelids. The owner noticed that the bird was also scratching and rubbing its head along the perch, indicating the presence of pruritus and/or irritation to the eyelids. Although the bird did not show other signs of generalized illness, it did appear to be a bit less active.

Throughout its life, the bird had been housed on its own in a standard-sized cage, which was placed in the living room of the owner. It had been fed an all-seed diet supplemented with some fruits and vegetables. Because of this, the referring veterinary surgeon had initially advised conversion to a pelleted diet and gave a multivitamin injection, but this did not result in resolution of the clinical signs.

Clinical examination

Upon physical examination, a severe bilateral swelling, ventral to the eye, was identified. The bird sneezed, producing a clear, serous nasal discharge. A distension of the cervicocephalic air sac and some mild dyspnoea was noted. The bird was otherwise found to be healthy and in good condition, with no other abnormalities identified.

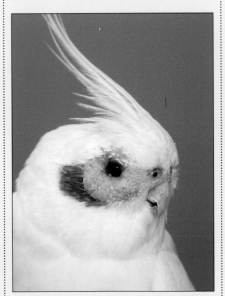

(© Yvonne van Zeeland, Utrecht University)

Sampling

A nasal flush and fine-needle aspirate of the sinus yielded no material. The sinuses were opened surgically, revealing the swelling to consist of solid, white tissue, with no caseous or purulent exudate present. Biopsy samples were collected for histopathology, which revealed the presence of a xanthoma.

Therapy

The bird was started on treatment with carprofen and trimethoprim-sulfa, pending sample results. Due to the size of the swellings, surgical debulking or excision was not considered an option. Therapy was, therefore, expectative, with advice to maintain the bird on a proper diet.

Outcome

Over several months, the clinical signs progressed and the bird was eventually euthanased due to progressive dyspnoea.

Case example 3: Gyrfalcon with dyspnoea and stridor

Presentation and history

A 4-year-old male hybrid Gyrfalcon was presented with a history of sneezing, nasal discharge, swollen eyelids, yawning and progressive dyspnoea, and exercise intolerance. These signs had been present for several weeks.

The bird came from a falcon breeding facility, where approximately 150 birds were kept in pairs. The falconer had noted similar signs in other birds at the facility, particularly in younger falcons, of which several had died. Although pathology had been performed on many of these birds, no aetiological cause had been identified.

Clinical examination

Tail bobbing and open-beak breathing were noted on observation of the bird from a distance and, upon physical examination, the bird was found to be in poor condition. Mucus nasal discharge and conjunctivitis were present. During restraint, the bird became progressively dyspnoeic. A gargling sound, sneezing and tracheal stridor were also noted. Upon oral inspection, a swelling and erythema of the glottal rim were noted.

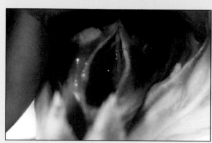

(© Yvonne van Zeeland, Utrecht University)

Sampling

A full haematological and biochemical profile was conducted, with all values considered to be within normal limits. Bacterial and fungal culture of material collected from the trachea (swab) and nasal cavity (flush) showed no growth of pathogens. Testing for the presence of *Chlamydia psittaci* (PCR and immuno-fluorescent antibody test of a conjunctival/choanal/cloacal swab) was negative. A biopsy sample was collected from the swollen mucosa of the glottis for histopathology, which revealed that *Cryptosporidium* spp. was present, definitively diagnosed as *Cryptosporidium baileyi* by PCR.

Therapy

Treatment was initiated with azithromycin for 3 days. As this treatment did not have any effect, the bird was subsequently switched to a therapy with paromomycin for 2 weeks, however, there was no clinical resolution of the signs following treatment with this drug either.

Outcome

Due to the lack of response to therapy and the bird's clinical condition, the prognosis was considered poor and the bird was euthanased.

An approach to the swollen avian eye

David Williams

A bird arriving with what the owner considers as a swollen eye might indeed have an enlarged globe resulting from an increase in intraocular pressure (IOP) or as a result of abnormal enlargement while having a normal IOP. However, much more likely in birds is that the patient has a periocular swelling related to infection and inflammation of the periocular sinuses or, if somewhat less marked, a chemotic swollen conjunctiva. Remember that the periocular space also includes the retrobulbar area. Less commonly, but still important to be aware of, the bird may have a neoplasm either within the eye or in the periocular region causing periocular swelling or even exophthalmos. In some instances, nothing may be enlarged at all except for the pupil – an optical illusion makes an eye with a widely dilated pupil appear larger. So a simple presentation of 'swollen eye' could be the result of a panoply of diseases. Most of these conditions are difficult to treat and management, rather than treatment, may be required.

Ophthalmic examination

Any bird presented with a swollen eye should undergo an ophthalmic examination. Assessing the visual capability of the eye in any species requires a menace response (reflex blinking in response to an approaching object) but this can be difficult in the bird. As described in Chapter 10, the use of a direct ophthalmoscope to examine the retina, lens and cornea on 0, 10 and 20 dioptres is mandatory, and, if available, an indirect ophthalmoscopic view of the fundus of the eye allows excellent assessment of whether the retina and the pecten are normal or damaged.

It might seem at first glance easy to distinguish an abnormality of the globe from swelling in the periocular region. In birds, the infraorbital sinus has extensive communication around much of the periocular region. Variations in the aetiology of infraorbital sinus swelling, as well as the gross appearance of swellings, sometimes complicate immediate diagnosis.

Infection is the most common cause of infraorbital swelling (see below), although repetitive swelling can be seen associated with respiratory changes in cases of obstructive breathing patterns. Infraorbital sinus swelling can also occur in conjunction with globe pathology.

Adnexal changes can lead to globe pathology through ocular surface exposure or leave the eye itself unscathed. The key in every case is to perform a full evaluation of the eyelids, the conjunctiva, the cornea and the intra-ocular structures. A checklist for ocular examinations:

- Check for head symmetry
- Palpate the periocular region to assess whether any swelling is firm or soft
- Evaluate the nostrils and choanal slit for discharge
- Listen for upper respiratory noise, both grossly and via auscultation
- Perform an ophthalmic examination, followed, if the instrumentation is available, with:
  - Measurement of the IOP
  - Schirmer tear test (although reference ranges vary dramatically between species. Practitioners are encouraged to research current literature)
  - Ultrasonography of the eye and periocular region
- Other tests include:
  - Cytology of the conjunctiva
  - Aerobic and anaerobic bacteriological culture and sensitivity.

Fortunately, in ophthalmology, so much can be gained from a thorough physical examination that this often provides quite sufficient information for diagnosis.

A key question is whether the swelling involves the globe itself or is limited to the periocular region. If the swelling is confined to a discrete area dorsal or ventral to the globe, an infraorbital sinusitis is the most likely diagnosis. If the swelling extends further around the globe, a wider inflammatory process involving other parts of the periocular sinus system may be involved.

Alternatively, the swelling may be extra-sinus and represent an inflammatory reaction or cellulitis in subcutaneous tissues. While trauma may be responsible (Figure 21.1), another common cause is a reaction to tick bites (Figure 21.2). In some cases the tick may still be present while in others the tick may have already detached, leaving clinical appearance and history as means of diagnosis. Therapy involves broad-spectrum antibiosis, fluid support and short-acting corticosteroids (this is one of the very few indications for corticosteroids in avian medicine). Prompt recognition and therapy is essential as death can result.

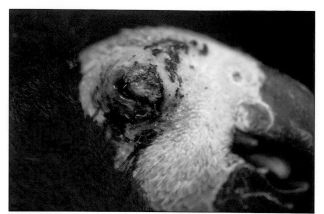

21.1 Generalized swelling of the ocular region in an African Grey Parrot. Trauma caused by another bird resulted in laceration of the third eyelid and a retrobulbar abscess. The globe was unaffected. (© John Chitty)

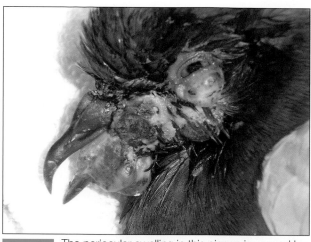

21.3 The periocular swelling in this pigeon is caused by avian poxvirus infection.

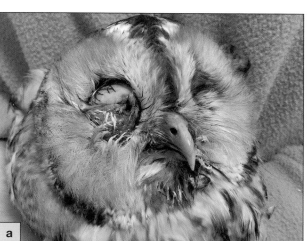

a

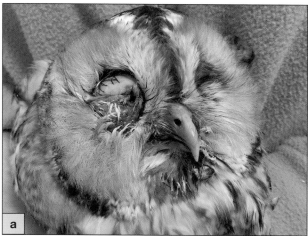

b

21.2 **(a)** Tick bite reaction in a Tawny Owl. **(b)** A localized tick bite reaction in the lower lid of a Harris' Hawk. (© John Chitty)

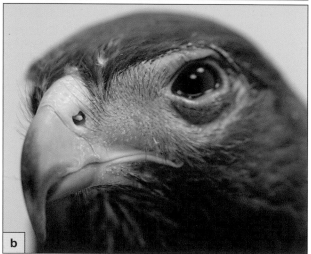

21.4 Infraorbital sinus neoplasia is uncommon; lymphoma is the most frequent type, as there is a large amount of lymphoid tissue in this region. The solid bilateral swellings in this African Grey Parrot were diagnosed as lymphoma by examination of fine-needle aspirates. (© John Chitty)

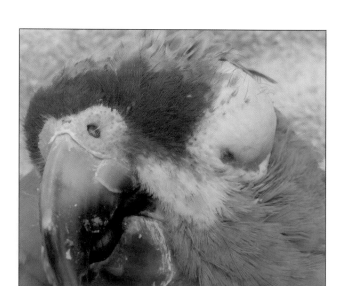

21.5 Fluid swelling on the dorsal part of the infraorbital sinus in an Amazon parrot. (© John Chitty)

Poxvirus can cause significant periocular swelling, although this is usually associated with scabbing and has quite a characteristic appearance (Figure 21.3).

If, however, the swelling is confined to the conjunctiva, then a conjunctivitis may be the sole problem or the only sign of systemic disease or even infectious/zoonotic disease (e.g. *Chlamydia psittaci*; see Chapter 19). If the swelling is firm, a chronic sinusitis (or, more rarely, neoplasia; Figure 21.4) may be the cause, while a soft fluctuant swelling may be fluid (Figure 21.5) or merely air (Figure 21.6), where the sinus is abnormally inflating because a plug of mucus or similar is acting as a valve and allowing air into the sinus but not letting it out. The anatomy of the sinus system is described in Chapter 2, which shows how such swelling may occur.

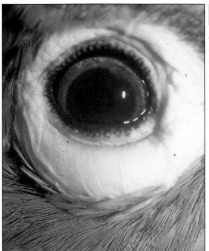

21.6 Amazon parrot with air-filled periocular swelling and cervicocephalic air sac obstruction.

Causes of ocular/periocular swelling

- Buphthalmos (uncommon)
  - Glaucoma
  - Uveitis
  - Developmental blindness
  - Neoplasia
- Exophthalmos/strabismus
  - Retrobulbar swelling
    - Abscessation
    - Neoplasia
    - Haematoma
  - Head/ocular trauma
  - Periorbital swelling (see below)
- Periorbital swelling
  - Infraorbital sinus
    - Infection (bacterial/fungal)
    - Inflation (usually associated with blockage in sinus/air sac drainage or severe dyspnoea)
    - Haemorrhage, including coagulopathy
    - Trauma
    - Neoplasia (uncommon)
  - Skin
    - Viral infections including poxvirus
    - Generalized dermatitis (bacterial/fungal)
    - Cnemidocoptic mange
    - Irritation from other external parasites including ticks/flies
    - Age-related skin changes (e.g. Galahs, other cockatoos)
    - Trauma
    - Neoplasia
- Conjunctiva/eyelids
  - Viral infections including poxvirus
  - Bacterial infections including *Chlamydia* and *Mycoplasma* spp.
  - Trauma including haematoma/bruising
  - Foreign bodies
  - Neoplasia

An approach to infraorbital sinusitis

It might be quite possible, as noted above, to come to a provisional diagnosis of infraorbital sinusitis (Figure 21.7) quickly, but treatment is a significantly more taxing task. Often the sinus fills with a solid caseous mass because the heterophils (which characterize avian pus) do not contain granules with oxidative and degradative enzymes, which result in the fluid pus of a mammalian abscess populated by neutrophils. A fine-needle aspirate biopsy will aid in assessing quite how viscous the purulent material is, and indeed whether the diagnosis of infraorbital sinusitis was the correct one in the first place. While this may be done on a conscious patient, it requires confidence and excellent restraint. Many practitioners prefer to anaesthetize their patients for safety. Positive contrast sinography (see Chapter 18) or an ultrasound scan (using a 12 MHz probe with a very small footplate), will aid in defining the extent of the sinus involvement and, if possible, further diagnostic imaging, such as magnetic resonance imaging (MRI) or computed tomography (CT) scanning, can prove particularly illuminating. The difficulty comes not so much in diagnosing the problem as in treating it. Many sinus lesions are so hard that the only way of removing them is by sharp dissection (Figure 21.8; see Chapter 17), while a small number can be resolved by flushing the cephalic sinus system (Figure 21.9; see Chapter 20), although in more complex or recurrent cases the bird will benefit from referral to a specialist centre.

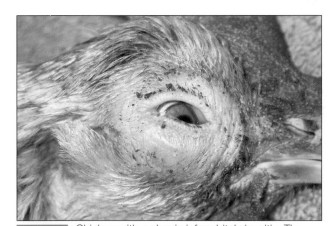

21.7 Chicken with a classic infraorbital sinusitis. The globe appears normal but vision is impeded by the swelling below the eye.

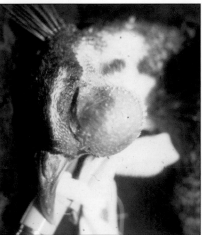

21.8 The severe infraorbital sinusitis in this peahen has formed a fibriscess where surgical removal of the inflammatory mass is necessary.

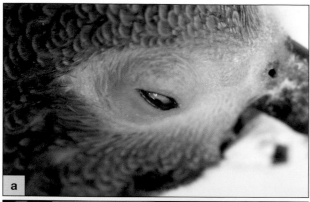

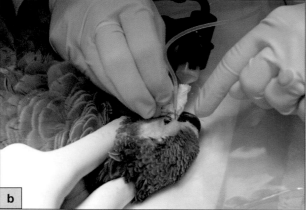

21.9 **(a)** The periocular swelling in this African Grey Parrot with sinusitis has been identified early enough that **(b)** flushing can alleviate the signs.

An approach to conjunctivitis

An eye where the conjunctivae are swollen and red is likely to have conjunctivitis (Figure 21.10) associated with infection. This could involve viruses (e.g. influenza or Newcastle disease), bacteria (e.g. *Chlamydia* or *Mycoplasma* spp.) or parasites (e.g. trematodes) (see Chapter 19). Cytology and bacteriology are essential diagnostic steps in the full evaluation of such conditions, although in many psittacine cases bacteriology fails to identify a specific agent, even where cytology shows a heterophilic infiltrate characteristic of bacterial infection. It is also the case that many cases are not primarily infectious and bacterial invasion is secondary to irritation (e.g. cigarette or wood smoke), allergy or hypovitaminosis A.

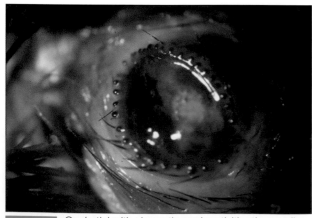

21.10 Cockatiel with chemotic conjunctivitis; the swollen conjunctiva severely impedes vision. This condition is responsive to topical antibiotic drops.

In cases of suspected chlamydiosis (psittacosis) or mycoplasmosis, polymerase chain reaction (PCR) testing of the sample obtained can give a diagnosis even when culture does not show a live organism; culture is unreliable with these agents.

Differentiating globe enlargement and exophthalmos

Where the eye appears to have an increased size it can be difficult initially to differentiate between globe enlargement and exophthalmos. The best method of differentiating between these two clinical entities is an ultrasonographic scan, with which the exact size of the globe can be measured and any retrobulbar swelling can also be appreciated. In birds the globe is much more closely apposed to the orbital wall than in the mammals practitioners are more used to dealing with, so a small amount of retrobulbar swelling can produce a more pronounced proptosis. Generally, also glaucoma is much less common in birds than in dogs and cats, so frank globe enlargement is lower down the differential list. Having said that, it can occur and is covered in more detail below.

Causes of globe enlargement

The sclera of most birds is thinner than that of a comparably sized mammal so a rise in IOP can produce globe enlargement or buphthalmos. Primary glaucoma has been diagnosed in one group of Snowy Owls (Rayment and Williams, 1997) but, much more commonly, an increase in IOP occurs secondary to intraocular inflammation or uveitis. Generally, uveitis results in a reduced IOP, since a prostaglandin-mediated increase in unconventional aqueous drainage occurs, not giving fluid outflow through the iridocorneal angle but rather through newly opened drainage pathways in the choroid. This happens when inflammatory debris blocks the iridocorneal angle, preventing aqueous drainage through the conventional outflow pathways. Even when this does occur, the increase in unconventional outflow may not be sufficient to overcome the inflammatory obstruction of aqueous drainage and thus glaucoma can occur secondary to fibrin production in an anterior uveitis, thus resulting in globe enlargement.

Another cause of globe enlargement in young birds can be compensation for a vision defect. The growth of the posterior segment of the normal developing eye is controlled by a feedback pathway involving the visual stimulus. It is in this manner that the growing eye remains emmetropic, correctly focusing the image on the retina. Obscuring vision in chickens results in a globe enlargement, not through increased IOP, but by abnormal growth of sclera in the posterior part of the eye. This has become an important model for the development of emmetropia in the human eye and also for understanding why a young bird with a visual deficit develops an abnormally large eye, which may be confused with one becoming buphthalmic through an increase in IOP. Similarly, birds kept in dark environments develop enlarged eyes.

It is assumed that the normal IOP in an avian eye is 15–20 mmHg, as in the companion mammals more commonly dealt with, but there is actually little evidence if that is the case. An evaluation of the IOP in

100 backyard chickens by the author showed the IOP to be 11.4 ± 1.2 mmHg as measured with the Tonovet® rebound tonometer, but this varied from 12.7 ± 1 to 10.6 ± 0.9 mmHg in birds of 1 and 7 years, respectively (Williams, in production). One study examining the IOP in over 100 3-week-old chicks found an IOP of 17.5 ± 0.1 mmHg using the Tonovet® rebound tonometer (Prashar et al., 2007). It is difficult to know how this figure relates to the lower values observed in older birds and indeed what relevance such data has to IOPs in different species of birds with eyes of extremely varied size and morphology (e.g. owls with wide iridocorneal angles compared to sparrows with very much smaller outflow structures).

Barsotti et al. (2013) and Reuter et al. (2011) both looked at IOP values in raptors (Figure 21.11). Both studies report substantially different values between species; differences between values for the same species may be explained by factors such as body position and time of day (Reuter et al., 2011). Another report documented IOP for ostriches measured using a Tonopen® applanation tonometer as being 18.8 ± 3.5 mmHg for all birds; IOP in juvenile ostriches measured 19.7 ± 3.6 mmHg and in adult birds 16.9 ± 2.9 mmHg, so there are differences between birds of different ages as well as different species (Ghaffari et al., 2012). The tonometric measurement is influenced by corneal thickness as well as by IOP, potentially explaining the intraspecies differences. In albino mutant quails, IOP of 19.6 ± 1.6 mmHg was found, compared with a pressure of 16.3 ± 1.4 mmHg in normal quails. The difference may not seem large but the mutant birds were glaucomatous, with ganglion cell loss and blindness (Takatsuji et al., 1986).

To date there is very little information on IOP in passerines or parrots; therefore, in a bird with unilateral ocular pathology, the unaffected eye should be used as a comparison where glaucoma is suspected. Alternatively, the IOPs from normal birds of the same species in the same environment can also be used as a comparison.

Species	Intraocular pressure
Hawks	
Common Buzzard	17.2 ± 3.53 mmHg[a] 26.9 ± 7.0 mmHg[b]
Eurasian Sparrowhawk	15.5 ± 2.5 mmHg[b]
Northern Goshawk	18.3 ± 3.8 mmHg[b]
Red Kite	13.0 ± 5.5 mmHg[b]
Falcons	
European Kestrel	8.53 ± 1.59 mmHg[a] 9.8 ± 2.5 mmHg[b]
Peregrine Falcon	12.7 ± 5.8 mmHg[b]
Eagles	
White-tailed Sea Eagle	26.9 ± 5.8 mmHg[b]
Owls	
Barn Owl	10.8 ± 3.8 mmHg[b]
Little Owl	9.83 ± 3.41 mmHg[a]
Long-eared Owl	7.8 ± 3.2 mmHg[b]
Tawny Owl	11.21 ± 3.12 mmHg[a] 9.4 ± 4.1 mmHg[b]

21.11 Intraocular pressure of raptors. [a]Barsotti et al., 2013; [b]Reuter et al., 2011.

There is even less data on the effects of anti-glaucoma medications normally used in mammals on the normal or glaucomatous avian eye. Carbonic anhydrase is an enzyme central in the production of the aqueous humour across mammals and birds; therefore, carbonic anhydrase inhibitors (e.g. dorzolamide) might be expected to act in a similar method in birds as in mammals. There is less certainty about the presence of receptors, such as those upon which the prostaglandin analogue latanoprost acts in dogs and primates. Timolol, a beta-adrenergic antagonist, reduces the IOP in chickens with experimental myopia (Schmid et al., 2000). Timolol and pilocarpine both reduced IOP in light-induced avian globe enlargement (Lauber et al., 1985), but the relevance to glaucoma in other avian species is unclear.

Exophthalmic globe

If the size of the globe is not increased but rather the eye is being pushed forward, then a retrobulbar space-occupying lesion is most likely to be the cause of the problem. Infection, of either the orbit or the periorbital sinuses, might be responsible, but in these cases one is more likely to see concurrent periocular swelling rather than merely a protrusion of the globe. Although rare, orbital neoplasms are more likely to be the cause of a straightforward globe exophthalmos than infectious aetiologies. Orbital adenomas and adenocarcinomas have been reported; pituitary neoplasms, which are a relatively common cause of exophthalmos in Budgerigars, have been described as long ago as 1954 but recently investigated in more detail (Dezfoulian et al., 2011; Langohr et al., 2012).

Enucleation and evisceration

Where globe enlargement occurs and the eye is blind with corneal exposure and ulceration, enucleation may be considered the best therapeutic option. Complete globe removal is a considerably more complex operation in birds than in mammals, because of the relative globe size in the avian head and the presence of scleral ossicles (bony plates) immediately behind the cornea, which preclude collapse of the globe in many cases. A better surgical option may be evisceration, where the globe contents are removed after opening the cornea (Dees et al., 2011; Murray et al., 2013). The resulting scleral shell is then packed with haemostatic felt or a similar substance and the eyelids closed across the face of the globe. This has the advantage of keeping the weight of the affected side of the skull roughly equivalent to the side with the remaining eye, as well as being a much easier and more rapid surgery.

Enucleation

This is more involved than in mammals due to the:

- Small overall size of the eye, but very large in relation to the rest of the head
- Extremely thin bone behind the eye meaning damage is easily done
- Extremely short optic nerve and blood vessels; iatrogenic damage to the rostral brain is more likely
- Little peribulbar tissue within the cavity
- Very muscular third eyelid with rich blood supply.

Enucleation is always performed under general anaesthesia (Figure 21.12):

1. The peribulbar area is prepared aseptically.
2. The eyelid margins are resected.
3. The third eyelid is located and retracted.
4. The margins of the globe are exposed and the eye incised at the junction of the cornea and sclera.
5. The contents of the eye are removed.
6. The sclera is removed piece by piece.
7. The optic nerve and blood vessels may be located and ligated. However, it is more usual to leave these *in situ*, attached to a very small piece of sclera in order to avoid excessive trauma.
8. The third eyelid is resected.
9. The cavity is closed in 2–3 layers using simple continuous sutures with 1 or 1.5 metric (5/0 or 4/0 USP) absorbable material.

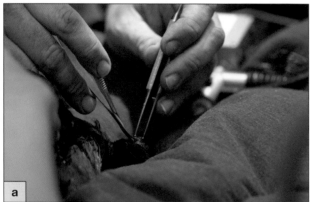

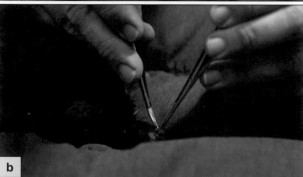

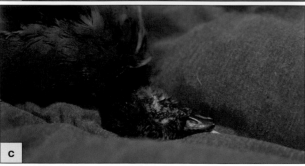

21.12 **(a–b)** Having prepared the eye aseptically and debrided the eyelid margins, the eye is dissected free by means of cutting the muscular attachments. **(c)** Having removed the eye (usually piecemeal), the third eyelid is removed and the lid edges opposed using two layers of simple continuous sutures. (© John Chitty)

References and further reading

Bailey TA, Nicholls PK, Wernery U *et al.* (1997) Avian paramyxovirus type 1 infection in houbara bustards (*Chlamydotis undulata macqueenii*): clinical and pathologic findings. *Journal of Zoo and Wildlife Medicine* **28(3)**, 325–330

Barsotti G, Briganti A, Spratte JR, Ceccherelli R and Breghi G (2013) Schirmer tear test type I readings and IOP values assessed by applanation tonometry (Tonopen® XL) in normal eyes of four European species of birds of prey. *Veterinary Ophthalmology* **16(5)**, 365–369

Dees DD, Knollinger AM and MacLaren NE (2011) Modified evisceration technique in a golden eagle (*Aquila chrysaetos*). *Veterinary Ophthalmology* **14(5)**, 341–344

Dezfoulian O, Abbasi M, Azarabad H, Nouri M and Kiani K (2011) Cerebral neuroblastoma and pituitary adenocarcinoma in two budgerigars (*Melopsittacus undulatus*). *Avian Diseases* **55(4)**, 704–708

Erickson GA, Maré CJ, Gustafson GA *et al.* (1977) Interactions between viscerotropic velogenic Newcastle disease virus and pet birds of six species. I. Clinical and serologic responses, and viral excretion. *Avian Diseases* **21(4)**, 642–654

Fernández-Juricic E, Moore BA, Doppler M *et al.* (2011) Testing the terrain hypothesis: Canada geese see their world laterally and obliquely. *Brain, Behavior and Evolution* **77(3)**, 147–158

Ghaffari MS, Sabzevari A, Vahedi H, Golezardy H (2012) Determination of reference values for intraocular pressure and Shirmer tear test in clinically normal ostriches (*Struthio camelus*). *Journal of Zoo and Wildlife Medicine* **43(2)**, 229–232

Grodio JL, Ley DH, Schat KA and Hawley DM (2013) Chronic *Mycoplasma* conjunctivitis in house finches: host antibody response and *M. gallisepticum* VlhA expression. *Veterinary Immunology and Immunopathology* **154(3–4)**,129–137

Gustafson CR, Cooper GL, Charlton BR and Bickford AA (1998) *Pasteurella multocida* infection involving cranial air spaces in White Leghorn chickens. *Avian Diseases* **42(2)**, 413–417

Langohr IM, Garner MM and Kiupel M (2012) Somatotroph pituitary tumors in budgerigars (*Melopsittacus undulatus*). *Veterinary Pathology* **49(3)**, 503–507

Lauber JK, McLaughlin MA and Chiou GC (1985) Timolol and pilocarpine are hypotensive in light-induced avian glaucoma. *Canadian Journal of Ophthalmology* **20(4)**, 147–152

Molina-Lopez RA, Ramis A, Martin-Vazquez S *et al.* (2010) *Cryptosporidium baileyi* infection associated with an outbreak of ocular and respiratory disease in otus owls (*Otus scops*) in a rehabilitation centre. *Avian Pathology* **39(3)**, 171–176

Murakami S, Miyama M, Ogawa A, Shimada J and Nakane T (2002) Occurrence of conjunctivitis, sinusitis and upper region tracheitis in Japanese quail (*Coturnix coturnix japonica*), possibly caused by *Mycoplasma gallisepticum* accompanied by *Cryptosporidium* sp. infection. *Avian Pathology* **31(4)**, 363–370

Murray M, Pizzirani S and Tseng F (2013) A technique for evisceration as an alternative to enucleation in birds of prey: 19 cases. *Journal of Avian Medicine and Surgery* **27(2)**, 120–127

Nakamura K, Ohta Y, Abe Y, Imai K and Yamada M (2004) Pathogenesis of conjunctivitis caused by Newcastle disease viruses in specific-pathogen-free chickens. *Avian Pathology* **33(3)**, 371–376

Prashar A, Guggenheim JA, Erichsen JT and Morgan JE (2007) Measurement of intraocular pressure (IOP) in chickens using a rebound tonometer: quantitative evaluation of variance due to position inaccuracies. *Experimental eye research* **85(4)**, 563–571

Rayment LJ and Williams D (1997) Glaucoma in a captive-bred Great Horned Owl (*Bubo virginianus virginianus*). *Veterinary Record* **140**, 481–483

Reuter A, Müller K, Arndt G and Eule JC (2011) Reference intervals for IOP measured by rebound tonometry in ten raptor species and factors affecting the IOP. *Journal of Avian Medicine and Surgery* **25(3)**, 165–172

Schmid KL, Abbott M, Humphries M, Pyne K and Wildsoet C (2000) Timolol lowers IOP but does not inhibit the development of experimental myopia in chick. *Experimental Eye Research* **70(5)**, 659–666

Shivaprasad HL and Phalen DN (2012) A novel herpesvirus associated with respiratory disease in Bourke's parrots (*Neopsephotus bourkii*). *Avian Pathology* **41(6)**, 531–539

Simova-Curd S, Richter M, Hauser B and Hatt JM (2009) Surgical removal of a retrobulbar adenoma in an African grey parrot (*Psittacus erithacus*). *Journal of Avian Medicine and Surgery* **23(1)**, 24–28

Takatsuji K, Sato Y, Iizuka S, Nakatani H and Nakamura A (1986) Animal model of closed angle glaucoma in albino mutant quails. *Investigative Ophthalmology and Visual Science* **27(3)**, 396–400

Watson VE, Murdock JH, Cazzini P *et al.* (2013) Retrobulbar adenocarcinoma in an Amazon parrot (*Amazona autumnalis*). *Journal of Veterinary Diagnostic Investigation* **25(2)**, 273–276

Williams D (in production) Ophthalmological (ocular) and otic (ear) disorders. In: *BSAVA Manual of Backyard Poultry*, ed. G Poland and A Raftery. BSAVA Publications, Gloucester

Case example 1: Conure with squamous cell carcinoma

Presentation and history

A female Green-cheeked Conure of unknown age was presented with a mass on the right eyelid. The bird had been purchased 1 week before with little history, and the new owner noticed a mass. The bird was bright and alert, and in reasonable body condition. There was a mild heart murmur present.

Diagnostic work-up

The bird was anaesthetized with isoflurane and oxygen, and an incisional biopsy of the mass was taken. Recovery was normal.

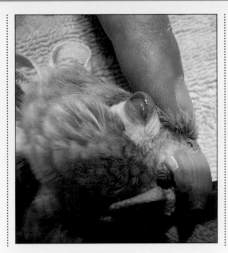

Therapy

The bird was placed on co-amoxiclav and meloxicam postoperatively. The histopathology results were consistent with a squamous cell carcinoma with incomplete margins.

Outcome

The bird survived 10 more months, before quality of life issues necessitated euthanasia.

Case example 2: Budgerigar with a retrobulbar mass

Presentation and history

A 7-year-old Budgerigar was presented with a sore-looking eye. Clinical examination revealed an exophthalmic left eye, with erythema, chemosis and a fixed dilated pupil.

Outcome

A retrobulbar mass was suspected and the owner elected for euthanasia without any further diagnostic tests.

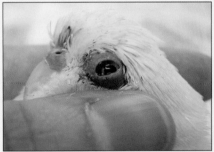
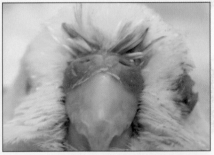

In a larger bird, if authorized, diagnostic testing may have included ultrasonographic examination and a possible attempt at fine-needle aspiration of the mass (dependent on size and access) with subsequent cytology. The prognosis of avian retrobulbar masses is poor.

Case example 3: Magpie with avian poxvirus

Presentation and history

A wild Australian Magpie presented with scabby, raised lesions in the periocular and perioral skin. These were consistent with avian poxvirus, and the case coincided with many wild birds being presented with similar signs.

Therapy and outcome

The bird was placed into care with a registered wildlife rehabilitator, and was

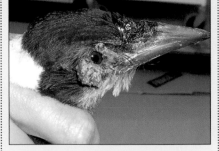

released when the lesions were fully healed, around 3 weeks later.

Cutaneous avian poxvirus is a common disease of wild passerines in Australia, and is usually self-limiting, provided there is no secondary bacterial infection. If the lesions are large, or interfere with vision or prehension of food, the birds may come into care. There is some concern about the contagious nature of the infection, which occurs through abraded skin, and some carers will not take on afflicted individuals for that reason. Nonetheless, given supportive care and feeding, most birds will recover and maintain a transient immunity.

Lower respiratory tract disease

John Chitty and Deborah Monks

Lower respiratory tract disease (LRTD) is common in parrots, raptors and passerines. However, it can be difficult to recognize because presenting signs are often non-specific and frequently not obviously respiratory. For the purposes of this chapter, the lower respiratory tract refers to the lungs and air sacs; investigation of disease in other parts of the respiratory system is described in Chapter 20.

Anatomy

The relevant anatomy and physiology of the avian lower respiratory tract is described in Chapter 2. The differences between birds and mammals explain some of the main reasons why respiratory signs are not always obvious in birds with LRTD and why clinical examination does not always pinpoint this system (Figure 22.1).

Anatomical feature	Effect
Fixed lungs with air capillaries	As birds lack alveoli, and the lungs do not expand/contract with breaths, there are no lung sounds to be heard on auscultation of the normal bird. Lung sounds may be produced in disease, but only in severe cases
Air sacs	The large volume of residual air and the time spent by air in the air sacs makes these susceptible to infection and/or irritation by airborne agents/materials. Again, minimal movements result in fewer audible sounds on auscultation. Those sounds that are heard tend to originate from the air sacs rather than the lungs (see above)
Respiratory movements	Breathing is by means of keel movements that may be almost imperceptible on observation. Large respiratory movements are only seen in severe cases. As a result of the body movements needed for increased effort, tail bobbing is the main sign of increased effort
Lack of exercise and respiratory reserve	Because of the air capillary system, birds have a very efficient gas exchange. Few captive birds, other than falconry birds, will exercise as they would in the wild, meaning that respiratory reserve is rarely reached except in advanced disease. Similarly, lack of exercise will result in obesity impinging on air sac volume, and reduced air movements in the air sacs further increasing the likelihood of infection/irritation

22.1 Effects of avian anatomy and physiology on clinical signs of lower respiratory tract disease (LRTD). (continues)

Anatomical feature	Effect
Plumage	Weight loss is often a feature of LRTD. Weight loss is not evident without keel palpation until it is extreme, because of the plumage covering the keel area.
Pneumatized bones	May allow entry of infection from limb injuries.

22.1 (continued) Effects of avian anatomy and physiology on clinical signs of lower respiratory tract disease (LRTD).

Clinical signs

The clinical signs of LRTD may be respiratory or non-specific.

Respiratory signs of LRTD

- Increased respiratory movements; tail bobbing; increased sternal movement (Figure 22.2).
- Open-beak breathing; extended head and neck.
- Altered voice.
- Respiratory noise.
- Cough (note: in parrots most coughing is owner-imitation; it is always worth checking this when taking a history).
- Reduced exercise tolerance and increase in time before normal breathing post-exercise.

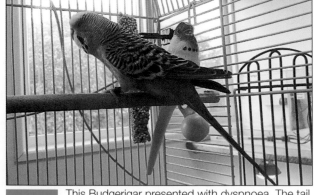

22.2 This Budgerigar presented with dyspnoea. The tail was bobbing with each breath and the bird's posture on the perch shows its neck and body extended to ease respiration.

Non-specific signs of LRTD

- Weight loss.
- Failure to gain weight (especially in raptors).
- Reduced exercise tolerance/hunting performance.
- Fluffing/weakness/collapse.
- Bird generally described as 'not right' (see Chapter 23).

One difficulty that may affect the urgency with which a patient is seen and the type of investigation carried out, is distinguishing LRTD from upper respiratory tract disease (URTD) (Figure 22.3). While both may be seen together (especially LRTD and tracheal disease), it is relatively unusual (see Case example 2). Aside from tracheal blockage, URTD is generally non-urgent while LRTD is always urgent.

Features of upper respiratory tract disease

- Nasal and/or ocular discharge
- Sinus swelling
- Distortion of nares
- Head shaking
- Head irritation
- Altered voice
- Cough (tracheal disease)
- Open-beak breathing (tracheal/glottal disease)
- Weight loss rare unless concurrent disease
- Respiratory noise on auscultation is referred noise
- Unusual to see systemic inflammatory reaction on haematology/electrophoresis

Features of lower respiratory tract disease

- No discharges
- No sinus swelling
- Nares not distorted
- No head shaking
- No head irritation
- May have altered voice
- Occasionally may cough
- Open-beak breathing unusual unless severe disease
- Weight loss common
- May have respiratory noise, especially if severe disease
- Expect to see inflammatory response on haematology/electrophoresis

22.3 Characteristic clinical signs distinguishing lower respiratory tract disease from upper respiratory tract disease.

Immediate life-saving measures

Some cases will present as emergencies and, while all cases of breathing difficulty should be treated as urgent, the following signs should indicate that the bird needs seeing as an absolute emergency:

- Open-beak breathing
- Collapse/extreme weakness
- Ataxia
- Rasping sounds when breathing.

See also Chapter 8 for first aid advice for owners.

When the bird is presented in a collapsed or weakened state, especially if it is also open-beak breathing, then it is most important to stabilize it before taking a history or performing a full clinical examination. In all cases where respiratory disease is suspected, the bird should be examined with an oxygen supply and mask close to hand. Some birds may collapse while being handled or just after, and owners should be warned accordingly.

Stabilization of the collapsed bird

1. Prepare all equipment likely to be needed.
2. Towel wrap the bird as quickly and gently as possible.
3. Supply oxygen via a facemask for 1 minute before adding isoflurane at 1–2%. Alternatively, midazolam may be given at 2 mg/kg intranasally or 1 mg/kg i.m.
4. As soon as possible, perform a tracheoscopy (see Editors' note).
5. Intubate and provide ventilation (either mechanical or very careful manual ventilation).
6. Perform the clinical examination.
   - If tracheal obstruction is noted, fit an air sac tube. Unless the bird is moribund, this will require an anaesthetic (see Chapter 17).
   - If ascites is noted, perform an ultrasound examination and take a sample of ascitic fluid. Full drainage can be performed if a large volume of fluid is noted. Obvious ascites can be carefully drained without ultrasound guidance.
   - If no obstruction is identified, take radiographs and blood samples.
7. Medicate as indicated; if there is no immediate diagnosis, give antibiosis (e.g. marbofloxacin), non-steroidal anti-inflammatory drugs (NSAIDs; meloxicam or carprofen) and subcutaneous fluids.
8. Reduce isoflurane and allow the bird to recover if the breathing pattern improves.
9. Nebulize (e.g. 1:250 dilution F10SC).
10. Hospitalize the bird in a heated humidified unit; ideally this should be in a dark quiet ward.
11. History can be taken during recovery.

Editors' note

Throughout this volume the emphasis has been on providing care for these species without recourse to specialized equipment. However, tracheoscopy is mandatory when examining and stabilizing the severely dyspnoeic bird. If this is not available then the bird should be referred to the nearest avian veterinary facility as soon as possible and ideally be sent directly to this facility for stabilization. However, basic rigid endoscopy equipment (2.7 mm rigid telescope and portable cold light source) can be purchased online for minimal outlay.

Stabilization of the dyspnoeic but not collapsed bird

1. Observe the bird and take its history from the owner.
2. Perform the clinical examination; in particular, assess body condition. If thin, then disease is likely to be long established and the bird has probably developed compensatory mechanisms, meaning that, although the long-term prognosis is less certain, it is more likely to be stable in the short term than the acutely dyspnoeic bird in good body condition.
3. Give subcutaneous fluids, antibiosis and NSAIDs before nebulizing (as above).
4. Hospitalize (as above) and reassess after 1–2 hours.
   - If the breathing improves, perform diagnostic investigations (see later) under general anaesthesia.
   - If the breathing worsens, treat as for a collapsed bird (see above).
   - If the breathing is unchanged, leave for a further 1–2 hours before performing diagnostic investigations.

Diagnostic techniques and indications

History

See Chapter 10 for basic history questions. Figure 22.4 lists specific areas of importance when investigating suspected LRTD.

Clinical examination

The timing of the clinical examination depends on the severity of the problem (see above and Chapter 10). In all cases, handling must be as smooth and gentle as possible and the bird should always be held upright (not flat) with its head raised. If the bird goes quiet or becomes distressed, the examination must be stopped, the bird released and, if necessary, provided with oxygen (see above). The owner should not be present during the examination and should be warned of the dangers associated with handling dyspnoeic birds.

In addition to a normal full examination, particular attention should be paid to:

- Mucus membranes. Cyanosis is rare, though inflammation may be noted
- Check nares, choana and glottis for discharges
- Auscultation (ideally a good-quality paediatric or infant stethoscope should be used):
  - Pectoral region – listen to the heart (rate/rhythm/presence of murmurs). Electrocardiography is indicated where there are rhythm disturbances
  - Abdominal air sac sounds – should be very quiet/non-existent. If there are rasping noises or 'dead' areas then suspect LRTD. This must be distinguished from referred upper respiratory noise

- Dorsum over lungs – assess respiratory noise through lungs; there should be minimal sounds. Lung sounds must be distinguished from referred sounds.
- Abdominal palpation – to assess the presence of ascites, presence of eggs and possible organomegaly
- Body condition (see Figure 22.1)
- In finches, tracheal transillumination should be performed looking for air sac mites (see Chapter 20).

Diagnostic investigation

LRTD signs indicate a need for a thorough diagnostic investigation. Many of these investigations require anaesthesia. These cases are, obviously, high-risk anaesthesia cases. As such, good facilities and technique are required and, ideally, mechanical ventilation. In the absence of such facilities, referral should be discussed with the client.

In all cases, the risks of anaesthesia should be discussed with the owner and balanced with the potential benefits of accurate diagnosis.

Anaesthesia of dyspnoeic birds

Where simple non-invasive tests are to be performed (e.g. blood sampling, radiography), sedation with midazolam (2 mg/kg) + butorphanol (1–2 mg/kg) can be given intranasally. If required, this can be reversed with intranasal flumazenil at 0.1 mg/kg divided between both nostrils. Supplemental oxygen should be given via tracheal intubation (preferably) or mask. Otherwise, the bird should be preoxygenated before mask induction with isoflurane. Isoflurane should be added by increments (i.e. 1% for 1 minute, then 2% for 1 minute, etc.) until sufficient anaesthetic depth is achieved to allow intubation and ventilation.

History	Comments
Signalment	Some species are more susceptible to aspergillosis (see 'Common causes and differential diagnoses'). Older birds are more susceptible to cardiovascular disease.
Environment	<ul><li>Are there any smokers in the house? Many will say they smoke, but not with the bird. Transference of material from the hands and clothes of smokers to the plumage has been associated with increased disease susceptibility in birds</li><li>Are there any airborne irritants used: air fresheners; sprays; solid fuel burners; incense burners; cooking fumes?</li><li>Is the bird kept in the kitchen? If yes, there is increased exposure to cooking fumes and, potentially, polytetrafluoroethylene (e.g. Teflon® pans)</li><li>Does the home have central heating?</li><li>Has there been any recent building/DIY work? This increases the chance of irritant dust; potential increased exposure to *Aspergillus* spores</li><li>Is the bird kept in an aviary? What substrate is used? Is there potential exposure to *Syngamus* spp.?</li><li>What is the recent disinfectant use/cleaning history for the cage/aviary?</li></ul>
Diet	Ideally, the owner should bring some feed in for assessment.<ul><li>Dusty seed and peanut/sunflower husks may increase exposure to *Aspergillus* spores</li><li>High-seed diets may predispose to obesity and atherosclerosis</li></ul>
Carrying box	For trained raptors: When was the box last cleaned? And how dirty was it? Uncleaned boxes (or those cleaned just before the bird is transported) may increase exposure to *Aspergillus* spores
Exercise	Exercise tolerance and current activity levels (especially raptors)
Clinical signs	<ul><li>How long present?</li><li>Changes in severity</li><li>Changes in signs</li><li>Relapsing episodes/previous respiratory problems?</li><li>Other birds affected?</li></ul>
Owner disease history	Are there clinical signs in the owner? Although zoonotic/anthronotic disease is extremely unusual, the most common reason for a coughing parrot is mimicry of the owner

22.4 Important considerations when investigating lower respiratory tract disease.

It is particularly important that all likely equipment needs are prepared prior to anaesthesia so the anaesthetic time is reduced as much as possible (see Chapter 16). During anaesthesia, particular importance should be given to maintaining body temperature and maintaining air sac perfusion (especially if ventilating); ideally, capnography should be used to monitor anaesthesia.

Diagnostic testing
Figure 22.5 lists potential diagnostic tests with their indications and comments on technique.

Common causes and differential diagnoses
Figure 22.10 lists the most common differential diagnoses for lower respiratory tract disease signs.

Species particularly sensitive to aspergillosis
- Parrots:
  - Grey Parrots
  - Macaws, especially Green-winged.
- Raptors:
  - Gyrfalcon
  - Goshawk
  - Snowy Owl
  - High-altitude eagles, such as Golden Eagles.

Aspergillosis is unusual in passerines, but note that this disease can be seen in any bird that is exposed to a sufficient quantity of environmental spores and/or immunocompromised

Diagnostic test	Indications	Comments
Radiography (Figures 22.6 and 22.7)	All cases	Lateral and ventrodorsal views should be taken. Can be used to detect: ■ Air sac and lung lesions: soft tissue densities; diffuse thickening; lung congestion; air sac wall thickening ■ Ascites ■ Organomegaly, including splenomegaly (indicating systemic inflammatory response) ■ Proventricular enlargement.
Haematology	All cases	Assessment of inflammatory response and immune status
Biochemistry	All cases	Assessment of liver/kidney function in organomegaly or in potential toxin-producing infections (e.g. aspergillosis)
Electrophoresis	Inflammatory disease/aspergillosis	Sensitive means of assessing inflammatory response. In aspergillosis, immune status is important in assessing prognosis; lack of response where there are obvious lesions indicates a guarded prognosis
Ultrasonography	Ascites (Figure 22.8) Cardiomegaly	Small footplate and high image turnover are more important than probe frequency, where a 7.5–12.5 MHz range is ideal. Normal values can be found in Krautwald-Junghanns et al. (2010)
Coelioscopy (Figure 22.9)	Air sac/pulmonary disease. No abnormality detected on radiography	Allows direct assessment of lesions. Coelioscopy can detect lesions too small or undeveloped to be seen on radiography: ideally, radiography should be used to determine the route of coelioscopy and to rule out contraindications (e.g. ascites, some organomegalies, extreme proventricular dilatation). Also allows for biopsy of lesions and/or air sacs/lungs. As described earlier with tracheoscopy, endoscopic evaluation is indicated in virtually all cases (birds larger than Cockatiels). If rigid endoscopy is not available then referral is indicated if possible

22.5 Potential diagnostic tests for lower respiratory tract disease.

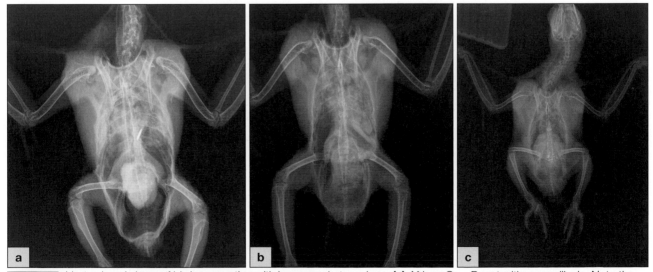

22.6 Ventrodorsal views of birds presenting with lower respiratory signs. **(a)** African Grey Parrot with aspergillosis. Note the granuloma in the left side just caudal to the lungs. The caudal air sacs are clear and slightly distended showing respiratory obstruction. **(b)** African Grey Parrot with a large aspergilloma filling the left-sided air sacs. In cases such as these, surgery is often required (after stabilization and initial antifungal therapy) to remove the fungal granulomas. **(c)** Obese Amazon parrot. Dyspnoea was caused by a combination of hepatomegaly and large fat deposits compressing air spaces.

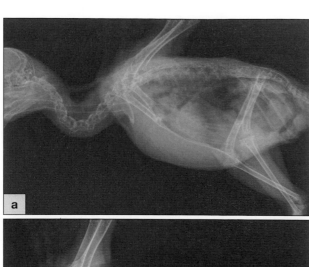

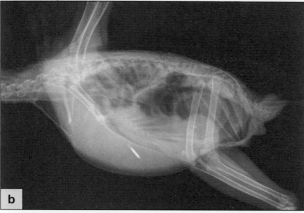

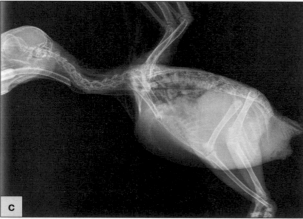

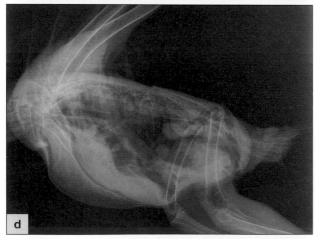

22.7 Laterolateral views of birds presenting with lower respiratory signs. **(a)** African Grey Parrot with splenomegaly and diffuse inflammation of the air sacs. **(b)** African Grey Parrot with granuloma formation in the air sacs and congestion of the lungs. **(c)** Ascites and cardiomegaly in an African Grey Parrot. **(d)** Parrot with splenomegaly, lung congestion (loss of definition) and thickening of the *septum horizontale* (air sac wall) indicating air sacculitis.

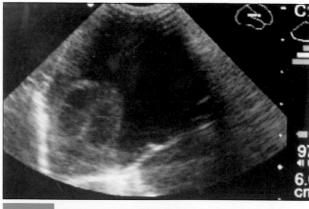

22.8   Enlarged heart and ascites on ultrasonography.

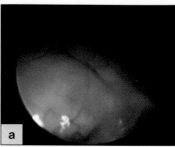

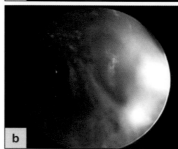

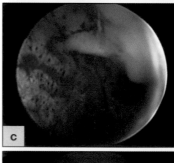

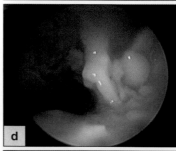

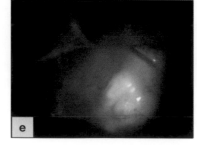

22.9

Coelioscopic views of *Aspergillus* lesions. **(a)** Granuloma formation; a thickened wall with a large vessel indicating host inflammatory response. Nebulization therapy is unlikely to penetrate such lesions. **(b)** Fungal lesion (right) invading pulmonary tissue. The lungs are inflamed and congested. Biopsy in this case revealed primary inflammatory disease; the fungus was a secondary invader. **(c)** Fungal lesion with host inflammatory response visible in lung tissue surrounding the lesion. **(d)** Extensive fungal lesion. Given the extent of the fungal development there is little or no granuloma formation and blood examination indicated a poor host immune response. **(e)** Old fungal lesion with walling-off and fibrin tags formed round a granuloma.

Category	Diseases	Comments
Infection	Bacterial air sacculitis/pneumonitis	Extremely common in all species; may occur secondary to inflammatory disease
	Aspergillosis – granulomas in lungs and/or air sacs	Extremely common, especially in certain species
	Mycoplasmosis	Potentially common, but hard to diagnose definitively
	Chlamydiosis	Unusual to see dyspnoea unless secondary to hepatomegaly
Aspiration pneumonia	Foreign body effects; bacterial infection	Especially in chicks being fed semi-liquid formulae Also seen as iatrogenic following crop tubing
Parasitic disease	Air sac mite (*Sternostoma*)	Very common in passerine birds, especially Lady Gouldian finches
	Gapeworm (*Syngamus trachea*)	Direct and indirect lifecycles Common in softbills and insect-eating raptors; occasional in parrots Seen in birds kept in soil- or turf-based aviaries
	Air sac worm (*Serratospiculum*)	Not seen in the UK; common in raptors in the Middle East
Primary inflammatory disease	Irritation; allergy/asthma	Especially in parrots (Amazons, Grey Parrots, macaws) May predispose to secondary bacterial or fungal infection Irritation more common with typical history of exposure to airborne irritants Lungs may appear congested Some birds are apparently asthmatic with repeated dyspnoeic episodes
Toxicity (Figure 22.11)	Especially polytetrafluoroethylene (PTFE; Teflon®)	Very common – often present dead unless very small doses inhaled – these generally present as acute dyspnoea/collapse History suggests exposure
Cardiovascular disease	Atherosclerosis; cardiomyopathy	Increasingly diagnosed in parrots and older raptors
Syringeal obstruction	Aspergillosis; foreign bodies	See Chapter 20
Ascites	Cardiac disease; neoplasia; hypoproteinaemia; egg-related peritonitis	See relevant sections
Extra-respiratory pressure	Organomegaly; proventricular dilatation	Hepatomegaly is a common cause of respiratory signs in Budgerigars and Cockatiels
Obesity	Not applicable	Especially in Amazon parrots

22.10 Potential differential diagnoses for lower respiratory tract disease.

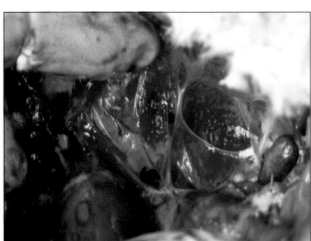

22.11 Post-mortem view of the lungs of a parrot that died following polytetrafluoroethylene (PTFE; Teflon®) inhalation. Note the extreme congestion and redness.

Therapeutics

Therapy depends on diagnosis. Figure 22.12 lists some of the most commonly used drugs, routes and indications.

Nebulization

Nebulization is commonly used in inflammatory airway disease, particularly in respiratory infections. In birds with respiratory irritation or asthma, providing steam (e.g. by placing the cage in a steamy bathroom for 30 minutes twice daily) will often assist greatly in acting as an expectorant and/or hydrating mucous membranes.

In respiratory infections, nebulization is anecdotally proposed as a means of introducing antimicrobials directly to lesions. In non-granulomatous lesions, this may be effective, although there is little evidence showing penetration or effectiveness of such agents when nebulized. In granulomatous disease, nebulization cannot penetrate lesions. However, clinical experience suggests that the expectorant and hydration effects of nebulization do benefit the patient in addition to any direct therapeutic effects.

When choosing an agent for nebulization it must:

- Be stable
- Be non-irritant
- Be non-toxic to the bird and handler (some absorption occurs from the lungs and air sacs as well as likely preening from feathers). Handlers are likely to inhale agents when removing the bird from the nebulization chamber
- Show some activity against likely infectious agents (see above).

A jet-type nebulizer should be used rather than an ultrasonic nebulizer as more drugs are stable when given with these and, in general, jet nebulizers produce a smaller droplet, allowing increased airway penetration.

Type of drug	Drug	Dose/route	Indications	Comments
Antibacterial	Marbofloxacin	10 mg/kg i.m., orally q24h	Bacterial infections	A reliable choice in many cases Daily dosing increases client compliance
	Enrofloxacin	10–15 mg/kg i.m., orally q12h	Bacterial infections	As for marbofloxacin, although increased tissue irritancy and twice daily dosing reduce its usefulness Licensed drug in the UK
	Doxycycline	100 mg/kg i.m., q5–7d	Bacterial infections, especially *Mycoplasma* or *Chlamydia* spp.	Vibravenos currently unavailable but may become available via a special import certificate Excellent drug for chlamydiosis, but very tissue irritant Vetafarm doxycycline available as compounded injection in Australia
Antifungal	Itraconazole	10 mg/kg orally q12–24h	Aspergillosis	Daily dosing used for prophylaxis when training susceptible raptor species; twice daily used in therapy Can be hepatotoxic and Grey Parrots seem particularly susceptible; if possible its use should be avoided in this species (if no alternative, may be used at 5 mg/kg q24h, although toxicity may still be seen at this level) May take 5–7 days to achieve therapeutic levels but is generally effective; typically, treatment of advanced aspergillosis takes 9–12 months
	Terbinafine	15 mg/kg orally q12h	Aspergillosis	Apparently safer alternative to itraconazole Appears effective but requires same treatment length as itraconazole
	Voriconazole	15 mg/kg orally q12h	Aspergillosis	These authors' drug of choice in aspergillosis. Although very expensive, it appears to have fewer side effects than itraconazole and treatment time is typically 2–4 months with apparently more rapid onset of action
Anti-inflammatory	Carprofen	5 mg/kg i.m., q24h	Inflammatory airway disease	
	Meloxicam	0.2–0.7 mg/kg orally q12h	Inflammatory airway disease	May assist in longer-term treatment
	Methylprednisolone sodium succinate	15 mg/kg i.v.	Inflammatory airway disease PTFE toxicity – **emergency use only!**	Use i.v. in acute asthma attack. **Do not use unless infectious disease ruled out in emergency situation.** Only use ultra-short-acting preparations
Bronchodilator	Aminophylline	5 mg/kg orally q12h	Inflammatory airway disease	
Antiparasitic	Ivermectin	200 µg/kg orally/percutaneous	Air sac mites Gapeworms	May not alleviate signs as dead parasites may also cause obstruction. Allow 6 weeks to clear parasites and must combine with environmental control
Cardiac drugs	Furosemide	2 mg/kg i.m., orally q12h		Care needed in dehydrated birds
	Enalapril	1.25 mg/kg orally q12h		
	Pimobendan	0.25 mg/kg orally q12h		

22.12   Drugs commonly used for the treatment of lower respiratory tract disease in birds.

It is simple to make a nebulization chamber by placing a small cage or carrying box inside a large plastic bag. This author recommends using F10SC at a 1:250 dilution for 30 minutes twice daily using such a setup.

References and further reading

Krautwald-Junghanns M, Pees M, Reese S and Tully T (2010) *Diagnostic Imaging of Exotic Pets: Birds, Small Mammals, Reptiles.* Schlutersche, Hannover

Case example 1: Glossy Black Cockatoo with clinical chlamydiosis

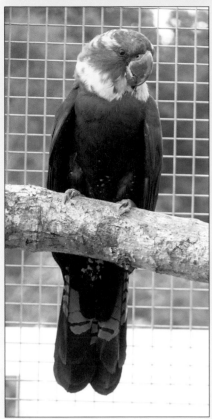

(Courtesy of Eliza Read)

Presentation and history

A 6-year-old Glossy Black Cockatoo hen presented with a history of being quieter than normal for a few weeks. She was acutely ataxic on the morning of presentation, and had moderate tachypnoea and mild dyspnoea on handling. She was housed in an aviary, with a cock bird.

Clinical examination and diagnostic investigations

On examination, the bird was found to be emaciated, with harsh lung sounds on auscultation. Coelomic palpation was unremarkable. Grossly, her droppings showed biliverdinuria, although faecal cytology was unrewarding.

Haematological examination demonstrated anaemia (packed cell volume 31%; normal 45–55%), leucocytosis (white blood cell count 25.5 x 10⁹/l ; normal 9–21 x 10⁹/l) and marked toxic changes in the heterophils. The heterophil numbers were within normal limits, and there was mild relative and absolute monocytosis (4%, normal <2%,

and 1.02 x 10⁹/l, normal 0–0.65 x 10⁹/l). The owner declined biochemical testing; samples were taken for *Chlamydia psittaci* testing, but were not immediately available.

Therapy

The bird was admitted into hospital for supportive care, including feeding and warmth. A depot doxycycline injection was given (75 mg/kg i.m.). The staff were instructed to use facemasks when handling this bird, and she was placed in the isolation ward.

Outcome

Over the next week, the bird's respiration gradually improved. She gained weight, and her haematological parameters returned to normal. *Chlamydia* serology was consistent with clinical chlamydiosis. She was discharged from hospital, and treated for a further 5 weeks with intramuscular doxycycline injections (administered by a local veterinary surgeon (veterinarian)). The owner was counselled as to the zoonotic implications of this disease, which resulted in his acutely, extremely unwell 8-year-old daughter being diagnosed with clinical psittacosis.

Case example 2: Green-winged Macaw with aspergillosis and *Escherichia coli* infection

Presentation and history

A 6-month-old female Green-winged Macaw presented with a chronic, several-week history of intermittent sneezing and acute mild to moderate dyspnoea.

Clinical examination and diagnostic investigations

There was mild mucoid nasal discharge, which showed clumps of homogenous, dividing Gram-positive cocci on cytology. Auscultation revealed crackles, centred over the cranial air sacs. Coelomic palpation was normal.

The bird was anaesthetized with isoflurane for venepuncture and radiology. Haematological analysis showed a leucocytosis of 36.2 x 10⁹/l (normal 4.2–10.8 x 10⁹/l) with a marked

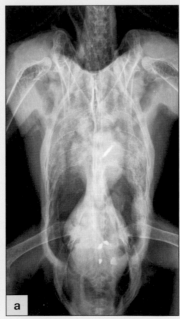

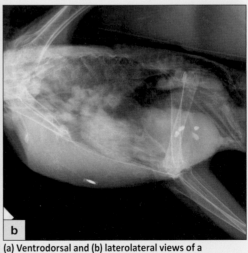

(a) Ventrodorsal and (b) laterolateral views of a Green-winged Macaw, showing multiple densities throughout the lung fields.

toxic relative and absolute heterophilia (90%, normal 45–65%; 32.59 x 10⁹/l, normal 1.5–5.7 x 10⁹/l). Radiographs showed multiple radiopaque densities within the lung fields, with several surrounding the syrinx.

Therapy

The bird was started on oral itraconazole at 5 mg/kg once daily and co-amoxiclav at 125 mg/kg twice daily, and admitted into hospital.

Two days later, she became acutely severely dyspnoeic, and was again anaesthetized. Tracheoscopy was performed, which demonstrated a rough, yellow mass in the syrinx. Swabs were taken for culture. Radiographs were repeated, which showed similar changes to those previously identified. An air sac breathing tube was surgically placed into the left caudal thoracic air sac, which markedly eased the bird's respiration. Tenacious mucus (3 ml) was drained from her air sac after placement of the tube. This was also sent for bacterial and fungal culture. Cytology revealed a homogenous

population of Gram-negative small rods, so enrofloxacin at 10 mg/kg twice daily was added to the treatment regimen. Itraconazole was ceased in favour of voriconazole, and amphotericin B was used intratracheally once daily.

Outcome

Treatments continued for the next 3 days with minimal change to the bird's condition. She was found dead in her cage on the fourth day. The culture results confirmed the presence of *Aspergillus* spp., with secondary *Escherichia coli* infection.

Case example 3: Thin Cockatiel with dyspnoea

Presentation and history

An 8-year-old female Cockatiel presented with moderate to severe dyspnoea. She had been exercising less for several weeks, and had stopped flying completely in the last week. She was thin on palpation (body condition score of 2/5).

Clinical examination and diagnostic investigations

The bird was preoxygenated prior to handling, but still became severely dyspnoeic during physical examination. Auscultation revealed mild gurgling on inspiration. The coelom was markedly distended. Coelomocentesis yielded 10 ml of turbid yellow fluid, consistent with ascites. Cytology of this fluid showed crenated leucocytes, some heterophils and macrophages. Haematological examination demonstrated a normal total white cell count, with a marked

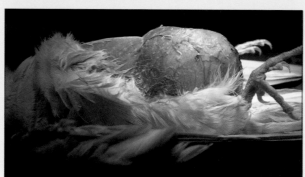

Cockatiel hen with marked ascites, being prepared for surgery. (Courtesy of Adrian Gallagher)

relative heterophilia. The absolute heterophil count was normal, although there were mild toxic changes on morphological assessment. The diagnostic coelomocentesis reduced the dyspnoea considerably.

The coelomic distension returned by the next day, and the owner consented to exploratory laparotomy to gain a diagnosis. Radiography was discussed, but discounted due to the likelihood of the fluid obscuring abdominal detail. Ultrasonography was not available.

The bird was anaesthetized with isoflurane and oxygen, after preoxygenation. An intraosseus catheter was placed in the distal ulna. A midline incision was made, and the coelom was explored after draining more ascitic fluid.

Outcome

A large multinodular mass was found in the ovarian and uterine region, adherent to multiple structures. Resection was impossible and the bird was euthanased on the table. The likely diagnosis was ovarian adenocarcinoma.

Case example 4: Foreign body ingestion in an African Grey Parrot

Presentation and history

A 3-month-old male African Grey Parrot was observed to ingest a feeding tube during hand feeding. The bird had been assessed by a local veterinary surgeon, who was not able to retrieve the feeding tube. Contrast radiography, using barium, had been

performed, after which the bird had become acutely dyspnoeic.

Clinical examination and diagnostic investigations

On presentation, the bird was in good body condition, but was moderately

dyspnoeic at rest. He decompensated somewhat on handling, becoming more dyspnoeic for up to 10 minutes afterwards. Auscultation showed severe harsh lung sounds. Radiographs were re-taken, which clearly showed aspiration of the barium, outlining the trachea, lungs and air sacs. The feeding tube could also be seen outlined within the proventriculus. ▶

Case example 4 *continued*

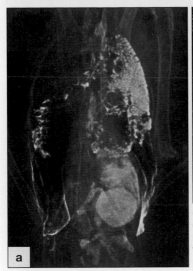

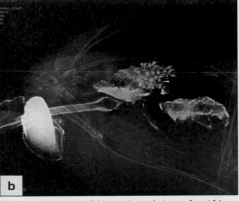

(a) Ventrodorsal and (b) laterolateral views of an African Grey Parrot with barium ingestion. Barium can clearly be seen outlining the trachea, the lungs and the air sacs. The outlined ingested feeding tube is visible in the proventriculus. (Courtesy of Adrian Gallagher)

Therapy

The bird was stabilized for 24 hours, with meloxicam (0.5 mg/kg orally q12h). Antibiosis was commenced with co-amoxiclav at 125 mg/kg orally q12h. Hand feeding was continued.

The next day, respiration had stabilized, and the bird only minimally decompensated after handling. Anaesthesia was induced with isoflurane and oxygen. An endotracheal tube was placed, and intermittent positive pressure ventilation was begun. An intraosseous catheter was placed, and surgical fluids were begun at 10 ml/kg/h. An ingluviotomy was performed, which allowed endoscopic retrieval of the tube.

Outcome

The bird made an uneventful recovery, and was discharged from hospital 3 days later.

The sick bird

Richard Jones

The vast majority of the avian species seen in practice have evolved as 'prey species', with even many raptor species being hunted by larger birds of prey or mammalian predators. Such predators have evolved to recognize the slightest weakness in an individual, indicating an easier meal, therefore prey species have developed an incredible capacity to disguise debilitation or underlying disease, in order to avoid predation.

As such, by the time a bird is displaying obvious outward clinical signs of illness (e.g. depression, collapse, vomiting or respiratory distress), the patient is generally critically ill with a guarded prognosis.

Whenever a client claims their bird is 'not right', especially if it has been observed over a few days, they should be taken seriously; reasons for this description can range from relatively benign behavioural issues due to environmental changes or the onset of sexual maturity, through to advanced systemic disease (Figure 23.1).

Diagnostic work-up

A systematic approach, starting with a detailed clinical and management history and clinical examination (as described in Chapter 10) is essential. In this author's experience, wherever possible a minimum of a 30-minute appointment is required to make any useful assessment.

History taking

A good history will provide clues and alert the veterinary surgeon (veterinarian) to potential problems even before the bird is examined and allow them to focus on the likely possible differential diagnoses, refining the rest of the diagnostic approach.

Signalment and source

- **Species:** certain conditions are more common in certain species, for example, aspergillosis appears to be overrepresented in Grey Parrots and Goshawks, and hypocalcaemia is overrepresented in Grey Parrots.

- **Age:** as a general rule, juvenile birds are more likely to suffer from infectious, developmental and nutritional deficiencies, whereas adult birds may have higher incidences of neoplasia, chronic malnutrition, reproductive disease and degenerative conditions.
- **Time in owner's possession:** birds that have been with the owner for many years are less likely to have infectious disease (as long as there has been no contact with other birds, e.g. at a show).
- **Source:** with experience, the clinician may be able to identify 'problem sources'.
- **Hand-reared or parent-reared:** it has been observed that hand-reared birds, without the benefits of natural parent nurturing, may be more prone to developmental abnormalities (e.g. osteodystrophy) and behavioural problems arising from 'imprinting' on humans. Parent-reared birds, on the other hand, may be more difficult to tame and, in certain species (e.g. Goshawks), are more prone to stress-related illnesses such as aspergillosis.

Husbandry and nutrition

- **Day-to-day management:** is the patient an aviary bird, breeding bird, companion bird or used for flying display, pest control or hunting in the case of falconry birds? A full assessment may best be covered by requesting in detail what happens to the bird (i.e. where is it, what does it eat and what does it do from the time it wakes up to the time it goes to sleep at night?). It is also important to establish possible exposure to infectious disease via contact with other birds, or to toxins in the environment, such as Teflon®, cigarette smoke or household plants.
- **Nutrition:** it is essential to gather information on what the bird actually eats (not just what it is offered), how the food is stored and prepared, and if any vitamin/mineral supplements are offered. Poor quality and inappropriately stored seeds may contain significant amounts of fungal spores, increasing the risk of aspergillosis, for example, and, in the case of raptors, any food item that has been shot may pose a risk of lead toxicity.

BSAVA Manual of Avian Practice: A Foundation Manual. Edited by John Chitty and Deborah Monks. ©BSAVA 2018

Clinical sign	Differential diagnosis
Off food or reduced intake	▪ Pain ▪ Mouth/beak trauma/lesion ▪ Systemic disease
Increased appetite	▪ Endoparasitism, avian gastric yeast ▪ Diabetes mellitus ▪ Exocrine pancreatic insufficiency
Weight loss	▪ Non-specific sign of illness ▪ Normal weaning process ▪ Increased exercise ▪ Reduced food intake
Change in colour/ consistency of faecal portion of droppings (see Chapter 24)	▪ Bacterial/viral/parasitic enteritis ▪ Proventricular dilatation disease (parrots) ▪ Chlamydiosis ▪ Liver disease ▪ Toxicosis (e.g. heavy metal) ▪ Dietary change
Blood in droppings (see Chapter 24)	▪ Reproductive disease (e.g. egg binding) ▪ Cloacal inflammation, neoplasia, cloacolith ▪ Endoparasitism (e.g. coccidiosis) ▪ Intestinal foreign bodies
Change in urate colour	▪ Hepatic/renal disease/haemolysis (green) ▪ Renal disease/lead toxicity (pink) ▪ Vitamin B injections, inappetence, yolk coelomitis (yellow)
Polyuria/polydipsia	▪ Stress/fear ▪ Renal/hepatic/pancreatic disease ▪ Diabetes mellitus ▪ Toxicosis (e.g. heavy metal, salt, aflatoxins) ▪ Pituitary adenoma (Budgerigars) ▪ Physiological in egg-laying females ▪ Recent conversion to pelleted diet
Fluffed-up posture	▪ Non-specific sign of illness
Tail bobbing (see Chapters 20 and 22)	▪ Physical exertion ▪ Primary upper/lower respiratory disease ▪ Increased coelomic pressure (e.g. ascites, egg binding, internal organ enlargement)
Wing droop (see Chapter 29)	▪ Weakness if bilateral ▪ Trauma, soft tissue/orthopaedic ▪ Degenerative/septic arthritis ▪ Neoplasia ▪ Developmental abnormality
Floor dwelling	▪ Non-specific sign of illness ▪ Leg/spinal injuries ▪ Inability to fly ▪ Egg binding ▪ Toxicosis (e.g. heavy metal) ▪ Weakness due to systemic disease
Neurological signs (ataxia, fitting, paralysis, paresis) (see Chapter 32)	▪ Toxicity (e.g. heavy metal, organophosphate, pyrethrin) ▪ Head trauma ▪ Hypocalcaemia ▪ Hypoglycaemia ▪ Weakness due to systemic disease ▪ Central nervous system lesions (encephalitis, proventricular dilatation disease, neoplasia, cerebrovascular incident) ▪ Cardiovascular disease
Lameness/leg paresis	▪ Injury ▪ Renal/testicular/ovarian enlargement (e.g. neoplasia) ▪ Pododermatitis ('bumblefoot') ▪ Osteodystrophy/developmental abnormality ▪ Degenerative/septic arthritis ▪ Gout ▪ Spinal pathology

Clinical sign	Differential diagnosis
Feather loss/ abnormalities (see Chapter 30)	▪ Psittacine beak and feather disease ▪ Feather destructive disorder ▪ Dermatitis ▪ Ectoparasites ▪ 'Normal' bald areas on crown of head in lutino Cockatiels, axillae and brood patches of incubating females ▪ Environmental trauma ▪ Malnutrition, systemic disease ▪ 'Stress bars' (stress, illness or administration of medications, e.g. fenbendazole, during feather growth)
Skin texture/colour changes	▪ Malnutrition ▪ Dermatitis ▪ Bruising (green) ▪ Subcutaneous fat, lipomas, xanthomas (yellow) ▪ Self-mutilation of shoulder/patagium (lovebirds)
Swellings	▪ Neoplasia ▪ Feather cysts ▪ Trauma ▪ Obesity ▪ Ascites ▪ Infection
Beak overgrowth/ abnormalities	▪ Trauma ▪ Psittacine beak and feather disease ▪ Congenital disorder (scissor beak/ prognathism) ▪ Malnutrition ▪ Limited access to abrasive surfaces ▪ Liver disease ▪ Cnemidocoptes infestation
Nares/cere disorders	▪ Chronic respiratory disease ▪ Cnemidocoptes infestation ▪ Cere hypertrophy (hyperoestrogenism in Budgerigars) ▪ Choanal atresia (Grey Parrots)
Ocular disorders	▪ Conjunctivitis/sinusitis (bacterial, viral, chlamydial, mycoplasmal) ▪ Eyelid abnormalities (congenital, scarring post-inflammatory disease, neoplasia) ▪ Corneal changes (lipidosis, ulceration) ▪ Cataracts ▪ Retinal detachment/inflammation
Enlarged abdomen	▪ Obesity ▪ Hepatomegaly ▪ Internal neoplasia (renal/gonadal) ▪ Egg binding ▪ Oviductal enlargement ▪ Yolk coelomitis ▪ Ascites (heart and/or liver disease) ▪ Hernia
Subcutaneous emphysema	▪ Trauma ▪ Chronic respiratory disease
Voice change/loss	▪ Syringeal trauma/inflammation/foreign body ▪ Depression due to underlying systemic disease
Poor performance (falconry birds)	▪ Respiratory disease ▪ Endoparasitism ▪ Musculoskeletal disease/trauma ▪ Weakness
Crop stasis/ regurgitation	▪ Generalized illness with ileus ▪ Bacterial/yeast/parasitic ingluvitis ▪ Foreign body obstruction ▪ Viral disease (e.g. polyoma)

23.1 Birds presented as 'not right' may have a wide range of clinical signs with many possible differential diagnoses.

Clinical examination

In this author's experience, in addition to the history, a minimum database should include bodyweight and condition score, thorough physical examination (as discussed in Chapter 10), faecal parasitology (especially for falconry birds) and, ideally, on-the-spot evaluation of packed cell volume, total solids and a stained blood smear.

Further diagnostics may be indicated in many cases (Figure 23.2).

Summary

Birds described as 'not doing right' may be suffering from a diverse range of physical, nutritional, environmental and behavioural conditions. Such cases require a methodical, systematic approach, combining a detailed clinical and environmental history with full physical examination and appropriate and carefully selected diagnostic tests, in order to establish the underlying cause.

It is only once a diagnosis is made that appropriate therapy can be instigated in order to offer the very best chance of resolution.

Diagnostic test	Indications
Blood biochemistry, haematology and electrolytes	Most sick birds
Radiography	Most sick or injured birds once deemed stable enough to sedate/anaesthetize
Endoscopy and endoscope-guided biopsy	Particularly useful to investigate respiratory disease, gastrointestinal disease and further evaluate soft tissue lesions evident radiographically
Toxicology (e.g. blood lead, zinc)	As deemed appropriate based on history and clinical examination
Microbiological investigations (e.g. culture and sensitivity testing, viral testing)	Suspected infectious disease cases and/or samples from inflammatory lesions
Ultrasound examination	Generally only useful in avian cardiac cases and in the ascitic patient
Advanced imaging (computed tomography, magnetic resonance imaging)	Neurological cases, chronic sinusitis

23.2   Indications for diagnostic tests in the sick bird.

Case example 1: Goshawk with aspergillosis

Presentation and history

A 1-year-old hand-reared male Goshawk presented with a history of reduced performance over a period of a week (putting less effort into chasing quarry than usual), as well as loss of 'voice' and respiratory noise following physical exertion. During the hunting season, the bird was kept tethered on a bow perch (see Chapter 3) in the owner's garden and at night it was kept on a tall perch in a wooden outbuilding. Its recent diet had consisted of day-old turkey poults and wild-caught rabbits.

The hawk was bright, alert and responsive, in good body condition, and although auscultation of the lungs, air sacs and trachea confirmed increased respiratory noise when restrained, physical examination was otherwise unremarkable.

Diagnostic work-up

The bird was admitted for further diagnostics and supportive therapy. In-house bloodwork revealed normal packed cell volume and total solids, although there was an apparent heterophilia and monocytosis evident on a blood smear, consistent with active, possibly granulomatous, inflammation. Faecal analysis was negative for intestinal parasites. Whole body ventrodorsal and

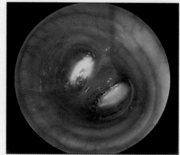
Syringeal granulomas in a Goshawk.

lateral radiographs were unremarkable, as was coelomic endoscopy, although tracheoscopy demonstrated bilateral syringeal granulomas obstructing approximately 80% of the airway. A sample was collected using endoscope-guided biopsy forceps and cytology demonstrated granulomatous inflammation with the presence of fungal elements consistent with aspergillosis.

Therapy

- Antifungal therapy: voriconazole at 12.5 mg/kg orally q12h for 21 days.
- Antimicrobial therapy: marbofloxacin at 10 mg/kg orally q24h for 10 days.
- Non-steroidal anti-inflammatory drugs: meloxicam at 0.5 mg/kg orally q12h for 10 days.
- Nebulization: F10 (1:250 dilution) for 1 hour q12h for 21 days.

- Advice on reducing exposure to further *Aspergillus* spores by avoiding contact with decaying organic materials (e.g. compost, bark chippings or hay) and ensuring good ventilation and hygiene in housing.

Outcome

Respiratory noise began to improve within 3 days of commencing therapy and was not audible by 10 days. Repeat endoscopy performed 3 weeks post-admission demonstrated marked improvement with minimal evidence of active inflammation at that point. The bird was rested for a further month and gradually introduced back into exercise. The owner reported a return to full fitness and hunting capacity, although there appeared to be a permanent loss of voice, presumably due to scarring of the syringeal membranes.

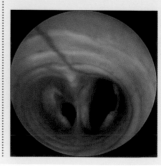
Syrinx 3 weeks post-admission.

Case example 2: African Grey Parrot with hypocalcaemia

Presentation and history

A 5-year-old, normally extremely talkative, male African Grey Parrot presented when his owner reported he was not as 'chatty' as usual. Appetite, respiration and stools were normal with no overt signs of clinical disease. The bird's bodyweight was stable at 460 g. The owner reported that the bird was on a 'varied' diet of a 'parrot seed mix', fruit and vegetables, although further questioning revealed he was particularly fond of sunflower seeds and peanuts. He was an indoor bird with no access to full-spectrum lighting or an outdoor aviary.

Diagnostic work-up

Physical examination was unremarkable but bloodwork revealed a moderate to marked hypocalcaemia: although total calcium was within the normal range at 1.8 mmol/l, ionized calcium measured 0.62 mmol/l (normal range: 0.95–1.2 mmol/l). Both haematology and biochemistry otherwise appeared essentially normal. Based on the above, it was decided to delay any further diagnostics, including radiography and coelioscopy, due to the increased anaesthetic risk posed by the severe hypocalcaemic state.

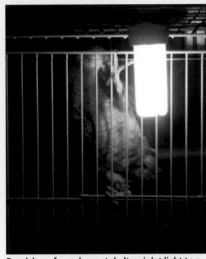

Provision of supplemental ultraviolet light to a hypocalcaemic African Grey Parrot.

Therapy

- Injectable calcium gluconate 10% at 10 mg/kg s.c. q12h for 3 days.
- An avian-specific calcium and vitamin D_3 supplement and a ultraviolet-B emitting 'bird lamp' were prescribed in the short term, with a view to convert the bird to a recommended commercial pelleted diet.

Outcome

Within 2–3 weeks the bird returned to his normal vocal self and repeat bloodwork confirmed a normocalcaemic state (ionized calcium 0.98 mmol/l). No further diagnostics were pursued and the bird was successfully converted on to a commercial extruded pellet diet.

Case example 3: Lanner Falcon with spondylosis

Presentation and history

A 14-year-old male Lanner Falcon presented with his owner describing this normally very aerial and dynamic falcon as 'not himself'; he was spending less time on the wing during flying displays, preferring to land on a nearby telegraph pole or roof before coming back in to the falconer to be fed. No other significant findings or observations were reported. During the flying season the bird was kept tethered on a block during the day and on a shelf perch indoors at night. Out of season he was 'free lofted' in an aviary and fed a diet of day-old chicks and adult mice.

Diagnostic work-up

The bird was bright, alert and responsive, of good bodyweight, in excellent feather condition, and physical examination was unremarkable. Bloodwork was essentially normal, although radiography revealed spondylosis of the lumbosacral junction.

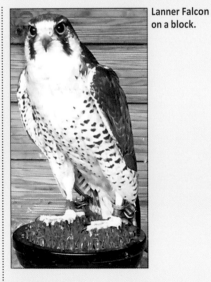

Lanner Falcon on a block.

Therapy and outcome

Although spondylosis can be an incidental, age-related finding, in this case the bird responded immediately to non-steroidal anti-inflammatory drug therapy (meloxicam at 0.5 mg/kg orally q12h) and deteriorated again when treatment was withheld, leading to the assumption that musculoskeletal pain was indeed the cause of reduced activity in this falcon. The bird was placed on long-term meloxicam therapy with intermittent 'tailing off' of therapy by gradually reducing the dosage as deemed appropriate based on performance, and continued to fly in display for another two seasons before being retired.

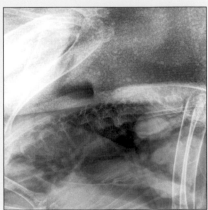

Spondylosis in a Lanner Falcon.

Case example 4: Peregrine Falcon with a coccidia burden

Presentation and history

A 3-year-old male Peregrine Falcon presented with a history of 'not doing right' and reduced performance. This was a falconry bird whose method of hunting, when released by the falconer, was to climb with rapid wing beats up to a height of several hundred feet until, using gravity, he would dive ('stoop') at flushed quarry. During the previous week, although appearing in peak physical condition with no change in appetite, bodyweight stable and no overt clinical signs, the bird's performance had deteriorated markedly: flight was now lacklustre and, rather than rapidly climbing as usual, he would glide on fixed wings and often land on a distant perch until retrieved by the falconer.

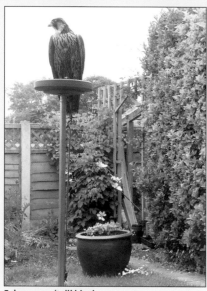

Falcon on a 'tall' block.

During the hunting season the bird was housed on a 'tall' falcon block on the lawn during the day, and a falcon block on a shelf in a brick outbuilding at night. Diet consisted of day-old turkey poults, quail and partridge. Shortly before presentation (around 2–3 weeks previously), the bird had been to a 5-day falconry field meeting where numerous birds were tethered on the same weathering lawn.

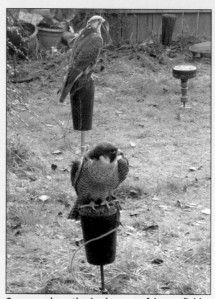

Communal weathering lawn at a falconry field meeting.

Diagnostic work-up

Physical examination and bloodwork were unremarkable, although examination of pooled faecal samples collected over 48 hours revealed a heavy coccidia burden.

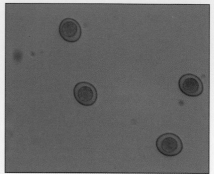

Coccidial oocysts (*Caryospora* sp.) in a faecal sample from a Peregrine Falcon.

Therapy and outcome

The bird was rested, with 10 mg/kg diclazuril administered orally on days 1, 3 and 10. A repeat faecal sample at 2 weeks was negative for intestinal parasites. The environment and equipment were thoroughly cleaned and all droppings collected on paper and disposed of daily to avoid re-infection. Within 2–3 weeks the falcon was back to peak performance.

Abnormal or loose droppings

Jean-Michel Hatt

Abnormal droppings, and a decreased appetite, are probably the most frequent first clinical signs of gastrointestinal tract disease. Birds typically excrete their wastes from the gastrointestinal and the urinary tracts together. Therefore, the term 'dropping' in this chapter refers to the excreta ('mute' in raptors) and special emphasis is given to a systematic differentiation of the parts of excreta (faeces, urates and urine) and possible variations that can be found. Abnormal droppings are often erroneously referred to as 'loose droppings'. Abnormal droppings may be due to changes in colour such as from cloacal haemorrhage. The term loose droppings refers to an increased water content of the excreta. However, it should be noted that the origin of the additional water may be polyuria or true diarrhoea. The former is a result of an imbalance in the urogenital tract, the latter results from disordered water and electrolyte transport in the intestine. In this chapter the main focus will be on diarrhoea and the diagnostic approaches.

To correctly diagnose the aetiology of loose droppings, the avian veterinary surgeon (veterinarian) must have a good understanding of the anatomy and physiology of both the avian gastrointestinal and urogenital tracts (see Chapter 2). For further information, the reader is also referred to Duke (1997).

Normal appearance of droppings

It is crucial to be aware of the normal appearance of excreta. Whereas this may be rather trivial for a practitioner dealing with mammals, it may be a challenge when working with birds. Owners rarely recognize true diarrhoea in a bird and will typically present the bird because of other clinical signs, such as depression or inability to fly (see Case examples). The large number of avian species and their range of nutritional strategies and gastrointestinal tracts results in a variety of appearances of excreta. Birds typically defecate several times a day. During the day the excreta may vary, as shown in Figure 24.1. Hens sitting on eggs will defecate less frequently and this will result in larger amounts per defecation and the typical form of the faecal part of excreta may change, which may be confused with diarrhoea. Figure 24.2 lists the typical appearance of excreta in birds commonly encountered in avian practice. In general, granivorous birds have a more compact faecal part of the excreta with a clearly separated uric acid fraction. The amount of urine will vary, with species originating from more arid climates (e.g. Budgerigars) having less urine and tropical species (e.g. Amazon parrots) producing more urine. Frugivorous birds such as Mynah birds have a higher amount of water in their excreta compared with granivorous birds. For the novice, the excreta of frugivorous birds may easily be interpreted as diarrhoea. In carnivorous birds, excreta are not clearly formed and the faeces, urates and urine will be combined. Also, it should be noted that diurnal birds of prey, such as the Common Buzzard, will expel excreta horizontally backwards (Figure 24.3), rather than letting the excreta fall as in seed-eating birds, which can make analyses of faeces more challenging.

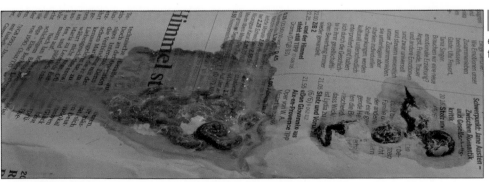

24.1 Normal (right) *versus* abnormal excreta (left) from a Blue-fronted Amazon.

Feeding type	Typical species	Colour of faeces	Consistency	Amount of urine
Granivores	Most parrots and passerines	Green	Formed faeces; uric acid clearly separated from faeces	Dependent on habitat; Budgerigars less than macaws
Frugivores	Mynah birds, Toucans	Brown to green	Loose faecal component; undigested chunks of food are frequently passed; loose droppings are difficult to diagnose	Large amount
Nectarivores	Lories and lorikeets	Brown	Loosely formed	Larger amount than granivores
Carnivores	Birds of prey	Different tones of dark brown to green	Soft; faeces in centre surrounded by chalky white urates; yellow faeces when feeding high-fat or light meat, green faeces normal before bird is fed	Moderate

24.2   Normal appearance of excreta in birds according to feeding strategy.

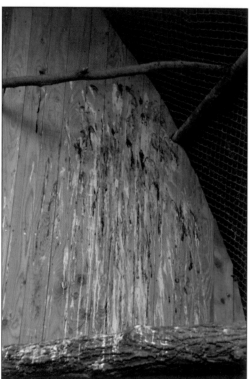

24.3   Diurnal birds of prey typically expel excreta horizontally backwards.
(Courtesy of Andreas Lischke)

Diagnostic approach

History

Diagnosis of the aetiology of loose droppings must follow a systematic approach starting with a thorough history, followed by distant examination and physical examination. Figure 24.4 summarizes important questions for the owner. The clinician should also try to find out about additional clinical signs of diseases that typically result in loose droppings (Figure 24.5). To save critical time and money, always consider typical diseases based on the age and species (Figure 24.6), so that the most efficient approach can be taken.

During history taking, observe the bird for clinical signs such as straining, because during distant examination stress may preclude the display of clinical signs.

Distant examination

The distant examination focuses on the bird and the cage or transport box with its contents. It is important to start with the distant examination during history

- How long have the droppings been loose? (Are the changes acute or chronic?)
- Is this the first time that loose droppings have occurred?
- Does the bird have access to free flight or is it confined to a cage? (Is there a risk of ingestion of toxins?)
- How many birds are affected?
- Have there been any changes in the bird's diet?
- How is the diet prepared? (Especially thawing of meat for raptors, hand-feeding of chicks)
- Are any multivitamins added? (May change the colour)
- Have there been any changes in management (e.g. addition of new bird to the collection, use of antibiotics)?
- Has the bird been egg laying recently?
- Other signs observed (e.g. regurgitation, bleeding, straining)
- Does the owner have an idea of what might be causing the loose droppings?
- Have any tests been carried out so far?
- Has the bird been treated and if so with what success?

24.4   Important questions to ask clients presenting a bird with loose droppings during history taking.

Disease	Typical clinical signs and/or species affected	Typical changes in the droppings
Chlamydia psittaci	Regurgitation; central nervous signs; respiratory signs	Lime-green to yellow-green urates
Salmonella spp.	Swollen joint (particularly in pigeons)	Lime-green to yellow-green urates
Mycobacterium spp.	Shifting leg lameness	Undigested food
Clostridium spp.	Regurgitation	Pseudomembranous casts; blood
Proventricular dilatation disease (avian bornavirus, ABV)	Central nervous signs, such as paresis, paralysis or blindness	Undigested food
Trichomonas spp.	'Wet around beak' due to regurgitation (especially Budgerigars)	Undigested food; watery droppings
Giardia sp.	Feather picking (particularly Cockatiels)	Undigested food
Coccidia	Especially in young falcons	Undigested food; pseudomembranous casts (*Caryospora* spp.)
Capillaria spp.	Granuloma in the oral cavity (particularly in diurnal birds of prey)	Undigested food

24.5   Loose droppings are often accompanied by additional clinical signs indicating disease.
(continues)

Disease	Typical clinical signs and/or species affected	Typical changes in the droppings
Candida albicans	White plaque in the oral cavity (particularly in young parrots)	Undigested food
Renal disease	Polydipsia	Granular consistency of droppings
Hepatic disease	Central nervous signs, such as torticollis	Blood; lime-green to yellow-green urates; watery green diarrhoea
Lead intoxication	Regurgitation, reduced crop emptying time, paresis of legs (particularly in diurnal birds of prey), kinked neck	Blood
Dehydration	Sunken eyes, increased refill time in the ulnar vein	Granular consistency of droppings
Cloacal papilloma	Particularly Amazon parrots, macaws, Hawk-headed Parrots	Blood
Cloacal prolapse	Especially cockatoos	Blood

24.5 (continued) Loose droppings are often accompanied by additional clinical signs indicating disease.

Age	Cause
Young parrot	Bacterial, viral, fungal, environmental (e.g. temperature, food)
Adult, small parrot	Parasitic (e.g. *Trichomonas* spp., *Giardia* spp.)/ fungal (e.g. *Candida* spp., *Macrorhabdus ornithogaster*)/viral, bacterial, toxin (e.g. lead), hepatic disease
Adult, large parrot	Viral, bacterial, toxin (e.g. lead), hepatic disease

24.6 Typical causes of loose droppings in parrots.

taking because some clinical signs, such as straining or picking around the vent, are not likely to be shown when the bird is feeling observed. As with every part of the clinical examination, it is important to remain systematic, with the distant examination carried out cranial to caudal. It is important to also observe the general behaviour of the bird (e.g. birds with proventricular dilatation disease will often also show clinical signs related to the central nervous system such as incoordination). Even if clinical signs appear obvious and may tempt the clinician to focus on a specific organ, it is nevertheless very important to carry out a complete general examination. Loose droppings may be part of a systemic disease or might be only one part of the problem.

Special attention during distant examination should be given to the plumage around the vent. Staining of the feathers with excreta is often observed with enteritis or with pathologies of the cloaca (Figure 24.7).

After the distant examination of the bird, the cage and its contents must be carefully investigated. The fact that birds defecate many times a day makes it most likely that excreta will be found even if the bird is brought in a transport box. The excreta may have been trampled upon, and this should not be confused with loose droppings. It should also be noted that excreta in

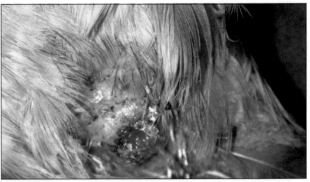

24.7 Vent of an African Grey Parrot with staining and tissue protruding from a neoplasia.

the transport box will often contain a higher amount of water as a result of stress; stress-induced polyuria is frequently seen in the transport box. In cases where the excreta cannot be evaluated adequately, the bird can be kept in a cage for up to three hours on a clean floor lined with white paper. A time-saving alternative may be to ask the owner to put white paper on the bottom of the cage floor before transportation so it can be used during the examination. Figure 24.8 summarizes abnormal droppings and the diseases that are commonly associated with them.

As with the distant examination of the bird, the distant examination of the excreta must be done systematically. First it is important to note the amount and the localization of the excreta within the cage. For this, it should be known that Budgerigars will produce excreta approximately 25 to 50 times per day, compared with macaws, which defecate 10 to 25 times per day (Hillyer, 1997) and birds of prey even less often. A reduced frequency of excreta production is normal in a female bird while sitting on eggs.

The location of defecation within the cage may be of importance. A depressed bird will be more prone to defecate always at the same place in comparison to a healthy bird that is moving around, which will lead to a more evenly distributed dispersal of excreta.

The next step is to inspect the excreta themselves. First, the general impression should be evaluated. For this it is important to know what the excreta look like in a healthy bird. Care must be taken to inspect the three different parts (urine, uric acid (urates) and faeces; see Chapter 10) of the excreta individually.

- Urine:
  - The clinician should especially evaluate the amount and the colour of urine produced; the urine, which is not as concentrated as in mammals, is usually colourless
  - The most frequent change in colour that occurs is biliverdinuria, which is typically considered a sign of hepatic diseases (see Case example 3)
  - Colour changes in urine can be associated with disease either within the urogenital tract or other organs
  - Some topical medications and food colourings will be excreted in the urine (e.g. topical proflavine can give yellow urates or beetroot can give purple colouring) (Harcourt-Brown, 2009).
- Uric acid portion (the urates):
  - The normal appearance is white to creamy (Figure 24.9)

Clinical appearance	Typical disease	Comments
Puffy droppings	<ul><li>Exocrine pancreas affected (acute necrosis especially in Quaker Parrots), chronic pancreatic necrosis due to Paramyxovirus-3 especially in *Neophema* spp., zinc intoxication)</li><li>More voluminous faeces may be due to a complete diet, which is higher in fibre</li></ul>	Check for amylase levels, >1500 U/l appears to be associated with pancreatitis (Doneley, 2001)
Bloody droppings	<ul><li>Lead intoxication</li><li>Herpesvirus infection (e.g. Pacheco)</li><li>Adenovirus (e.g. haemorrhagic disease of turkeys),</li><li>Paramyxovirus 1 (Newcastle Disease)</li><li>*Clostridia* spp.</li><li>*Macrorhabdus ornithogaster*, no fresh blood but dark faeces due to haemorrhage in the (pro-)ventriculus</li><li>Liver disease resulting coagulopathy</li><li>Cloacal disease (papilloma, cloacitis)</li><li>Prolapse (oviduct, cloaca)</li><li>Egg laying</li></ul>	Blood lead levels >0.2 ppm (20 pg/dl) are suggestive of lead toxicosis. Levels >0.5 ppm (50 pg/dl) are diagnostic for lead toxicosis
Undigested food in droppings	<ul><li>Proventricular dilatation disease</li><li>Bacterial or parasitic gastroenteritis (e.g. mycobacteria, *Giardia*, coccidia)</li><li>*Macrorhabdus ornithogaster*</li><li>*Candida albicans*</li><li>Grit impaction or lack of grit</li></ul>	
Pseudomembranous casts	<ul><li>*Caryospora* spp. (coccidia)</li><li>*Clostridium perfringens*</li></ul>	
Mucoid droppings	<ul><li>*Cryptosporidium* (parrots)</li><li>Wasting syndrome in Peregrine Falcons</li></ul>	
Watery green diarrhoea	<ul><li>*Spironucleus columbae* (in pigeons)</li><li>Paramyxovirus-1 (Newcastle disease)</li></ul>	Check wet mount microscopy of faeces for the detection of *Spironucleus columbae*
Watery droppings	<ul><li>*Hexamita* spp. (particularly in pigeons)</li><li>Nervousness</li><li>High salt or mineral intake</li></ul>	
Dry yellow droppings	<ul><li>*Campylobacter jejuni* (particularly in tropical finches)</li></ul>	
Granular consistency of droppings	<ul><li>Dehydration</li><li>Cloacal urolith</li><li>Renal disease (particularly in birds of prey)</li></ul>	
Lime-green to yellow-green urates	<ul><li>Herpesvirus infection (e.g. Pachecos disease)</li><li>*Chlamydia psittaci*</li><li>*Salmonella* spp.</li><li>General liver dysfunction</li></ul>	Important to identify aetiology

24.8 The gross appearance of excreta may indicate the likelihood of certain diseases (see Appendix 4).

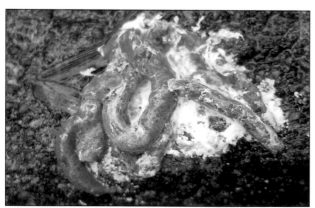

24.9 Normal excreta in a granivorous bird, the urates are white and creamy.

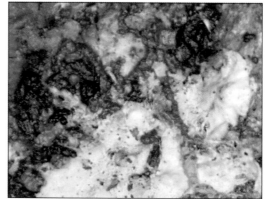

24.10 Normal excreta of a Great Horned Owl. Note the large amount of urates.
(Courtesy of Andreas Lischke)

- In granivorous birds, the urates represent a rather separate part of the excreta but they might mix with the faeces in diarrhoea
- In carnivorous birds, faeces are in the centre surrounded by chalk white urates (Figure 24.10)
- Due to the white colour of the urates, fresh blood from the cloaca or renal tract is more easily recognized in the uric acid portion than in the faeces
- Colour changes in the urates can be associated with disease either within the urogenital tract or in other organs. Light green to dark green urates

indicate a hepatitis; green to bronze urates can occur after trauma and bruising and can also be caused by hepatitis.

- Faeces:
  - Special emphasis is given to the volume, consistency and colour of the faeces
  - In most birds, the faeces are green (e.g. seed-eaters) to brown or black (e.g. carnivores)
  - Voluminous faeces can be normal and occur in situations where there is a high vegetable or fluid content in the diet. However, any cause of malabsorption (e.g. gastrointestinal disease, pancreatitis, parasitism, peritonitis, renal disease or neoplasia, or liver disease) can also cause an increase in bulk (Jones, 2009)
  - A creamy-clay colour of faeces with a puffy appearance indicates pancreatic disease
  - Faeces that are darker than normal may indicate haemorrhage in the small or large intestine, but a darker colour can also be the result of ingestion of berries such as blackberries. Blood from the more proximal intestinal tract will result in a dark coloration of faeces. Haemorrhagic diathesis can also occur as a result of starvation, especially in small birds such as passerines. Depending on the site of the haemorrhage, faeces will be either darker (upper intestinal tract) or fresh blood can be seen as part of the excreta (lower intestinal tract). Changes in colour can also occur due to dye in the newspaper on the cage floor (Harrison and Ritchie, 1994)
  - A more compact consistency is found in granivorous birds, with the exception of aquatic birds and carnivorous birds
  - Hens sitting on eggs will defecate less often, but will produce larger amounts of faeces with a softer appearance, which might be confused with loose droppings
  - Certain conditions can result in mucoid diarrhoea, such as the recently described wasting syndrome in Peregrine Falcons (Jones et al., 2013)
  - An increased consistency of faeces might also be seen as a sign of dehydration
  - It is also important to note any undigested food, especially seeds or other abnormal parts (e.g. nematodes) (Figure 24.11)
  - Absence of nematode larvae; however, this does not necessarily mean the absence of nematodes altogether

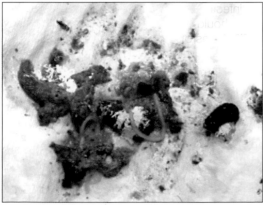

24.11 Ascarids in the loose droppings of an Amazon parrot.

- Infections with *Macrorhabdus ornithogaster* or avian bornavirus (proventricular dilatation disease) frequently result in the passing of undigested food but other causes might be vitamin E and/or selenium deficiency, lack of grit or excess oil in the diet
- Beware to differentiate undigested seeds in the faeces from seeds that have fallen on the faeces. The latter typically cover the faeces and are not stained with faeces (Figure 24.12)

Besides inspecting the excreta, it is also important to note any other abnormalities in the cage, such as regurgitated food. However, the clinician should be aware that regurgitation may, in some birds, occur as a result of travelling to the clinic.

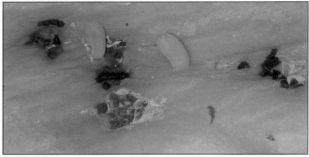

24.12 Seeds that have fallen on to the excreta might be mistaken for undigested seeds, as seen with certain diseases such as proventricular dilatation disease.

Physical examination

Following distant examination, the bird is handled for physical examination (see Chapters 9 and 10). It is important to note that, compared with other classes of animals, avian physical examinations must be carried out systematically and within a short timeframe. When investigating loose droppings the veterinary surgeon may already have decided to collect specific samples, such as cloacal swabs or blood, during the initial physical examination; therefore, it is important to have a list of differential diagnoses ready, based on the history and the distant examination of the patient. Typically, weighing, temperature measurement and auscultation of the heart and the lower airways are performed as part of the general physical examination. Body condition status is assessed in most birds based on the palpation of the pectoral musculature. For the evaluation of loose droppings, this parameter is also of importance as it may give information regarding the differentiation of acute *versus* chronic disease.

Special attention during the physical examination of birds with loose droppings is given to the cloaca. Staining of the feathers around the cloaca is an important finding. The cloaca itself and the surrounding tissue should be inspected for the occurrence of masses, blood or any other abnormalities. Papillomas are often associated with Amazon parrots, macaws and Hawk-headed Parrots. Prolapsed tissue from the cloaca, due to idiopathic straining or excessive sexual behaviour, occurs in cockatoos (Hadley, 2005).

For a cloacal swab, a sterile moistened swab is used to collect a sample from the coprodeum (representative for gastrointestinal disease). If a mass is visible around the cloaca, an impression smear is recommended (Monks, 2005).

Diagnostic techniques

A multitude of diagnostic techniques exist which aid in determining the cause of abnormal droppings. The techniques should be used based on the results of the clinical examination, likelihood of the disease in the species and the expectations of the owner. The following methods are listed in order of importance in relation to loose droppings. A special focus is given to faecal microbiology, especially bacteriology and parasitology (see Chapter 12).

Although analyses such as microscopy and culture are essential for the investigation of loose droppings, other analyses such as blood testing and diagnostic imaging may be used according to additional clinical signs and the owner's expectations.

Wet mount faecal microscopy

Mix a small amount of excreta (about the size of the head of a match; 1–2 mm³) with a drop of water or saline on a microscope slide. Mix the drop with a circular motion until the specimen is approximately 1 x 1 cm on the slide add a coverslip and examine under the microscope, starting at low magnification up to X400 magnification for the presence of parasites, such as nematode eggs (e.g. ascarids in parrots or *Capillaria* spp. in birds of prey) or protozoans (e.g. *Giardia* spp. in Cockatiels, *Trichomonas* spp. in Budgerigars, coccidia and *Cochlosoma* spp. in passerines). It is important to perform the microscopic examination without delay as ciliate protozoans will quickly lose their motility and will be less easy to identify.

To better visualize protozoal cysts (e.g. *Giardia* spp.) put two drops of iodine solution on the edge of the coverslip. This will stain cysts and increase their visibility. Live protozoans are usually visible at a magnification of X200. Motility seen at higher magnification should be differentiated from Brownian motion, which is a random motion of particles suspended in fluids. Brownian motion does not result in a net movement.

Native examination will often also allow the visualization of fungal infection such as *Candida* spores and the large bacilli-like *Macrorhabdus ornithogaster*, which often affects Budgerigars but may also be found in other species. Their visibility can be improved by adding a drop of lactophenol blue at the edge of the coverslip.

It is important to note that absence of infectious organisms, especially parasites, does not rule out the disease, as excretion may only occur intermittently.

Fixed staining techniques for faecal examinations

For the diagnostic evaluation of loose droppings it is also recommended that a Gram stain of excreta or material from a cloacal swab is performed. Typically, this examination will be carried out in conjunction with microbiological cultures and sensitivity testing. The great advantage of the microscopic examination is that the clinician may immediately have a result and the findings will help in more rational decision-making for initial therapy, while awaiting culture results.

The examination is carried out at high-power magnification (oil immersion X1000) and allows the differentiation of groups of bacteria and their number. Although some controversy exists regarding the bacterial flora of birds, there is clear evidence that in parrot faeces only small amounts of Gram-negative bacteria (e.g. Enterobacteriaceae) will be found. The majority of bacteria are Gram-positive cocci and rods (e.g. *Bacillus*, *Corynebacterium*, *Lactobacillus*, *Staphylococcus* and *Streptococcus* spp.). Clostridia are considered abnormal in the faeces of parrots, but can be found in the faeces of birds of prey. The latter also tend to have more Gram-negative bacteria in their faeces compared with parrots, especially if they are fed chicken (Bangert *et al.*, 1988).

Gram stain will also stain fungi such as yeasts (*Candida* spp.) and *Macrorhabdus ornithogaster* (Figure 24.13). Primary fungal infections of the intestinal tract are rare and often should be considered a secondary problem. The finding of a few yeasts or *Macrorhabdus ornithogaster* in a clinically healthy bird is generally not considered a reason for treatment, although the bird may be infectious to other birds. Large numbers of *Macrorhabdus* organisms, or a bird with consistent signs, would indicate treatment is required. It should also be noted that diet might influence the bacterial composition (Glünder, 2002; Fischer *et al.*, 2006).

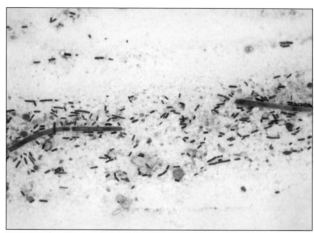

24.13 Gram stain of the faeces of a Budgerigar, showing overgrowth of Gram-negative bacteria and two *Macrorhabdus ornithogaster* organisms.

The diagnosis of Macrorhabdus leaves the clinician balancing contradictory issues of infectious disease control and social welfare. While many infected birds are asymptomatic, some birds will develop clinical disease, and some birds will die from this condition. Conversely, advising social isolation of any positive bird is a significant welfare concern, especially given the relative insensitivity of testing (some birds may be positive but undiagnosed). One option is to maintain cages of 'already infected' birds, while another is to have birds in adjacent cages with the opportunity to mutually head preen but prevent faecal access.

Besides infectious agents, the presence of inflammatory cells should also be noted, as they are not present in the faeces of a healthy animal.

Although less commonly used, additional staining techniques exist. Acid-fast organisms such as *Mycobacterium* spp. can be stained with the Ziehl–Neelsen technique; for the clinical practice, fast stains exist. Macchiavello or Giemsa stains are used for the detection of *Chlamydia* spp. If a cytological examination is needed, rapid stains such as Diff-Quik® or Hemacolor®, are frequently used by clinicians.

Parasitological examination

In case of suspected parasitological disease, it is recommended to perform a flotation and possibly a sedimentation. Flotation can easily be performed in the veterinary practice by mixing a small amount of excreta with a flotation solution. Commercial flotation solutions are available which typically contain zinc sulphate. Homemade flotation solutions can be made by dissolving 454 g of sugar in 355 ml of tap water or 400 g of salt in 1 l of tap water. Sugar solutions are preferred to salt solutions as they tend to result in less distortion of nematode ova. A simple method to perform a flotation is to mix a small amount of excreta with flotation solution in a test tube. Fill the tube until a slight positive meniscus is formed and place a coverslip over it. Wait for 10 to 20 minutes and remove the coverslip straight upwards and place it on a microscopy slide for further examination.

The clinician should always be aware that absence of parasites in a sample is not diagnostic, as parasites are often shed intermittently, and ideally samples collected over several days should be investigated. In birds fed whole prey, parasites might originate from the prey food and be only transitory.

Microbiological culture

Even though microscopy, especially with Gram stains, can give an indication as to which bacterial organism is involved in causing the diarrhoea, and this can be an important guide regarding the choice of treatment while awaiting culture results, it cannot replace bacterial culture. Culture is performed on the basis of a swab from fresh excreta or a cloacal swab, and should include aerobic and anaerobic cultures. *Salmonella* spp. should always be checked for in the culture in cases of diarrhoea. It should be noted that a cloacal swab is unreliable for the detection of salmonellae in birds, as they are excreted intermittently and in low numbers (Fanelli *et al.*, 1971). In birds of prey, *Salmonella* infection tends to result in acute disease *versus* more chronic disease in pigeons. Other typical pathogens causing loose droppings are *Campylobacter* sp., *Clostridium* spp., and *Yersinia pseudotuberculosis* (Dorrestein, 1997). Furthermore, *Escherichia coli*, *Pseudomonas* spp., *Aeromonas* spp. and *Pasteurella multocida* can all cause enteritis and diarrhoea.

Whenever possible, sensitivity testing should follow culture not only to allow the use of an active antibiotic, but also to make a sensible choice of antibiotic according to the increasing risk of development of multidrug resistance. When interpreting results of microbiology, the clinician should be aware of physiological differences regarding intestinal flora. The culture of *E. coli* in a bird of prey or a frugivorous bird is not surprising, whereas in a granivorous bird this could be a cause of concern, especially when linked to disease. In general, it can be said that if a bacterium is isolated from a bird with loose droppings in a pure or almost pure culture in the absence of another aetiological agent, then it may be considered significant.

Blood tests

A large number of parameters can be investigated in the blood and the clinician must always make a choice regarding the differential diagnoses of the case. Additional testing for toxins or infectious agents (antigen or antibodies) may be necessary. Blood analysis is also of importance to evaluate the loss of minerals (especially sodium, chloride, potassium and bicarbonate) which often occurs as a result of diarrhoea.

Diagnostic imaging

The choice of diagnostic modalities is constantly increasing and generally their use is very much defined by availability and readiness of the owner to pay for the costs. Traditionally, radiography has been used in avian medicine, followed by endoscopy. More recently, ultrasonography, computed tomography (CT) and magnetic resonance imaging (MRI) have also been applied. With the exception of radiography, it should also be noted that often a referral to a specialized clinic or university setting may be necessary for further diagnostic imaging. Typically, diagnostic imaging necessitates general anaesthesia, which owners may be reluctant to allow due to potential risks.

Radiography: Radiography can provide important information for the diagnosis of loose droppings. In cases of suspected hepatitis (e.g. green-stained urates, elevated bile acids), an increased liver size may be suspected in the radiographic images. Foreign bodies such as excessive grit or lead can also be recognized. Findings in relation to loose droppings can also be gas in the intestine or dilatation of parts of the gastrointestinal tract (e.g. proventriculus; Figure 24.14). Gas in the intestine can occur as a result of bacterial enteritis, tube feeding, gaseous anaesthesia, dyspnoea, proventricular dilatation disease, ileus or intestinal parasites (Rupley, 1999).

The use of oral barium sulphate (30–60%, 20 ml/kg) for contrast radiography is a good method of gaining further information from radiographic images, especially when performed at different time intervals (Figure 24.15). It is important to note that contrast radiographs are always made following plain radiographs. When

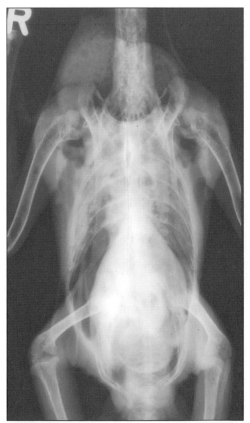

24.14 Macaw with proventricular dilatation disease. The crop and the proventriculus are severely distended and filled with gas.

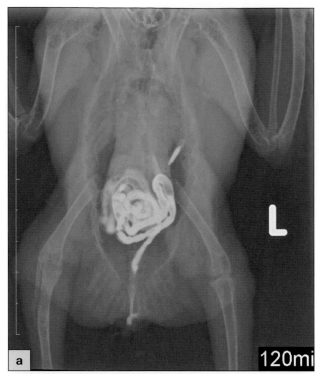

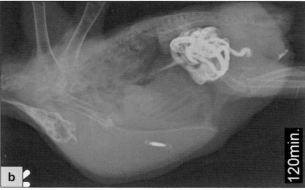

24.15 (a) Ventrodorsal and (b) laterolateral views showing contrast radiography with barium sulphate which has been performed at different time intervals to reveal a reduced gastrointestinal transit time.

using contrast radiography, the clinician must always be aware of the physiological gastrointestinal transit time of the species involved.

Factors such as diet, stress and time of day can also influence gastrointestinal transit time. Based on the transit time and the anatomical structure to be evaluated, the time post contrast medium application for the radiography is defined (see also Chapter 18). Information that can be gained from contrast studies include the transit time, abnormalities of the filling of the intestinal lumen (e.g. due to mucosal thickening as it occurs with mycobacterial infections or dilatation of the proventriculus) and changes in the position of the gastrointestinal tract (e.g. due to a mass effect outside the gastrointestinal tract). If further information on gastrointestinal motility is needed, contrast fluoroscopy is a useful tool (Beaufrère *et al.*, 2010; Kubiak and Forbes, 2012). Fluoroscopy can be performed repeatedly without handling while the awake animal is perching in a box.

Endoscopy: The endoscopic evaluation of the gastrointestinal tract can involve the oesophagus, crop, proventriculus and ventriculus, or the cloaca up to the distal part of the colon. Typically, rigid endoscopy is used in the avian practice, although flexible endoscopy can be of use as well, especially in large birds, to reach the ventriculus.

For the diagnosis of loose droppings, investigation of the cloaca and distal colon appears most useful. An endoscopic evaluation of the cloaca is recommended, especially when fresh blood is found on the faeces or the feathers around the cloaca are covered with faeces or blood. Typical findings are papillomas, cloacoliths or a retained egg, all of which might not always be visible radiographically (e.g. soft-shelled egg).

Coelioscopy can be recommended in cases where extra-intestinal causes are suspected to be causing loose droppings. Hepatitis is an example that can result in diarrhoea. The major advantages of endoscopy over other diagnostic imaging techniques are the direct visualization of the organ and the possibility of biopsy sampling for histology or microbiological culture.

Ultrasonography: The use of ultrasonography for the diagnostic evaluation of loose droppings in birds is limited compared with the evaluation of organs such as the heart. In avian medicine, important limiting factors for ultrasonography are the small window for ultrasonography of the coelomic cavity and the presence of air sacs, which have a negative effect on image quality. For the typical pet bird, with a bodyweight of up to 500 g, a convex or linear transducer of 5.5–14 MHz has been used. For the examination of the coelomic cavity plucking of feathers may not always be necessary. Fasting pigeons and quails for 12–18 hours followed by instillation of water in the crop and the cloaca prior to the examination had a positive influence on visualization and the image quality (Krautwald-Junghanns *et al.*, 2002; Pees *et al.*, 2006). Structures of the gastrointestinal tract that can be well visualized are the crop, ventriculus, intestines (especially the duodenal loop) and the cloaca. Indications for ultrasonography with regard to loose droppings are suspicion of ileus, foreign bodies, neoplastic conditions, extra-intestinal masses that influence gastrointestinal function (e.g. dystocia, enlarged liver) or inflammatory processes in the intestine (Figure 24.16).

Problem	Possible ultrasonography findings
Inflammatory lesions	■ Increase of intestinal diameter ■ Increased thickness of wall ■ Less homogeneous liver echogenicity and focal heterogeneous areas ■ Dilatation of hepatic blood vessels
Obstruction	■ Hyperechoic surface of foreign body with distal acoustic shadowing ■ Increased filling of intestinal loops
Ileus	■ Increase of intestinal diameter ■ Abnormal intestinal motility ■ Accumulation of anechoic fluid
Neoplastic conditions	■ Focal asymmetrical thickening of intestinal wall ■ Hypomotility
Intussusception	■ Abnormal intestinal motility ■ 'Onion ring' layers
Extra-intestinal mass	■ Enlargement of organ (e.g. liver, kidney, salpinx) ■ Thin- or soft-shelled egg ■ Abnormal location of intestinal landmarks such as ventriculus or duodenum

24.16 Investigation of loose droppings using ultrasonography.

Computed tomography and magnetic resonance imaging: The availability of CT and MRI has significantly increased in the last 10 years. However, costs are often prohibitive and the use of these modalities for the diagnostic investigation of loose droppings in birds is still an exception. Indications for CT and MRI are similar to ultrasonography and include mechanical or paralytic ileus, neoplasia and extra-intestinal masses that influence gastrointestinal function (e.g. dystocia, enlarged liver). The advantages of CT and MRI are the possibility for additional analyses of the images once the examination has taken place and the lack of superposition of organs, hence a more detailed evaluation of organs, compared with ultrasonography and radiography. A disadvantage, besides cost, is the need for general anaesthesia and the duration of the examination, especially when MRI is used. It therefore has to be emphasized that the referring veterinary surgeon and the institution performing the CT or MRI need to have a firm indication for the procedure and confidence that they can interpret the results.

Infectious agent testing: The aetiology of loose droppings often is an infectious agent. An increasing number of these infectious agents can be diagnosed by antibody or antigen testing. Diseases that will require such testing are *Chlamydia psittaci*, avian bornavirus and herpesvirus, but adenovirus, influenza virus and paramyxovirus also need to be considered as potential aetiologies for enteritis and diarrhoea. Details on the choice of tests and the sampling are given in Chapter 19.

Treatment

The treatment of loose droppings will typically be initiated by supportive treatment aimed at replacing lost fluid and electrolytes, and an increased ambient temperature. An increased environmental temperature is especially important in most pet birds due to their small size and high metabolic rates, which quickly result in a life-threatening condition if not supported.

Rehydration, typically with crystalloid fluids, should be provided via the intravenous, intraosseous or subcutaneous route (see Chapters 11 and 15). If possible, an indwelling intravenous or intraosseous catheter for continuous support is recommended in critical cases.

Supportive feeding should be given, if necessary by gavage feeding of specialized mixes (e.g. Emeraid® Nutri-Support, Roudybush™ Careline Acute Care, Harrison's Recovery Formula, Oxbow's Carnivore Care, Hill's® Prescription Diet a/d). Every step should be taken to increase the voluntary uptake of fluids and solids by the bird. When providing supportive treatment, provision of electrolytes should be secured, especially as loose droppings typically result in a loss of sodium, chloride, potassium and bicarbonate. The use of probiotics such as *Lactobacillus* spp. may be beneficial for the recovery of the intestinal flora.

In addition to supportive treatment, specific treatment will be given, which may include antifungals (e.g. amphotericin B against yeast or *M. ornithogaster*), antibiotics, antiparasitics (e.g. metronidazole against *Trichomonas* or *Giardia* spp., but also clostridia) and/or anti-inflammatory and analgesic drugs. With antibiotic drugs, it is recommended to treat whenever possible based on culture and sensitivity. While awaiting laboratory results, a broad-spectrum antibiotic can be administered, such as co-amoxiclav (which is also active against anaerobes) or trimethoprim/sulphonamide combinations. If chlamydiosis is suspected, treatment should be started with doxycycline or enrofloxacin. In cases of regurgitation, the author has had good results in psittacine birds by giving an antiemetic drug such as ondansetron at 1–2 mg/kg orally q12h for 3–4 days.

When treating infectious agents, attention must be given to prevent reinfestation. Treatment of the entire flock might be necessary and cleaning of cages and cage contents with an appropriate product should be advised.

Acknowledgements

The author is grateful to Mr Andreas Lischke for providing Figures 24.3 and 24.10.

References and further reading

Bangert RL, Ward ACS, Stauber EH *et al.* (1988) A survey of the aerobic bacteria in the feces of captive raptors. *Avian Diseases* **32**, 53–62

Beaufrère H, Nevarez J, Taylor WM *et al.* (2010) Fluoroscopy study of the normal gastrointestinal motility and measurement in the Hispaniolan amazon parrot (*Amazona ventralis*). *Veterinary Radiology and Ultrasound* **51**, 441–446

Doneley RJT (2001) Acute pancreatitis in parrots. *Australian Veterinary Journal* **79**, 409–411

Dorrestein GM (1997) Bacteriology. In: *Avian Medicine and Surgery*, ed. RB Altman, SL Clubb, GM Dorrestein *et al.*, pp. 255–280. WB Saunders, Philadelphia

Duke GE (1997) Gastrointestinal physiology and nutrition in wild birds. *Proceedings of the Nutrition Society* **56**, 1049–1056

Fanelli MJ, Sadler WW, Franti CE *et al.* (1971) Localisation of salmonellae in the intestinal tract of chickens. *Avian Diseases* **15**, 366–375

Fischer I, Christen C, Lutz H *et al.* (2006) Effects of two diets on the haematology, plasma chemistry and intestinal flora of budgerigars (*Melopsittacus undulatus*). *Veterinary Record* **159**, 480–484

Glünder G (2002) Influence of diet on the occurrence of some bacteria in the intestinal flora of wild and pet birds. *Deutsche Tierärztliche Wochenschrift* **109**, 266–270

Hadley TL (2005) Disorders of the psittacine gastrointestinal tract. *Veterinary Clinics of North America: Exotic Animal Practice* **8**, 329–349

Harcourt-Brown NH (2009) Psittacine birds. In: *Handbook of Avian Medicine, 2nd edn*, ed. TN Tully, GM Dorrestein and AK Jones, pp. 138–168. Saunders Elsevier, Philadelphia

Harrison GJ and Ritchie BW (1994) Making distinctions in the physical examination. In: *Avian Medicine: Principles and Application*, ed. BW Ritchie, GJ Harrison and LR Harrison, pp. 144–175. Wingers Publlishing, Lake Worth

Hillyer EV (1997) Physical examination. In: *Avian Medicine and Surgery*, ed. RB Altman, SL Clubb, GM Dorrestein *et al.*, pp. 125–141. WB Saunders Company, Philadelphia

Jones AK (2009) The physical examination. In: *Handbook of Avian Medicine, 2nd edn*, ed. TN Tully, GM Dorrestein and AK Jones, pp. 56–76. Saunders Elsevier, Philadelphia

Jones R, Forbes N, Stidworthy MF *et al.* (2013) An emerging wasting syndrome in peregrine falcons (*Falco peregrinus*), *International Conference on Avian, Herpetological and Exotic Mammal Medicine* pp. 235–237. *1*. Wiesbaden, Germany

Krautwald-Junghanns M-E, Stahl A, Pees M, Enders F and Bartels T (2002) Sonographic investigations of the gastrointestinal tract of granivorous birds. *Veterinary Radiology and Ultrasound* **43**, 576–582

Kubiak M and Forbes NA (2012) Fluoroscopic evaluation of gastrointestinal transit time in African Grey parrots. *Veterinary Record* **171**, 563–564

Monks D (2005) Gastrointestinal disease. In: *BSAVA Manual of Psittacine Birds, 2nd edn*, ed. N Harcourt-Brown and J Chitty, pp. 180–190. BSAVA Publications, Gloucester

Pees M, Kiefer I, Krautwalt-Junhghanns M-E *et al.* (2006) Comparative ultrasonographic investigations of the gastrointestinal tract and the liver in healthy and diseased pigeons. *Veterinary Radiology and Ultrasound* **47**, 370–375

Rupley AE (1999) Diagnostic techniques for gastrointestinal diseases of psittacines. *Seminars in Avian and Exotic Pet Medicine* **8**, 51–65

Case example 1: African Grey Parrot with green, malodorous, voluminous faeces

Presentation and history

An 18-year-old female African Grey Parrot presented with a 2-week history of not perching and of green, malodorous and more voluminous faeces. She was eating well, on a diet of seeds, pellets and fruits, and was kept indoors and outdoors in a cage, together with a male African Grey Parrot.

The bird was presented in sternal recumbency, but was able to use its feet, appearing moderately depressed, with a body condition of 3/5 and an empty crop.

Diagnostic work-up

- Faecal examination (wet mount): no abnormalities
- Faecal examination (Gram stain): increased number of Gram-negative rods
- Haematology: mildly reduced packed cell volume
- Chemistry: mildly reduced ionized calcium, moderately increased creatine kinase, mildly increased uric acid
- Radiography: crop mildly filled with gas and proventriculus possibly mildly enlarged
- Lead: within normal limits
- *Chlamydia psittaci* (polymerase chain reaction, PCR): negative
- Avian bornavirus (PCR): positive.

Diagnosis: Proventricular dilatation disease.

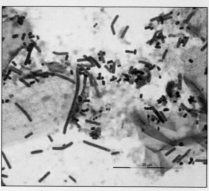
Increased number of Gram-negative rods.

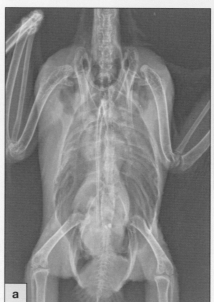
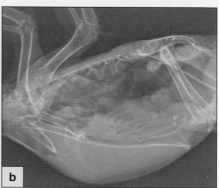
(a) Ventrodorsal and (b) laterolateral views show a mildly enlarged proventriculus.

Therapy

While awaiting laboratory results, supportive treatment with subcutaneous fluids, calcium gluconate, lactulose and broad-spectrum antibiotics (enrofloxacin) and butorphanol should be administered.

Outcome

No improvement of the bird's condition. Due to the diagnosis of proventricular dilatation disease and the grave prognosis, the owner elected for euthanasia. The partner bird tested negative for avian bornavirus (PCR).

Case example 2: Hawk-headed Parrot with haematochezia

Presentation and history

An adult Hawk-headed Parrot of unknown age and sex was presented. The bird had been purchased the year before from a private breeder and kept as a single bird in a cage on a diet of seed mixture, fruits, vegetables and nuts. The owner also chews some of the food (bread, pasta, sometimes cheese) and feeds the parrot from his mouth.

The owner found the parrot on the bottom of the cage 5 days prior to presentation; the bird could not move its right leg, did not want to eat and was making a lot of noise. The parrot was presented to a private practitioner. There

was no fracture palpable and the bird was discharged and prescribed oral treatment with meloxicam. There was no improvement and the bird was referred for a second opinion.

Diagnostic work-up

On clinical examination, lameness of the right leg with soft tissue swelling on the tibiotarsus was identified, with moderate depression, nutritional condition 3/5, anorexia, and diarrhoea with traces of fresh blood.

- Haematology: mild leucocytosis, moderate heterophilia, monocytosis and lymphopenia

- Biochemistry: severely elevated uric acid, aspartate aminotransferase and creatine kinase
- Faecal examination (wet mount): ciliates
- Faecal examination (Gram stain): increased number of Gram-negative rods
- Faecal culture and sensitivity testing: +++ *Escherichia coli* (enrofloxacin sensitive)
- Radiography: soft tissue swelling in the right tibiotarsus
- Ultrasonography: hyperechoic zone in the kidneys suggestive of renal fibrosis. Differential diagnosis: renal mineralization (e.g. gout, other nephropathy).

▶

Case example 2 *continued*

Diagnosis: nephropathy, endoparasites, bacterial enteritis, soft tissue swelling on right tibiotarsus (possibly soft tissue trauma).

Therapy

Intravenous and subcutaneous fluids, metronidazole, enrofloxacin, itraconazole and meloxicam were prescribed and the bird was force-fed. The itraconazole was used due to concern that the monocytosis may have been linked to the presence of a fungal granuloma.

Outcome

The therapy continued for 3 weeks with regular blood checks until the uric acid and other blood values were within normal limits. The paresis/paralysis resolved within 10 days. The bird was subsequently discharged without further therapy and with instructions for the owner not to feed the animal with pre-chewed and/or table food. There was recurrence of diarrhoea 5 months later. Haematology revealed a similar pattern of moderate leucocytosis, heterophilia, monocytosis and lymphopenia, and a mild elevation in the creatine kinase values. *Chlamydia* testing (PCR) of a

swab from the conjunctiva, choana and cloaca was negative; faecal bacteriology was again positive for *E. coli*. Ultrasonography showed a small cystic formation cranial to the kidney of unknown origin. The therapy was repeated with a change of the antimicrobial to co-amoxiclav for 3 weeks. No recurrence was noted.

Case example 3: Cockatiel with biliverdinuria

Presentation and history

A 10-year-old male Cockatiel was presented with a 2-day history of depression and no flying. The bird was housed together with 12 other Cockatiels indoors, with daily free flight. Diet consisted of a seed mixture, millet spikes, salad and, occasionally, fruit.

On examination, the bird was sitting on the floor of the cage, appeared depressed and had moderate torticollis. Severe biliverdinuria was obvious in the mildly loose droppings. Feathers around the cloaca were stained with faeces and the crop was full. The bird had a nutritional condition of 2/5.

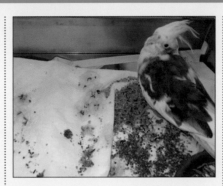

Diagnostic work-up

- Haematology: moderate leucocytosis, with heterophilia, monocytosis and lymphopenia
- Biochemistry: severely elevated bile acids, aspartate aminotransferase (AST) and mild elevation of creatine kinase (CK)
- Faecal examination (wet mount): no abnormalities

- Faecal examination (Gram stain): 60% Gram-positive and 40% Gram-negative bacteria
- *Chlamydia* testing (complement fixation): negative
- Owner declined additional examinations for heavy metal intoxication, and culture and sensitivity testing of faeces.

Diagnosis: hepatoencephalic syndrome (consider hepatitis), enteral dysbacteriosis.

Therapy

Subcutaneous fluids, enrofloxacin (while awaiting *Chlamydia* testing results), lactulose, multivitamin and probiotics.

Outcome

Treatment was continued for 14 days and no recheck was carried out, but the owner reported that the bird was fine.

Egg retention

Stefka Curd

Egg retention, or post-ovulatory stasis, is the failure of an egg to pass through the oviduct at a normal rate (delayed oviposition, 'egg binding').

A further and more advanced sign is dystocia. Dystocia is a condition where the egg is the reason for a mechanical obstruction of the caudal oviduct and/or cloaca, impairing the function of the caudal gastro-intestinal tract. This can lead to cloacal impaction or cloacal prolapse.

Causes of egg retention vary in different species and are often multifactorial. They include nutritional deficiencies and hypocalcaemia (often seen in Grey Parrots due to malnutrition and/or lack of ultraviolet exposure); smooth muscle functional deficiency of the oviduct and/or uterus; infection or mechanical tears/damage of the oviduct (in the smaller species); obesity and inadequate exercise; and stress factors such as hypo- or hyperthermia and inappropriate housing and nesting conditions.

In the author's experience, small birds (e.g. finches, canaries) which lay for the first time often have an inadequate-sized egg; Budgerigars and, especially, Cockatiels, on the other hand, are prone to excessive egg laying, which can lead to fatigue of the oviduct with subsequent systemic disease processes.

Clinical signs

Because egg binding and dystocia are clinical signs which can have different underlying causative reasons, the owner must be made aware that initial treatment is of the clinical sign (egg retention/dystocia) and that finding the causative reason for this sign is not always straightforward. Underlying, secondary complications may also be present.

Smaller species, such as finches, canaries, Budgerigars and Cockatiels, are usually more severely affected than larger species, which could be due to a poorly supplemented diet (seed diets alone are generally low in calcium) or species characteristics (e.g. many pet Cockatiels can lay up to 20 eggs per year). Often, clinical findings include acute onset of depression, dyspnoea, ruffled feathers (Figure 25.1), and an abdominal mass palpated on clinical examination. In smaller birds, occasionally sudden death occurs.

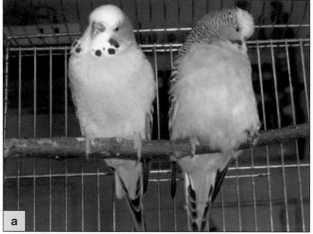

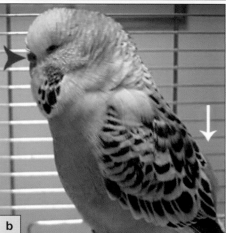

25.1 **(a)** Comparison of a healthy Budgerigar (left) and a Budgerigar with abdominal distension and wide perching stance. **(b)** Budgerigar showing depression and fluffed-up feathers. Note the hypertrophic cere often seen in female budgerigars (arrowhead) and the protrusion of the back (arrowed) often seen with abdominal distension and dyspnoea.

Larger species may still be perching but with a wide stance or, more often, they will be sitting on the bottom of the cage and may show signs of leg lameness and/or uni/bilateral paresis of the legs. Less frequent and larger volumes of faeces may be passed, which is often noted by the owner. Some degree of respiratory difficulties may be seen as well.

Diagnostic tests

Often, diagnosis of egg binding is based on clinical signs noted by the owner, their duration, taking a thorough history of the bird, physical examination and supportive diagnostic tests, including blood examination, radiography and ultrasonography (Figure 25.2).

In ratites 'uterine contractions' can be seen via ultrasonography during normal egg laying, and lack of contractions is considered a sign for egg binding in these species. Such contractions have not been observed in parrot species, but ultrasonography is an invaluable tool in differentiating an enlarged coelom where no egg can be palpated.

Clinical approach

1. If the bird is distressed and shows any sign of dyspnoea, place the bird together with its cage in a large warm oxygen-supplied box or incubator (Figure 25.3), before taking the history from the owner. This will give the bird a chance to recover from the journey to the surgery.
2. After taking the history from the owner, and when the bird is more stable, continue with the physical examination. It is useful to know when the last egg was laid. As a general guideline, parrots lay an egg every other day. Take care when removing the bird from its cage. Often, placing a towel over the bird is a gentle restraint and minimizes stress while a quick but thorough physical examination can be performed. An enlarged cloaca may be seen with a distended abdomen and an egg may be palpated in the ventral coelomic area.
3. Stabilize the patient: give fluids (the author prefers giving 5% glucose: saline at a ratio of 1:1), either intravenously or subcutaneously (see Chapter 15). Give analgesia (e.g. butorphanol at 1–2 mg/kg i.m.).
4. Give a bolus of calcium at 100 mg/kg either as calcium borogluconate or calcium gluconate subcutaneously together with the fluids. Alternatively, a bolus of high-calcium powder (e.g. 200 mg/g) could be mixed with a small amount of

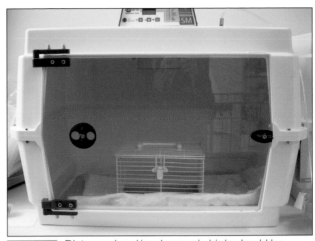

25.3 Distressed and/or dyspnoeic birds should be placed in an oxygen box or incubator to recover before examination.

baby parrot food or other powdered cereal-based baby food, and given into the crop with a crop tube. A dose of 100 mg/100 g bird given this way is usually sufficient for the bird to stand, and the egg is usually passed.
5. Place the bird immediately back into a warm, humid and oxygenated environment (e.g. incubator). If possible, place the bird in a dark and quiet area or cover the incubator with a towel. Leave the bird in the incubator for about 15–20 minutes prior to further examination.
6. Perform further clinical tests, depending on the severity of the case:
   - Radiography (see Chapter 18 for positioning). It is important that at least a straightforward whole body radiograph is performed (Figure 25.4). Take note of the size of the egg, if is it only one, how thick the shell is and if there are concurrent conditions. Pay attention to the bird's bone density. If it is an egg-laying hen, expect increased bone density (medullary bone in most long bones). Well developed medullary bone suggests adequate calcium reserves for egg production. If the egg is a normal shape, the

Diagnosis	Clinical signs	Diagnostic features	Therapy
Soft-shelled egg	Distressed bird Often good general condition Signs persist more than a week without general change in clinical condition	Clinical examination: enlarged coelom, no egg on palpation Radiography: displacement of the ventriculus (see Figure 25.5) Ultrasonography: visualization of the egg (see Figure 25.8)	Surgery
Soft-shelled egg with concurrent salpingitis	Bird displays signs of egg laying for a long time Recent rapid deterioration	Clinical examination: enlarged coelom, no egg on palpation Haematology: often elevated white blood cell count (with or without toxic heterophils) Radiography: see Figure 25.7 Ultrasonography: presence of soft-shelled eggs with excessive fluid accumulation in the salpinx (see Figure 25.8)	Surgery Antimicrobials
Egg-yolk peritonitis	Decreased egg production History of recent egg laying Depression Anorexia Poor condition	Haematology: elevated white blood cell count with toxic heterophils Radiography: loss of detail (see Figure 25.10) Ultrasonography: presence of egg yolk in the coelomic cavity outside salpinx (see Figure 25.11)	Long-term parenteral antimicrobials Stabilization Surgery
Coelomic hernia	Straining Abdominal distension Good general condition	Often chronic egg layers Radiography: better visualization of the displaced intestinal loops using contrast (e.g. barium sulphate)	Surgery

25.2 Differential diagnoses for egg retention.

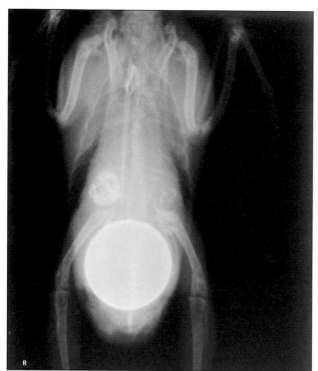

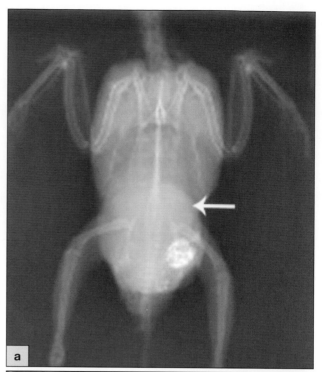

25.4 Radiograph of an egg-bound bird. Note the size and the thickness of the egg: it is far too big for the size of the bird and the shell is quite thick. These are signs that the egg has been in the uterus for a while.

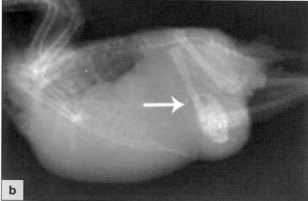

25.5 (a) Ventrodorsal and (b) lateral views of a bird with a shell-less egg. (a) A soft tissue opacity can be seen dorsal to the ventriculus (arrowed). (b) There is ventral and lateral displacement of the ventriculus (arrowed).

shell is not thickened, the bird has good bone density and is in a good general condition, conservative therapy should be considered. The shell production happens in the uterus and the passing of the egg from this point is less than 1 day. Therefore, the time between diagnosing the egg on the radiograph and normal egg deposition should not exceed 24 hours

- If there is no radiopaque egg shell to be seen, but there is a displacement of the ventriculus caudally on a ventrodorsal radiograph and ventrally on a lateral radiograph (Figure 25.5), further investigations such as ultrasonography should be performed (see Figure 25.2)
- Take a blood sample for haematology and blood chemistry with protein electrophoresis (including ionized calcium) if possible (for sample techniques and interpretation, see Chapter 12).
  - Hypocalcaemia is a frequent cause of egg binding. The reason could be secondary to low-calcium diets, high-fat diets, aberrant calcium metabolism (lack of sunlight) and hypomagnesaemia (Grey Parrots). Radiographs of birds with no medullary bone formation support this diagnosis.
  - Elevated uric acid levels could be a sign of impaired kidney function (due to compression of the renal circulation by the egg) and/or dehydration and indicates a higher risk while operating. It is preferable, if the condition of the bird allows, to place an intravenous/intraosseous catheter (see Chapter 15) and give aggressive fluid therapy.
  - Elevated white blood cell count with toxic heterophils would be an indication for a concurrent infection, which will require antimicrobials as well.

Therapy

The choice of therapy is largely indicated by the severity of the clinical signs and the patient's condition. Generally, guidelines include stabilizing the patient, fluid therapy, parenteral calcium and heat, which are often adequate for minimally depressed patients (see 'Clinical approach').

Topical application of prostaglandin

Topical application of prostaglandin E2 or dinoprostone gel has been described. The gel should be applied at the entrance of the reproductive tract to the cloaca, at a dose of 1 ml/kg bodyweight. This procedure should be considered as an option before the 'manual' delivery of the egg. The contractions that are produced are quite strong and the egg should be expelled within 15 minutes. The application of prostaglandin E2 should be performed only if the general condition of the bird is good, the uterus is intact and free of disease and neoplasia, the egg is not adhered to the oviduct and its size is normal relative to the body size of the bird.

The use of prostaglandin F should be avoided at all costs, as it promotes generalized smooth muscle contractions without specifically relaxing the utero-vaginal sphincter.

Some older literature describes the use of oxytocin, but more recent studies show that oxytocin does not have the desired effect and can dangerously compromise the cardiovascular system, and therefore should be avoided.

Manual delivery of the egg

If the bird is still in good clinical condition after first aid therapy but 24 hours have passed and the bird has still not laid the egg, further intervention should be considered. The choice of intervention is mostly dependent on the radiological evaluation of the egg. If there is a visible egg with a normal shell and the bird is still stable, consider helping the bird to 'deliver' the egg manually. For this procedure the author recommends general anaesthetic using isoflurane and butorphanol at 2 mg/kg as analgesia. After the bird has been anaesthetized, the cloaca is lubricated using sterile gel (Intrasite® or KY® jelly) and the vagina is slightly dilated using cotton buds or a small haemostat. Palpate the egg through the coelomic wall and apply a constant gentle digital pressure until the egg is visible (Figure 25.6). Take care not to induce oviduct or cloacal prolapse in the process. If prolapsed tissues are present, cleaning and repair of the significant lacerations should be performed.

In small birds (Budgerigars, finches), it is possible to perform a form of 'episiotomy'. This is done if the egg is lodged in the caudal oviduct, or urodeum, and if its size is big relative to the size of the bird. Often the egg is visible through the cloaca, but it is not possible to deliver it using gentle pressure; episiotomy is the method of choice in order to avoid oviduct or cloacal prolapse under these circumstances. A small incision of the ventral wall of the cloacal sphincter is made to enlarge it and the egg can then be expelled using light pressure. The cloacal sphincter is closed using simple interrupted sutures of 1.5 metric (4/0 USP) monofilament material (Monocryl®, Monosyn®, PDS®).

If the egg shell is thickened (the egg has been in the oviduct for too long) and the egg appears too big for the size of the bird (see Figure 25.4), it is not necessary to wait for 14–24 hours before intervening. If the patient appears calmer and generally more stable 30 minutes after placement in an incubator/oxygen box, general anaesthesia can then be performed before manual delivery of the egg. In this case, the egg is obviously too big to be expelled whole so ovocentesis (aspiration of the egg contents with a large needle) is warranted. After surgical preparation, apply digital pressure as described above until the tip of the egg can be seen through the opening. The safest way to perform ovocentesis is transcloacally.

Following aspiration, the firm egg shell can be collapsed, which is done with slight fingertip pressure. All shell pieces should be removed very gently as the sharp shell pieces can cause uterine damage and any retained fragments pose an infection risk .

Transcoelomic ovocentesis has also been described. This procedure may be used for soft-shelled eggs, because they can pass easily after aspiration. Complications, such as secondary coelomitis due to the leakage of egg contents, should be considered (the author has never performed this method).

Surgical removal via ventral coeliotomy and hysterotomy/hysterectomy

This is the method of choice if the egg is severely adhered to the wall of the oviduct; there is radiographic/ultrasonographic evidence of changes in the egg shell or evidence of a soft-shelled egg (Figure 25.7) or shell-less egg (Figure 25.8); and if the uterus is ruptured or the egg is ectopic. This surgery should only be performed by an experienced avian surgeon (see Chapter 17).

Post-dystocia, longer-term reproductive control is essential to prevent recurrence (see Chapter 4).

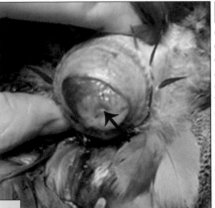

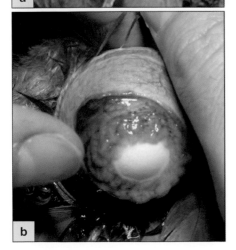

25.6 (a) Lubricating the cloaca and uterine opening (arrowed) and (b) applying gentle pressure at the proximal part of the egg can help to deliver it. (Courtesy of the Clinic for Zoo Animals, Exotic Pets and Wildlife, University of Zurich)

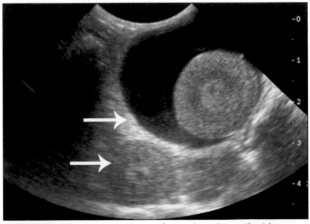

25.7 Ultrasonography performed on the patient in Figure 25.5. There are two eggs (arrowed) visible in the coelom. (Courtesy of the Clinic for Zoo Animals, Exotic Pets and Wildlife, University of Zurich)

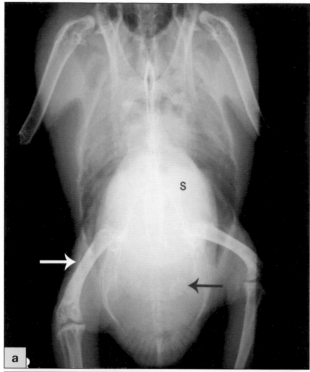

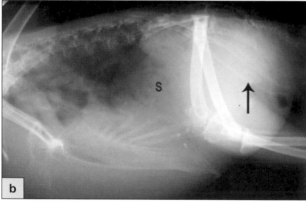

25.8   **(a)** Ventrodorsal view of a bird with a shell-less egg and concurrent salpingitis. The soft tissue structure (S) and a small almond-shaped structure, the shell-less egg (black arrow), are visible. Note the increased radiopacity in both femora (white arrow). **(b)** Plain lateral view of the same bird. The soft tissue structure (S) and the almond-shaped structure, shell-less egg (arrowed), can again be seen. (Courtesy of the Clinic for Zoo Animals, Exotic Pets and Wildlife, University of Zurich)

Complications

Prolapsed tissue

Prolapse of the cloacal tissues (Figure 25.9), vagina, uterus or oviduct can occur as a result of dystocia, normal egg deposition, manual delivery of the egg or further pathophysiological conditions of the gonadal tissues. Predisposing factors include malnutrition, salpingitis, and cloacitis in connection with a soft-shelled or abnormal egg. Differentiation between oviduct and rectal prolapse can be difficult and endoscopy may be needed.

Prolapse of the cloaca often occurs after chronic straining, poor muscle tone or sexual frustration. Any tissue that is prolapsed can devitalize quickly and become a source of infection. Therefore, before any attempt to replace the tissue, take a sample for culture

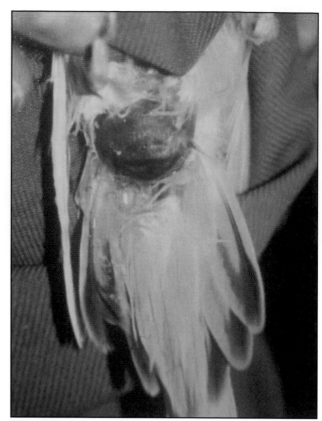

25.9   A 7-year-old Budgerigar with cloacal prolapse. Note the feather loss around the vent and the slight protrusion of the cloaca due to straining.

and sensitivity testing. If the tissue looks swollen, flushing with sterile saline will not be sufficient. A small gauze moistened with a mixture of sterile saline and 50% glucose solution 1:1 applied to the prolapsed tissue will help to decrease the oedema. After this, using gentle pressure and moist cotton buds, the prolapsed tissue is replaced. A single horizontal mattress suture, using 1.5 metric (4/0 USP) synthetic absorbable material, should be placed on both sides of the vent (depending on the bird's size). This will help the tissue to revitalize and to reduce in size, but also leave an opening for the faeces and urine to pass. Recurrence is common. If the cloaca prolapses repeatedly, cloacopexy should be performed.

Birds presented with larger tissue prolapse (oviduct, intestine) are often in shock, and must be stabilized initially (see Chapter 11).

As with intestinal prolapse, when uterine/oviduct prolapse is present there is often intussusception. Pushing the offending organ back through the cloacal opening and placing a suture will not lead to a satisfactory outcome. Surgery with coeliotomy and removal of the intussuscepted material or hysterectomy should be performed once the patient is stabilized.

Egg-related peritonitis

Egg-related peritonitis or egg yolk peritonitis is a term describing the presence of egg yolk in the coelomic cavity outside the salpinx. Egg yolk peritonitis can be septic or non-septic. This condition, if septic, is often fatal and the prognosis is better if the condition is discovered in the early stages. Non-septic egg yolk peritonitis has a better prognosis because the yolk causes a mild histiocytic response and is gradually reabsorbed.

The causes of egg yolk peritonitis include reversed peristaltic or ectopic ovulation, salpingitis, metritis, ruptured oviduct and neoplasia.

Clinical signs include cessation of egg production, depression, anorexia and a history of recent egg laying.

Coelomic swelling is often noted on clinical examination. Acute egg yolk peritonitis often causes a massive increase in the white blood cell count. Radiography (Figure 25.10), ultrasonography (Figure 25.11) and abdominocentesis are helpful diagnostic aids.

The choice of therapy depends on the severity of the clinical signs and laboratory findings. Where infection is present, long-term parenteral antibiotics based on culture and sensitivity results, as well as supportive care, are needed. The coelomic pressure can be reduced using coelomocentesis to relieve breathing. The severity of the pathological process in the coelomic cavity can be assessed later. If there is an excessive amount of yolk or adhesions, surgery with ventral coeliotomy and flushing of the coelomic cavity is indicated.

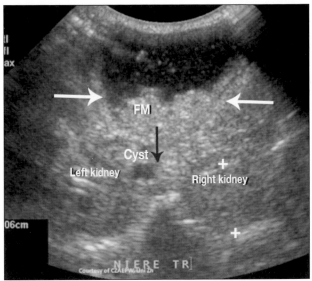

25.11 Ultrasonography performed on the same bird as in Figure 25.10 with suspected egg yolk peritonitis. Note the cystic structure with thin wall and hyperechoic material (FM) floating inside (white arrows). The right kidney is marked with small white callipers and there is a small cystic structure arising from the region of the left kidney (black arrow). (Courtesy of the Clinic for Zoo Animals, Exotic Pets and Wildlife, University of Zurich)

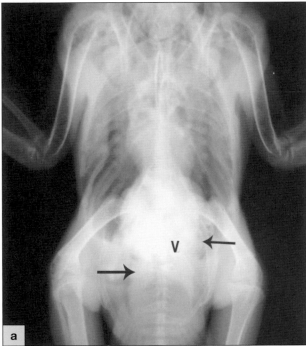

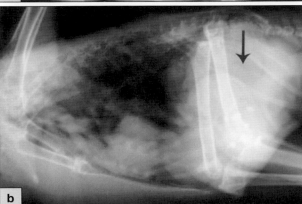

25.10 (a) Ventrodorsal and (b) lateral views of a bird with egg yolk peritonitis. In both, there is a loss of detail in the caudal coleom (arrowed). The kidneys could not be well differentiated and the ventriculus (V) is more caudally and ventrally displaced. Air sacculitis is also a possibility. (Courtesy of the Clinic for Zoo Animals, Exotic Pets and Wildlife, University of Zurich)

Prognosis is dependent on early detection and treatment. Most cases resolve with medical treatment. Only chronic egg-related peritonitis proves difficult to treat and is often a fatal condition in avian species.

Other syndromes associated with egg yolk peritonitis include egg-related pancreatitis, which can lead to temporary diabetes mellitus (often seen in Cockatiels and Budgerigars).

Periodically, a currently reproductively active hen will present with acute-onset neurological signs. These signs can include head tilt, head tremors, intention tremors, a wide-based stance, proprioceptive deficits and difficulty standing. In fatal cases, histopathology will sometimes demonstrate emboli within the blood vessels of the brain. It is assumed that the high circulating levels of fats in a reproductively active hen can lead to a stroke-like event. Often called a 'yolk stroke', it is not usually egg yolk per se that is the cause of the embolism. Blood tests will be consistent with a reproductively active hen. Characteristically, all but the worst affected hens will tend to show a gradual clinical improvement with adequate supportive nursing, although residual deficits are not uncommon. Many clinicians treat these cases with anti-inflammatory drugs. Most hens will recover to a sufficient extent that they are functional within a cage, although they may not be capable of breeding and rearing chicks in the future. It is possible, although unusual, for hens to have a second embolic event, with associated second acute deterioration.

Excessive egg laying

For more information on excessive egg laying, see Chapter 4.

Coelomic hernia

Coelomic hernias are often seen in obese female birds, especially Psittaciformes (cockatoos and Budgerigars).

Hernias are often related to breeding, hormonal disturbances (chronic egg laying) or space-occupying abdominal masses. High-energy diets serve as a driver for egg production and lead to obesity. In birds, it is often not a true hernia (with separation of the aponeurosis of the abdominal muscles at the ventral midline) but a dilatation in the coelomic wall due to general thinning of the muscles. Aetiology is a weakening of the connective tissue due to hyperoestrogenism. Coelomic hernias may also occur in male birds with hormone-producing testicular tumours. It has been suggested that, in birds with chronic egg laying due to alterations in calcium metabolism, the muscles of the abdominal wall become weakened (muscular atony). The muscle distension is often seen in the caudal coelomic region close to the cloaca. Small hernias are of little clinical consequence; where there is distension and not a tear in the muscle wall, there is little risk of organ entrapment. Even with a hernia, birds can continue to pass urates and faeces. Diagnosis is based on the history and clinical examination.

On palpation, the hernia often has a soft consistency and intestines can be felt close to the abdominal wall. Chronic hernias may cause a yellowing of the skin (xanthomatosis) (Figure 25.12).

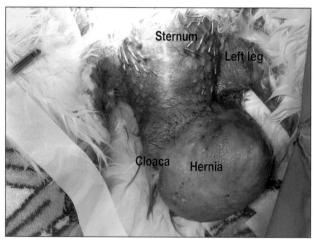

25.12   An 8-year-old Sulphur-crested Cockatoo with coelomic hernia, exhibiting signs of egg laying. The hernia is well visible to the right and close to the cloaca. Note the yellow discoloration of the skin (xanthomatosis).

Radiography is always recommended for determining the course of treatment (Figure 25.13). A contrast radiograph helps to identify organs from the gastrointestinal tract (intestines or/and ventriculus). In female birds with hyperoestrogenism, there is an increased radiopacity in the long bones. In male Budgerigars with hormone-secreting gonadal tumours, a change in the colour of the cere (from blue to brown) can be observed.

The therapy chosen depends on the severity of the hernia and the possible underlying cause (e.g. chronic egg laying). Prior to any consideration of surgery, the quality and quantity of the food given should be considered. Whenever possible, if on a seed diet, the bird should be converted to a more balanced pellet or fresh food diet, exercise must be enforced and weight

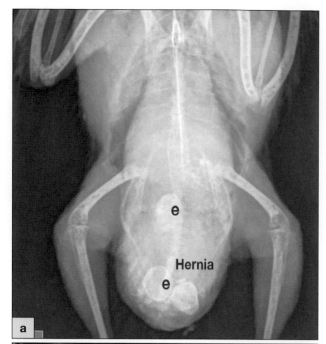

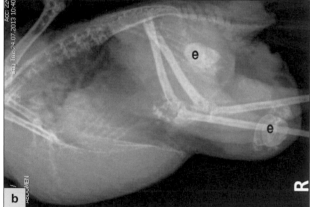

25.13   (a) Ventrodorsal and (b) lateral views of a bird with a hernia. Note the radiopaque structures in the coelom (e); these are old eggs. The bird exhibited signs of egg laying according to the owner but nothing was produced.

reduced slowly. Salpingohysterectomy at the time of hernia repair is also advised. If there is no evidence of egg production (easily seen on ultrasonography), placement of a 4.7 mg deslorelin acetate implant should be considered as an alternative, with advice to the owner about when this should be replaced (which may have species or individual variation).

In avian species it is often not possible to tuck the musculature while repairing the hernia, and sometimes an additional mesh implant is advisable. When chronic large hernias are removed, there is a risk of respiratory compromise due to compression of the abdominal air sacs and blood returned to the heart. If there is already a xanthomatosis of the skin covering the hernia, it should be excised as far as possible. The skin in this region is very fragile and special care should be taken while healing.

Case example 1: Budgerigar with distension of the caudal abdomen

Presentation and history

A 6-year-old female Budgerigar was presented with signs of broodiness and a progressive distension in the caudal abdomen. The change in behaviour had been observed by the owner for 1 week, with the bird mostly on the bottom of the cage, but no eggs had been laid so far. The bird had laid eggs in the past regularly; according to the owner, she laid up to 20 eggs last season and not always in the provided nest box. The owner had always removed the eggs immediately after they had been laid. The bird lived in an aviary with three more Budgerigars, one female and two males. They were fed an all-seed diet *ad libitum*.

Diagnostic work-up

On presentation the bird was perching in the cage and the distended coelom was clearly visible. Physical examination showed a bird of good weight (46 g) with a distended lower abdominal region and a hard structure palpated within the cloaca. There was xanthomatous change of the ventral coelomic region. Radiography confirmed an egg and changes in the bones consistent with polyostotic hyperostosis and hyperoestrogenism. Hernia was also suspected.

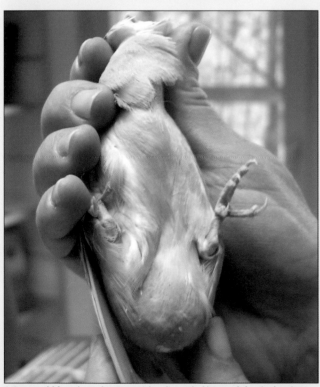

A 6-year-old female Budgerigar with a distended lower abdominal region, and yellow discoloration of the skin (xanthomatosis). Hernia is also suspected.

Therapy

The bird was given 0.5 ml calcium 10% gluconate plus 1 ml glucose/saline solution s.c. and a bolus of 0.5 ml glucose/saline in the right jugular vein. Hens presented with dystocia are often dehydrated and therefore the fluid deficiency should be calculated and added to maintenance fluids of 2–3 ml/kg/h i.v. It was suspected that the bird was hypocalcaemic (due to the history of continuous egg-laying behaviour) but blood tests were not performed.

After the injection, the bird was placed in a small oxygen box where the temperature was maintained at 31°C and humidity at about 55%. No perching was provided and the food was placed on the floor as well. The bird was eating well.

After 30 minutes, with the help of a sterile cotton bud, a small amount (size of a small pea) of dinoprostone gel (prostaglandin E2) was applied directly around the palpable egg (vaginal opening). The egg was not expelled within 60 minutes after the application of the gel, so surgical intervention was necessary.

Butorphanol at 2 mg/kg was given i.m. and the bird was anesthetized with isoflurane. The bird was positioned in dorsal recumbency. After applying gentle pressure to the caudal part of the abdomen, the egg could be visualized in the cloaca.

With a gentle massage and application of sterile KY® gel around the egg, it was expelled with light pressure. A parenteral injection of gonadotropin-releasing hormone (GnRH; depot) and agonist (leuprolide acetate at 100 µg i.m.) was given at the end of the operation.

Outcome

The hernia was resolved surgically. The recovery was uneventful.

Recommendations to the owner for reducing the broody behaviour and continuous egg laying were:

- Reduce the length of daylight experienced (8–10 hours maximum)
- Place the cage in a different environment (e.g. a different room)
- Remove the nest box
- Reduce the amount of food and change to a more balanced diet
- The removed eggs should be replaced with artificial ones
- GnRH implant (4.7 mg deslorelin implant) every 6–8 months or leuprolide acetate every 4 weeks.

The hernia resolved with the removal of the xanthomatous changed skin, 3 months later.

Salpingohysterectomy was advised but not performed (owner's non-compliance).

Cloacal, uterine and rectal prolapse

Angela Lennox and Amber Lee

Anatomy

Cloacal anatomy is discussed in detail in Chapter 2.

Clinical signs

Depending on the length and severity of prolapse and the tissue affected, birds presented can vary from showing no other apparent signs of illness to depressed and moribund. History and physical examination findings may include only the presence of a variably sized prolapse, or may include tenesmus, haematochezia, increased respiratory rate and effort, pelvic limb paresis/paralysis and self-mutilation of the vent area. Female birds with prolapse related to the reproductive tract may have a history of recent oviposition. In some cases, prolapse may be intermittent.

The size of the prolapse can vary widely, from a small swelling to the presence of the entire oviduct or large portions of the lower gastrointestinal (GI) tract. Coelomic palpation may reveal the presence of a mass or fluid. Often the feathers around the vent are soiled with faeces, urates or blood. In birds with secondary cloacitis, Clostridium infections can produce diarrhoea with gas and a fetid odour.

In all cases, a thorough history should be obtained to include information regarding the age, sex, diet and housing conditions, along with reproductive status and activity, to help ascertain the potential underlying cause of a prolapse.

Differential diagnosis

Prolapse may be the result of primary disease of the cloaca itself, or be secondary to disease conditions involving structures that terminate in or are near the cloaca.

Primary diseases of the cloaca contributing to cloacal prolapse

Primary diseases of the cloaca include infectious or inflammatory cloacitis, neoplasia, trauma, haematoma, strictures, adenomatous polyps and, in certain species, disease of the phallus (Figure 26.1). Infectious diseases include bacterial cloacitis (typical bacteria

Primary diseases of the cloaca
■ Infectious disease
– Bacterial, including mycobacteriosis
– Viral (avian bornavirus, herpesvirus-related papillomas)
– Fungal
– Parasitic/protozoal, including *Sarcocystis*
■ Trauma
■ Neoplasia
– Lymphosarcoma
– Squamous cell carcinoma
– Haemangioma
– Fibrosarcoma

Secondary diseases of the cloaca
■ Diseases of the reproductive tract
– Dystocia
– Salpingitis
– Chronic hormone stimulation
– Chronic oviposition
– Neoplasia
■ Diseases of the urinary tract
– Cloacoliths
– Urolithiasis
■ Diseases of the gastrointestinal tract
– Bacterial, fungal and parasitic enteritis
– Intussusception
– Obstruction
– Hypermotility disorders
■ Cloacal atony due to nerve injury
■ Other coelomic masses or space-occupying lesions

26.1 Diseases that may result in prolapse in birds.

and mycobacteriosis), fungal infections, viral infections (herpesvirus) and parasitic infections (including *Sarcocystis* spp.).

New World parrots, in particular Green-winged Macaws, appear to be predisposed to herpesviral-related papilloma (Rosen, 2012). Clinical presentation usually involves one or more fleshy masses that may intermittently prolapse (Figure 26.2). Papillomas occur throughout the entire GI tract and can appear in the oral cavity as well. An association between papillomas and the formation of intestinal, bile duct or pancreatic adenocarcinomas has been discovered, therefore bloodwork and radiographs for the assessment of liver function and hepatomegaly should be performed.

Primary neoplasia of the cloaca has been reported in numerous species, including both parrots and

BSAVA Manual of Avian Practice: A Foundation Manual. Edited by John Chitty and Deborah Monks. ©BSAVA 2018

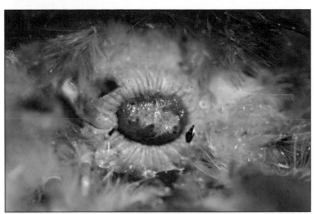

26.2 Cloacal papilloma in a Green-winged Macaw. (Courtesy of B Doneley)

passerines. The most common primary neoplasm is adenocarcinoma followed by lymphosarcoma, squamous cell carcinoma, haemangioma and fibrosarcoma.

In a series of over 500 cases, cloacal biopsy revealed the incidence of cloacitis to be approximately 40%, cloacal papillomas 20% and a variety of other neoplasms comprised approximately 14% (Reavill, unpublished data).

Secondary diseases of the cloaca contributing to cloacal prolapse

Prolapse, as a result of diseases of tissues terminating in the cloaca, is more common than primary disease of the cloaca. In many cases, the physiological cause of the prolapse is excessive straining (see Figure 26.1). Causes of straining include:

- Chronic behavioural maladaptation and inappropriate bird–human bonding (see Chapters 4 and 5)
- Dystocia or other disease of the reproductive tract
- Disease of the lower intestine
- The presence of cloacoliths or ureteroliths
- Cloacal atony due to chronic vent trauma or spinal cord trauma
- The presence of other coelomic masses or space-occupying lesions.

In all cases it is important to perform a full diagnostic work-up to ensure that the underlying cause is identified, and to prevent diagnostic and treatment omissions.

The most common cause of cloacal prolapse, due to secondary underlying disease, is that relating to the reproductive tract in female birds. Any potential primary disease of the reproductive tract might result in prolapse, including infectious/inflammatory disease and neoplasia. Many cases of reproductive-related prolapse are directly associated with oviposition. Malnutrition, obesity and general debilitation from chronic egg laying can contribute. Reproductive-related disease is covered in more detail in Chapter 4.

Cockatoos appear to be overrepresented as a species for developing cloacal prolapse. Intestinal prolapse is usually attributed to diseases that cause tenesmus, including enteritis, intussusception, and other intestinal obstructions or masses. Rectal prolapse, secondary to hypermotility or infection, has been reported in juvenile macaws.

A case of megacloaca in a Moluccan Cockatoo has been reported in the literature (Graham *et al.*, 2004) and the underlying cause appeared to be chronic osteomyelitis of the synsacrum and caudal vertebrae with a likely secondary *Clostridium* spp. cloacitis. The bird was treated surgically by reducing the diameter of the coprodeum and then remained on medical therapy of metronidazole and *Lactobacillus* supplementation to minimize the recurrence of malodorous faeces and faecal retention.

Cloacoliths are firm concretions of urates found within the cloaca. These have been reported in few species of birds and their exact aetiology is unknown. It is suspected that they may be related to previous incidents of egg binding, infectious cloacitis or neurological disease of the cloaca leading to changes in the microflora of the cloaca that alter the solubility of uric acid, allowing it to precipitate out in solid form. Ureteroliths are even less commonly reported in birds and their cause is unknown. In poultry, incidence may be related to vitamin A deficiency, excess dietary calcium, other dietary electrolyte imbalances and infectious bronchitis virus. Other space-occupying intracoelomic masses including tumours, enlarged organs or granulomas also have the propensity to cause cloacal prolapse.

Approach

Initial patient management

At the time of presentation, a careful history is acquired, including age, sex of the bird (if known), history of oviposition and/or reproductive-related behavior, diet including supplementation, along with information on acquisition, exposure to other birds and clinical signs (see Chapter 10).

The patient must be carefully evaluated, and appropriate supportive care delivered even prior to diagnostic work-up and primary treatment. For the patient that is bright, alert and responsive (often with a smaller prolapse), initial therapy may include warmth, fluids and gentle cleansing and lubrication of the prolapse with sterile lubricant to prevent further damage and desiccation. However, some patients present moribund or in shock due to septicaemia, blood loss, other underlying disease conditions, or (in cases of a formed egg or space-occupying mass) compression of the caudal coelomic nerves and vasculature. These patients require emergency management and shock therapy (see Chapter 11).

Diagnostic work-up

Ideal initial diagnostic work-up includes a complete blood count (CBC), biochemistry panel and radiographs in two views. In each case, clinical judgment must be used to determine the patient's ability to undergo diagnostic testing. The authors have found low-dose sedation (midazolam at 0.5–1 mg/kg and butorphanol at 1–3 mg/kg) extremely useful to reduce anxiety and discomfort, and allow diagnostic testing that might be dangerous with manual restraint and struggling, or with general anaesthesia.

CBC and biochemistry values give information on the overall condition of the bird, and the presence of other complicating factors such as anaemia, systemic infection and renal failure. Radiographs may give information on the cause of the prolapse itself. Significant radiographic findings include the presence of a shelled egg, fluid or other masses, or changes suggesting hormonal stimulation, including hyperostosis of bones (see Chapter 18) (Figure 26.3). Contrast radiography is extremely useful for suspected disease of the GI tract, or to provide information on other masses or abnormalities that may affect the position of the GI tract. Cloacal contrast studies can be useful, as retroperistalsis allows the flow of contrast into the colon, which may outline masses within the cloacal lumen.

Ultrasonography is a quick, non-invasive method to evaluate a large prolapse or the coelomic cavity. Ultrasonography has been shown to be superior to radiography for detection of eggs or egg product without mineralized shell. Ultrasonography can also aid in the diagnosis of salpingitis and differentiate between oviductal masses and other caudal coelomic masses. The size of some birds may make ultrasonography more difficult.

Examination of the cloaca itself is often helpful, especially for diagnosis of primary cloacal disease. In medium- to large-sized birds, portions of the mucosa of the vent and proctodeum may be viewed by gently everting the vent with a lubricated cotton-tipped applicator. Indirect visualization may be attempted with an otoscope and sterile cone, but gives only a partial view of the cloaca. Cloacoscopy is ideal, and provides maximal visualization and flexibility. Most descriptions of cloacoscopy recommend use of a 2.7 or 1.9 mm rigid endoscope equipped with a diagnostic sheath for gentle insufflation of warm sterile fluid to expand the vent and enhance visualization (Figure 26.4). The diagnostic sheath also allows introduction

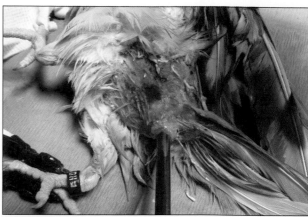

26.4   Use of a rigid endoscope with diagnostic sheath and fluid insufflation for cloacoscopy to visualize the cloaca.

of biopsy forceps or other instruments for collection of diagnostic samples. The endoscope is passed through the vent while the operator holds the lips of the vent around the sheath of the endoscope, creating a seal, and then saline is infused to dilate the cloaca and allow a view of all three chambers. The entire surface of each chamber should be examined. Care must be taken when collecting mucosal biopsy samples to sample only a superficial piece of tissue without going full thickness and thus avoid perforation of the cloaca.

Other diagnostic testing includes biopsy and histopathology of masses or other abnormal-appearing tissue, and culture and sensitivity testing. There are specific pathogen tests available for avian bornavirus and avian herpesvirus (see Chapter 19).

Treatment of cloacal prolapse – general approach

Treatment is based upon the following goals:

1. Initial protection of the prolapsed tissue from further damage and desiccation.
2. Supportive care of the patient, which may include shock therapy, general fluid support, antibiotics, analgesia and nutritional supplementation.
3. Resolution of the prolapse based upon identification and treatment of the cause.

Initial protection of the prolapsed tissue

Initial treatment includes gentle cleansing, irrigation and lubrication. If the prolapse is small and no egg or mass is palpable, it may be gently replaced into the cloaca with or without the placement of stay sutures for further protection pending diagnostic work-up and definitive therapy. A small prolapse can be gently replaced with a lubricated cotton-tipped applicator. With the applicator in place, two lateral horizontal mattress sutures are placed on either side of the vent. The resultant opening must be small enough to prevent re-prolapse, but large enough to allow withdrawal of the cotton-tipped applicator (see Case Example 1) and normal passage of faeces. Careful monitoring will determine if adjustments in suture placement need to be made. Very large prolapses, or those with necrotic or devitalized tissue, should not be managed with simple replacement. In these cases consider referral to an avian specialist.

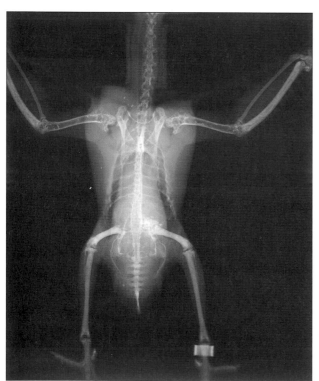

26.3   Ventrodorsal view of a female Cockatiel with chronic oviposition that ultimately resulted in a prolapse. Note the hyperostosis of the ulnas, femurs and tibiotarsi consistent with chronic hormone stimulation. Widening of the hepatic/proventricular silhouette may suggest organ enlargement, which could include the reproductive tract.

Supportive care

Supportive care of the critical patient is described in Chapter 11. In addition to warmth, fluids and nutritional support, some patients with primary or secondary infectious diseases benefit from antibiotic therapy. Prolapse likely produces discomfort. Analgesic choices include topical lidocaine (2–3 mg/kg) or bupivacaine (1–2 mg/kg), butorphanol (1–3 mg/kg), fentanyl (0.2 mg/kg s.c.), and, in the well hydrated patient without evidence of renal dysfunction, meloxicam (0.5–1 mg/kg). Some conditions may be a result of a nutritional disorder, including deficiencies of calcium. Specific nutrient supplementation may be beneficial.

Resolution of the prolapse

Even in cases of small prolapses that are easily replaced, all attempts should be made to determine the cause and provide definitive treatment. It is rare for simple replacement alone as a sole therapeutic modality to provide permanent resolution. The authors have treated numerous referral cases of prolapse that were addressed with replacement alone and resulted in serious or life-threatening complications weeks to months later. More common causes of prolapse and suggested therapies are listed below.

Treatment of cloacal prolapse – specific approaches

Dystocia

Chapter 4 includes a discussion of dystocia management (see also Chapter 25). Eggs contained within a larger prolapse can be carefully manipulated out of the oviduct after flushing and lubrication of the tissue. The egg should 'crown' through the oviductal orifice of the urodeum and/or through the uroproctodeal fold. If the egg is inadvertently delivered through the wall of the oviduct or cloaca, the defect should be repaired. After removal, small prolapses of pink, normal-appearing tissue may heal with replacement and placement of stay sutures (see Case example 1). However, replacement of necrotic or devitalized prolapsed tissue is not recommended, and is associated with a high incidence of disease and death due to coelomitis and septicaemia. In these cases, coelomic surgery and salpingectomy are highly recommended. Coelomic surgery is challenging, but techniques are well described.

Birds presenting for reproductive-related prolapse, are likely to prolapse again if oviposition resumes. Therefore, all attempts must be made to decrease hormone stimulation and discourage reproductive behaviour. Both husbandry changes and specific medications may be useful. Husbandry changes are designed to reduce environmental stimuli, and may include decreasing photoperiod, removing nesting material and reducing the actions or presence of other birds, humans and/or objects perceived as a mate. A careful examination of the bird–owner bond may reveal interactive behaviours contributing to hormonal stimulation (see Chapter 5).

A number of pharmacological agents have been used to alter reproductive status in birds. Drugs currently used and recommended are long-acting gonadotropin-releasing hormone (GnRH) analogues. These include leuprolide acetate and deslorelin acetate, which initially stimulate the release of luteinizing hormone (LH) and follicle-stimulating hormone (FSH) from the anterior pituitary gland and then down-regulate GnRH receptors in cells, which produce these hormones via negative feedback mechanisms. While there is a great deal of work to be done on the effects of these drugs in individual bird species for specific indications, leuprolide injections have been reported to decrease hormone concentrations for approximately 2 weeks. In quail, deslorelin was reported to have an effect as early as 2 weeks post-implantation and appeared to have individual variable efficacy for up to 70 days.

Chronic hormone stimulation

Vent prolapse may be a result of chronic hormonal stimulation and masturbation; however, all other causes of prolapse must be identified or ruled out first. Treatment is similar to that described above to decrease oviposition with the inclusion of behavioural modification (see Chapter 5) or hormonal therapies. In some chronic cases, the cloacal wall and sphincter are damaged and flaccid, resulting in leakage of droppings, foul odour and repeated cloacal prolapse. These birds may benefit from reconstructive surgeries, including cloacopexy and ventplasty, which are described below. If the underlying reproductive problems are not addressed with behavioural and environmental changes then the straining may continue and lead to failure of the surgery.

Cloacitis

Treatment is aimed at identifying the underlying cause, if possible. Empirical antimicrobial treatment may be beneficial pending results of culture and sensitivity testing or biopsy.

Papillomatosis

Herpesvirus has been associated with the formation of papilloma-like lesions throughout the GI tract and has been linked to the formation of bile duct carcinoma. The diagnosis of papillomas can be confirmed with cloacal biopsy; alternatively, acetic acid may be applied to the mucosa and if blanching of the tissue occurs then papillomatosis can be suspected. Numerous treatments have been advocated, including debulking using cryotherapy, electrocautery or chemical cautery, or an attempt at complete removal with dissection or 'cloacal stripping' techniques. All aggressive treatments of cloacal mucosa incur risk of stricture formation. Surgical approaches for the removal of papillomas have included both vent eversion and a ventral midline cloacotomy. It should be noted that papillomas have been found to regress as well as recur spontaneously after surgical resection. For this reason some practitioners recommend no treatment unless there are clinical signs of prolapse, pain and/or haematochezia.

Cloacoliths and ureteroliths

Diagnosis of cloacoliths may occur from palpation on physical examination or be confirmed radiographically. Cloacoliths can often can be removed endoscopically, fragmented into pieces and flushed away. Patients require continued monitoring with survey radiographs every 6–12 months as cloacoliths can recur. Although uncommon in veterinary medicine, a case of ureterolithiasis in an Amazon parrot has been reported in the literature (Dennis and Bennett, 2000). Excretory ureterography confirmed the location of the stones within the ureters, and surgery was performed for removal but the technique was difficult, with multiple surgeries and different surgical approaches required.

Neoplasia

The diagnosis of neoplasia may be suspected from physical examination, radiographs or diagnostic endoscopy; however, biopsy of affected tissue is required for definitive diagnosis. Both primary neoplasia of the cloaca and primary coelomic tumours can lead to prolapse. Treatment of cancer depends on the location and type of neoplasia, which necessitates biopsy and histopathology for diagnosis. For primary intestinal or cloacal neoplasms such as adenocarcinoma, adenomas and sarcomas, complete surgical excision is the gold standard of treatment. Adjunct therapies, including chemotherapy and radiotherapy, may be considered for full resolution.

For coelomic tumours involving the GI or reproductive tract, information from radiographs and ultrasonography may be suggestive, but endoscopic or surgical biopsy is required for definitive diagnosis. Lymphoma, adenocarcinoma, leiomyosarcoma, leiomyomas, adenomas and granulosa cell tumours have been reported. In cases of uterine adenocarcinoma, surgical hysterectomy is indicated. Ovarian carcinomas are more difficult to treat, as complete ovariohysterectomy is challenging. Anecdotally, these may respond to partial ovariectomy and chemotherapy (carboplatin); two cases of ovarian adenocarcinoma in Cockatiels were managed medically with deslorelin implants.

Intestinal diseases

In cases where enteritis results in intestinal prolapse, culture and sensitivity testing and faecal examinations should be performed to reveal the infectious aetiology. After replacement of the affected tissues, antimicrobials, antifungals or antiparasitics should be instituted as indicated. If any of the prolapsed tissue has sustained sufficient trauma that it becomes devitalized, intestinal resection and anastomosis is indicated. Intussusception is also treated surgically.

Selected surgical procedures

Anaesthesia and surgery in the avian patient require experience and familiarity with anatomy. Some cases may benefit from referral to an avian specialist.

Cloacotomy

When the internal mucosa of the cloaca cannot be fully visualized externally through the vent, incision through the coelom and into the cloaca is an alternative. This allows direct visualization of the cloacal lumen and then subsequent removal or biopsy of masses or abnormal tissue. The patient is anaesthetized and placed in dorsal recumbency, then the caudal coelom is prepared and an incision is made over the cloaca. It is often helpful to place a cotton-tipped applicator into the cloaca from the vent to aid identification. The shape and size of the incision depends on the size of the patient and the amount of exposure required. Subcutaneous tissues are dissected, the fat layer reflected, and the abdominal muscle wall incised. The cloacal serosa is incised full thickness, with care to avoid the ureters and reproductive tract openings.

From here, biopsy samples can be collected or papillomas and other masses resected. Tissue handling must be gentle, as often the cloacal mucosa is inflamed or infected. Closure of the cloacal wall is then performed with either interrupted or continuous inverting pattern sutures with absorbable suture material. The body wall and skin are closed routinely. Cloacopexy or ventplasty may be performed at the same time.

Cloacopexy

Cloacopexy surgery involves creating a permanent adhesion between the cloaca and the body wall with the aim of preventing further prolapse. A cotton-tipped applicator is placed inside the cloaca to ensure its position within the coelom, then a horizontal incision is made over the most anterior portion of the cloaca through the skin, being careful not to incise the thin cloacal wall. The fat pad present on the ventral aspect of the cloaca is reflected or removed. In more severe recurrent cases, two sutures are placed, one around the eighth rib on each side, and then each is passed through the cloacal wall full thickness. Each suture is tightened so that the cloacal wall is opposed to the rib. Another description of the procedure utilizes the ventral body wall as a secondary place of attachment for the cloaca (Forbes, 2002). Colonic entrapment within the cloacopexy site, adhesion formation and obstructions have been reported as potential postsurgical complications.

Colopexy

Colopexy in birds is challenging, and may benefit from referral to an avian specialist. This technique was reported in a male cockatoo that was suffering from chronic, recurrent colocloacal prolapse of presumed sexual aetiology.

Ventplasty

For more information about ventplasty, see Chapter 17.

References and further reading

Antinoff N, Hoefer HL and Rosenthal KL (1997) Smooth muscle neoplasia of suspected oviductal origin in the cloaca of a Blue-fronted Amazon Parrot (*Amazona aestiva*). *Journal of Avian Medicine and Surgery* **11(4)**, 268–272

Beaufrère H, Nevarez J and Tully Jr TN (2002) Cloacolith in a Blue-fronted Amazon Parrot (*Amazona aestiva*). *Journal of Avian Medicine and Surgery* **24**, 142–145

Bowles HL (2002) Reproductive diseases of pet bird species. *Veterinary Clinics of North America: Exotic Animal Practice* **5**, 489–506

Bowles H, Lichtenberger M and Lennox A (2007) Emergency and critical care of pet birds. *Veterinary Clinics of North America: Exotic Animal Practice* **10**, 345–394

Christen C and Hatt JM (2006) What is your diagnosis? *Journal of Avian Medicine and Surgery* **20**, 129–131

Crosta L, Gerlach H, Burkle M *et al.* (2003) Physiology, diagnosis, and diseases of the avian reproductive tract. *Veterinary Clinics of North America: Exotic Animal Practice* **6**, 57–83

Dennis PM and Bennett RA (2000) Ureterotomy for removal of two ureteroliths in a parrot. *Journal of the American Veterinary Medical Association* **217(6)**, 865–686

Detweiler DA, Carpenter JW, Kraft SL *et al.* (2000) Radiographic diagnosis: avian cloacal adenocarcinoma. *Veterinary Radiology and Ultrasound* **41(6)**, 539–541

Divers SJ (2010a) Avian diagnostic endoscopy. *Veterinary Clinics of North America: Exotic Animal Practice* **13(2)**, 187–202

Divers SJ (2010b) Avian endosurgery. *Veterinary Clinics of North America: Exotic Animal Practice* **13(2)**, 203–216

Echols MA (2002) Surgery of the avian reproductive tract. *Seminars in Avian and Exotic Pet Medicine* **11(4)**, 177–195

Forbes NA (2002) Avian gastrointestinal surgery. *Seminars in Avian and Exotic Pet Medicine* **11(4)**, 196–207

Graham JE, Tell LA, Lamm MG *et al.* (2004) Megacloaca in a Moluccan Cockatoo (*Cacatua moluccensis*). *Journal of Avian Medicine and Surgery* **18**, 41–49

Hadley TL (2005) Disorders of the psittacine gastrointestinal tract. *Veterinary Clinics of North America: Exotic Animal Practice* **8**, 329–349

Hadley TL (2010) Management of common psittacine reproductive disorders in clinical practice. *Veterinary Clinics of North America: Exotic Animal Practice* **13**, 429–438

Hillyer EV, Moroff S, Hoefer H *et al.* (1991) Bile duct carcinoma in two out of ten Amazon parrots with cloacal papillomas. *Journal of the Association of Avian Veterinarians* **5(2)**, 91–95

Johne R, Konrath A, Krautwald-Junghanns ME *et al.* (2002) Herpesviral, but no papovaviral sequences, are detected in cloacal papillomas of parrots. *Archives of Virology* **147**, 1869–1880

Keller KA, Beaufrère H, Brandão J *et al.* (2013) Long-term management of ovarian neoplasia in two Cockatiels (*Nymphicus hollandicus*). *Journal of Avian Medicine and Surgery* **27**, 44–52

King AS and McLelland J (1984) Cloaca and vent. In: *Birds: Their Structure and Function, 2nd edn*, pp. 187–199. Baillière Tindall, Bath

Morrisey JK (1999) Gastrointestinal diseases of psittacine birds. *Seminars in Avian and Exotic Pet Medicine* **8**, 66–74

Petritz OA, Sanchez-Migallon Guzman D, Paul-Murphy J *et al.* (2013) Evaluation of the efficacy and safety of single administration of 4.7 mg deslorelin acetate implants on egg production and plasma sex hormones in Japanese quail (*Coturnix coturnix japonica*). *American Journal of Veterinary Research* **74(2)**, 316–323

Pollock CG and Orosz SE (2002) Avian reproductive anatomy, physiology and endocrinology. *Veterinary Clinics of North America: Exotic Animal Practice* **5**, 441–474

Popovitch CA, Holt D and Bright R (1994) Colopexy as a treatment for rectal prolapse in dogs and cats: a retrospective study of 14 cases. *Veterinary Surgery* **23**, 115–118

Radlinsky MG, Carpenter JW, Mison MB *et al.* (2004) Colonic entrapment after cloacopexy in two psittacine birds. *Journal of Avian Medicine and Surgery* **18**, 175–182

Romagnano A (1996) Avian obstetrics. *Seminars in Avian and Exotic Pet Medicine* **5(4)**, 180–188

Rosen LB (2012) Topics in medicine and surgery: avian reproductive disorders. *Journal of Exotic Pet Medicine* **21**, 124–131

Schmidt RE (1999) Pathology of gastrointestinal diseases of psittacine birds. *Seminars in Avian and Exotic Pet Medicine* **8(2)**, 75–82

Styles DK, Tomaszewski EK, Jaeger LA *et al.* (2004) Psittacid herpesviruses associated with mucosal papillomas in neotropical parrots. *Virology* **325**, 24–35

Taylor M and Murray MJ (1999) Endoscopic examination and therapy of the avian gastrointestinal tract. *Seminars in Avian and Exotic Pet Medicine* **8(3)**, 110–114

van Zeeland YRA, Schoemaker NJ and van Sluijs FJ (2009) Novel surgical technique for treating colocloacal prolapse in a cockatoo. *Association of Avian Veterinarians Annual Conference Proceedings* 347–348

Wakenell PS (1996) Obstetrics and reproduction of backyard poultry. *Seminars in Avian and Exotic Pet Medicine* **5(4)**, 199–204

Case example 1: Female Cockatiel with cloacal prolapse

Presentation and history

An 8-year-old female Cockatiel presented for decreased activity and appetite over the previous few days, and the presence of pink tissue prolapsing from the vent. The bird had laid 10 eggs over the last 2 weeks; the last egg was laid 1 hour before presentation.

On physical examination the bird was bright and alert, and able to pass faeces. The coelomic space (between keel and pelvis) was widened, and there was a 1 cm pink mass protruding from the cloaca. There were no other significant clinical findings.

Diagnostic work-up

Considering the history of recent oviposition, the identity of the prolapsed tissue was likely cloaca, or part of the salpinx. As the bird was stable, diagnostic work-up commenced, and the tissue was covered with sterile lubricant.

Radiographs demonstrated polyostotic hyperostosis of the ulnas, femurs and tibiotarsi (see Figure 26.3), consistent with hormone stimulation, and widening of the hepatic/proventricular silhouette, which supports organ enlargement or the presence of a mass. There was no evidence of mineralized egg product

within the coelom, and a complete blood count and chemistry panel were unremarkable.

Therapy

The bird was sedated with midazolam and butorphanol, with supplemental oxygen provided via facemask, and the prolapse was gently flushed and replaced with a cotton-tipped applicator. With the cotton-tipped applicator in place, two horizontal mattress sutures were placed at both lateral aspects of the vent, allowing enough room to retract the applicator.

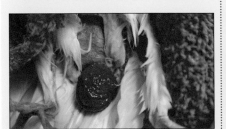

The history, plus the irregular appearance of this prolapse, suggested the identity of the prolapse was the uterus. Due to the acute presentation, the tissue was still pink and healthy in appearance.

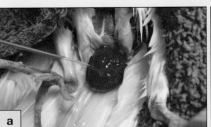

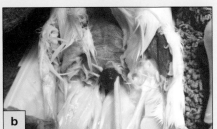

(a) The prolapse was gently irrigated and lubricated with sterile lubricant. (b) The prolapse was gently replaced with a lubricated cotton-tipped applicator.

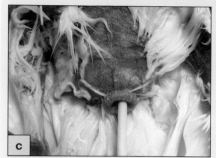

(c) Replacement was uncomplicated.

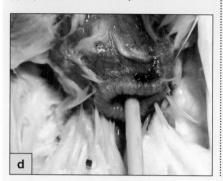

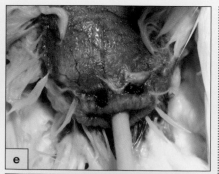

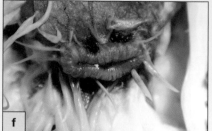

(d–f) With the cotton-tipped applicator in place, two horizontal mattress sutures were placed at both lateral aspects of the vent, leaving enough room to retract the applicator.

Outcome

As the history included the passage of 10 eggs over the last 2 weeks, a tentative diagnosis of chronic hormone stimulation and oviposition was made; however, the presence of reproductive pathology could not be ruled out. The owners were given written instructions on how to reduce hormonal stimulation, and the bird was administered leuprolide acetate every 2 weeks for three treatments. As recurrence is common, the owners were cautioned to monitor carefully for signs of returning reproductive behaviour.

Case example 2: Amazon parrot with papillomatosis

Presentation and history

A 25-year-old male Double Yellow-headed Amazon Parrot presented for straining during the passage of faeces for a few weeks' duration. The previous day, the owner noticed small spots of fresh blood on the newspaper at the bottom of the cage. There was no history of previous medical problems, and the bird was otherwise bright and alert, and eating and drinking normally.

On physical examination the bird was overweight based on pectoral muscle mass; otherwise there were no other significant findings. Upon gentle eversion of the cloacal mucosa with a lubricated cotton-tipped applicator, there was a slight 'cobblestone' appearance with small raised areas over the mucosal surface (see Figure 26.2).

Diagnostic work-up

Given the species predisposition, papillomatosis was considered the most likely cause for the straining, frank blood in the faeces and lesions seen on cloacal examination. Important differentials to consider included cloacitis, cloacoliths, trauma or primary neoplasia of the cloaca.

A complete blood count and chemistry panel were unremarkable, except for a mild leucocytosis. Radiographs did not reveal any space-occupying masses; however, the hepatic silhouette seemed slightly widened. Since the bird was otherwise stable, he was premedicated, then anaesthetized to obtain a cloacal mucosal biopsy sample. The results of the cloacal biopsy confirmed cloacal papillomatosis. The owner declined additional work-up beyond cloacal biopsy.

Therapy

As the papillomas were causing discomfort, the bird underwent cryosurgery to reduce the size of them. After the procedure, the bird was sent home with meloxicam to reduce pain and inflammation. At recheck, one week later, lesions were improved and the bird was no longer straining.

Outcome

After 2 years the bird presented with weight loss, inappetence and lethargy. The bird had a distended coelomic space, and radiographs confirmed marked hepatomegaly and ascites. A complete blood count revealed an elevated white blood cell count with heterophilia, and elevated aspartate aminotransferase (AST), creatine kinase (CK) and bile acids. He was treated in hospital with supportive care and antibiotics but died 2 days later. On post-mortem examination, he was found to have cloacal papillomas, bile duct carcinoma and pancreatic ductal carcinoma.

Case example 3: Umbrella Cockatoo with flaccid vent

Presentation and history

A 10-year-old male Umbrella Cockatoo presented for a wellness examination. There were no reported concerns; however, upon questioning, the owner reported the bird had become selectively bonded to the female owner, from whom he continually solicited attention and petting, and aggressive towards the owner's husband, other family members and visitors. He was also noted to rub his vent against his favourite toy.

On physical examination the bird was bright and alert, and there were no significant findings with the exception of a slightly flaccid-appearing vent with normal-appearing cloacal mucosa readily visualized through the lips of the vent.

Diagnostic work-up

History and physical examination findings suggested the most likely differential diagnosis to be inappropriate bird–human bonding and chronic hormonal stimulation with resultant reduced vent–cloacal tone, likely a result of constant straining during masturbation. Other important processes to consider included diseases of the reproductive tract (infectious, neoplastic), urinary tract (cloacoliths), GI tract problems (infectious enteritis, intussusception, obstruction), cloacal atony due to spinal nerve trauma, or other coelomic masses or space-occupying lesions.

Diagnostic testing was thorough and included complete blood count, radiographs and coelomic endoscopy. On radiographs there were no significant findings except for increased soft tissue opacity in the area consistent with the gonad. The bird underwent diagnostic endoscopy, revealing that the testes were enlarged and smooth in appearance. A biopsy specimen of testicular tissue was obtained, which revealed active but normal testicular tissue. As cloacal tissue was not truly prolapsed, and the vent was only slightly flaccid, no surgical therapy was proposed at that time.

Therapy

The owners of the bird went through behavioural counselling to decrease inadvertent hormone stimulation and encourage more social 'flock' behaviours. This included recommendations to reduce petting and intimate contact, handle the bird for transfers only (from cages to play-stands) and allow the bird on the hand only, not the shoulder. All desired behaviours were reinforced using a favourite treat as positive reinforcement. Recommendations also included removal of the favourite toy from the cage, establishment of night and day cages, decreasing light cycles, and teaching the bird to spend time foraging for food. GnRH agonist therapy was discussed as a potential option if behavioural modification alone was not effective.

Outcome

The owners were receptive to the changes and vigilantly practised their behavioural 'homework'. Over time, the bird became receptive to the husband and most newcomers to the household, and the vent and cloaca were no longer abnormal in appearance. The owners subsequently noted an increase in hormonal behaviour each spring, and elected to treat the bird with leuprolide acetate each March/April.

Vomiting and regurgitating bird

Thomas N. Tully, Jr

The gastrointestinal (GI) tract is commonly involved in many avian diseases, and vomiting and/or regurgitation (Figure 27.1) is a common presentation. For the veterinary surgeon (veterinarian), it is very important to know the difference between regurgitation and vomiting. By clearly defining and properly assessing all the clinical disease signs of an ill avian patient, the practitioner will be closer to determining a valid differential diagnosis list.

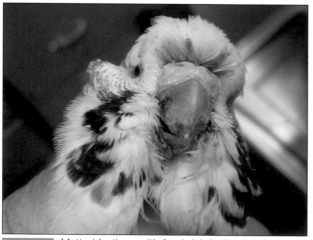

27.1 Matted feathers with food debris that has been regurgitated or vomited by a Budgerigar.

Vomiting is defined as the ejection of all or part of the stomach contents through the mouth; **regurgitation** is to return partially digested food from the mouth. Although the definitions sound very similar, vomiting is often a more violent act of involuntary spasms resulting in the ejection of food from the stomach through the mouth, while regurgitation is usually more passive and, in birds, food is usually expelled from the crop during and after the action of head bobbing. To understand abnormal disease conditions it is essential that one knows the normal anatomy of the GI tract involved in regurgitation and vomiting.

The avian beak is the opening into the oral cavity. The beak is used to bring food into the mouth and, in some species (e.g. parrots), may actually prepare the item for digestion by mechanically breaking it into smaller pieces. There are salivary glands in the oral cavity of many avian species, but digestion is not initiated in this area as the glands primarily secrete mucus. Food is swallowed into the cervical oesophagus and, as the food bolus moves caudally in the oral cavity, the choanal opening is reflexively closed by muscular action to prevent aspiration into the infraorbital sinus through the choana. When drinking, most birds accumulate the fluid on the ventral aspect of the oral cavity, after which the bird raises its head and allows the water to go down the oesophagus primarily through gravitational flow. The ingluvies, or crop, is at the terminus of the cervical oesophagus and is anatomically located at the thoracic inlet of most avian species. It is very important for veterinary surgeons to know where the crop is located for external physical assessment and surgical procedures. The crop can be used as a storage organ for food if the ventriculus is full. The inability of a bird to move food through the crop in a timely manner can be the result of a disease process or can cause disease. When the body is ready to digest the food in the crop, it moves through the thoracic oesophagus into the proventriculus, or true stomach.

The proventriculus lies in the left dorsoventral area of the coelomic cavity of most bird species. The ventriculus is composed of four semi-autonomous masses that work in union to mechanically break down ingested food material. Gastric proteolysis occurs primarily in the ventriculus; the formation of casts in raptor species also occurs in the ventriculus. The expulsion of casts from the oral cavity of birds demonstrates the ease and normal function of material being moved from the more caudal locations of the stomach into the oesophagus and finally out of the mouth. Normal retrograde movement of material from the stomach and crop includes the expulsion of casts (e.g. in raptors) and feeding of young (e.g. in parrots, pigeons).

Examination

As with any patient that presents with clinical disease signs, the vomiting/regurgitating patient requires a thorough external physical examination. The essential first step in determining a definitive diagnosis is obtaining a thorough history of the bird's health condition from the owner. As important is gathering information

BSAVA Manual of Avian Practice: A Foundation Manual. Edited by John Chitty and Deborah Monks. ©BSAVA 2018

on the environment where the bird lives, its enclosure and diet. It is important to remember that asking the right questions and being specific during history-taking will gain more useable details toward developing an accurate differential diagnosis list. An example of asking the proper question is not just asking what the bird is *fed*, but extending the question to what the bird actually *eats*.

Important questions to ask clients presenting a regurgitating or vomiting bird

- When did the owner first notice the animal regurgitating/vomiting? (Approximation of chronicity should be given)
- Are there any apparent predisposing factors associated with the condition?
- What does the regurgitated material look like?
- For how long does the bird regurgitate or vomit?
- Has the owner ever noticed this problem with other birds in the cage, if there are any?
- Have any new birds recently been introduced into the house?
- Has the patient ever been noted to regurgitate/vomit in the past? If so, what were the associated conditions? What was done when the bird previously exhibited this behaviour?
- Does the regurgitated material smell?
- What is the bird's behaviour after the regurgitating/vomiting event?
- What is the bird's appetite? (If this can be determined)
- Have there been any new toys, perches or furniture added to the cage?
- Has the bird chewed/torn up any toy, perch or anything else in the house?
- Has the cage been painted or is it new?
- How long has the bird been living in the cage?
- What is the bird fed? Treats? Favourite foods?
- What does the bird normally eat on a daily basis?
- Where does the drinking water come from? What type of container is the drinking water placed in for the bird to access?

Important initial criteria to evaluate when examining a regurgitating or vomiting bird

- Check feathers around the beak and eyes for matting of regurgitated material due to head shaking after the event
- Check the choanal slit for inflammation, eroded lateral papillae and oedema, which may denote chronicity of the problem
- Feel for the crop at the thoracic inlet. Is it full? Can a foreign body be palpated?
- Feel the pectoral muscles to determine body condition
- Visually examine the faeces; is it normal based on the owner's and/or veterinary surgeon's evaluation?
- Weigh the bird
- Evaluate the bird's attitude. Is it bright, alert or depressed?

After obtaining the full history of the patient, a physical examination should be performed. It is important to weigh the bird and ascertain the general body condition of the patient to determine how much blood can be safely collected for diagnostic testing. The general rule of thumb for collecting blood from a healthy avian patient is 1 ml per 100 g bodyweight. It is reasonable to assume that birds in poor body condition or significantly affected by illness will not withstand having the maximum amount of blood removed. Once blood has been collected for diagnostic testing, the samples can be prepared for submission, and the patient examined.

Unless there is a life-threatening condition upon presentation, the bird should receive a thorough examination from beak to tail. At any point during the examination a finding may be linked to the presenting complaint, in this case vomiting/regurgitation. Especially for upper GI disease, the external physical examination will focus on the oral cavity, palpation of the oesophagus and crop, and determining the body condition of the patient.

The oesophagus can be visualized when collecting blood from the right jugular vein. Food may be detected in the oesophagus during the physical examination through palpation. When palpating the crop, it should be determined whether the bird has been eating or, if hand-fed, if the formula is not passing through in a normal manner. Food in the crop can be an indication of crop stasis (or that the bird has recently been fed).

Feeling the pectoral muscles on flighted birds is the best way to determine body condition. The pectoral musculature comprises approximately 20% of a flighted bird's bodyweight. The amount of muscle mass is directly correlated to the patient's body condition: the less muscle mass and more prominent the keel bone, the poorer the body condition. One can safely assume that if the patient is in poor body condition then the disease process is more chronic than acute. Body condition scores range from 1 to 5, with 1 being thin and 5 obese. A score of 3 is considered a perfect body condition score (see also Chapter 10).

Other tests that may aid in diagnosing the underlying disease condition are bacterial culture (oral cavity, crop), crop cytological examination, radiography, contrast radiography, fluoroscopy and endoscopy. The initial selection of diagnostic tests is dependent on the history, clinical disease signs, patient's condition and physical examination findings; the results allow determination of an initial differential diagnosis list. The top differential diagnoses can guide the selection of specific diagnostic tests for confirmation and development of an initial treatment plan (Figure 27.2) (Mayer, 2013).

Once the bird is stabilized and gains strength, secondary diagnostic testing can be performed (e.g.

Extra-gastrointestinal conditions	Primary gastrointestinal conditions
- Behavioural - Stress, motion sickness, recovery from inhalant anesthesia - Intoxication - Obstruction - Systemic disease	- Viral disease - Bacterial disease - Fungal disease - Parasitism - Obstruction - Irritation - Reaction to ingested food/plants

27.2 Important differential diagnoses for regurgitating/vomiting avian patients.

radiography, fluoroscopy and endoscopy). Many veterinary practices do not have fluoroscopy or endoscopy equipment or the expertise to apply this technology in avian species. Birds requiring advanced diagnostic techniques should be referred to a practice where the procedure can be performed. By reducing the number of diagnostic tests, this diminishes the owner's financial investment in the healthcare provided to their animal, reduces stress to the patient and focuses the attention on the disease problem affecting the patient. Once a definitive diagnosis is determined the proper treatment can be initiated or continued.

Diagnostic work-up for birds presented for regurgitation and vomiting

- Direct choanal smear – identify pathogenic bacteria, commensal yeast organisms, *Candida albicans*
- Culture and sensitivity testing of crop swab – identify pathogenic bacteria and which antimicrobial agents the organism(s) is/are sensitive to
- Crop cytology – identify *Macrorhabdus ornithogaster*, granulomatous disease
- Plain radiographic images – visualize enlarged proventriculus, metallic foreign bodies, some space-occupying masses
- Contrast radiographic images – visualize space-occupying masses, radiolucent foreign bodies
- Fluoroscopy – determine GI movement; if dysfunctional, possible condition associated with proventricular dilatation disease
- Rigid/flexible endoscopy – examine crop, ventriculus, proventriculus; biopsy samples of upper GI tract; removal of ingested foreign bodies

---

Diseases and conditions that cause vomiting and/or regurgitation

There are a number of diseases that cause vomiting and regurgitation in avian species. It is important to determine if the vomiting or regurgitation is a normal or abnormal condition. Normal behaviours of birds that result in vomiting and/or regurgitation include stress, post-anaesthesia recovery, mating behaviour, feeding of young, after administration of oral medication or nutritional supplementation, production of casts in raptor species, and when riding in a vehicle.

Stress

Whether the bird is in its normal or an unfamiliar environment (Figure 27.3), a stressful event can result in it regurgitating recently ingested food. When regurgitating food, the bird will start bobbing its head up and down to bring the food from the stomach and/or crop until the food is expelled from the beak. When stress is the underlying basis of regurgitation there is often a specific cause and effect noted in the patient's history by the clinician: a preceding event that is uncommon to the bird at which time the animal may appear agitated (e.g. a physical examination, grooming procedure) that causes the bird to regurgitate food. This

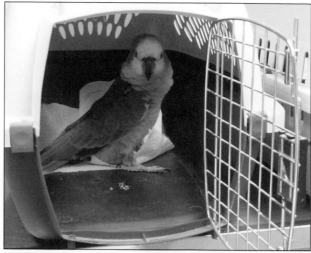

27.3 Travel is stressful for many birds and may result in the patient regurgitating ingested food.

condition is transitory; having an informed owner, knowledgeable of this behaviour, will help reduce the incidence of placing the animal in stressful conditions and understand that this is a normal process when the animal is under duress.

Post-anaesthesia

Most birds that are treated at veterinary hospitals, have a relatively rapid GI transit time. In the author's practice, contrast media was noted at the cloaca 45 minutes after being placed in the crop of a Blue and Gold Macaw. As avian species have a high metabolic rate and require a high level of energy to maintain normal physiological function, recommendations for fasting an avian patient prior to general anaesthesia generally range between 2 and 3 hours, but this is not always possible. Even if the bird has been fasted or if an emergency procedure is required while the patient is under general anaesthesia, the bird may regurgitate during or after the event while recovering (Figure 27.4).

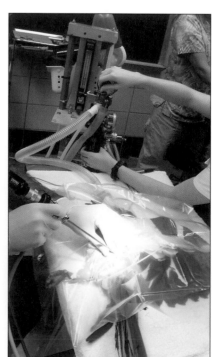

27.4

The avian patient may regurgitate/vomit during recovery from a surgical procedure in which general anaesthesia was performed, even if properly fasted.

An endotracheal tube should be placed after the bird has been anaesthetized to reduce and/or prevent the risk of aspiration of food material into the trachea through an open glottis. The oral cavity should be monitored on a regular basis for evidence of regurgitated food material. If food is present within the patient's oral cavity while under general anaesthesia, it should be removed with a cotton bud as soon as possible. Usually, if the bird regurgitates following recovery, after the endotracheal tube has been removed, it will be able to clear the glottis and oral cavity without assistance, but should be closely monitored. Restraining the bird and attempting to remove regurgitated material may stress the bird further and increase the risk of aspiration, so it is normally advised to allow the bird to recover without interference.

Mating behaviour

It is not uncommon for parrot species to regurgitate food as a sign of affection to a mate or perceived mate (e.g. human owner, reflection of the bird in a cage mirror). The act of regurgitation begins with head bobbing, after which the bird extends its neck and brings food out of its mouth by opening its beak and pushing the material out with its tongue. The act of vomiting or regurgitation can also involve head shaking, during which food material is scattered over a wide area in front of the bird. In most cases, when birds, especially parrots, regurgitate as a show of affection to a mate or perceived mate, the action is usually associated with feeding behaviour. The act is deliberate and focused in an attempt to feed the other bird, human or reflection in the mirror the food in its mouth directly into the oral cavity of its real or imagined mate. This behaviour may be appalling to a human owner, when first witnessed, and result in an emergency veterinary visit. Often a veterinary surgeon can determine the cause of regurgitation through affection during history-taking. It is not uncommon for male birds to masturbate on or around an owner for whom they are regurgitating and view as their mate.

Vomiting/regurgitation manifestations and associated causes/conditions

- Violent shaking and flinging food over the head feathers:
  - Crop infection
  - Reaction to ingested material
  - Reaction to therapeutic agent
  - Sharp foreign body ingestion
- Head/neck bobbing and flow of regurgitated food out of beak:
  - Affection to mate, owner or its reflection in the cage mirror
  - Young bird during feeding or after feeding
  - Post-anaesthetic recovery
  - Motion sickness (e.g. during/after a car ride)

Feeding of young

Parrots feed their young by regurgitating previously ingested food into the mouths of their chicks. This is a relatively straightforward diagnosis and the concerned owner is likely to be observing adults feeding young for the first time. An informed owner who understands the normal feeding habits of adult birds when raising young, will help reduce the concern of this behaviour with future clutches.

Medication or nutritional supplementation

It is not uncommon for avian patients to regurgitate after giving them oral medication or nutritional supplementation, either directly in the crop using a stainless steel gavage needle or by oral administration using a dosing syringe. The immediate reaction of the patient to the medication or nutritional supplementation is not difficult for the clinician to diagnose. Birds have a tendency to regurgitate after oral treatment, therefore it is imperative that the oral treatment always be performed immediately prior to placing the patient back into its enclosure. The patient should not be restrained for any period of time after administering oral treatment. Continuing to restrain a struggling bird that has regurgitated, will result in aspiration and possible death. If the bird regurgitates in its cage, it will shake its head, throwing food and/or medication in an attempt to clear its mouth; rarely are there problems associated with the bird clearing its own oral cavity, and it will usually swallow any remaining material after the initial event.

The patient should be monitored to make sure there is an uneventful recovery from the treatment response. More vigilance should be exercised in weaker or more debilitated patients if they regurgitate after oral treatment. The veterinary surgeon must assess the reason behind the patient's response to treatment, which could include weakness, adverse reaction to the medication or overfeeding with the nutritional supplementation. Trimethaprim-sulfa, D-penicillamine suspension, levamisole, ketoconazole, itraconazole and metronidazole suspension, among other medications, frequently cause regurgitation in avian patients immediately after oral administration.

Production of casts in raptors

In birds of prey, a normal part of the digestive process is the formation of casts in the ventriculus, which are removed from the digestive system through the mouth. The casts consist of indigestible material (bones and fur) and are compressed as pellets to a size that can move backwards through the proventriculus, oesophagus/crop, and out of the mouth without difficulty.

Casting in raptors (Forbes, 2014)

- Raptors should not generally be provided food with casting material until they are >12 days old, >20 days in some species
- Young birds may have difficulty casting some material such as fur; proventricular obstruction may occur
- The ovarian follicles and swollen oviduct of breeding females may cause a reduction in coelomic space and result in obstruction
- Raptors usually cast 8–16 hours after a meal
- Indigestible matter (e.g. grass, soil) that is consumed with food may cause intestinal blockage
- Ingested foreign bodies brought up with the cast may cause obstruction or laceration
- Ingestion of oversized food items can cause GI blockage
- Overeating may cause delayed ingestion and/or crop infection

---

Motion sickness

Many bird owners have reported that their birds have regurgitated/vomited while riding in a car or aeroplane. It is often difficult to determine if the animal is responding to the motion of the vehicle or the stress of being removed from a familiar environment or having the knowledge that it is going to the veterinary clinic. If there is a history of regurgitation/vomiting occurring when the bird is transported in a vehicle, then the owner should be told to fast the bird for 1–2 hours prior to journeys, if possible. For small caged birds weighing <100 g (e.g. finches, Budgerigars, Canaries) fasting for only 30 minutes prior to the trip may be required.

Disease

Although there are a number of normal and iatrogenic causes of vomiting and regurgitation in birds, there are far more disease conditions that cause the same signs. Diseases that contribute to avian patients vomiting and regurgitating will be classified in this chapter as infectious (bacterial, viral, parasitic, fungal and yeast) and non-infectious.

Infectious disease

Bacterial infections

Bacterial infections that result in inflammation of the oral cavity (stomatitis), oesophagus (oesophagitis), crop (ingluvitis) and proventriculus/ventriculus (gastritis), can result in irregular episodes of vomiting and regurgitation. The severity and number of events is dependent on the location and extent of the infection. Contributing problems associated with upper GI infections include, but are not limited to, anorexia and secondary infections from commensal organisms (e.g. *Candida albicans* – see 'Fungal organisms'). Inadequate nutrition, increasing impact of the primary infection, secondary infections and concurrent immunosuppression are the complexities involved with GI bacterial infections in avian patients that necessitate a quick identification of the primary bacterial pathogen(s).

Diagnostic work-up: Avian patients that present with clinical signs of regurgitation and vomiting often have concurrent problems such as anorexia and depression. As with all cases, a thorough history and physical examination are required. Where bacterial infection of the upper GI tract is suspected, the objective is to confirm the diagnosis by identifying the pathogens and antibiotics to which they are sensitive. A quick assessment of the severity and possible chronicity of the illness can be determined through assessing body condition, submission of a blood sample for a complete blood count (for overall assessment, a plasma chemistry panel may be included), and oral and/or crop culture/sensitivity testing and oral and/or crop cytology.

Therapy: Bacterial infections are best treated with medications to which the organism is proven sensitive. It is important to assess the patient's condition and ability to take oral medications before this form of therapy is prescribed. If the patient has crop stasis or difficulty in maintaining the therapeutic agent within the upper GI tract after administration, then other forms of antibiotic therapy must be selected (e.g. intramuscular injections). Supportive care is essential to maintain the patient's general condition and aid in recovery. Fluid therapy is important to replace fluid loss and sustain normal hydration. If inflammation is associated with the infectious process, mucosal protective agents (e.g. sucralfate) may be required. For pain management and anti-inflammatory properties it is imperative that the veterinary surgeon consider the potential side effects that non-steroidal anti-inflammatory drugs may have on the already diseased GI tract. Secondary GI disease conditions (e.g. candidiasis, parasites) must be treated at the same time as the primary bacterial disease.

Viruses

Although a number of viruses may be listed as potential causes of vomiting and/or regurgitation, only a few are of primary concern to avian practitioners. Viruses that have been associated with vomiting and/or regurgitation include falcon herpesvirus, pigeon herpesvirus, duck plague virus, papillomatosis (unknown aetiology but a virus is suspected), proventricular dilatation disease (definitive aetiology unknown but bornavirus is suspected to be involved with the disease process), psittacine beak and feather disease (circovirus), avian polyomavirus and adenovirus.

The viral infection in which regurgitation and/or crop stasis most commonly occur, is avian polyomavirus infection, particularly in non-Budgerigar parrot species (Figure 27.5). Infected chicks and young birds often show clinical signs; infection in birds over 16 weeks of age is usually subclinical. The first young birds presented with regurgitation and crop stasis associated with polyomavirus are usually the largest and fastest growing; clutchmates that have been exposed are possibly infected but as yet subclinical. Unfortunately, supportive care and treatment of secondary disease conditions (e.g. bacteria, candidiasis) is usually unsuccessful. If the bird presents with clinical GI signs associated with a polyomavirus infection, death usually occurs within 24 hours. Clutchmates will usually succumb to the viral infection within the week. Vaccination of exposed birds does not appear to have an impact on preventing the disease.

While the other viruses listed may be the underlying cause of vomiting and/or regurgitation, they rarely occur with this clinical sign. It is not uncommon for birds to develop ingluvitis or proventriculitis as a result of a bacterial infection due to dysfunction of the GI tract caused by the viral disease. Moreover, bacterial infections are much more likely in birds that are immunosuppressed as a result of a viral infection.

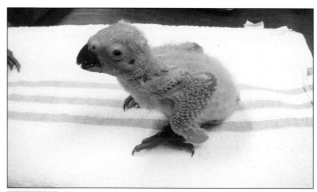

27.5 Young birds, such as this African Grey Parrot, are very susceptible to polyomavirus if exposed. One of the first clinical signs associated with polyomavirus in birds of this age is crop stasis or regurgitation. Note: the pictured chick is healthy.

Diagnostic work-up: There has been a significant improvement and proliferation of ante-mortem avian diagnostic tests for viral diseases. These advancements have occurred mainly in conjunction with scientific discoveries in the field of molecular biology, especially as it pertains to PCR technology. While there are many diagnostic PCR tests available today for avian viral diseases that may cause vomiting/regurgitation, pathology is still the gold standard to definitively diagnose viral infections. The best chance of getting a true positive in birds that are infected with a viral disease is in individuals that are showing clinical signs consistent with that particular infectious process; this is particularly true for polyomavirus and bornavirus testing (see also Chapter 19).

Therapy: At the time of publication, there is no specific antiviral treatment available for diseases that cause vomiting and regurgitation in birds. Supportive care can be provided but generally the viral diseases are uniformly fatal in birds that present with disease signs. The best way to combat viral disease in avian species is to have disease-free birds, maintain good quarantine procedures for new birds being introduced into an aviary and to vaccinate when possible.

Parasites

There is a number of different parasites that can cause disease to various portions of the avian GI tract and result in vomiting and/or regurgitation. In many GI parasite cases, the birds present with many disease signs, including anorexia, cachexia and diarrhoea. *Capillaria* spp., *Dispharynx* spp., *Syngamus* spp., *Spiropter* spp. and *Ascaris* spp. are nematodes that cause primary disease in the GI tract that will cause a bird to regurgitate. These nematodes usually affect the lower GI tract or stomach; *Syngamus* spp. are found in the trachea. Inflammation and a heavy worm burden may cause a bird to develop upper GI disease signs, such as crop stasis, anorexia and regurgitation. Young peafowl are very susceptible to *Capillaria* spp. infections and are usually presented moribund and extremely emaciated. Birds infected with *Syngamus* spp. can have a frothy blood-tinged discharge in and around the oral cavity. *Syngamus* spp. will also cause birds to cough and gag, which may result in regurgitation of ingested food.

Protozoal parasites, such as *Trichomonas* spp., are found in the oral cavity, oesophagus and crop, while *Giardia* spp. and *Histomonas* spp. are commonly located in the intestinal tract. Regardless of where the protozoal parasites are located, they can cause regurgitation in infected birds. The obvious clinical signs associated with *Trichomonas* spp. infections are ulceration and diphtheritic necrotic areas within the oral cavity and on the oesophagus.

Cestodes, trematodes and *Plasmodium* spp. are other classes of parasites that can cause upper GI disease problems due to intestinal blockage (cestodes) or systemic illness (trematodes and *Plasmodium* spp.).

Diagnostic work-up: In most cases of GI parasites a direct faecal examination or faecal flotation will identify either the organism, as is the case for protozoan parasites, or eggs, for ascarids, trematodes and cestodes. *Plasmodium* spp. are identified in blood smears since they are a haemoparasite. To identify *Trichomonas* spp., a direct swab of lesions identified in the oral cavity or oesophagus will be needed and subsequently placed on a slide for direct examination. Although *Syngamus* spp. are found in the trachea and respiratory system, the eggs laid by the adult worms will be coughed up and swallowed by the avian host. The swallowed double-operculated eggs can then be identified through a faecal flotation examination. To increase one's chances of seeing and identifying a protozoal parasite when examining a direct faecal smear, it is suggested to warm the slide prior to placing the faecal sample and to use dilute iodine solution as a contrast agent. Protozoal parasites are hard to identify and may not be present in large numbers, therefore diagnostic aids (Lugol's staining of the slide) used for identification are recommended.

Therapy: Treatment of parasites that may cause vomiting/regurgitation is based on first identifying the parasite that is causing the disease problem. Once identified, there are specific treatments recommended for protozoan parasites (e.g. metronidazole), ascarids (e.g. fenbendazole) and cestodes (e.g. praziquantel). Often the initial treatment for these parasites is unsuccessful and a second round or more of treatment is required. If direct exposure is associated with the lifecycle of an identified parasite, then environmental cleaning and separation of infected from non-infected birds are required. Re-examinations of diseased birds are required to ensure a treatment success.

Fungal organisms

The primary disease organism that is associated with upper GI tract dysfunction is *Candida albicans*, which is considered 'normal' flora in low numbers, but can contribute to the disease process as an opportunistic organism. Candidiasis can be observed in the oral cavity or upper oesophagus as whitish plaque lesions and may extend into the crop. Mucormycosis is another opportunistic organism that can cause granulomas within the digestive system of birds. *Aspergillus* and *Penicillium* spp. are most often associated with respiratory infections in birds. Rarely, *Aspergillus* or *Penicillium* spp. can become generalized and cause GI infections similar to candidiasis.

Macrorhabdus ornithogaster (or megabacteriosis) is a common cause of regurgitation/vomiting in Budgerigars, small psittacine species and passerines. Birds are commonly presented in very poor body condition with a history of anorexia, regurgitation/vomiting, diarrhoea, matted feathers around the head and a pasty vent. A common description among bird owners for this GI fungal infection is 'going light', which is a common phrase to describe birds in very poor body conditions.

Diagnostic work-up: Using cotton-tipped swabs and collecting samples of lesions within the oral cavity or on the oesophageal mucosa will yield material that can be placed on a slide for examination for *C. albicans*. The swab can be inserted through the oral cavity and past the cervical oesophagus into the crop to collect samples for direct evaluation of fungal organisms. A Gram stain can be used to help identify *Candida* spp. organisms. As with other infectious diseases, a pathology examination from harvested tissue samples of a dead bird or histopathological evaluation of affected tissue will yield fungal evidence of disease if present.

M. ornithogaster can be identified by swabbing the crop or obtaining a stool sample and performing a Gram stain on the sample. The very large rod-shaped organism can be identified as Gram positive if stained in this manner through microscopic examination of the slide. The large microorganism can also be easily identified when viewing a direct wet smear of a crop swab or stool sample from an infected bird. If a post-mortem examination is performed, the organism is best identified through swabbing the isthmus between the proventriculus and ventriculus. The swabbed material is then placed on a slide to be stained and examined under a microscope. *M. ornithogaster* organisms are also identified through histopathological examination of affected GI tissue samples (e.g. crop, proventriculus, isthmus, ventriculus) collected during the gross post-mortem examination procedure.

Therapy: Treatment of *C. albicans* can be achieved by using nystatin and/or fluconazole. Nystatin is only effective if it comes into direct contact with the organism; fluconazole provides systemic therapy. Currently itraconazole or voriconazole are the treatment options of choice for aspergillosis. If *C. albicans* is found in the budding form and not the hyphal growth phase, treatment is often successful. The outcome of treating GI aspergillosis or mucormycosis is much more guarded and requires a much more aggressive long-term therapy. The veterinary challenge of treating candidiasis is finding out what the primary disease condition is, since this organism is an opportunistic organism. The animal is immunosuppressed if candidiasis is identified, and ultimately successful treatment of this mycotic organism is dependent on treating the underlying cause of the primary disease process.

Treatment for *M. orithogaster* is uniformly non-rewarding regarding a 'cure', but improved patient condition is possible with therapeutic intervention. Treatment recommendations at this time include amphotericin B at 100 mg/kg orally q12h for 30 days. Although sodium benzoate has been recommended as a potential treatment for *M. ornithogaster*, there is no scientific evidence of its effectiveness as a therapeutic option in clinically ill birds. Therefore, at this time sodium benzoate should not be considered a treatment option for birds diagnosed with *M. ornithogaster*.

Toxicity

Heavy metals

It is not uncommon for birds to present with heavy metal toxicity. The most common heavy metal toxins are lead, zinc, copper and mercury. Mercury is common in fish-eating wild birds and is not considered a problem for companion avian or cage bird species. Although there are several clinical signs associated with heavy metal toxicity in birds due to the effects on various body systems, the GI tract is a primary target area due to the presence of the ingested metal. Anorexia, gastroenteritis, diarrhoea, vomiting, bradycardia, cardiovascular effects, non-regenerative anaemia and regurgitation are often observed in birds diagnosed with heavy metal toxicity. With lead toxicity, birds will develop diarrhoea, bright green urates, ± frank blood and/or haematuria in the droppings (Figure 27.6). Often the primary clinical sign associated with lead toxicity in birds is considered to be neurological. While central

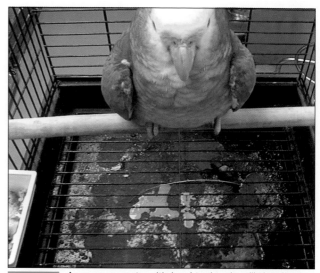

27.6   Amazon parrots with lead toxicosis will develop gastrointestinal disease including haematuria, diarrhoea and regurgitation/vomiting.

nervous anomalies are frequently noted, the GI system may be affected as much or more.

Regurgitation is the most common clinical sign noted in birds diagnosed with zinc toxicity (Figure 27.7). Zinc is a nutrient required by the bird's body, unlike lead, therefore extreme amounts must be ingested for clinical disease to occur. Self-induced feather picking has anecdotally been associated with zinc toxicosis, but GI signs, primarily regurgitation, are the recognized pathological effect of this disease.

Diagnostic work-up: If heavy metal toxicosis is suspected, then blood samples should be submitted for a complete blood count and blood metal levels prior to the initiation of treatment. The complete blood count will determine if the patient has a non-regenerative

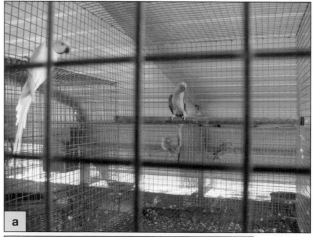

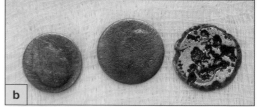

27.7   **(a)** Zinc wire typical of cages used to house birds both as pets and in an aviary setting. **(b)** Coins removed from a goose that was regurgitating due to zinc toxicosis associated with the metallic objects.

anaemia, which is a common consequence of chronic heavy metal toxicosis. Radiographic images are also required to determine if any ingested metal remains in the GI tract, particularly the ventriculus. Even if there is no evidence of ingested metal in the bird's GI tract, the possibility of toxicosis still exists through the animal's ingestion of very small particles or dissolved particulates. This is why the definitive diagnostic test for heavy metal toxicosis is the measurement of blood levels for the toxins.

Treatment: Treatment with a chelating agent, such as calcium EDTA or dimercaptosuccinic acid (DMSA), should begin immediately if heavy metal toxicosis is suspected. The benefits of initiating treatment prior to a definitive diagnosis far outweigh the risks. As mentioned previously, blood should be collected for heavy metal levels prior to the commencement of treatment. Although oral D-penicillamine has been recommended as an option for treatment, it must be compounded from a capsule for administration in avian patients. Unfortunately, the smell and taste of this compounded drug is repulsive and often results in the patient vomiting and regurgitating after administration. If D-penicillamine is used to treat heavy metal toxicity in birds, only the capsule form should be administered, therefore only very large birds would benefit from this drug.

Even if blood levels of the toxic metal are reduced successfully, a further challenge is to remove any ingested metal from the digestive tract. This is a more difficult problem if the metal is located in the ventriculus. Mineral oil, peanut butter and psyllium have all been recommended to try to speed the movement of metal particles from the bird's ventriculus. A magnet glued to the open end of a red rubber tube can be passed down the oesophagus to remove magnetic metal foreign bodies from the crop, ventriculus and proventriculus (Figure 27.8). Lead, as well as some other metals (e.g. lead shot), cannot be removed in this way. There have been studies that have found that feeding the patient grit will increase the rate of passage of metal particles from the ventriculus (Lupu and Robins, 2009). Supportive care of the bird undergoing treatment is important because secondary anaemia, anorexia, dehydration and stress to body organs (e.g. kidney) can and will affect the ability of the animal to recover.

Pesticides, insecticides and household chemicals

Products located around a house that may induce regurgitation and/or vomiting include pesticides, insecticides and household chemicals. Examples of pesticides that may have toxic GI effects in birds include organophosphate compounds, organochlorines, carbamates, rotenone, arsenicals and nitrates. As with heavy metal toxicosis, the ingestion of these products will cause a variety of clinical disease signs, most notably affecting the nervous system and the function of body systems. Household chemicals that may be ingested include chlorine, detergents and disinfectants. The cause for regurgitation may be associated with an adverse reaction of the GI mucosa and/or an acute inflammatory response to the compound. It would be a rare case if an avian patient ingested an undiluted pesticide, insecticide or household chemical. The danger for exposure comes with dilution either in an enclosed area that has been cleaned or outdoors where water pools after product application.

Diagnostic work-up: Diagnosis can be difficult for ingested pesticides, insecticides and household chemicals. Smell may be helpful if the bird has regurgitated shortly after ingesting the compound, and the patient's history provided by the owner may uncover exposure to one of the toxic compounds. With organophosphate toxicity, birds will often present with rear leg paresis and acetylcholinesterase levels will aid in determining a definitive diagnosis of disease associated with these products. Routine blood diagnostic testing is effective in determining the patient's overall health status and direct treatment protocol for stabilization and supportive care.

Therapy: Once the overall health status of the patient is determined, treatment can continue with a more focused effort. Initially, if the ingestion event was acute, flushing of the crop will help remove excess material prior to absorption into the body. There is an ongoing clinical debate on the effectiveness of oral administration of activated charcoal to reduce the absorption of ingested toxin and bind material through the digestive tract to prevent exposure. If there is a possibility of recent toxin ingestion, activated charcoal should be considered as a treatment option.

Atropine is the treatment of choice if organophosphate toxicity is diagnosed or suspected. Acetylcholinesterase levels should be tested on blood collected prior to initiation of atropine therapy. As with all avian patients suffering from debilitating disease, supportive care is warranted, including fluid therapy, nutritional support, and hospitalization in a critical care unit may be necessary.

Food and plants

Although uncommon, a bird may regurgitate or vomit after eating a plant or a specific food item. Birds appear to have (based on clinical observation) a keen taste, but will on occasion eat a toxic plant or food that will cause an adverse GI reaction. Chocolate, salt, philodendron, dieffenbachia, poinsettia, and berries from lariope grass are a few foods and plants that have been implicated in birds regurgitating or vomiting.

Diagnostic work-up: A history of the disease condition, provided by the owner, will often provide information leading to a definitive diagnosis. Often the owner will be able to provide a sample of the plant or food for identification or flushing of the crop for ingested contents may provide some remnants. In many cases, the owner will actually see the bird eat the plant or feed the bird food that causes the animal to regurgitate.

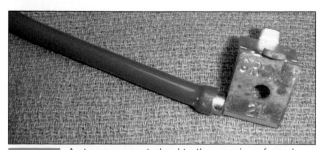

27.8 A strong magnet glued to the opening of a red rubber catheter can be used to remove metallic foreign bodies from the crop, ventriculus and proventriculus.

Therapy: Treatment of a bird that eats a toxic plant or food is supportive and based on what is identified as the definitive disease-causing agent. The patient's crop and/or proventriculus can be flushed along with providing fluid therapy and placing the animal in a critical care unit. Anti-inflammatory medication, GI protectants, activated charcoal and nutritional support are recommended based on the patient's diagnosis and condition.

Foreign bodies and gastrointestinal obstructive lesions

If there is an obstruction blocking normal passage of food through the GI tract, the bird may vomit or regurgitate. Obstructive lesions (Figure 27.9) include foreign bodies, neoplasia, granulomas, intussusceptions, volvulus or ileus. A foreign body (e.g. wood chip, plastic toy fragment, rope thread) can be located in any part of the digestive system and still cause regurgitation either through complete or partial blockage or mucosal irritation. Unfortunately, there are no guidelines or requirements to manufacture 'bird safe' toys or label them for appropriate bird size. Therefore, many owners purchase toys that are acceptable for small birds (<100 g) and place them in the cage of larger birds (>400 g). Moreover, rope, raw hide, electronic equipment, plastic, cane, painted wood and painted metal toys are manufactured for birds with no oversight (Figure 27.10). Cotton rope is a popular material for bird toys and is placed in many cages for the animals to play with. The author has treated a Galah, among others, that suffered from an intestinal obstruction due to ingested cotton rope fragments from a destroyed toy in its cage. The bird ultimately died despite extreme surgical and medical intervention to try to save its life.

Diagnostic work-up: Diagnosis of foreign bodies and GI obstructive lesions is best made by using traditional or contrast radiographic imaging techniques. If the affected area is in the upper GI tract (i.e. oesophagus to the ventriculus), endoscopic examination may be helpful to observe the material in question. Fluoroscopic and sonographic imaging modalities are other diagnostic imaging options.

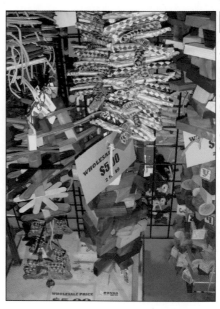

27.10

Unregulated bird toy manufacture results in material being used that can lead to ingested foreign bodies that cause gastrointestinal obstruction.

Therapy: Recommended treatment is removal of the foreign body or GI obstructive lesion. For neoplastic obstructive lesions, radiation and/or chemotherapy may reduce the size of the tissue mass. Surgical removal is always an option and is often used for lower GI lesions. Upper GI foreign bodies may be removed through the use of a rigid or flexible endoscope. If an endoscope is used, a flexible endoscope is often preferred over a rigid instrument due to the greater length of the former. Also, the flexible endoscopes often have fluid flow capabilities and an instrument channel within the diameter of the scope that provides many more grasping instrument options.

Summary

Vomiting and regurgitation can occur in birds due to organ and metabolic dysfunction. Haemochromatosis, hepatotoxins, hepatic neoplasia, visceral gout and renal disease are some of the disease processes that can result in a patient that vomits or regurgitates. There are relatively few disease conditions that result in vomiting and/or regurgitation being the only clinical sign exhibited by a bird. It is likely that the bird is exhibiting a normal behaviour if vomiting or regurgitation is the only clinical sign noted on the physical examination and all diagnostic testing results are normal. There are some exceptions, such as infectious ingluvitis, therefore the veterinary surgeons must be astute in their medical evaluation of each case that presents with these clinical signs. A rapid definitive diagnosis, effective treatment protocol and supportive care will often result in successful case resolution of vomiting or regurgitating patients.

References and further reading

Forbes NA (2014) *Practical raptor nutrition* [online]. Available at: www.afvp2.com/IMG/pdf/Practical_Raptor_Nutrition_Neil_Forbes.pdf/

Lupu C and Robins S (2009) Comparison of treatment protocols for removing metallic foreign objects from the ventriculus of budgerigars (*Melopsittaus undulatus*). *Journal of Avian Medicine and Surgery* **23**, 186–193

Mayer J (2013) Clinical algorithms. In: *Clinical Veterinary Advisor: Birds and Exotic Pets*, ed. J Mayer and TM Donnelly, p. 664. Elsevier Saunders, St Louis

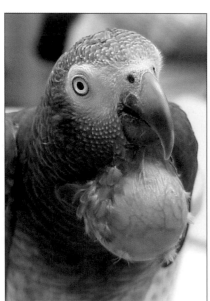

27.9

Submandibular abscess in an African Grey Parrot can stimulate vomiting/regurgitation.

Case example 1: Regurgitating/vomiting Umbrella Cockatoo

Presentation and history

A 3-year-old Umbrella Cockatoo was presented with a 2-day history of regurgitation/vomiting of clear fluid mixed with ingested food. On physical examination the bird was in good body condition, bright and alert, and had a normal stool.

Diagnostic work-up

Diagnostic testing performed included a complete blood count, plasma chemistry panel and crop swab cytological examination. The only abnormality noted in the blood tests was an increased total white blood cell count. On the crop swab cytological examination, a number of Gram-negative organisms (35%) were noted along with Gram-positive cocci and rods (65%) as well as one or two Candida spp. per oil immersion field.

Therapy

The bird was prescribed ciprofloxacin (10 mg/kg orally q12h for 12 days) and released to the owners' care to return in 7 days for re-examination.

The owner called 3 days after the examination and stated that the treatment did not appear to be effective and the bird continued to regurgitate. Upon presentation for the second time, the bird still appeared in good condition but was regurgitating during the physical examination. After the second physical examination no external abnormalities were noted except a fluid-filled crop. A crop swab was submitted for aerobic culture and sensitivity testing. A gamma-haemolytic Streptococcus spp. was isolated from the crop and was resistant to third generation penicillins, third generation cephalosporins, aminoglycosides and fluoroquinolones. The organism was sensitive to trimethoprim-sulfa and doxycycline. The bird was prescribed doxycycline (25 mg/kg orally q12h for 14 days).

Outcome

The owner reported that the bird ceased regurgitating 1 day after treatment started and upon re-examination 14 days later, no signs of the original presenting problem were present.

Bacterial ingluvitis is not uncommon in psittacine species. Although there is an overwhelming amount of published material denoting the pathogenicity of Gram-negative organisms adversely affecting the GI tract of birds, Gram-positive organisms can cause disease as well. The antimicrobial-resistant nature of the isolated organism shows the importance of culture and sensitivity diagnostic testing when selecting treatment options for ingluvitis cases which present with vomiting/regurgitation.

Case example 2: Blue and Gold Macaw with zinc toxicosis

Presentation and history

A 6-year-old Blue and Gold Macaw presented with a 4-day history of regurgitating clear fluid on an irregular basis. The owner stated that the bird was rather destructive and it was not uncommon for it to tear up items within the house since it was maintained out of its cage for most of the day. On physical examination, there were no external abnormalities noted except for a fluid-filled flaccid crop.

Diagnostic work-up

Diagnostic tests performed on the patient after the physical examination included a complete blood count, plasma chemistry panel, crop swab cytological examination and full body radiographic imaging due to the history of the bird being destructive and having free access to household items. No abnormalities were noted from the diagnostic test results and the bird was anaesthetized for radiographic examination.

The radiographic images revealed two small metallic foreign bodies in the ventriculus. When the owner was informed, she mentioned that the bird had played with a small metal motorcycle toy that belonged to her son and broke off pieces. At that time, blood was collected to determine zinc levels. The results came back as elevated and a diagnosis of zinc toxicosis was made.

Therapy

With zinc toxicosis, if the source of zinc is removed, the body will successfully resolve the elevated levels to the point of resolving the problem. If the source cannot be immediately removed, as with this case, chelation therapy should be implemented and the foreign body removed in the manner possible. Chelation therapy was initiated with calcium EDTA at 35 mg/kg i.m. q8h for 4 days and psyllium orally q24h to try to remove the foreign body from the ventriculus. After the initiation of chelation therapy the bird ceased to regurgitate and behaved in a normal manner. After 4 days of treatment, full body radiographic images were acquired and revealed that the ventricular foreign bodies had passed through the GI tract. Chelation therapy was continued for 3 more days, after which a blood zinc test showed normal levels.

Outcome

The bird was released from the hospital and did not have any recurrence of regurgitation. The owner was instructed to provide increased supervision and reduce exposure to objects that the bird can destroy and ingest.

While radiographic images will provide evidence of ingested heavy metals, this diagnostic test is not the definitive manner to diagnose heavy metal toxicosis. The recommended method to definitively diagnose heavy metal toxicosis in avian species is measurement of toxic blood levels. Birds can be suffering from heavy metal toxicosis and not have any radiographic evidence of ingested metal in the GI tract.

Case example 3: Budgerigars with *Macrorhadbus ornithogaster*

Presentation and history

Three adult Budgerigars were presented with a 12-day history of regurgitation and vomiting, matted feathers around the head and pasty vents. The birds were from a Budgerigar breeding facility where birds were bought and sold on a regular basis, in an effort to generate different colour mutations and show birds. The birds were in extremely poor body condition and the owner elected to have the birds euthanased for full body post-mortem examination.

Diagnostic work-up

When examined grossly, the birds were in poor body condition and had fluid-filled GI tracts. No other gross abnormalities were noted. A swab of the upper GI tract was collected from each bird and examined with a light microscope. *Macrorhabdus ornithogaster* was identified and confirmed on histopathological examination of GI tissue sections.

Outcome

Unfortunately, at this time, treatment for *M. ornithogaster* is uniformly unrewarding. Treatment recommendations for large groups of birds include amphotericin B at 100 mg/kg orally q12h for 30 days or sodium benzoate at 1 teaspoon (5 ml)/l drinking water for 5 weeks. However, intense aviary management and bringing in disease-free birds is recommended.

The thin bird

28

Elisa Wüst and Michael Lierz

In avian practice, loss of body condition is a common presentation. It is a clinical sign of many diseases that regularly occur in companion animals and is therefore very non-specific. Usually, a loss of bodyweight is a sign of a chronic disorder, as it takes some time for the bird to lose condition. The rate of loss of body condition is faster in smaller birds due to their more rapid metabolic rate. Additionally, a lower than required energy intake (starvation) also results in thin birds that do not have any other pathological condition. Body condition is also influenced by the environmental temperature; a lower temperature increases metabolism, resulting in a more rapid loss of weight. This appears particularly in birds kept outside in winter (especially in species originating from tropical areas). Nearly every medical condition that affects the general condition of a bird can lead to emaciation due to loss of appetite. In juvenile birds, a constant bodyweight is also pathological and comparable with weight loss in fully grown birds, as these growing birds should have a daily increase in bodyweight.

Emaciation can be diagnosed in the living bird and is defined as severe weight loss, especially the loss of subcutaneous fat and muscle tissue. Emaciation is an extension of general weight loss, and is a non-specific sign. Emaciation usually occurs in two phases:

- In the first phase, mostly fat and carbohydrate depots (liver glycogen) are consumed
- In the second phase, depletion of proteins is dominant. This can be seen clinically by the depletion of skeletal muscles.

In comparison, cachexia is usually diagnosed at post-mortem examination, and is a weakness and wasting of the body due to severe chronic disease or starvation.

- In a cachectic bird, there is not only the loss of subcutaneous fat but also of intra-abdominal and cardiac depots.
- Cachexia is accompanied by muscle and internal organ atrophy and organ failure.
- The bone marrow also alters in consistency.

Where a bird is already cachectic, the chances of recovery are very low. Intensive care and supplementation of energy and proteins are vital. In general, birds with weight loss must always be treated as emergencies, as such a condition may quickly lead to death.

Birds are regularly only presented in end-stage conditions when they show abnormal behaviours such as fluffing up, excessive sleeping and anorexia. Weight loss is often not recognized by the owner as the plumage covers the decrease in muscle mass. As a result, monitoring a bird's weight is a very useful method to detect potential disease prior to the demonstration of clinical signs. Physical examinations should always include a combination of bodyweight measurement, pectoral muscle palpation and examination of subcutaneous fat depots (Figure 28.1). Only a combination of these results will allow an accurate assessment of the patient's body condition.

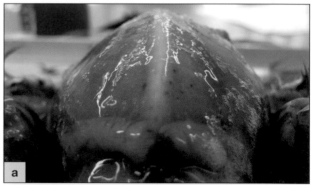

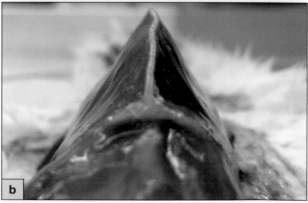

28.1 **(a)** The chest muscles of a bird should be as high as the sternum. **(b)** An emaciated bird demonstrates a clearly visible and palpable sternum with reduced chest muscle.

28

Aside from the clinical appearance of a thin bird, some histological findings also point towards emaciation. The most common histological finding in emaciated or cachectic birds is liver atrophy, also called 'starvation liver'. Birds that have a negative calorie balance or are chronically diseased usually have a decreased rate of red cell production or an increased rate of red cell absorption. As a result, iron accumulates in phagocytic cells in the liver, as well as the spleen and kidney, causing a haemosiderosis (Figure 28.2). This is a reversible alteration and not directly associated with liver disease. Prolonged caloric deficiencies might additionally lead to pancreatic atrophy (Figure 28.3). Macroscopically, this alteration is not usually visible, but in the histopathological examination an acinar epithelial atrophy associated with normal islets of Langerhans is detectable. A hyperplasia of the thyroid gland may also be a sign of a catabolic metabolism. Histologically, the size of the epithelium of the thyroid may be visibly increased, with or without reduction of the colloid (Figure 28.4). Oedema may occur concurrently to emaciation or cachexia. This is caused by a decreased intravascular osmotic pressure due to the reduction of albumin levels in the blood. Albumin is either used for energy production or lost due to kidney or gastrointestinal disease. In cases of nutritional imbalances and starvation, a severe energy deficit causes histological signs of emaciation and oedema without further alterations such as inflammation.

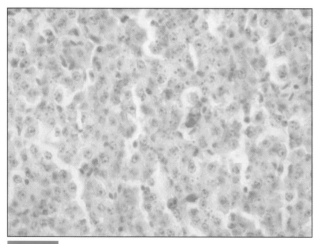

28.2   Haemosiderosis in the liver. (Courtesy of H Pendl)

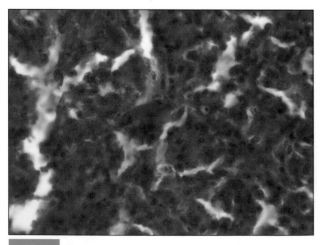

28.3   Pancreatic atrophy. (Courtesy of H Pendl)

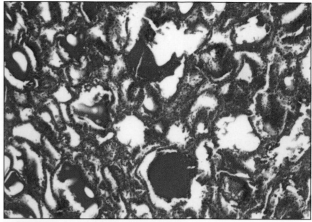

28.4   Hyperplasia of the thyroid gland. (Courtesy of H Pendl)

Causes of weight loss

The causes of weight loss and emaciation in birds can be broadly divided into three categories (Figure 28.5):

- **Nutrient deficiency:** qualitative or quantitative malnutrition due to lack of sufficient food, imbalanced nutrients or problems in the feeding method
- **Endogenous deficiency:** an insufficient use of nutrition, with normal absorption from the digestive tract. Endogenous deficiency is caused by an increased action of the catabolic metabolism instead of the normal anabolic metabolism. Causes include chronic infections, neoplasia, chronic internal organ insufficiency (liver, kidney, endocrine pancreas deficiency) or hormonal disorders (e.g. hyperoestrogenism)
- **Absorption deficiency:** a malnutrition due to anorexia or disease of the intestinal tract such as maldigestion and malabsorption, which includes exocrine pancreatic deficiency. The inability to swallow and problems related to motility caused by toxins or disease are other potential factors.

The cause of weight loss and emaciation for a particular case can be determined with a detailed history and clinical examination, but in some cases histological findings may support the diagnosis. Figure 28.6 illustrates the wide range of causes of emaciation and cachexia in birds.

Nutritional weight loss

Nutritional weight loss due to insufficient energy supply is very rare in captive pet birds. Most owners feed too much; obesity is the most common nutritional aberration. In severe cases, chronic obesity causes accumulation of fat cells in the liver and displacement of healthy liver cells (Figure 28.7).

Steatosis, the process of abnormal retention of lipids within a cell, has an adverse effect on the normal processes of synthesis and elimination of triglyceride fat. Excess lipid accumulates in vesicles that displace the cytoplasm. Large accumulations can damage cell elements and, in severe cases, the liver cell may even burst. This stage is mostly unrecognized by the owner as the bird shows almost no obvious clinical signs.

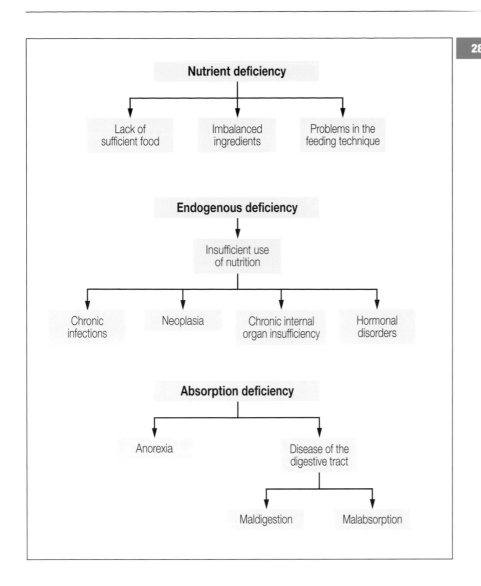

28.5   Broad categories of causes of weight loss and emaciation.

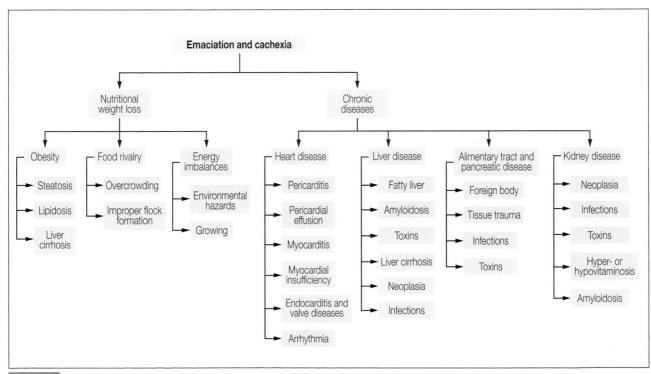

28.6   Overview of potential causes of emaciation and cachexia.

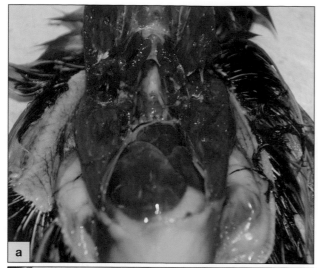

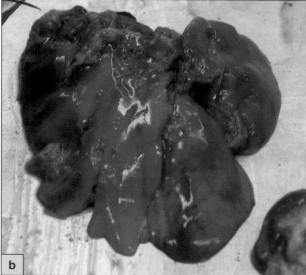

28.7   **(a–b)** Post-mortem views of a fatty liver.

However, in some cases the **fatty liver** may cause **lipidosis**, especially if fat deposits are mobilized due to anorexia, stress or metabolic imbalances caused by bodyweight reduction. In some cases this may lead to loss of muscle tissue and wasting of the bird. In severe cases it may cause anaemia, blood coagulation disorders and hepatoencephalopathy.

Over time, such liver disorders may lead to **liver cirrhosis** and therefore should be treated as early as possible to avoid irreversible effects.

- Cirrhosis is the end-stage of chronic liver aberrations and is irreversible.
- Physiological structures are infiltrated with fibrotic tissue involving usually more than 50% of the total liver tissue.
- This causes severe circulatory problems of the liver and likely further necrosis of the tissue.
- Clinical signs at this stage are ascites, blood coagulation disorders, hepatic encephalopathy, hepatic coma and death (Jones and Orosz, 1996).
- An elevation of alanine transaminase and glutamate dehydrogenase along with bile acids may be seen either simultaneously or separately.
- Creatine kinase is usually not elevated in liver disease and this assists in distinguishing the elevated values from other diseases.

- Triglycerides and cholesterol are elevated in fatty liver syndrome.
- In the blood cell count, non-regenerative anaemia might be present.
- Final diagnosis can be made by ultrasonographic or endoscopic evaluation and biopsy of the liver.

Birds that are kept in outside aviaries, in collections of larger flocks or that are still growing are more susceptible to nutritional weight loss. Lower-ranked birds in flocks may be kept away from feed by superior conspecifics and, even if enough food is provided by the owner, single birds may starve. Outside aviaries are more prone to falling temperatures, resulting in higher energy requirements of the birds, especially in species that originate from tropical climates; they are unable to eat enough to fulfil their requirements (particularly true of smaller species).

Bird keepers do not always adjust the amount or energy content of feed to meet the changing requirements of birds. During colder temperatures, high-energy food should be provided. Juvenile birds also have a higher energy requirement not only to grow properly but also to maintain body temperature when they are less than fully feathered. Growing birds usually increase their bodyweight by around 10% per day and in cases where no growth is recorded for more than 1–2 days, a detailed examination and feeding regime analysis is required.

Chronic diseases

Heart
Heart diseases in birds are still underdiagnosed because they are not on the list of differential diagnoses of many veterinary surgeons (veterinarians). However, heart disorders are regularly detected, especially in birds with chronic emaciation, in particular in cases without obvious other infections or pathologies.

Pericarditis: Acute weight loss and apathy may be caused by pericarditis. Pericarditis is regularly a consequence of systemic bacterial infections, such as granulomatous pericarditis (caused by trichomonosis in pigeons) or exudative pericarditis, or due to systemic degenerative processes such as uraemic pericarditis (caused by gout). Diagnosis is usually made by radiography (via identification of a dense, irregular heart shadow) or ultrasonography (where the thickened pericardium can be measured). In pericarditis caused by gout, elevated uric acid in the blood chemistry might be present. In every case of pericarditis elevation of the white blood cell count is prominent. Treatment of pericarditis is dependent on the underlying cause.

Pericardial effusion: Acute anorexia, weight loss and apathy may be also caused by pericardial effusion. This is most commonly a consequence of exudative pericarditis or increased back pressure due to a heart insufficiency. In some cases it follows a traumatic incident. Compared with a usually clear fluid in the pericardium, a more dense bloody fluid appears after trauma. In rare cases, neoplasia, especially of the heart base, might also lead to pericardial effusion. In some cases, the effusion is accompanied by an ascites, especially in cases of increased blood pressure. On radiography the heart shadow is massively enlarged and in the case of additional ascites the coelomic cavity demonstrates a diffuse shadowing. In ultrasonography, the effusion can be seen as a hypoechogenic rim around the heart. Therapy focuses on the fast elimination of the effusive fluids and can be done by puncture or centesis. As an alternative, furosemide (0.5–1 mg/kg q12–24h) may be used to increase renal excretion of fluids. Care should be taken in dehydrated birds and furosemide should not be used in hyperuricaemic birds.

Myocarditis: Myocarditis in birds may be acute but is more often a chronic process, which is usually secondary to an underlying cause. The cause may be infectious, toxic (e.g. lead intoxication), metabolic (e.g. gout, diabetes mellitus) or neoplastic. These birds are presented with a history of losing weight with normal food intake and general depression. Sometimes dyspnoea occurs as well. Radiography and ultrasonography show a dense and enlarged heart silhouette and ultrasonographic aberrations of the heart muscle. Blood chemistry shows a significant elevation of alanine transaminase, lactate dehydrogenase and creatine kinase. In some cases, depending on the underlying cause, uric acid, calcium, potassium and sodium levels are altered. Additionally to the treatment of the underlying cause, basic treatment includes angiotensin-converting enzyme (ACE) inhibitors and electrolytes.

Myocardial insufficiency: The most common reason for chronic weight loss caused by cardiac disease is myocardial insufficiency. Myocardial insufficiency is commonly caused by valve defects and pulmonary hypertension originating from chronic aspergillosis, lung fibrosis or atherosclerosis. It may also be a consequence of infectious disease or intoxication (e.g. lead). Myocardial insufficiency is also described in cases of haemochromatosis in mynahs. In addition to reduced body condition, dyspnoea and weakness are common clinical signs. Patients with myocardial insufficiency demonstrate a heart murmur during auscultation. Radiography will show enlargement of the heart shadow as well as an enlarged liver silhouette. In some cases the underlying cause can be seen as well (e.g. dense lung tissue or atherosclerotic plaques in the aorta). Usually cardiac ultrasonography is the diagnostic method of choice and is also the safest approach for the bird. Heart measurements, cardiac efflux, valve and ventricle aberrations can be measured as well as swirling flow in ventricles and vestibules. Therapy usually involves ACE inhibitors (enalapril at 0.5–2.5 mg/kg q12–24h) and calcium sensitizers (pimobendan at 0.15–0.3 mg/kg q12h), furosemide (0.5–1 mg/kg q12–24h) (if required) and treatment of the underlying cause.

Endocarditis and valve diseases: Chronic inflammation and metabolic dysfunction may lead to endocarditis and valve diseases. Most findings described in birds are idiopathic but some are consequences of cardiac compensation (especially in the left atrioventricular valve) or systemic bacterial infections (e.g. *Streptococcus* spp., *Staphylococcus* spp., *Pasteurella multocida*, *Erysipelothrix rhusiopathiae*). Affected birds often demonstrate chronic wasting, oedema and sometimes dyspnoea. Endocarditis can be detected by auscultation or Doppler as it produces a 'clunk' noise. Diagnosis is made by ultrasonography demonstrating the dysfunction of the valves. Birds usually react well to treatment with ACE inhibitors and calcium sensitizers in addition to treatment of the underlying cause.

Arrhythmia: Arrhythmia is commonly found in emaciated birds. However, it is difficult to distinguish if the arrhythmia is the cause for emaciation or if the emaciation caused the arrhythmia due to a severe electrolyte imbalance. Hypocalcaemia is a common cause, especially in African Grey Parrots. Arrhythmia may also be caused by septicaemia or intoxication with organophosphates or other drugs. Birds presented in this condition must immediately be treated as heart failure can occur any time. Further clinical signs include sudden disorientation and opisthotonos, seizures or coma. Arrhythmia is simply diagnosed with auscultation. The patient should be handled with care to avoid stress; in some cases sedation might be necessary. Electrocardiography (ECG) may help to evaluate the kind of arrhythmia, but evaluation is often difficult in birds as they will not lie still without heavy sedation or anaesthesia. ECG probes for small mammals fit most birds without problem. Clips can be a problem because of the thin skin of birds, but needle electrodes work well. Therapy might involve calcium sensitizers and ACE inhibitors for long-term treatment. If the patient is in immediate severe distress, glycosides (digoxin at 10–20 µg/kg q12h) and atropine (0.5 mg/kg i.v.) can be used for immediate short-term treatment.

Liver

The liver is the central organ of metabolism. It has a wide range of functions, including detoxification, protein synthesis and production of biochemicals necessary for digestion. The liver participates in almost every metabolism in the body and is crucial for the function of other organs. Therefore, liver diseases result in poor body condition and weight loss, either by an altered metabolism or due to anorexia. Because of its multidimensional functions, the liver is prone to many diseases. The most common are bacterial, viral and parasitic infections (e.g. herpesvirus, mycobacteriosis, salmonellosis, chlamydiosis, ascarids), fatty liver disease, cirrhosis, neoplasia and drug effects. Many other diseases (e.g. aspergillosis, diabetes mellitus, gout) also interfere with liver function due to indirect effects. Other chronic inflammation, stress or constant exposure to antigens such as aspergillus spores, might lead to the production of amyloid AA proteins, which are deposited in the liver cells, impairing their function. The deposition causes amyloidosis, which is a chronic disease leading to severe emaciation of the bird, despite eating. Chronic liver diseases are common in birds, as the first signs of dysfunction are usually overlooked by the owner. Additionally, in many cases, the liver shows clinical signs only after extensive loss of function; therefore, birds presented are mostly in the end-stage of liver disease.

Green urates accompany many diseases of the liver as a main clinical sign. The green colour is caused by biliverdin, which is excreted with the uric acid. Other obvious clinical signs include anorexia, biliverdinuria, dyspnoea and ataxia, as well as coagulopathies. Liver diseases may be diagnosed by imaging (radiography, ultrasonography), where the silhouette of the liver is larger in diameter than the silhouette of the heart.

Blood chemistry analysis is a very helpful tool. In birds, the elevation of bile acids, aspartate transaminase, alanine transaminase and glutamate dehydrogenase alongside a normal creatine kinase level indicates liver disease (note: creatine kinase may be slightly elevated due to handling stress; this is not to be falsely interpreted as muscle damage). Additionally, the reduction of plasma cholinesterase is a sign of a reduced metabolic capacity of the liver. Triglycerides and cholesterol are elevated in fatty liver syndrome (Figure 28.8). Tuberculosis affects the liver severely but, interestingly, birds do not have a reduced appetite; therefore, a common presentation is a thin bird with a diagnostically affected liver that is still eating normally.

It is important to remember that the liver has a great capacity to regenerate. Treatment should include supplementation of amino acids as well as a dietary change. To support liver metabolism and prevent ammonaemia, milk thistle (15 mg/kg q24h) and lactulose (0.2–1 ml/kg q8–12h) may be supplemented. Birds that are already anorectic should be force-fed with high-protein food to avoid lipidosis.

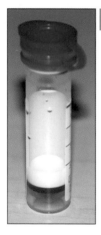

28.8 Severe lipaemia.

Alimentary tract

Oral cavity and crop: Foreign bodies and tissue trauma in the oral cavity and/or crop may lead to sudden unwillingness to ingest food. **Stomatitis** regularly occurs as a consequence of burns after the ingestion of food that is too hot (e.g. crop burn in hand-reared chicks) or caustic agents. Some infections, such as candidiasis, trichomonosis and herpesvirus, may cause stomatitis-like plaques in the upper alimentary tract. Ingluvitis (inflammation of the crop) with dilatation and stasis can be caused by candidiasis, especially in juvenile birds. Other infections, including viral or bacterial, septicaemia, peritonitis, liver or kidney failure, pancreatitis and intoxication with lead or zinc, hyperoestrogenism and neoplasia, are able to cause crop motility disorders as well. These birds are presented with clinical signs such as regurgitation, apathy and anorexia; in most cases the dilatation of the crop can be seen and palpated. Treatment should be chosen according to the origin of the disease. In some cases antiemetics such as metoclopramide (0.3–2 mg/kg q8–24h) can be helpful, although they should be used with care when foreign body obstructions are suspected.

Proventriculus and ventriculus: Disorders of the proventriculus and ventriculus (gizzard) are multifactorial and mostly chronic. In some cases foreign bodies (e.g. rope or cotton fibres) can lead to obstruction and infection. Some foreign bodies (e.g. fibres) are not visible in radiographs and contrast radiography is necessary. Ulceration and inflammation of the proventriculus and ventriculus with hyper- or hypomotility are associated with many infections (e.g. *Macrorhabdus ornithogaster*). In cases of hypomotility, dilatation of the proventriculus is common. This can be caused mechanically (pressure caused by food congestion) or may be infectious (avian bornavirus, candidiasis) or toxic (aflatoxicosis, lead and zinc intoxication). In cases of avian bornavirus, the hypomotility is caused by a neurological inflammation of the ganglia and therefore the proventriculus wall gets very thin and ruptures may occur (Figure 28.9). Birds are presented with clinical signs such as emaciation or cachexia due to the maldigestion. Additionally, fluffed-up feathers, apathy and sometimes undigested food in the faeces are common. Affected birds have a normal appetite despite a constant weight loss. Treatment should include highly digestible food with high protein and fat, as well as the treatment of the underlying cause.

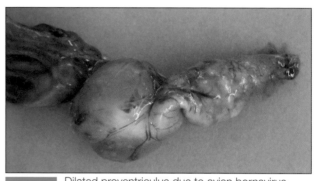

28.9 Dilated proventriculus due to avian bornavirus. Ingested food is visible through the thin wall.

Enteritis: Enteritis is commonly caused by the ingestion of decayed food or poor hygiene management that leads to infection with bacteria such as *Clostridium* spp., *Salmonella* spp., *Yersinia* spp., *Escherichia coli*, *Klebsiella* spp. or *Mycobacterium* spp.. Fungal infections with *Candida* spp. and *Macrorhabdus ornithogaster* should also be considered and, especially in outdoor aviaries, parasitic infection. Commonly, nematodes such as *Capillaria* spp. and *Ascarides* spp., coccidia and *Cryptosporidium* spp. are detected, whereas cestodes are rarely seen in captive birds. Viral infections of the intestine, for example, rotavirus and coronavirus, occur but are difficult to diagnose as the virus quickly disappears once clinical signs develop. Usually, birds with enteritis are presented with alterations in the consistency of the faeces. They are watery or mucilaginous with changes in colour and odour. As a result of the accelerated passage and malabsorption, the bird becomes emaciated and cachectic. In severe cases with intense loss of water and electrolytes, the bird becomes dehydrated with acute clinical signs prior to emaciation. The diagnosis is usually made via faecal analysis, including microbiology and parasitology. In suspected cases of enteritis, microbiological tests, including electron microscopy to detect viral agents, might be helpful. Treatment should include highly digestible food, with high protein and fat, parenteral supplementation of amino acids and electrolytes, and treatment of the underlying cause.

Pancreas

The pancreas is a primary organ for the production of different hormones and enzymes involved in the metabolism. Therefore, pancreatic disorders lead to many different diseases depending on which part is affected. However, all disorders affect parts of the metabolic pathways, resulting in maldigestion or, as in the case of diabetes, metabolic malabsorption and, therefore, emaciation and poor body condition of the bird. Though acute pancreatic disorders may occur, in most cases they are chronic in nature and presented at a late stage to the veterinary surgeon.

Chronic pancreatitis usually involves disorders of enzyme function, in particular trypsin; this leads to maldigestion and malabsorption, in particular of fat. Chronic pancreatitis may be caused by chronic bacterial infections (*Chlamydia*, *Salmonella*, *E. coli*), viral diseases (herpesvirus) or high zinc levels in the diet. Inherited factors may also play a role. Predispositions are obesity, diabetes mellitus and chronic egg laying due to high triglyceride levels in the blood.

Birds presented with chronic pancreatitis have a history of polyphagia with severe weight loss. The faeces are voluminous, soft, grey and fatty; they can be tested using Lugol's solution for undigested starch and with Sudan-II stain for fat. Blood chemistry shows elevation of lipase and amylase and low calcium levels. Treatment should include highly digestible food with high protein, parenteral supplementation of amino acids and electrolytes, as well as oral pancreatic enzymes.

Kidney

The kidney is the main organ for the excretion of nitrogenous products and regulates many trace elements. Kidney diseases are often secondary to many other diseases and kidney failure is commonly a result of other problems. Intoxication often leads to kidney problems. The kidney has an enormous capacity to compensate functional loss and it is estimated that around 70% of function may be lost before clinical signs occur. Therefore, obvious kidney problems are regularly indicative of end-stage disease. Depending on the loss of function, kidney disorders can lead to the loss of water, protein and trace elements. In most cases they are chronic, and constant weight loss of the bird occurs. Additional clinical signs are often non-specific and include emaciation, cachexia, polyuria and polydipsia as well as sometimes oliguria or anuria. End-stage neoplastic cases are sometimes presented with dyspnoea and lameness due to the expansive kidney mass.

Kidney disorders are difficult to diagnose in birds. Few blood chemistry values are specific for the kidney; levels of uric acid, urea, as well as calcium, phosphorus and potassium can be helpful in combination with aspartate transaminase. Only severe kidney damage will be detectable by blood chemistry therefore, diagnostic imaging, especially endoscopy involving a kidney biopsy with subsequent histopathology, is a priority in the diagnosis of kidney disease. Severe enlargement of the organ will be detectable on radiographs as well. Sometimes contrast radiography might be beneficial, and could involve either barium sulphate to highlight the intestine or intravenous iodine contrast to highlight the kidney and excretional function. In some cases kidney cysts and neoplasias are detectable by ultrasonography. For specific diagnosis of amyloidosis (Figure 28.10), the kidney biopsy sample is stained with

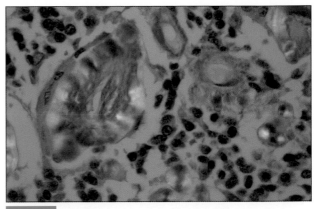

28.10 Amyloidosis in the kidney. (Courtesy of H Pendl)

Congo red. Treatment of kidney disorders involves extensive diuresis to restore kidney function. Electrolytes should be balanced and rechecked often to prevent other metabolic functions from being impaired. Tyrode solution (electrolyte solution with 0.8% sodium chloride (NaCl), 0.02% potassium chloride (KCl), 0.02% calcium chloride (CaCl$_2$), 0.01% magnesium chloride (MgCl$_2$), 0.005% monosodium phosphate (NaH$_2$PO$_4$), 0.1% glucose and 0.1% sodium bicarbonate (NaHCO$_3$) should be provided to increase renal function followed by sodium-reduced drinking water. Additional therapy should focus on the underlying cause.

Neoplasia: Neoplasia originating from the kidney is very common in elderly Budgerigars. Adenocarcinoma, cystadenocarcinoma and nephroblastoma are most common.

Inflammation: Inflammation is the most common kidney disorder in birds. It can be histopathologically divided into nephritis and glomerulonephritis. Inflammation may be caused by general infections with bacteria (*Chlamydia* infections are specifically described). Some systemic viral diseases are also known to cause kidney inflammation (e.g. polyomavirus, herpesvirus). Kidney-specific coccidia cause granulomatous nephritis in some species. Chronic nephritis can cause nephrosis, a non-inflammatory nephropathy, which is a degenerative disease of the renal tubules.

Nutritional kidney disease: Nutritional kidney diseases are often seen in birds on non-formulated diets or seed-only diets. High-protein and calcium levels and deficiency of vitamins A, D$_3$ and B in the diet, as well as irregular water intake, can cause gout. In some cases a genetic heritage is suspected. Gout frequently occurs in combination with other medical problems such as obesity, hypertension, abnormal lipid levels, lead poisoning, renal failure and haemolytic anaemia. All these conditions lead to high levels of uric acid in the blood, which is the underlying cause of gout and its signs. Gout may affect the kidney only or involve the serosal membranes as well (Figure 28.11). In such cases death occurs quickly. In some cases articular gout occurs, resulting in inflammatory arthritis, which is usually recognized early by the owner.

Hypervitaminosis D$_3$: Hypervitaminosis D$_3$ and high calcium levels can lead to calcification of the kidney with non-specific clinical signs and is described especially in large macaws.

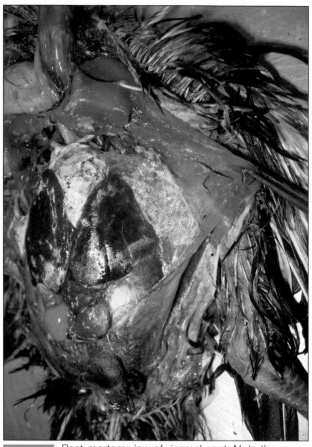

28.11 Post-mortem view of visceral gout. Note the powder-like coating of the serosa.

Common primary infectious diseases causing weight loss in birds

- **Bacterial:**
  - *Mycobacterium avium* spp. (*Mycobacterium avium* complex (MAC))
  - *Clostridium* spp. (e.g. *Clostridium perfringens*)
  - *Salmonella* spp.
  - *Escherichia coli*
  - *Klebsiella* spp.
  - *Yersinia* spp.
  - *Chlamydia* spp.
- **Fungal:**
  - *Candida* spp.
  - *Macrorhabdus ornithogaster*
  - *Aspergillus* spp.
- **Viral:**
  - Papillomaviruses
  - Herpesviruses
  - Avian adenovirus
  - Avian paramyxoviruses APMV-1 (Newcastle disease) and APMV-3
  - Avian bornavirus
- **Parasitic:**
  - *Trichomonas gallinae*
  - *Giardia* spp., *Hexamita* spp., *Cochlosoma* spp.
  - Coccidia
  - *Cryptosporidium* spp.
  - *Atoxoplasma* spp.
  - *Ascaridia* spp.
  - *Capillaria* spp.
  - Cestodes

(For description of the agents, see Chapter 19)

Amyloidosis: Amyloidosis is often seen in birds with chronic inflammatory diseases or constant activation of the immune system by external factors (e.g. high loads of *Aspergillus* spores, toxins) or stress. It is characterized by the deposition of the protein amyloid AA in the kidney cells, resulting in a loss of organ function.

Treatment of the emaciated patient

In avian practice, most patients are an emergency, especially if they are in poor condition with weight loss. Birds tend to mask ill health in order to keep themselves safe from predators. Therefore, owners usually only become aware of clinical signs at an advanced stage of the disease process.

Fluid therapy

Usually patients that are emaciated or cachectic are also dehydrated; fluid therapy is essential for recovery. In severe cases, circulation may be already affected due to shock. The typical signs of shock are low blood pressure, rapid heartbeat and poor end-organ perfusion. Fluids applied subcutaneously are poorly absorbed; therefore, to achieve a fast recovery, the preferred initial action should be intravenous administration. Fluids can be supplied as a bolus at 5 ml/kg or as a constant rate infusion. In larger birds, an intravenous catheter can be placed in the brachiocephalic or femoral vein. In smaller patients it is recommended to place an intraosseous catheter in the ulna or the tibiotarsus (Figure 28.12; see Chapter 15).

The rate of the infusion depends on the condition of the bird:

- For a short period of time (emergency): up to 20–40 ml/kg/h
- For maintenance: 2 ml/kg/h is sufficient, set at constant for several hours (see Chapters 11 and 15)
- For acute liver support and instant energy: a mixture of Ringer's solution and 5% glucose at a ratio of 1:1 can be used.

For short-term emergency management the Ringer's solution and glucose mixture can also be administered to carnivorous species, but for maintenance only glucose-free solutions should be given to carnivorous species. Glucose is the general metabolic agent that can be metabolized by any cell and is the fastest correction tool in the metabolic response to starvation. For support of liver function and restocking of the depots for protein synthesis, parenteral amino acids should be administered.

In birds without circulatory distress and for long-term administration, fluids can be given subcutaneously at 20–100 ml/kg once or twice daily, depending on the rate of dehydration. In birds with unknown, or questionable, renal function care must be taken at the high end of the dose range given, as hypervolaemia can occur.

Fluid replacement:

dehydration (%) x bodyweight (kg) x 1000 ml = fluids (ml)

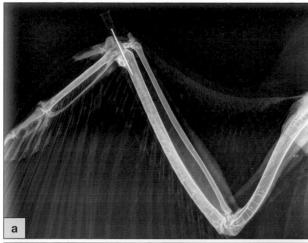

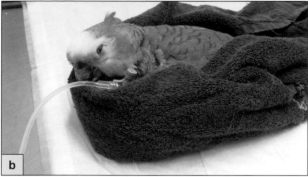

28.12 Intraosseous catheters. **(a)** Radiographic view. **(b)** Patient with an intraosseous catheter in the ulna is wrapped in a towel during intensive care treatment.

Heat therapy

In cachectic birds, loss of body protein affects the function of important organs. To reduce the loss of further energy and help stabilization, it is highly recommended that the patient is warmed. Birds can be placed into custom-made clima-boxes (Figure 28.13). Inside these boxes, the regulation of temperature and air humidity ensures that the bird will not overheat (which can happen quickly in weak birds under heat lamps as they are unable to move away from the heat to self-regulate temperature). In emergency cases, infrared light or similar heat sources are sufficient, but the patient needs to be monitored closely and a thermostat should be used (see also Chapter 11).

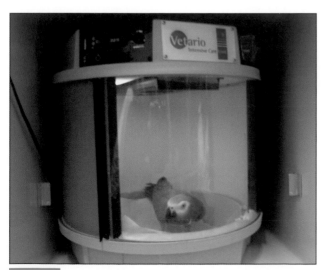

28.13 Custom-made clima-box for heat therapy.

Nutrition

If the bird is stable enough and there is no risk of regurgitation, the emaciated patient should be force-fed as soon as possible with highly digestible food, consisting of high protein and fat in small portions (not more than approximately 2–5% of bodyweight per feed). The absorption of fat in birds is up to 98–99%. There are many critical care formulations available, depending on whether the bird is a seed-eater, insectivore or carnivore (see also Chapters 6 and 11).

Oral omega-3 fatty acid supplements such as fish oil improve appetite and bodyweight. Fatty acids can be used directly as an energy source by most tissues in the body. L-carnitine is required for the transport of fatty acids from the cytosol into the mitochondria during the decomposition of lipids for metabolic energy. Therefore, oral formulations of L-carnitine (1000 mg/kg per feed) should be added to the diet.

In birds presented with digestive problems or pancreatitis with maldigestion of fat, enzymes should be supplemented to the food for better absorption. For long-term success, birds should be switched to a formulated diet (especially herbivorous birds) (see Chapter 6).

Blood transfusion

In severe cases of emaciated, and therefore very weak, birds, and in patients with kidney and liver diseases, anaemia and/or coagulopathy is commonly present. In these cases, a blood transfusion is indicated to overcome the critical stage. A slow bolus of 5 ml/kg of fresh blood mixed with citrate at a ratio of 5:1 can be given intravenously. If one bolus is not enough, the treatment can be repeated some time later to avoid circulatory distress. Preferably, the donor blood should be from the same species as the recipient, but in emergencies it can be taken from other species as well. The rule of thumb is that the closer the recipient and donor species are, the longer the erythrocytes live. If a second blood transfusion is necessary days later, a cross-matching test between both birds (if the same species) should be performed prior to transfusion; if a different species' blood was used in the first transfusion, then the second transfusion should be from another different species. Vitamin B and iron should be supplemented because they are crucial for the synthesis of red blood cells. For coagulation disorders, an additional injection of vitamin K (0.2–2.5 mg/kg q6–12h) is recommended.

Summary of treatment of the emaciated patient

- **Fluid therapy**
  - Initial intravenous bolus (5 ml/kg; 1:1: Ringer's solution and 5% glucose) OR
  - Constant rate infusion (initially 20–40 ml/kg/h; maintenance 2 ml/kg/h) OR
  - Subcutaneous fluids (40–100 ml/kg once or twice daily)
- **Heat therapy**
  - Custom-made clima-boxes with temperature and humidity management (see Figure 28.13)
  - Other heat sources require careful observation
- **Nutritional therapy**
  - Glucose for rapid energy
  - Fatty acids for direct tissue energy; fat can be absorbed at 98–99%
  - L-carnitine for transport
  - Enzymes in cases of maldigestion
  - Amount of food should not exceed 2–5 % of bodyweight per feed (Figure 28.14)

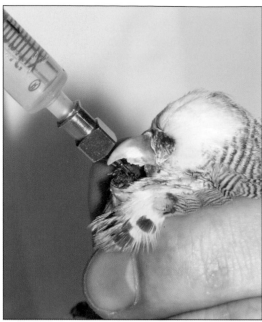

28.14 A crop cannula can be used for force-feeding or to provide oral medication.

References and further reading

Camus AC and Heatley J (2001) What is your diagnosis? *Journal of Avian Medicine and Surgery* **15**, 54–57

Christen C (2011) Klinische Untersuchung. In: *Leitsymptome bei Papageien und Sittichen*, ed. M Pees, pp. 6–10. Enke Verlag, Stuttgart

Doneley B, Harrison GJ and Lightfoot TL (2006) Maximizing information from the physical examination. In: *Clinical Avian Medicine Volume I*, ed. GJ Harrison and TL Lightfoot, pp. 153–154. Spix Publishing, Palm Beach

Dubé C, Dubois I and Struthers K (2011) Intravenous and intraosseous fluid therapy in critically ill birds of prey. *Journal of Exotic Pet Medicine* **20(1)**, 21–26

Gerlach H (2001) Megabacteriosis. *Seminars in Avian and Exotic Pet Medicine* **10**, 12–19

Harrison GJ and McDonald D (2006) Nutritional considerations. In: *Clinical Avian Medicine Volume I*, ed. GJ Harrison and TL Lightfoot, pp. 85–108. Spix Publishing, Palm Beach

Henderson GM, Gulland FMD and Hawkey CM (1988) Haematological findings in Budgerigars with megabacterium and trichomonas infections associated with 'going light'. *Veterinary Record* **123**, 492–494

Honkavouri KS, Shivaprasad HL, Williams BL *et al.* (2008) Novel bornavirus in psittacine birds with proventricular dilatation disease. *Emerging Infectious Diseases* **14**, 1883–1886

Jones MP and Orosz SE (1996) Overview of avian neurology and neurological diseases. *Seminars in Avian and Exotic Pet Medicine* **5(3)**, 150–164

Kistler AL, Gancz A, Clubb S *et al.* (2008) Recovery of divergent avian bornaviruses from cases of proventricular dilatation disease. Identification of an candidate etiologic agent. *Virology Journal* **5**, 88

Kradin RL and Mark EJ (2008) The pathology of pulmonary disorders due to *Aspergillus* spp. *Archives of Pathology and Laboratory Medicine* **132(4)**, 606–614

Krautwald-Junghanns ME and Kummerfeld N (2011) Kapitel: Erkrankungen des Herzens und der großen Blutgefäße. In: *Kompendium der Ziervogelkrankheiten*, ed. EF Kaleta and ME Krautwalk-Junghanns, pp. 169–177. Schlütersche Verlagsgesellschaft, Hannover

Lennox AM and Lichtenberger M (2011) Advanced fluid support for birds. In: *Scientific Proceedings of the Association of Avian Veterinarians 2011*, pp. 185–190. Association of Avian Veterinarians, New Jersey

Lichtenberger M (2004) Principles of shock and fluid therapy in special species. *Seminars in Avian and Exotic Pet Medicine* **13(3)**, 142–153

Lichtenberger M (2004) The avian cardiovascular system: anatomy and physiology for the clinician. In: *Proceedings of the 25th Annual Association of Avian Veterinarians Conference and Expo, Avian Specialty Advanced Program*, pp. 11–23. Association of Avian Veterinarians, New Jersey

Lierz M (2005) Avian renal disease: pathogenesis, diagnosis and therapy. In: *Veterinary Clinics of North America – Clinics Collection: Exotic Animal Practice*, ed. AE Rupley, pp. 241–260. WB Saunders, Philadelphia

McGavin MD and Zachary JF (2007) *Pathologic basis of veterinary disease, 4th edn.* Mosby/Elsevier, St Louis

Orosz SE (2004) The avian cardiovascular system: anatomy and physiology for the clinician. In: *Proceedings of the 25th Annual Association of Avian Veterinarians Conference and Expo, Avian Specialty Advanced Program*, pp. 3–10. Association of Avian Veterinarians, New Jersey

Pees M and Krautwald-Junghanns ME (2009) Cardiovascular physiology and diseases of pet birds. In: *Veterinary Clinics of North America: Exotic Animal Practice, Cardiology* **12(1)**, 81–97

Rinder M, Ackermann A, Kempf H *et al.* (2009) Broad tissue and cell tropism of avian bornavirus in parrots with proventricular dilatation disease. *Journal of Virology* **83**, 5401–5407

Rosenthal K, Miller M, Orosz S and Dorrestein GM (1997) Cardiovascular system. In: *Avian Medicine and Surgery*, ed. RB Altman, SL Clubb, GM Dorrestein and K Quesenberry, pp. 489–500. WB Saunders, Philadelphia

Schmidt RE, Reavill DR and Phalen DN (2003) *Pathology of Pet and Aviary Birds*. Iowa State Press, Ames

Wang T, Hung C and Randall D (2006) The comparative physiology of food deprivation: from feast to famine. *Annual Review of Physiology* **68**, 223–251

Case example 1: African Grey Parrot with chronic weight loss and acute seizures

Presentation and history

A 26-year-old African Grey Parrot presented with chronic weight loss (slow weight loss over a several-month period with normal appetite) and a recent history of short sudden seizures with unconsciousness during the day.

Clinical examination

On examination the bird was found to have:

- Slightly unbalanced movements
- Blue skin around the eyes
- Poor body condition with loss of muscle; bodyweight 356 g (species reference: 450–500 g)
- Muffled heart sounds with arrhythmia; indicative of cardiac syncope on auscultation.

Diagnostic work-up

- Blood chemistry: elevated creatine kinase (980 IU/l; reference: 50–850 IU/l); low calcium (0.51 mg/l; reference: 0.8–1.4 mg/l)
- Complete blood count: elevated haematocrit (60%; reference: 35–45%), moderately elevated estimated white blood cell count with heterophils (28 x 10⁹/l; reference: 10–25 x 10⁹/l)
- Radiography: enlarged heart shadow, enlarged vessels
- Ultrasonography under sedation: pericardial effusion, enlarged right ventricle, decreased contractility, indicative of cardiac syncope

▶

Case example 1 continued

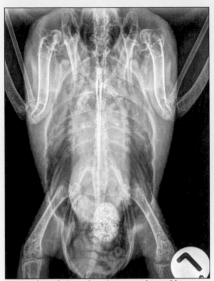

Ventrodorsal view showing an enlarged heart shadow.

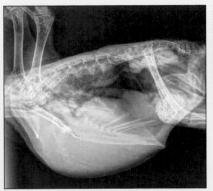

Laterolateral view showing enlarged vessels.

Therapy

The bird was diagnosed with pericardial effusion, dilatative cardiomyopathy and syncope and treated with:

- Enalapril at 0.5 mg/kg q12h
- Pimobendan at 0.3 mg/kg q12h
- Furosemide at 0.2 mg/kg q24h
- Fluids at 100 ml/kg

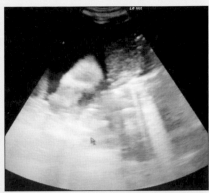

Ultrasonogram of the pericardial effusion.

Outcome

Therapy improved the health of the bird significantly. The bird was stable under life-long therapy with enalapril and pimobendan.

Case example 2: Blue-fronted Amazon with liver fibrosis

History and presentation

A 10-year-old Blue-fronted Amazon was presented with anorexia, sudden weight loss and apathy.

Clinical examination

On examination the bird was found to have:

- Severe loss of muscle tissue
- Depots of body fat under the skin
- An enlarged abdomen
- Respiratory distress during examination
- Severe apathy, reacting only when touched.

Diagnostic work-up

- Plasma highly lipaemic
- Blood chemistry: elevated blood ammonia (255 mmol/l; reference: 35–60 mmol/l), elevated aspartate aminotransferase (1500 IU/l; normal: 130–350 IU/l), elevated triglycerides (13 mmol/l; reference: 1–2 mmol/l), elevated cholesterol (25.2 mmol/l; reference: 3–7 mmol/l)
- Radiography: enlarged liver silhouette
- Ultrasonography: highly irregular liver tissue, liver and bile ducts enlarged
- Endoscopy: enlarged liver, yellow-green colour on biopsy
- Histology of the liver biopsy sample: anisokaryosis, anisocytosis, liver fibrosis

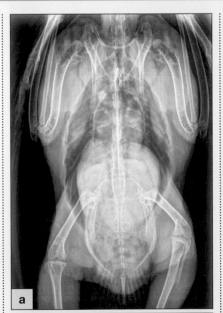

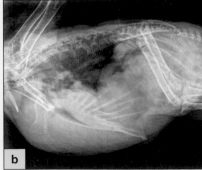

(a) Vendrodorsal and (b) laterolateral views of an enlarged liver silhouette.

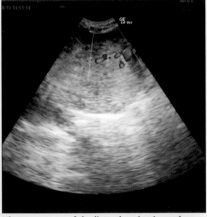

Ultrasonogram of the liver showing irregular tissue and enlarged bile ducts and vessels.

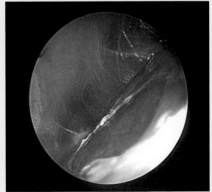

Endoscopic image of the yellow-green discoloration of the liver.

Therapy

The parrot was diagnosed with acute lipidosis due to anorexia and former obesity and chronic liver fibrosis.
Acute lipidosis therapy:

- Intravenous fluid therapy with Ringer's solution and glucose (ratio 1:1) at 2 ml/kg/h
- Force-feeding with high-protein food and lactulose after stabilization.

Chronic liver fibrosis therapy:

- Formulated diet
- Injection of vitamin B_{12} at 25 μg/kg s.c.

once weekly (for 4–6 weeks)
- Omega-3 and omega-6 fatty acids (fish oil) at 1 ml/kg
- Silimarin at 125 mg/kg.

Outcome

The bird recovered with therapy. After changing its diet the bird returned to health.

Case example 3: Golden Parakeet with avian bornavirus

Presentation and history

A 4-year-old Golden Parakeet was presented with a 4-week history of making baby feeding sounds, rocking behaviour, severe weight loss with normal food intake, and decreased frequency of droppings that, when present, included undigested seeds.

Clinical examination

On examination the bird was found to have:

- Poor body condition (190 g; species normal: 250 g)
- Poor general condition
- Neurological signs (swaying, rocking, difficulty perching).

Diagnostic work-up

- Complete blood count: decreased haematocrit (26%), elevated estimated white blood cell count (36 x 10^9/l)
- Blood chemistry: low calcium (0.42 mg/l; reference: 0.8–1.4 mg/l); high creatine kinase (1800 IU/l; reference: 50–850 IU/l)
- Crop and cloacal swabs negative for yeast and Gram-negative bacteria
- Radiography: enlarged proventriculus
- Avian bornavirus polymerase chain reaction (PCR): parrot bornavirus positive (ct:15.4)
- Avian bornavirus serology: 1:2,500

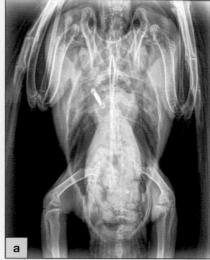

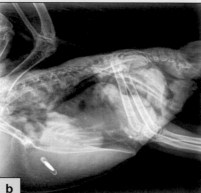

(a) Ventrodorsal and **(b)** laterolateral views of an enlarged proventriculus.

Therapy

The parrot was diagnosed with avian bornavirus infection (proventricular dilatation disease; PDD), and had a poor prognosis. Palliative therapy was instituted:

- Formulated diet
- Fluid therapy at 40 ml/kg electrolyte solution
- Mineral and vitamin supplementation
- Non-steroidal anti-inflammatory drugs (celecoxib at 15 mg/kg q12h).

Outcome

At first the bird improved with therapy. The bird seemed to recover with constant non-steroidal anti-inflammatory drugs initially, but after 3 months, the bird had to be euthanased due to poor general condition and emaciation.

Wing and leg trauma

Brett Gartrell

The diagnosis and treatment of musculoskeletal injuries in birds (Figure 29.1) share much common ground with the approaches used in mammalian medicine. The same diagnostic modalities, principles of wound healing and methods of fracture stabilization apply. It is important to remember these fundamental principles when approaching such injuries in birds.

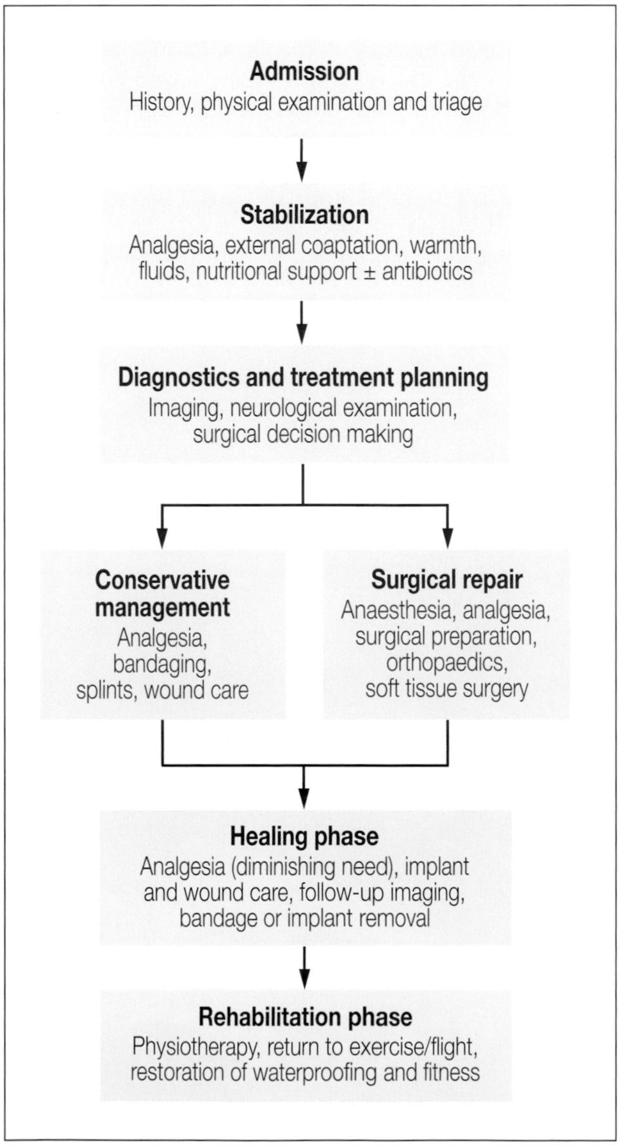

Admission
History, physical examination and triage

↓

Stabilization
Analgesia, external coaptation, warmth, fluids, nutritional support ± antibiotics

↓

Diagnostics and treatment planning
Imaging, neurological examination, surgical decision making

↓

Conservative management
Analgesia, bandaging, splints, wound care

Surgical repair
Anaesthesia, analgesia, surgical preparation, orthopaedics, soft tissue surgery

↓

Healing phase
Analgesia (diminishing need), implant and wound care, follow-up imaging, bandage or implant removal

↓

Rehabilitation phase
Physiotherapy, return to exercise/flight, restoration of waterproofing and fitness

29.1 Flow chart for the diagnosis and treatment of limb injuries.

> **Key points: anatomy (see also Chapter 2)**
> - Pneumatized bones connect to the respiratory system and have a periosteal blood supply that must be preserved during fracture repair
> - Avian bone is more brittle than mammalian bone and more likely to splinter when fracturing or during repair
> - Adaptations for flight have resulted in anatomical differences from mammalian anatomy, for example, the keel, coracoids and synsacrum
> - The primary wing feathers insert directly on to the periosteum of the ulna and primary tail feathers insert on to the pygostyle

Initial assessment

Triage of the patient and injury is best performed at an early stage. This requires a holistic assessment of the patient. A bird that has a poor prognosis for return of function may need to be euthanased. Indicators of a poor prognosis for return to function include: loss of nerve or blood supply below the injury; injuries close to or involving a joint; multiple injuries; and open contaminated wounds or fractures. While this chapter focuses on musculoskeletal injuries, a holistic appraisal of all body systems (see Chapter 10) should contribute to triage. For example, ocular injuries may limit return to function even if all musculoskeletal injuries can be repaired.

Having made an initial assessment of the injury, supportive care of the patient is critical. Fluid therapy, analgesia, thermal and nutritional support are all critical in any avian emergency. Fluid therapy is also critical for maintaining good blood perfusion to the limbs. For limb injuries, consideration should be given to initial wound care that supports soft tissues and minimizes desiccation and further contamination of wounds. This may include gentle plucking of wound edges, light debridement, lavage, sparing use of antiseptic or hydrocolloid topical agents and dressings. Fractures should be supported by appropriate external coaptation to provide analgesia, minimize further trauma to tissues and protect feathers from damage (see Chapter 17). Non-adhesive bandages are ideal for this purpose.

> ### Key points: first aid and triage (see also Chapter 11)
>
> - Control haemorrhage
> - Provide analgesia
> - Assess the neurological and vascular integrity of the limbs early and often
> - Stabilize fractured limbs with bandages or splints
> - Treat and prevent contamination of open wounds
> - Protect the feathers

In cases of severe trauma or with wild patients, having carried out this initial first aid and triage, a period of supportive care before proceeding with diagnostics is often advisable to allow a patient's condition to stabilize. This is counterbalanced by the need to provide timely surgical intervention. A period of stabilization of 12–24 hours is often beneficial in improving anaesthetic and surgical outcomes.

> ### Key points: feather care
>
> - Feathers are needed for flight, thermal insulation and waterproofing
> - Pluck feathers for surgical preparation, **do not clip**. Use minimal surgical margins to prevent heat loss
> - Feathers touching open wounds incite an inflammatory response and should be removed
> - Remove blood, exudates, faeces and urates from feathers with warm soapy water and rinse well
> - On feathered areas use non-adhesive bandages only
> - Provide perches or blocks
> - Put tail protectors on long-tailed perching birds and all raptors in hospital (see Chapter 9)

Diagnosis of musculoskeletal injury to the limbs

The key component for diagnosing and managing injuries to the limbs of birds is a careful and comprehensive physical examination, repeated at regular intervals throughout the course of the bird's treatment and recovery from injury. Observation will provide information about the carriage of the wings and weight-bearing on the limbs. When assessing wing carriage, look for symmetry between the wings, and look to see that the wings are folded close and comfortably to the body without drooping. The 'spring test' of stretching the wing and releasing it to see how it returns to resting position is a very useful test of wing function (see **Spring Test 1** and **2** clips on CD). With subtle injuries, observing the bird in flight can provide important information. For example, injuries to the keel and coracoids may result in a bird that appears clinically normal at rest but is unable to gain height in flight. Weight-bearing on the hindlimbs is ideally assessed at a walk. While stance at rest can be helpful, it is

important to take into account that birds have a tendon-locking mechanism in their legs that allows them to stand on one leg for prolonged periods without fatigue.

During the physical examination the limbs should be palpated for symmetry, muscle tone and evidence of injury, such as swelling, crepitus or laxity. It is best to work systematically from proximal to distal along the limb, using the contralateral limb for comparison. Careful palpation of the thoracic inlet can sometimes detect injuries to the coracoids, keel and clavicles. Alcohol can be used sparingly to part feathers along the limb to check for bruising and haemorrhage. Manipulate all joints to check for range of motion and discomfort. Carefully examine the plantar surfaces of the feet and nails for injury and inflammation.

The vascular integrity of the limbs is assessed by: examining the colour and warmth of soft tissues; needle pricks to draw blood spots from the distal limbs; and the filling time of the peripheral veins (brachial and ulnar veins in the wing, medial tarsometatarsal and saphenous vein in the legs). In medium to large birds, blood flow can be assessed by using Doppler monitors (Figure 29.2) and ultrasonography. Early indicators of vascular compromise include oedema of the distal tissues, darkening of the colour of the soft tissues and cooling of the limb. If these signs are detected, ensure that good fluid therapy is in place to maintain blood perfusion, keep the bird in a warm environment, use non-steroidal anti-inflammatory drugs such as meloxicam, or peripheral vasodilators such as isoxsuprine to reduce swelling, and ensure bandages do not restrict blood flow to the distal limb. The application of topical heat may be used to encourage blood flow in compliant patients.

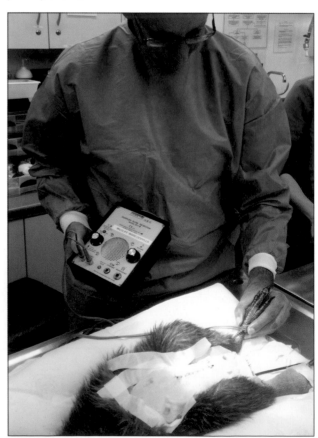

29.2   Using a Doppler monitor to assess limb blood flow.

Neurological examination of the limbs uses the principles of mammalian neurology adapted to the anatomy of the bird's limbs. For example, wheel-barrowing is inappropriate in avian patients. Withdrawal reflexes, proprioception, perception of painful stimuli and reflex arcs, such as the patellar reflex, are the simplest neurological tests to use. Following a detailed protocol for neurological examination of birds is recommended. Complete loss of neurological function associated with traumatic injury suggests a grave prognosis, whereas partial loss of function should be viewed more optimistically as return of neurological function after the resolution of swelling and inflammation is common. Complete loss of neurological function in the limb in the absence of other injury may suggest either spinal haemorrhage or contusion, or an avulsion of the brachial or inguinal plexus. Both of these have a poor prognosis. More advanced electroneurodiagnostics are available for assessing nerve function, but are often limited by a lack of basic biological information on avian neurophysiology.

All birds with suspected musculoskeletal injury to the limbs should be examined by radiography. A minimum of two orthogonal views of both the affected and unaffected limbs is required for an accurate assessment of limb injury. For conventional radiography, fine detail screens or mammography plates are needed to give good extremity detail. Computed tomography can be useful in the diagnosis of shoulder, pelvic and spinal fractures where the overlapping structures make conventional radiography difficult to interpret (see also Chapter 18).

More advanced diagnostic techniques such as magnetic resonance imaging and scintigraphy are available in referral centres but are generally not required for most cases.

Treatment principles and techniques

The basic principles of treatment of injuries to the wings and legs of birds broadly follow those in mammalian medicine, but are sometimes limited by the size of avian patients, the limited soft tissues on the distal limbs, the brittleness of avian bone and the differences in musculoskeletal anatomy.

Key points: treatment choices

- Fully assess all injuries before attempting surgical repair
- Loss of vascular supply below a fracture necessitates amputation of the limb or euthanasia
- Loss of neurological function can sometimes be temporary, due to inflammation and swelling; surgery is best postponed until severity and prognosis are more fully apparent
- Dislocations are emergencies; rapid resolution is critical to treatment success
- Fractures that involve the joint or come within approximately 10 mm of joint surfaces carry a poor prognosis for full return to function
- Contaminated compound fractures of pneumatized bones often result in refractory osteomyelitis and can progress to pneumonia and airsacculitis. Early and aggressive treatment is essential

---

Soft tissue wounds are best managed using surgical debridement and lavage followed by either primary or secondary skin closure where possible. The limited skin and soft tissue available, combined with the need to maintain feather alignment, means that many wounds are left to heal by second intention. Skin advancement flaps can be used in the upper areas of the leg and wing. Infection must be cleared from wounds before attempting closure. Once a clean wound bed is established, hydrocolloid gels and dressing are useful in promoting re-epithelialization.

Orthopaedic repair using external coaptation, internal fixation techniques (such as intramedullary pinning) and external fixator devices are commonly used in avian practice. Bone screws and plates are used more rarely in avian practice due to the brittleness of avian bone and the predisposition of the bones to crack. More information on bandaging and surgical techniques can be found in Chapter 17. A summary of the advantages and disadvantages of these commonly used techniques is provided in Figures 29.3 and 29.4. Ideally, postoperative radiographs should be taken to assess the success of surgery and guide postoperative care plans.

Bone grafting is often useful in the repair of malunions, delayed unions and fractures with large cortical defects in the bone. The principles of bone grafting include having rigid fixation of fracture ends, a good vascular supply, and the absence of infection at the grafting site. Suitable sites for harvesting bone grafts include the tibiotarsus, ribs and keel. Pneumatized bones are not suitable sites from which to harvest bone graft material; when grafting into pneumatized bones, care should be taken to ensure the graft comes into contact with periosteal blood supply to ensure vascularization of the grafted bone.

Amputation should be considered only as a salvage procedure when return of function to the limb cannot be achieved. Some indications for limb amputation include avascular necrosis, complete loss of neurological function, refractory osteomyelitis or arthritis. While difficult to confirm, phantom pain is likely to occur in avian patients, similar to that seen in humans and mammals. An amputation should occur only if the bird has a good quality of life post-surgery. Most wild birds will not be able to survive with an amputated limb. Some birds, such as macaws, will be unable to breed successfully with an amputation so careful consultation with owners is required before proceeding.

On the other hand, many companion birds have a good quality of life post-amputation of a wing or leg. With leg amputations, if a weight-bearing surface can be salvaged, such as the scaled skin of the hock, this can reduce postoperative complications of pressure sores and wound breakdown. Leg amputations should only go ahead if the contralateral limb is sound, and owners should be warned to watch for complications in the remaining leg such as pododermatitis and arthritis. Complications of leg amputation are more likely in larger birds, although definitive size limits have not been established (some sources state that birds >100 g are more likely to develop problems). Postoperative management of substrates and perches to provide clean and cushioned surfaces is important in reducing these complications. Padding of perches with non-fibrous material may also be useful in protecting the stump especially in heavier birds.

Site of injury	Anatomical considerations	Recommended treatment options	Common complications of the injury
Coracoid and keel	Pneumatized bones Close proximity to heart	Wing to body bandage Intramedullary pinning of coracoid fractures for precision flyers	Pulmonary haemorrhage Ankylosis of shoulder Cardiac damage
Clavicles; scapula	Thoracic inlet diameter Small, fragile bones	Wing to body bandage Cage confinement only	Ankylosis of shoulder Slow crop emptying
Shoulder joint	Complex tendon structures that enable flight	Luxation: ■ Stable after reduction – wing to body bandage ■ Unstable after reduction – surgical stabilization Fracture: ■ Wing to body bandage, poor prognosis	Ankylosis of shoulder Loss of flight Brachial plexus avulsion
Humerus	Pneumatized bone Fractures will displace and over-ride	Tied-in external fixator and intramedullary pin Intramedullary pin and wing to body bandage (small birds) Bone plate (very large birds)	Non-unions and malunions Osteomyelitis Pneumonia and airsacculitis Propatagium contracture
Elbow	Minimal soft tissues Fragility of nerve and blood supply	Luxation: ■ Stable after reduction – figure-of-eight bandage ■ Unstable after reduction – transarticular fixator Fracture: ■ Transarticular fixator, poor prognosis ■ Wing to body bandage, poor prognosis	Arthritis Chronic dislocations Joint ankylosis
Radius and ulna	Ulna is larger than radius Medullary bones Primary wing feathers insert on the ulna	Only one bone fractured – figure-of-eight bandage Both fractured – intramedullary pinning of both or external fixator of ulna	Propatagium contracture Joint ankylosis Synostosis leading to loss of wing pronation/supination
Carpus; carpometacarpus	Minimal soft tissues Fragility of nerve and blood supply	Splints and bandage to antebrachium Internal fixation/external fixators in large birds	Wing tip oedema Devascularization

29.3   Recommended treatment options for injuries of the forelimb of birds by injury location.

Site of injury	Anatomical considerations	Recommended treatment options	Common complications
Synsacrum	Fusion of hip and spine Proximity of kidneys Pneumatized bones Open ventrally	Cage rest	Loss of nerve function to tail, legs and cloaca Haemorrhage and contusion to spinal cord
Hip	Limited rotation compared with mammals Proximity of kidneys	Luxation: ■ Stable after reduction – cage rest, slinging or spica splint ■ Unstable after reduction – surgical stabilization Acetabular or femoral head fractures: ■ Femoral head excision (controversial in heavy birds)	Renal haemorrhage and infarction Chronic dislocations Arthritis Sciatic palsy
Femur	Pneumatized bone Fractures will displace and over-ride	Tied-in external fixator and intramedullary pin Intramedullary pins and spica splint (small birds) Plate in very large birds	Non-unions and malunions Osteomyelitis Sciatic palsy
Stifle	Minimal soft tissues Care with collateral ligaments	Luxation: ■ Stable after reduction – spica splint ■ Unstable after reduction – transarticular external fixator, or conjoined intramedullary pins (one in femur, one in tibiotarsus) Fracture: ■ Transarticular external fixator, poor prognosis	Chronic instability Arthritis Joint ankylosis
Tibiotarsus; tarsometatarsus	Medullary bones Lateral and medial vessels	External fixators (type 1b and 2 preferred) Intramedullary pin and Robert Jones bandage (small birds)	Joint ankylosis Osteomyelitis
Hock	Scaly inflexible skin Minimal soft tissues Care with collateral ligaments	Luxation: ■ Stable after reduction – half-cast splint or Robert Jones bandage ■ Unstable after reduction – type 1 transarticular fixator or half-cast splint Fracture: ■ Type 1 transarticular fixator or half-cast splint, poor prognosis	Chronic instability Arthritis Joint ankylosis
Pedal joint, foot and phalanges	Scaly inflexible skin Minimal soft tissues Medullary bones	Shoe splints for land birds Ball bandages for perching birds	Pododermatitis Arthritis Self-mutilation (parrots)

29.4   Recommended treatment options for injuries of the hindlimb of birds by injury location.

Postoperative care and rehabilitation

The surgical or conservative stabilization of limb injuries is only a step on the path to recovery. As much care and attention to postoperative care must be given as to the surgery itself if a successful outcome is to be achieved. This care consists of the postoperative period, physiotherapy and rehabilitative exercise aiming to return the limb to full function.

Postoperative care of patients with limb injuries involves good supportive care including species-specific husbandry, analgesia, prevention of infection and care of bandages and/or surgical implants. Cleaning and monitoring pin tracts for infection is vital to prevent osteomyelitis. Analgesia protocols vary widely as there are limited pharmacokinetic data to support clinical avian medicine. The author currently uses butorphanol at 4 mg/kg i.m. q6–12h in the pre-operative, intraoperative and immediate postoperative phases based on subjective assessments of the degree of pain. Following surgery, this analgesia is blended with meloxicam at 0.5 mg/kg orally q12h in conjunction with oral or intravenous fluid therapy. The response to analgesia of avian patients is highly variable and such decisions need to be based on an assessment of the stability of the injury repair, the behavioural responses to analgesia and withdrawal of analgesia, including appetite, demeanour and carriage of the injured limb.

Physiotherapy

The aim of physiotherapy is to maintain and restore limb function, in particular the mobility of joints and muscle tone and strength. It also aids in restoring proprioceptive function of the affected limb. Physiotherapy needs to start early in the recovery period but this is balanced by the need to maintain fracture stability. Physiotherapy should be introduced gradually, and a good physiotherapy protocol does not exhaust the patient or slow healing times. Rest days from physiotherapy are recommended. The simplest protocol for physiotherapy is to remove bandages on a weekly basis and do passive range of motion exercises to reduce joint ankylosis and muscle stiffness. In the early stages this is often done under general anaesthesia to minimize pain and stress and prevent excessive movement of fracture ends. As fractures heal and soft tissue injury diminishes, this can be done with the patient under mild sedation or fully conscious depending on the tractability of the patient.

A particular and unique issue of concern in wing fractures is contracture of the propatagium. The propatagium is the skin fold that runs between the shoulder and the carpus and supplies downward thrust during flight. It is essential to the function of flighted birds. A serious complication of wing bandages is contracture and fibrosis of the propatagium, which, if allowed to occur, will preclude flight even if the other wing injuries heal well. Physiotherapy to stretch and maintain the propatagium consists simply of a range of motion extensions of the wing and elbow. If propatagial contracture has occurred and is detected early, then gradually increasing the range of motion used in the physiotherapy can sometimes restore the wing to function. An early return to flighted exercise is vital.

Flighted exercise is the last stage of physiotherapy for the recovery of birds from wing injuries. There are two basic approaches used for this. One is to provide a safe area for flight and either simply allow the bird to make use of this space or encourage it to fly by placing desired items in elevated locations. For most birds, large circular aviaries allow the best use of space for flight. Aviary furniture should be limited to encourage free flight and nylon mesh can be used on interior walls to minimize injuries. The second approach used for flighted exercise in the recovery phase is to use falconry techniques. Rehabilitated wild birds of prey exercised in this fashion have higher fitness and better survival rates than aviary-exercised birds, but there are concerns about the habituation of the birds to humans that occurs with these techniques.

Physiotherapy for leg injuries should start with passive range of motion exercises but be extended to weight-bearing exercise as soon as possible. In ground-dwelling birds, treadmills are useful for promoting exercise, but practitioners should be aware that birds need to be gradually introduced to this exercise. For birds that use their feet to manipulate items, such as parrots and birds of prey, this should be encouraged as early as possible during recovery.

Feather care

Care of feather quality remains vital throughout the recovery phase from injury. A feather grafting technique known as imping may temporarily repair damaged primary feathers (see Chapter 15). It is common for birds in hospital to lose waterproofing through a combination of external agents soiling the plumage, lack of preening and poor nutritional condition. An important component of recovery is allowing birds the ability to restore their plumage. This can be highly species-specific, but the general principles are to encourage birds to preen by providing water for bathing or swimming, misting birds with water sprayers and providing a safe and secure retreat to allow time for daily preening. Severely soiled plumage may need to be washed to restore waterproofing; detailed protocols for bird washing have been developed as part of oiled wildlife response.

CD extras

Spring test 1
Spring test 2

Case example 1: Harrier Hawk with fractured wing

Presentation and history

A wild subadult male Harrier Hawk was presented after being found by the side of the road unable to fly, with a drooping right wing. On examination, there was a small open wound, swelling, crepitus and greenish bruising around the proximal third of the antebrachium. There was good vascular and neurological function below the fracture.

The bird's right wing was placed in a wing to body bandage to stabilize the fracture prior to diagnostic testing. Other supportive care included analgesia using butorphanol at 4 mg/kg i.m. q12h and oral fluids using lactated Ringer's solution at 40 ml/kg q12h. Limited pharmacokinetic studies suggest treatment with butorphanol q6h but the stress of increased handling in wild birds must be balanced with the analgesia frequency. A plastic tail protector was applied. The bird was placed in a darkened cage in a warm room overnight.

Diagnostic work-up

Radiographs taken under general anaesthesia showed a non-displaced oblique fracture of the right ulna. The radius was intact. There was associated soft tissue swelling.

Clinical pathology results were:

- Packed cell volume = 49%
- Total solids = 48 g/l
- Blood lead level: <0.01 mg/l.

Therapy

The bird's right wing was placed in a figure-of-eight bandage. Butorphanol at 4 mg/kg i.m. q12h was continued for 48 hours and then withdrawn. Meloxicam was started immediately after radiography at 0.5 mg/kg orally q12h and continued for 3 weeks in combination with oral fluid therapy using lactated Ringer's solution at 40 ml/kg q12h. The bird was kept in a small area to minimize flight.

Rehabilitation and outcome

After 23 days, the bandage was removed and the fracture was palpably stable with a good callus present. There was no evidence of patagial contracture or joint ankylosis on physical manipulation of the wing, so the bird was sent immediately to a rehabilitator and placed in a flight aviary. After another 4 weeks, it was flying well and was released back to the wild at the site of capture.

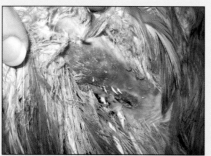

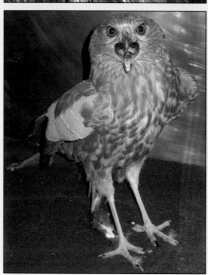

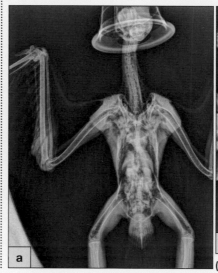

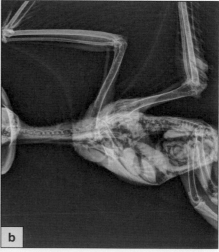

(a) Ventrodorsal and (b) lateral views of the fracture.

Case example 2: Brown Kiwi with fractured tibiotarsus

Presentation and history

A wild subadult (18-month-old) male Brown Kiwi was found on a routine check of its radiotransmitter to have a recent closed fracture of the right tibiotarsus. The bird was transported immediately to a local veterinary surgeon (veterinarian).

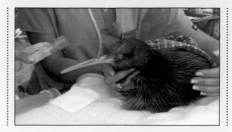

The local veterinary surgeon stabilized the fracture in a Robert Jones bandage and gave oral fluids and butorphanol at 4 mg/kg i.m. for analgesia. The bird was placed in a quiet darkened cage in a warm room and transported by air freight to a specialist hospital for surgical assessment the next day. ▶

Diagnostic work-up

Radiographs taken under general anaesthesia showed a comminuted midshaft fracture of the right tibiotarsus and fibula. There was a large butterfly segment present in the lateral aspect of the tibiotarsal fracture and moderate soft tissue swelling associated with the fracture.

Clinical pathology revealed a regenerative anaemia.

- Packed cell volume = 21%
- Total solids = 50%
- White blood cell count: 33.4 x 10⁹ cells/l; 10–20% reticulocytes and leucocytosis with a predominant lymphocytosis (heterophils 10.4 x 10⁹ cells/l, lymphocytes 21.7 x 10⁹ cells/l, monocytes 1.3 x 10⁹ cells/l).

The anaemia was likely due to traumatic blood loss but the cause of the lymphocytosis was not definitively determined.

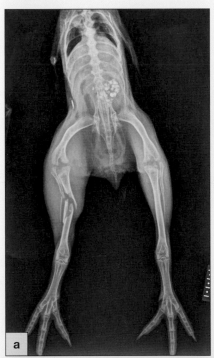

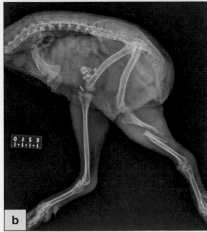

(a) Ventrodorsal and (b) lateral views of the fracture.

Therapy

An intravenous catheter was placed prior to surgery and, intraoperatively, a blood transfusion was given using 35 ml (20 ml/kg) of citrated blood from a captive Brown Kiwi. This was accompanied by intraoperative intravenous fluid therapy at 10 ml/kg/h using 0.9% saline with 2% dextrose, co-amoxiclav at 150 mg/kg i.v. and butorphanol at 2 mg/kg i.m. immediately preoperatively and again postoperatively. The fracture was repaired under general anaesthesia using two cerclage wires to reduce the loose butterfly fragment, and then a tied-in intramedullary pin and type 1 lateral external fixator. Postoperative radiographs showed acceptable stabilization of the fracture but it was noted that the upper lateral pin was placed very close to the stifle joint.

Immediately postoperatively, the soft tissues of the leg were more swollen and there were proprioceptive deficits and no

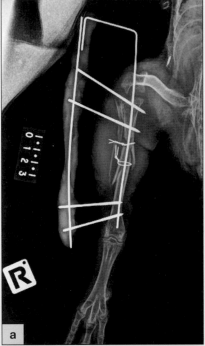

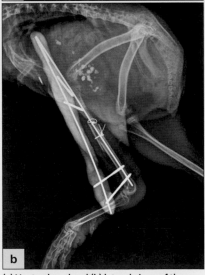

(a) Ventrodorsal and (b) lateral views of the fracture following repair.

withdrawal reflex. The vascular supply to the foot was intact. For 5 days postoperatively, cold compresses were used to reduce swelling at the surgery site and supportive care consisted of fluid therapy at 20 ml/kg orally q12h, co-amoxiclav at 150 mg/kg orally q12h, meloxicam at 0.5 mg/kg orally q12h and butorphanol at 4 mg/kg i.m. q12h. The pin tracts were cleaned daily with a 0.05% chlorhexidine solution. There was minimal discharge from the pin tracts, except for the upper pin, which drained synovial fluid. The neurological and motor function of the leg improved slowly over this period. Butorphanol was withdrawn after 5 days but was reintroduced at day 10 postoperatively, based on subjective assessments of behaviour and appetite.

The kiwi was kept in cage confinement and radiographs were taken 4 weeks after surgery and then every 2–3 weeks until the fracture had healed. The proximal pin was removed 48 days postoperatively due to continuous synovial fluid drainage, and antibiotics were withdrawn a few days later when this tract healed. The fracture callus was judged sufficiently stable to remove the intramedullary pin and fixator at 76 days postoperatively. At this time, all analgesia was withdrawn.

Rehabilitation and outcome

At the removal of implants, it was noted that there was disuse atrophy of the muscles of the right leg and osteoporosis of the tibiotarsus and tarsometatarsus compared with the contralateral limb. Physiotherapy was commenced, beginning with passive range of motion movements of the limb, encouraging walking in the enclosure and building up to forced walking on a treadmill. The bird regained strength and functional use of the limb and was released back to the wild 102 days after surgical repair of the fracture.

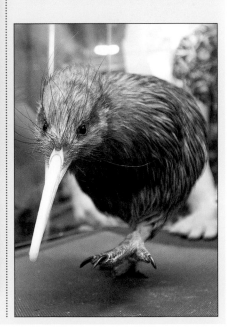

Case example 3: New Zealand Wood Pigeon with a fractured coracoid and clavicle

Presentation and history

A New Zealand Wood Pigeon was found underneath a window, unable to fly. The bird was bright and feisty but bright green urates were present in the droppings. On examination there was bruising over the left and right cranial pectoral muscles. The bird could lift both wings.

The bird was placed in a wing to body bandage. Other supportive care included analgesia using butorphanol at 4 mg/kg i.m. and oral fluids using lactated Ringer's solution at 40 ml/kg. The bird was placed in a small darkened cage in a warmed room overnight.

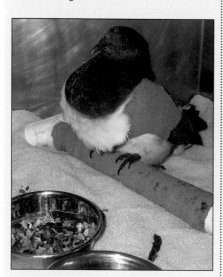

Diagnostic work-up

Radiographs taken under general anaesthesia showed a displaced distal diaphyseal fracture of the left coracoid and a mid-shaft fracture of the clavicle. There was bruising on the right pectoral musculature.

Clinical pathology results were within normal limits.

- Packed cell volume = 45%
- Total solids = 42 g/l
- White cell count: 19×10^9 cells/l (heterophils 14.25×10^9 cells/; lymphocytes 2.85×10^9 cells/l; monocytes 1.90×10^9 cells/l).

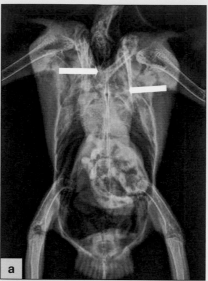

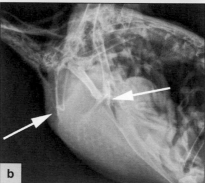

(a) Ventrodorsal and (b) lateral views of the fractures (arrowed).

Therapy

Initially, conservative treatment was planned for this bird; it was placed in a wing to body bandage and supportive care was continued with fluid therapy at 40 ml/kg orally q12h, meloxicam at 0.5 mg/kg orally q12h, butorphanol at 4 mg/kg i.m. q12h and crop feeding with a parrot hand-rearing mix at 20 ml/kg orally q12h. The green urates and bruising resolved over 5 days but the bird remained inappetent, had delayed crop emptying and was distressed in the bandage. After 5 days, intramedullary pinning of the coracoid was carried out under general anaesthesia. A threaded pin was driven retrograde into the coracoid and extended out of the shoulder. Intraoperative radiography was used to assess the placement of the pin in relation to the heart. A wing to body bandage was placed.

Postoperatively, the bird was maintained on the supportive care listed above with the addition of co-amoxiclav at 125 mg/kg orally for 5 days. The bird began eating 2 days after surgery and crop emptying was normal. Bandages were changed under general anaesthesia every second day for 2 weeks, with gentle passive range of motion exercise carried out on the affected wing. After this period, bandage changes and physiotherapy were carried out with the bird conscious. The intramedullary pin was removed 28 days after surgery.

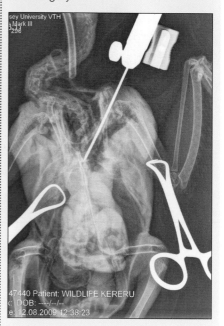

Rehabilitation and outcome

The bird went to a flight aviary and was encouraged to fly on a daily basis. After 3 months, the bird was released back to the area it had come from.

Feather loss

John Chitty

Feather loss is a common presentation in avian practice. This partly reflects the frequency with which such issues occur, but also reflects its obviousness, and importance, to owners. While few disorders resulting in feather loss are genuine emergencies, they are often perceived as such.

Just as in small animal practice, disorders of the integument often reflect internal disease, and there is a much higher frequency of behavioural disorders resulting in a feather destructive disorder (FDD) in birds with concurrent disease. In addition, issues with husbandry may also result in FDD or diseases of skin or feather. FDDs are a growing issue in raptor medicine, with the condition identified most frequently in Harris' Hawks (and, occasionally in the author's experience, kites and falcons).

Types of feather loss

For the veterinary surgeon (veterinarian), the first step is to distinguish the type of feather loss presented. This may be classed as feather dystrophy, FDD or true feather loss (Figure 30.1). In all cases, however, the clinician should remember that feathers grow in tracts and so some featherless areas are normal (Figure 30.2) and that brood patch development (featherless regions under the wings) may occur prior to egg incubation in some birds (see Chapter 2).

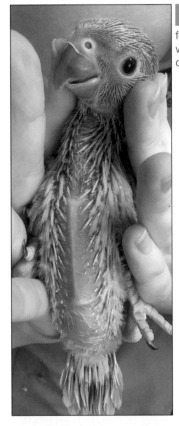

30.2 Physiologically normal featherless tract (apterium) well demonstrated on a chick. (© John Chitty)

Type	Clinical features	Historical features
Feather dystrophy	■ Feathers abnormally shaped ■ Abnormal colour ■ Stress marks (Figure 30.3) ■ Easily broken ■ Easily lost with abnormal 'pinching off' (Figure 30.4)	■ Sometimes broken feathers seen ■ Otherwise presented for abnormal feathering (or incidental finding)
Feather loss	■ Feathers missing from part or all of body; all areas may be affected including the head ■ Broken feathers unusual unless pruritic	■ Often sudden onset ■ May coincide with moult ■ Lost feathers may be found in or around housing ■ May be seen rubbing or scratching affected areas
Feather destructive disorder	■ Feathers missing or broken off over part of the body (NOT the head) ■ Abnormal downy feathers may be seen (Figure 30.5)	■ Bird may be seen plucking or chewing feathers ■ Bird may vocalize on plucking ■ Lost feathers may be seen in or around housing ■ May be sudden or chronic onset ■ Often cyclical

30.1 Determination of feather disease.

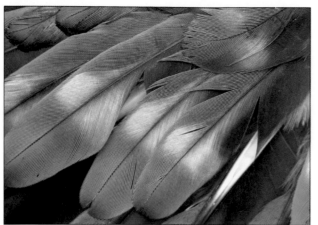

30.3 Fret marks often appear as lines or 'pinches' along feathers. In this young Green-winged Macaw a series of red or yellow (reduced pigment) marks appeared on all growing contour feathers after a stressful event (crop burn). Note also the diffraction pattern on the 'normal' parts of the feathers. (© John Chitty)

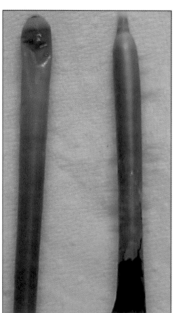

30.4 'Pinching off' in a hawk feather (right) compared with a relatively normal blood feather (left) from the same bird. Pinching off indicates a severe interruption to the growth of that feather. If localized, then trauma or infection should be suspected. If generalized, then systemic disease should be suspected. However, it should be remembered that this sign represents past issues during growth and may be historic at the time of examination. If damage to the feather follicle is severe, future feathers may also pinch off. (© John Chitty)

Skin mutilation

Skin lesions may be seen in conjunction with feather loss and may be investigated as described below and in Chapter 12. Skin mutilation, however, is an unusual sequel to feather damaging and is usually seen as a separate clinical entity (Figure 30.6). This is described in Chapter 5 and should be treated as urgent or an emergency depending on the depth of tissue damage. Otherwise, feather loss is rarely, if ever, an emergency presentation.

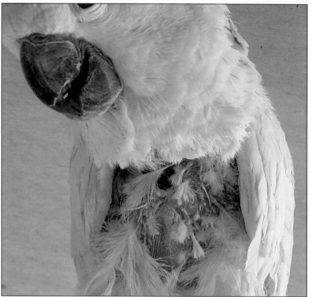

30.6 This Moluccan Cockatoo persistently mutilated the skin over the cranial keel region (a common site for mutilation in this species). There was also evidence of feather destructive disorder (FDD) in this region, although whether the mutilation progressed from FDD or *vice versa* (or the feather damage was simply 'collateral' damage) was impossible to determine. (© John Chitty)

Common causes

Once the type of feather loss is identified, a list of potential differential diagnoses can be compiled (Figures 30.7–30.14).

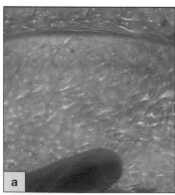
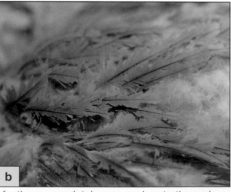
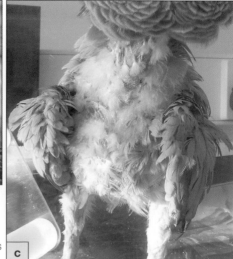

30.5 **(a)** Feather plucking with feathers completely removed; note the early regrowth from the follicles. **(b)** Feather destructive disorder (FDD) where the feathers have been trimmed. **(c)** A very common FDD presentation with downy feathers over the body. These are the plumulaceous barbules of the body feathers and are normally hidden under the plumage. In these cases the bird bites off the tips of the growing feathers, leaving just the downy bases. (© John Chitty)

Cause	History features	Clinical features
Removal by another bird	■ Housed with another bird ■ Nesting/bonding behaviours noted ■ May see one bird pluck the other	■ Feather loss can occur anywhere, but especially over the head ■ Feather regrowth will occur as soon as the pair are separated; this should be done whenever feather loss occurs in a paired/group-housed bird. The pair should be kept side by side but not so one can reach the other through the cage bars
Skin disease (varying aetiology)	■ May be pruritic	■ May be skin lesions present; these should be biopsied (Figure 30.8)
Nutritional disease	■ Poor-quality diet	■ More usually will result in broken feathers (feathers often more brittle than normal), altered colour, or FDD. Improve diet and assess effect
Secondary to FDD	■ History of plucking feathers (especially seen in rescue birds)	■ Long-term plucking may result in follicle damage or loss of follicles ■ Skin appears smooth with no evidence of trauma ■ Typical distribution of FDD is shown in Figure 30.9
Folliculitis	■ May be pruritic	■ Inflammation of feather follicles ■ Usually localized on the wings
Localized trauma	■ Sits next to wire (especially if the cage is small) ■ Feeder requires head to be stretched through a narrow gap	■ Persistent rubbing leads to feather damage or loss ■ Distribution corresponds to area rubbed
Parasites	■ Very unusual ■ Recent purchase ■ Contact with other birds ■ May be pruritic	■ Feather lice/mites seen ■ Swollen feather bulbs and/or debris around feather base or inside calamus (Figure 30.10) ■ Microscopy of such material should confirm diagnosis (Figure 30.11)
Localized or referred pain	■ Bird seen rubbing or pecking at single affected area	■ For example, arthritis or hepatopathy may lead to feathers broken or lost over affected area
Circovirus/polyomavirus	■ Budgerigars ■ Lorikeets	■ 'French moult' where young birds are produced with missing wing and/or tail or body feathers. The feathers lost (they do not regrow) correspond to the age at which the bird was infected (Figure 30.12) ■ In other birds, feather loss may accompany feather dystrophy (Figure 30.13)

30.7 Differential diagnoses for true feather loss.

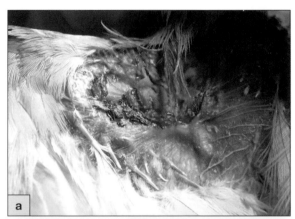
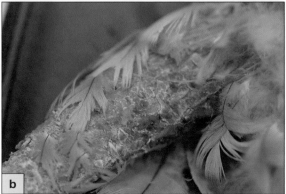

30.8 Skin lesions. **(a)** Dermatitis in a lovebird may be presented as feather destructive disorder or feather loss if the owner has not noticed the skin lesions. **(b)** Bacterial pyoderma in an African Grey Parrot causing feather loss and skin scaling/crusting over the legs. The bird was extremely pruritic. (© John Chitty)

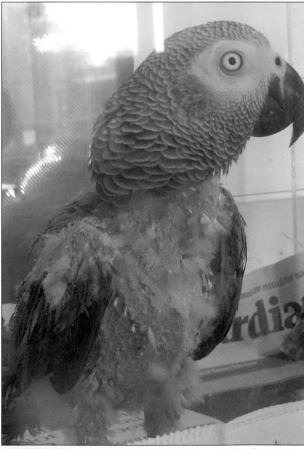

30.9 Typical feather destructive disorder distribution in an African Grey Parrot. Note the normal head feathers. (© John Chitty)

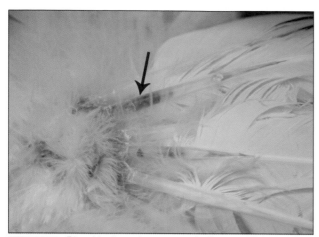

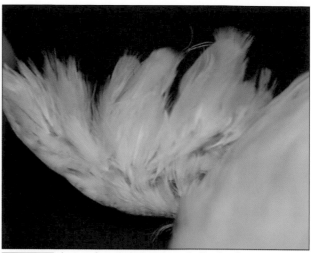

30.10 Blood in the calamus may indicate quill mite infection. Sampling of the material (see Chapter 12) in the case of quill mite infection will show mites and eggs (see Figure 30.11). However, in this case, the blood was due to the more common presentation of trauma during feather growth and past haemorrhage (arrowed). (© John Chitty)

30.12 Loss of remiges in a juvenile Budgerigar with French moult. (© John Chitty)

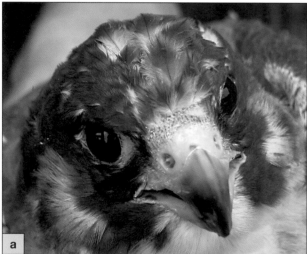

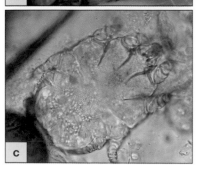

30.11 (a–c) Epidermoptid mite infestation of a Peregrine Falcon. A topical solution of 1:50 ivermectin:propylene glycol was applied to the lesions at twice-monthly intervals. (© John Chitty)

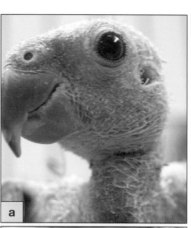

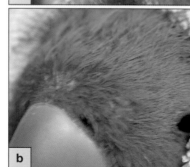

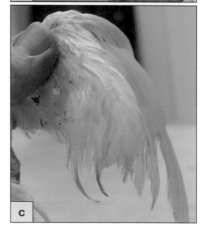

30.13 (a) Complete feather loss over the head of a parakeet with circovirus infection. (b) Signs of circovirus can occasionally be minimal, as in this male Eclectus Parrot. Such minimal signs are not pathognomonic for circovirus infection, and other differential diagnoses such as sinusitis should be investigated as well as performing specific tests for circovirus. (c) Loss and curling of wing feathers in a Cockatiel with circovirus infection. (© John Chitty)

Cause	Historical features	Clinical features
Circovirus	■ Progressive feather changes/loss with each moult; may wax and wane in some species (e.g. lorikeets) ■ Newly purchased bird (especially from market or pet shop) ■ Previous mixing with other birds (not necessarily recent)	■ Black shiny beak in cockatoos/Grey Parrots ■ Feathers may be abnormal in shape or show changed pigment; changes seen over whole body (most cases) ■ Cracked/broken beak in advanced cases
Polyomavirus	■ Particularly small psittacine birds	■ May see twisted feathers, often in conjunction with feather loss
Nutritional disease	■ Poor diet or period of anorexia/malnutrition	■ Generally loss of feather pigment ■ Can be broken feathers or stress marks and feathers can be more brittle
Liver disease	■ Typically poor diet	■ Usually secondary to hepatic lipidosis; obese birds (often Amazons) ■ Change/loss of feather pigment (Figure 30.15)
Localized trauma	See Figure 30.7	■ Feathers may be broken or curled (see Figure 30.7)
Folliculitis	See Figure 30.7	■ May cause easily broken feathers or stress marks (see Figure 30.7)
Feather cysts	■ Typically passerines	■ Large swellings containing feather material ■ Curled feathers may originate from the cyst (Figure 30.16)
Genetic	■ Passerines ■ Budgerigars ■ Grey Parrots	■ 'Feather duster' forms with curled feathers over body ■ Red feathers
Secondary to feather destructive disorder	■ History of plucking feathers	■ May see broken feathers or (more commonly) down covering areas of the body where the distal parts of the feathers have been pinched off ■ Long-term plucking may lead to production of depigmented feathers due to follicle damage
Systemic illness	■ History of illness	■ Can lead to production of stress marks in feathers growing at the time of illness ■ Typically generalized

30.14 Differential diagnoses for feather dystrophy.

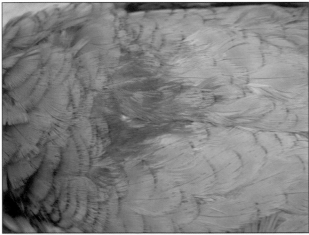

30.15 Yellowing of green body feathers in an Amazon parrot with hepatic lipidosis. (© John Chitty)

What causes red body feathers in African Grey Parrots?

Many African Grey Parrots are presented with red feathers intermingled with the normal grey body feathers. While some texts may describe this as pathognomonic for circovirus infection, there are many potential causes.

- **Circovirus infection:** affected feathers tend to be completely red (though not always) and more red feathers appear with each moult. The beak is normally black and shiny with loss of powder down.
- **Genetic:** these are the so-called 'King Greys'. Red feathers (either completely red or fringed with red) appear at first adult plumage and may or may not increase in number with each moult (Figure 30.17).
- **Chronic feather plucking:** feather follicles damaged by repeated plucking may produce red feathers.
- **Zinc toxicosis:** this has been reported as a cause of red feathering.

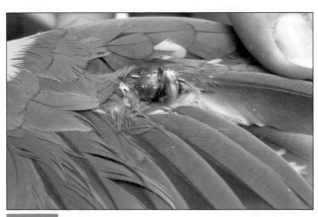

30.16 Feather cyst on an Amazon parrot. (© John Chitty)

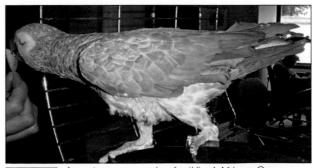

30.17 An extreme example of a 'King' African Grey Parrot. The bird tested negative for circovirus on both polymerase chain reaction blood testing and skin biopsy. (© John Chitty)

Feather destructive disorder

FDD is truly a complex and multifactorial syndrome with many possible differential diagnoses and frequently multiple factors implicated in each single case.

As such, it is often impossible to pin down a single cause in each case or even to determine which of a multiple of therapies/husbandry changes has been effective, and a complete medical and behavioural assessment is usually necessary.

Medical

Many systemic illnesses have been implicated in FDD (Figure 30.18). In particular, zinc toxicosis and malnutrition are often cited, though whether as primary or complicating causes is hard to assess. Hypothyroidism is often mentioned yet is extremely hard to confirm as few laboratories can accurately measure the low levels of total thyroxine found in birds. Empirical dosing with thyroid hormone is not recommended. FDD may also be associated with reproductive hormone fluctuations and particularly associated with reproductive-linked behavioural disease.

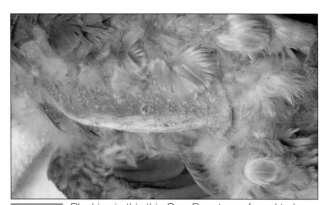

30.18 Plucking in this thin Grey Parrot was found to be secondary to proventricular dilatation disease. It was presumed that the bird was plucking over the affected stomach and intestine. (© John Chitty)

Dermatological

It is important to remember that ectoparasites are unusual in cage birds and an extremely unusual cause of FDD. More common causes include:

- Pruritus – possibly linked to irritation or allergy
- Dermatitis – infectious or irritant/allergic
- Feather pulpitis (Figure 30.19)
- Folliculitis (Figure 30.20).

Social/environmental

- Poor early socialization and development (see Chapters 4 and 5).
- Poor preening technique.
- Overtiredness (excessively long daylight hours).
- Lack of bathing.
- Dry atmosphere/low humidity.
- Poor cage position (see Chapter 3).
- Iatrogenic, especially poor wing-clipping technique.

Behavioural

Inappropriate pair bonding with the owner may result in:

- Attention-seeking behaviours
- Separation anxiety
- Anxiety-related disorders.

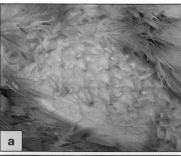
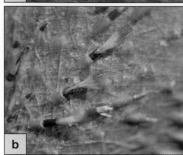
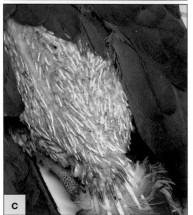

30.19 (a) Normal pin feathers emerging after a plucking incident. (b) The emerging pin feathers appear darker and slightly swollen compared with those in (a). This is typical in pulpitis. (c) Both normal and pulpitis feathers are evident here. Some of the inflamed pin feathers have been traumatized. It can be hypothesized that this bird is pruritic. (© John Chitty)

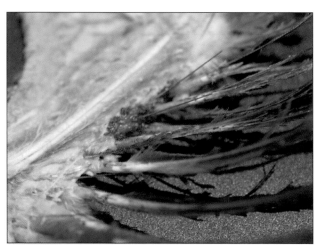

30.20 Feather destructive disorder and folliculitis in a Grey Parrot; note how the feathers have been chewed. (© John Chitty)

It is the author's view that FDD behaviours do not represent stereotypical behaviour (they are generally interruptible, and many 'examples' show more characteristics of learned or attention-seeking behaviours on closer examination) or obsessive-compulsive behaviour (it is impossible to prove that the bird cannot cope with the consequences of not plucking).

Feather destructive disorder in Harris' Hawks

The notes in the text refer, in the main, to FDD in parrots. However, FDD is becoming increasingly common in Harris' Hawks kept for falconry purposes (Figure 30.21). This species is unusual in being a social hunter which is a major factor in their popularity in falconry.

The approaches described in the text for parrots will be appropriate for assessing the problem in Harris' Hawks. However, the following may also be of relevance:

- Feather pulpitis appears very common in this species and the author has found evidence of pulpitis in all cases seen. It has not been determined whether it is a primary, secondary or perpetuating factor
- Many cases occur during the moult when not being flown. A return to training can assist
- Many cases appear in single-kept birds and moving to tethering near other hawks may help. However, cases have been seen in birds kept in aviaries in a breeding pair as well as in birds tethered in groups

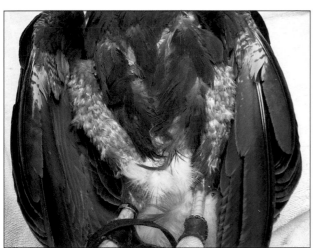

30.21 Typical distribution of feather destructive behaviour in a Harris' Hawk. (© John Chitty)

Diagnostic work-up

Feather loss and dystrophy

The causes of these syndromes are quite similar, so investigation can be carried out along similar lines.

History taking and clinical examination, as described in Chapter 10, are essential.

The bird's signalment and contact with other birds are particularly important as there is the potential for feather loss/dystrophy to be caused by infectious diseases.

It is also useful to ask the owners to bring in any abnormal feathers that have been moulted or broken off. Requesting them to bring photographs of the bird over the time owned may enable the clinician to see changes as they evolve.

The approach is summarized in Figure 30.22.

As stated earlier, these are difficult, time-consuming and complex cases. As such, suitable time and resources should be allocated to their investigation. Initially a minimum of a 30-minute appointment should be made, ideally at a quiet time of day. Where behavioural issues are suspected as many members of the bird's household as possible should be encouraged to attend the appointment. This will assist both in obtaining history and in explaining training and therapeutic techniques.

Most importantly, expectations must be managed. Full 'cure' is quite unusual and any resolution will require considerable owner and financial commitment (Figure 30.23). Without this, there is little chance of success and it may be more pragmatic to consider rehoming or even euthanasia of such cases. Potential outcomes should be discussed with the owner.

- **Resolution of FDD and behavioural 'contentment':** the ideal scenario, though unusual.
- **Behavioural 'contentment' and non-progressive FDD:** the feather damaging remains unresolved yet does not progress beyond the previous regions affected and normally only occurs at moult. This is the most common 'success' and is an acceptable outcome.
- **Behavioural 'contentment' and progressive FDD:** this is not common, as it implies a medical or dermatological cause of FDD, which are normally the most responsive cases.
- **Resolution of FDD but behavioural issues persist:** this is not an acceptable outcome as the bird is not happy and further issues are likely to manifest.
- **Failure to achieve resolution of FDD or behavioural issues:** this is not an acceptable outcome and rehoming or euthanasia should be considered in such cases.

History taking

A vital first step is to determine that feathers are being damaged by the bird (see Figure 30.14). A full history is essential (see Chapters 5 and 10).

- Signalment: including species, age, sex (if known) and source.
- Previous disease history.
- If a second-opinion consultation, details of previous investigations, therapies and responses to these are needed. Many owners will also have tried over-the-counter remedies and it is important to have details of these as well.
- Diet, including supplements and mineral blocks. The proportion of each part of the diet given and consumed by the bird should be estimated. Is grit provided?
- Environment, including details of the cage, perches and toys given (are the toys given in rotation?). Do the owners smoke? Do they use air fresheners/sprays near the bird? Is the bird kept near cooking fumes? It can be very useful to have pictures of the cage and where it is sited.
- Daily regime: how much time in/out of the cage? Does the bird go outside? If not, is ultraviolet light provided, and for how long? When does the bird 'go to bed'? For how long is the owner with the bird?

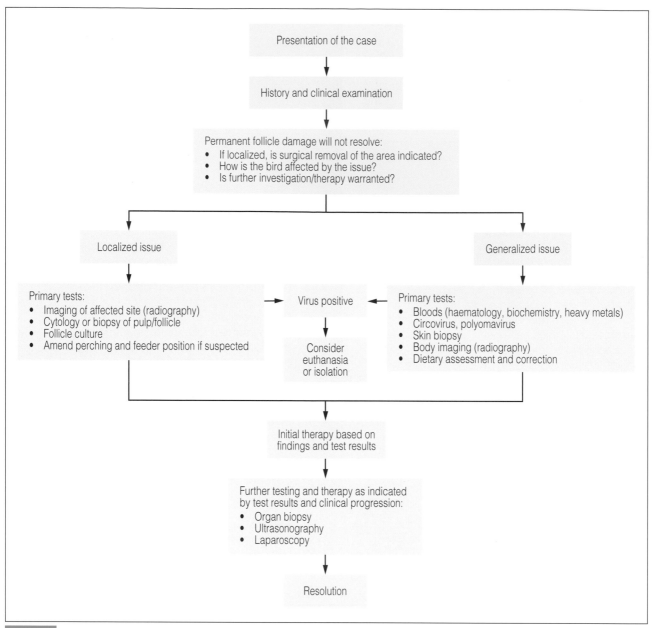

Presentation of the case

↓

History and clinical examination

↓

Permanent follicle damage will not resolve:
- If localized, is surgical removal of the area indicated?
- How is the bird affected by the issue?
- Is further investigation/therapy warranted?

Localized issue

↓

Primary tests:
- Imaging of affected site (radiography)
- Cytology or biopsy of pulp/follicle
- Follicle culture
- Amend perching and feeder position if suspected

Virus positive

↓

Consider euthanasia or isolation

Generalized issue

↓

Primary tests:
- Bloods (haematology, biochemistry, heavy metals)
- Circovirus, polyomavirus
- Skin biopsy
- Body imaging (radiography)
- Dietary assessment and correction

↓

Initial therapy based on findings and test results

↓

Further testing and therapy as indicated by test results and clinical progression:
- Organ biopsy
- Ultrasonography
- Laparoscopy

↓

Resolution

30.22   An approach to feather loss/dystrophy.

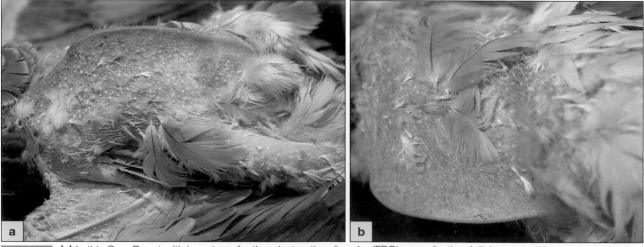

30.23   **(a)** In this Grey Parrot with long-term feather destructive disorder (FDD) some feather follicles can still be seen and feather regrowth is possible. **(b)** In this case of FDD, the skin over the keel is completely smooth and devoid of feather follicles. As such, there is permanent damage and no prospect of feather regrowth even if underlying causes are addressed and corrected. (© John Chitty)

When alone, is the radio or television left on? Are there other birds? If so, which species? Details of interactions between the birds and their disease history should be obtained.

- Is the bird sprayed or a bath provided each day? If so, are any products added to the water? Is the house centrally heated?
- Rearing history, i.e. is the bird hand- or parent-reared? If hand-reared, do the owners know when the bird was taken from the parents? Was it reared alone or with others?
- Relationship with owners; for example, is there a favourite owner? Is the bird male or female? Does the bird feed the owner, or make sexual displays to them? How does the owner handle/stroke the bird? Is the favourite owner away a lot? Have there been any changes or stresses within the family?
- Reproductive history; for example, have any eggs been laid? When?
- Moulting history: when did the bird last moult? How long for?
- Wing clipping: is the bird clipped? Has it ever been clipped?
- FDD history:
  - Is this the first incidence?

- If not, when did it happen before? For how long? Which feathers were affected? Did the bird re-feather completely before starting again? Details of therapies.
- When did the bird start plucking? For how long has the bird been plucking?
- Which feathers were affected first? Has the area affected changed or spread?
- How does the bird pluck/chew? Nibbling? Aggressive chewing? Does it chew its claws? (See Figure 30.20).
- Does the bird rub/scratch itself on the cage or perches?
- When does the bird pluck/chew? Are the owners present or not? If present, what is their response? Does the bird interrupt other behaviours to pluck/chew? If the bird does pluck, then videos of the bird's behaviour (including sound) are extremely useful.

Clinical examination
A full clinical examination is also required (see Chapter 10) with particular emphasis on the integument and plumage. The investigation is summarized in Figure 30.24.

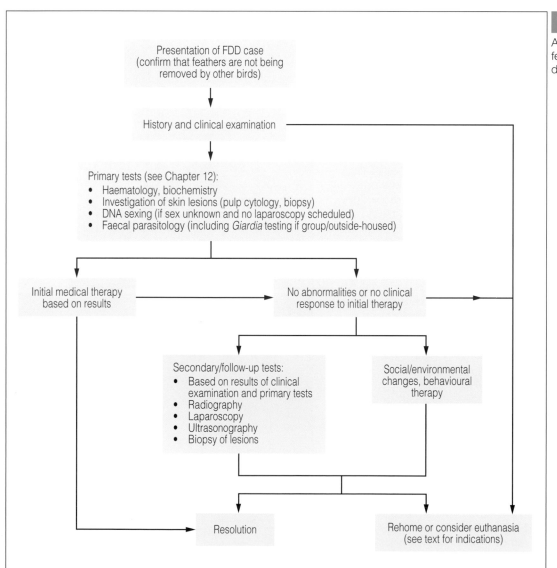

30.24

An approach to feather destructive disorder (FDD).

Areas of debate in feather loss examination and management

There are areas of investigation and management that can be controversial.

Allergy and intradermal testing

Allergy has frequently been described as a cause of feather picking/chewing. It may be suspected where there is one or more of the following:

- Pruritus
- Skin lesions/appropriate cellular changes on skin histopathology
- Seasonality
- Recurrent pyoderma/superficial infections
- Positive responses on intradermal skin tests
- Recovery after removal of suspected allergen and relapse on re-exposure.

The role of intradermal skin testing is controversial. The very thin skin of birds makes the technique extremely difficult and it will generally need to be performed under anaesthesia. Birds do not respond to histamine as a positive control (codeine phosphate is used). There is also argument about species differences, injection sites and dose rates of allergens. Although protocols have been described, this technique cannot currently be recommended, as positive responses should not be interpreted as diagnostic of allergy unless also indicated by the seasonality of the condition or confirmed by removal/re-exposure testing.

Diet and malnutrition

Malnutrion is frequently implicated in FDD. It is unlikely to be a primary cause, although a poor plane of nutrition may act as a stressor and/or restrict the ability of the bird to regrow plumage as well as affect skin integrity. The standard seed diets fed to many birds are often of poor quality and poorly balanced. Further deterioration may have occurred due to spoilage in transport/storage. Spoiled seed is a frequent source of fungal respiratory disease (aspergillosis). It is therefore advisable in all cases to improve the plane of nutrition. This may be done by converting the bird from seed to a good-quality pelleted ration (e.g. Harrison's Bird Foods) or to supplement with vitamin/mineral mixes. This may not need to be done immediately, as a change of diet (and ensuing stress) may not be advisable at a time when there are many other management changes being performed.

Use of collars

Collars to prevent chewing/plucking have often been advocated. Various forms are suggested.

- Elizabethan-type collars made from plastic or card (Figure 30.25a). These may be placed in the conventional manner (cone around the head) or inverted leaving the head free.
- Stultiens™ or extension collars (Figure 30.25b). Commercial screw-on versions are available or one may be made from foam pipe insulation and tape.
- Combination collars.
- Bubble collars (Figure 30.25c). These come in a variety of sizes and appear well tolerated. They are easy to apply and remove, yet extremely resistant to damage by the bird. However, care must be taken if using for extended periods as rubbing can occur.

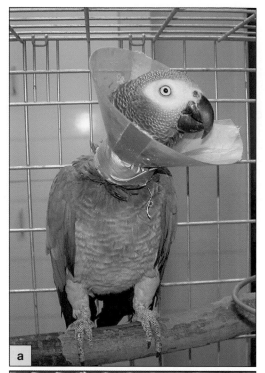

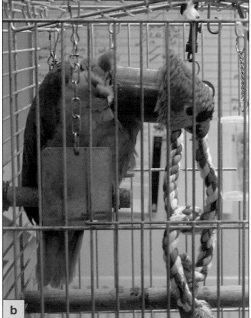

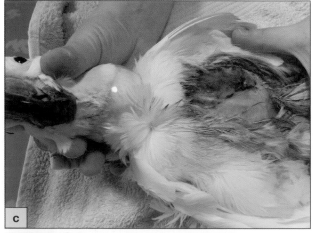

30.25 Collars to prevent chewing/plucking are advocated. **(a)** Elizabethan collar. **(b)** Extension collar. **(c)** Bubble collar applied to a self-mutilating cockatoo. (© John Chitty)

However, problems may be associated with these collars.

- They may not prevent the bird plucking or may mean that it starts plucking feathers it can reach.
- Destruction of the collar by the bird.
- Stress associated with the collar. In the author's experience this has resulted in the death of several birds due to the inability to feed (when not carefully monitored after placement) and in one case inability to raise the head. Remember that many of these birds may already be under stress.
- Collaring the pruritic bird is inappropriate.
- Inability to preen may actually result in dermatological disease or worsen existing disease.
- Poorly positioned collars or those with hard edges may result in pressure necrosis of skin and subcutaneous tissues.
- Inability to determine whether concurrent therapies are having any effect. It is not unusual for a collared bird to re-feather completely, only to resume plucking immediately on removal of the collar.

So, should collars be used at all? The author has not used one (except in self-mutilating birds that are causing severe life-threatening damage to themselves) in the last 5 years. However, they may be appropriate where the plucking is deemed to be due to habit following an identified trigger and where all other causes have been ruled out, environment and diet corrected, and therapies put in place to correct inappropriate behaviours.

References and further reading

Chitty JR (2003a) Feather plucking in psittacine birds. 1. Presentation and medical investigation. *In Practice* **25(8)**, 484–493

Chitty JR (2003b) Feather plucking in psittacine birds. 2. Social, environmental and behavioural considerations. *In Practice* **25(9)**, 550–555

Chitty JR (2005) Feather and skin disorders. In: *BSAVA Manual of Psittacine Birds, 2nd edn*, ed. N Harcourt-Brown and J Chitty. BSAVA Publications, Gloucester

Chitty JR (2008) Raptors: feather and skin diseases. In: *BSAVA Manual of Raptors, Pigeons and Passerine Birds*, ed. J Chitty and M Lierz. BSAVA Publications, Gloucester

Doneley B (2011) *Avian Medicine and Surgery in Practice*. Manson Publishing, London

Jenkins JR (2001) Feather picking and self-multialtion in psittacine birds. *Veterinary Clinics of North America: Exotic Animal Practice* **4(3)**, 651–667

Rupley A (1997) *Manual of Avian Practice*. Saunders, Philadelphia

Samour J (2008) *Avian Medicine, 2nd edn*. Elsevier, Philadelphia

Case example 1: Plucking in an African Grey Parrot

Presentation and history

A 2-year-old African Grey Parrot was presented with plucking of 1 month's duration over the cranial keel region and ventral neck. Plucking had begun in December and the bird had not plucked previous to this.

The bird was kept in a cage in the living room with the cage positioned in the window. The owner and their family rose at around 6 am and went to bed around midnight each day. During this time there was activity and light where the parrot was kept. The bird resented showering and so this was not performed.

Plucking occurred all the time, with the parrot plucking in front of the owners (to which they would respond by telling it to stop) and plucked feathers (entire) were found in the cage in the morning. The bird was eating and drinking normally (seed diet) and had normal droppings.

Diagnostic work-up

The bird was normal on examination barring a region with no feathers but a few swollen pin feathers.

Blood sampling revealed a monocytosis and ionized calcium of 0.91 mmol/l (normal range 0.96–1.25 mmol/l). The bird was sexed as male. Feather pulp revealed many white blood cells and bacteria.

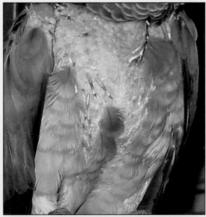

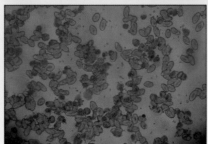

Therapy

- Antibiosis: marbofloxacin at 10 mg/kg orally q24h
- Calcium: vitamin D_3 supplementation in water
- Institution of a 12-hour light:12-hour dark cycle with the bird being taken to

roost in a covered cage in a quiet dark room for 12 hours each night.
- Daily warm water showering, with positive reinforcement techniques used to overcome initial fear of showering.
- Diet change to a pelleted ration and provision of foraging enrichment within the cage.
- Advice on training and handling to encourage the bird to be removed from the cage more frequently without building a pair bond (at 2 years old the bird is unlikely to be sexually active, but future issues can be averted by developing a healthy owner–bird relationship).
- Advice on not reinforcing the behaviour by ignoring feather removal and giving attention when not plucking.

Outcome

Plucking behaviour stopped after 10 days of therapy. Feather regrowth started 2 months later and the feathers were removed again, albeit over a smaller area. Again, there was an apparent response to antibiosis.

Over the next few years the pattern was repeated, with a small area over the crop being plucked after each moult. The area has not enlarged and the plucking does not appear progressive.

The bird is showing no other abnormal behaviours and appears to interact with its owners and environment in an expected manner, and there are no other apparent issues. Further clinical investigation has not been performed.

Case example 2: Dermatitis in an Amazon parrot

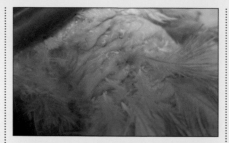

Presentation and history

A 7-year-old Blue-fronted Amazon Parrot was presented with feather loss over the head. The condition had started a week previously and progressed rapidly. The bird was eating and drinking normally and droppings were normal.

There was a loss of feathers over the head and the skin was thickened, especially at the oral commissures and ventral neck. The rest of the skin and plumage was normal. During the consultation the bird was observed rubbing its head.

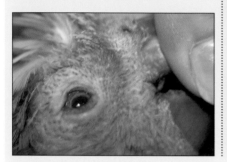

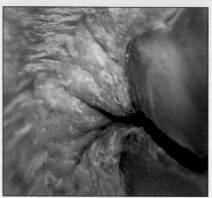

Diagnostic work-up

Blood sampling revealed a monocytosis and no other abnormalities. Skin scrapes revealed no parasites. Skin biopsy showed a marked inflammatory response and numerous budding yeasts.

Therapy

Itraconazole was given orally at 10 mg/kg q24h. Daily spraying with a 1:250 dilution of F10SC (Health & Hygiene Pty) was instigated.

Outcome

Therapy was continued for a month, during which time feather regrowth occurred over most of the affected area. The skin became less thickened.

There have been no relapses, though an underlying cause was not established.

Case example 3: Red feathers in an African Grey Parrot

A 10-year-old male African Grey Parrot was presented with red feathering over the body. These feathers had been appearing over the past 2 years and were now very numerous. The beak had recently become overgrown. The bird was apparently healthy and eating a pelleted ration.

The body plumage appeared normal other than many red feathers; some were completely red. The secondary wing feathers had been clipped. The beak was black and shiny. On further questioning, the owner recalled that it had previously been dusty. The beak was also thickened and overgrown. There were some feathers lost over the top of the head. There were no other abnormalities on examination.

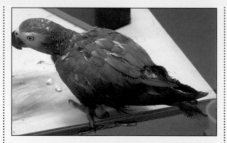

Diagnostic work-up

Blood sampling revealed no abnormalities. Zinc levels were in the normal range (<31µmol/l), circovirus polymerase chain reaction on blood was positive. Skin biopsy was not performed.

Therapy

Remedial beak correction was performed under general anaesthesia. The bird was kept as a single pet bird. Advice was given on avoiding contact with other birds.

Outcome

Over the next few years, feather loss started and the remaining feathers became more dystrophic. The beak continued to overgrow and was reshaped as required.

The bird died of a bacterial septicaemia several years later.

The sick baby bird

Deborah Monks

The sick baby bird is a commonly presented patient at any practice dealing with birds. Frequently presented as emergencies, sick chicks tend to decompensate faster than adult birds, which necessitates a quicker, more targeted approach to diagnosis and treatment. The practice must be able to supply appropriate hospitalization facilities for chicks, including the ability to provide heat up to 32°C. The practice may need to provide arrangements for out-of-hours feeding. As largely immune-incompetent individuals, chicks (Figures 31.1 and 31.2) must be able to be segregated from the main hospital, to minimize nosocomial disease.

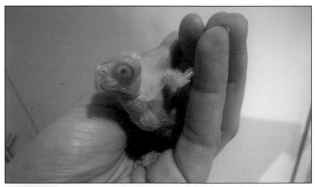

31.1 This young Cockatiel is totally dependent for warmth, feeding and care. (Courtesy of Dr M Cowan)

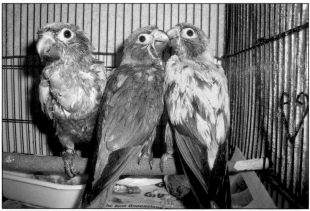

31.2 This clutch of Sun Conures are no longer reliant on human hand-rearers for warmth, but still require feeding.

History taking

A thorough history is absolutely crucial to avian paediatric medicine. In addition to the history-taking recommendations in Chapter 10, there are specific questions to be asked when the patient is a baby bird (Figure 31.3).

Many owners that hand-rear chicks are inexperienced, which leads to basic errors in hygiene and husbandry. Unethical vendors will sell chicks for new owners to 'finish off', claiming that the bird will have a better bond to the new owner if hand-reared by them. Such claims are not only erroneous, but often result in poor welfare outcomes for the chicks, and heartbreak for the new owners. Many behavioural maladaptations have their roots in inappropriate hand-rearing, leaving birds poorly equipped to integrate into human and/or avian life in the long term. Detection of disease often occurs late in the disease process.

Figure 31.4 provides a quick reference guide to common brooding temperatures and feeding schedules. See Chapter 4 for more detail about the different methods of hand-rearing, and the possible consequences. See Chapter 5 for more detail about behavioural problems in birds.

Clinical assessment of a sick chick

Chapter 10 covers the general physical examination of a bird. In addition, there are specific areas of physical examination of a baby bird that require closer attention.

The crop is an extremely distensible out-pouching of the oesophagus, designed to allow rapid filling and storage of food, then slower trickle-through to the proventriculus and ventriculus (see Chapter 2). In unfeathered birds, the crop is easy to examine. In feathered chicks, the feathers must be parted, and in some cases wet down, to visualize the crop appropriately. Surgical spirit can be used to facilitate examination; however, it can lead to evaporative cooling, so should be used cautiously. The crop must be assessed for the degree of filling, or the presence of foreign bodies. If the crop is full it must be palpated carefully as regurgitation and aspiration may occur. Any lesions, scabbing

Factor	Questions	Comments
Prenatal	<ul><li>Any pre-existing or known parental disease?</li><li>Are the parents known successful breeders (have they produced live chicks before)?</li><li>Have they successfully reared chicks to weaning?</li><li>How do the parents cope with human intervention?</li><li>How often is the nest box lining changed?<ul><li>Is there any smell in the nest box substrate?</li><li>Describe the cleaning regime for the nest and aviary/cage.</li></ul></li><li>How often are the parents given new food and water?<ul><li>Describe the cleaning regime for the food and water dishes.</li></ul></li><li>If hand-rearing this chick, why was it removed from its parents?<ul><li>At what age was this done?</li></ul></li></ul>	<ul><li>Parents chronically infected with disease may show poor fertility, have high incubation mortality or produce ill-thrifty chicks.</li><li>It is not common for minimally tame parents to traumatize the chicks as displacement behaviour during nest or aviary inspections.</li><li>Poor attention to the hygiene of the parents' enclosure is likely to lead to bacterially or fungally infected chicks. It may result in deaths in shell or to hatching of ill-thrifty chicks.</li></ul>
Incubation	<ul><li>Was this egg incubated by the parents?<ul><li>If so, how often was the egg checked?</li><li>How closely was the hatching process monitored?</li><li>Did the chick have any known problems hatching?</li><li>Any known problems with siblings?</li></ul></li><li>Was this egg incubated artificially?<ul><li>If so, what sort of incubator?</li><li>How were the temperature and humidity monitored?</li><li>How was the unit prepared for this season?</li><li>How long was it run prior to being used for eggs?</li><li>Have there been any electricity supply issues?</li><li>How often is the incubator sterilized?</li><li>Have there been problems with any other chicks?</li></ul></li></ul>	<ul><li>Poorly incubated chicks may die during the hatching process or show dehydration or oedema at hatch. Some may hatch with already established bacterial or fungal infections.</li></ul>
Hand-rearing	<ul><li>Is this bird being hand-reared (see Chapter 4)?</li><li>If so, which formula is being used?<ul><li>What is the expiry date of the formula?</li><li>How has it been stored?</li><li>Is the formula being prepared fresh for each feed?</li><li>At what temperature is it being fed?<ul><li>How is this checked?</li><li>Is it being well stirred to avoid hot spots?</li></ul></li></ul></li><li>What implements are being used for hand-feeding?<ul><li>Spoon/syringe/crop tube?</li><li>How are the hand-rearing implements being cleaned?</li></ul></li><li>What is the feeding regime?<ul><li>How many feeds are being given per day?</li><li>How many hours between each feed?</li><li>What volume is being fed at each meal?</li></ul></li><li>How much has the crop emptied between each feed?</li><li>How does the chick respond to being fed?<ul><li>Is it head bobbing?</li><li>Is it excited and calling for food?</li><li>Is it swallowing the food?</li></ul></li><li>How many chicks are being hand-reared?<ul><li>Are there separate implements for each individual?</li><li>Is there cross-contamination between chicks?</li></ul></li></ul>	<ul><li>It is recommended that feed is prepared fresh for each feed to prevent the risk of spoiling.</li><li>If a crop tube is used then the crop should be checked for perforations and bruising.</li><li>All feeding equipment needs to be cleaned after every feeding, with hot soapy water, followed by disinfectant, rinsing and being left to dry. This cleaning process includes flushing out crop tubes and syringes, followed by disinfection and rinsing. Poor hygiene during the hand-rearing process is a major cause of bacterial and fungal infections in chicks.</li><li>As a general rule, chicks should have their crops empty completely overnight, and be no less than one-quarter empty throughout the day. Feeding frequencies and volumes should reflect this. Depending on the species, approximately 10% of the chick's weight should be fed at each feed (see Chapter 4).</li></ul>
Brooding process	<ul><li>What sort of brooder is used?<ul><li>What is the substrate?</li><li>How often is it changed?</li><li>Is there any smell associated with the substrate?</li><li>Could the substrate be ingested?</li></ul></li><li>What sort of heating does the brooder have?<ul><li>How is it monitored?</li><li>What is the humidity?</li><li>How is the humidity maintained?</li><li>How is the humidity monitored?</li></ul></li></ul>	<ul><li>See Figure 31.4 for recommended brooder temperatures.</li></ul>
Infectious disease/ quarantine	<ul><li>How many breeding birds does the owner have?<ul><li>What species?</li><li>Any new introductions in the past year?</li><li>Where are new introductions housed relative to the parents of this bird?</li></ul></li><li>Does the owner only hand-rear birds that they have bred?<ul><li>If not, what is the source of the other baby birds?</li><li>Did they use the same breeder as previously?</li><li>Have they had any problems with this breeder before?</li><li>What sort of quarantine exists between the bought-in chicks and the home-bred chicks?</li></ul></li><li>Are any other chicks affected?</li><li>Do the chicks travel anywhere else (e.g. pet stores, bird shows)?</li><li>Does the owner handle any birds that are not their own?</li></ul>	

31.3   History taking for chicks.

Age	Brooding temperature (°C)	Feeding regime
Recent hatchlings	33–34	Every 2 hours, throughout night
Unfeathered chicks	32–33	Every 4 hours, stopping for 6 hours during night
Chicks with some pin feathers	29.5–32	Every 4–6 hours
Fully feathered chicks	24–29.5	Two to three times daily
Weaned chicks	20–24	Not needed

31.4 Common brooding temperatures and feeding schedules for baby birds.

as oedema or ascites. If possible, fluid should be aspirated and assessed cytologically. Occasionally, large aspiration events will result in food being deposited in the caudal air sacs. The change in compliance of the air sacs can occasionally be detected via palpation.

Musculoskeletal deformities are not uncommon in growing birds. Limbs should be thoroughly palpated, and joints assessed for appropriate range of motion. The spine and keel may have deviations, which can often be detected via palpation. Fractures, fracture calluses and metabolic bone disease may be detected. Skeletal abnormalities are more common when chicks are being reared on a homemade diet, or the parents only have access to poor nutrition (such as seed). The beak should be assessed for any misalignment (Figure 31.5).

A dehydrated chick shows shiny, reddened skin that tents on gentle pinching (Figure 31.6). The skin overlying the carina does not move as freely. Mucous membranes are tacky, which can be detected when trying to pass crop tubes or take oral smears. Crop contents are often doughy. Total solids and packed cell volume (PCV) estimations may be done to give more objective assessments. Be aware that chicks have a lower PCV and total solids than an adult of the same species.

Lastly, the faeces of a chick should *always* be assessed microscopically, using wet smears and Gram stains. Diff-Quik® is used by some practitioners to determine the morphology of the bacteria, although it fails to give as much information as a Gram stain (see Chapter 12). There is always a large fluid component to a chick's droppings, due to the high fluid content of their diet.

or fistulation should be noted, as should the presence or absence of muscular contractions. A healthy chick should have several muscular contractions per minute. A crop wash should be performed in all baby birds, and assessed initially as a wet smear, and then as a Gram stain if indicated. Inexperienced practitioners should always perform both a wet smear and a Gram stain.

Aspiration is not an uncommon event when birds are being hand-reared. Auscultation may detect harsh air movement or crackles.

Examination of the coelom may reveal masses or fluid accumulation. Although not common, coelomic masses are usually retained egg yolks (in very young chicks) or gastrointestinal foreign bodies that have progressed more distally within the gut. Occasionally organ enlargement, such as hepatomegaly, can be seen. Fluid accumulation needs to be further defined

---

Initial triage of a sick chick

1. **Is the chick alert?**
   - Yes. Go to 2.
   - No. Could the chick be:
     - Dehydrated? Treat for dehydration. Go to 2.
     - Cold? Place in age/temperature appropriate brooder immediately. Go to 2.
     - Hypoglycaemic? Check blood glucose, if possible. Cage-side glucometers can give a rough estimate of blood glucose levels. Treat for hypoglycaemia. Go to 2.
     - Infected/septicaemic? Take blood for haematological analysis, if possible. Treat for infection, if appropriate. Go to 2.
     - Potentially suffering from a viral disease? Ensure good biosecurity. Take appropriate samples. Go to 2.
2. **Is there food in the crop?**
   - Yes. Is it emptying?
     - Yes. Use oral fluids and feeding. Go to 3.
     - No. Treat for crop stasis.
   - No. Feed immediately. Go to 3.
3. **Are there any crop abnormalities?**
   - Yes. Is there a fistula present?
     - Yes. Treat for crop burn/crop trauma. Go to 4.
     - No. Are there palpable masses in the crop?
       - o Yes. Consider general anaesthesia and removal via the oral cavity or via ingluviotomy, assuming patient is stable. If not, stabilize patient first. Go to 4.
4. **Are there any musculoskeletal abnormalities?**
   - Yes. Could these be related to abnormal calcium homeostasis? Is there potential for hypocalcaemia?
     - Yes. Perform in-house ionized calcium test (if possible). Supplement with calcium promptly if suspicous of hypocalcaemia (hypocalcaemia may cause muscle weakness, including cardiac). Treatment is covered in Chapters 11 and 29. Go to 5.
     - No. Treat as indicated. Consider radiography to further diagnose the problem. Go to 5.
5. **Do any of these conditions require the use of antibiotics?**
   - Yes. Ensure coverage with prophylactic antifungal agents. Nystatin (at 300,000 IU/kg q12h, 20 minutes prior to feeding) is a good choice as it is not systemically absorbed

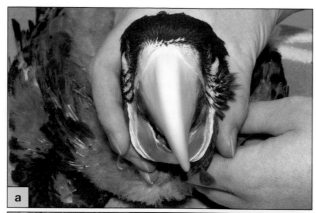

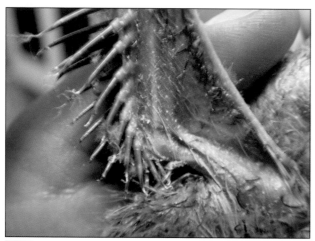

31.5   **(a)** A macaw chick with a scissor beak. **(b)** With correcting apparatus in place. (© John Chitty)

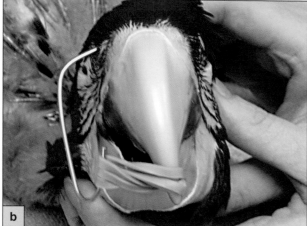

31.6   Dehydrated nestling with increased skin turgor demonstrated under the wing. (Courtesy of Dr Robert Doneley)

Specific conditions and treatments

Crop stasis

A baby bird's crop may cease moving for a number of reasons, including foreign bodies, gastrointestinal infection and viral infection. Husbandry issues may be involved (incorrect ambient temperature, incorrect feeding formula temperature, incorrect feeding formula consistency or concentration). However, regardless of the cause, static food and fluid in a crop, kept at over 40°C, will always become secondarily infected. So, even though bacterial and fungal infection present in a static crop must be treated, the owners need to be cautioned that there may be an underlying primary issue. 'Sour crop' is a term used in the avicultural industry to denote a static, infected crop, but it tends to be avoided by veterinary surgeons (veterinarians) as it does not denote the underlying cause of the problem.

Chicks with static crops may have sedimentation of the feeding formula (separation of the powder and more liquid components), and will have reduced ingluvial muscle contractions. The muscle contractions that do occur are often feeble. The owners may have noticed an increase in the level of begging for food by the chick, or a reduction in weight gain. As the condition advances, the chick may become depressed and dehydrated, or the feeding response may reduce. Diagnosis of the condition is by physical examination, crop wash (wet smear and Gram stain) and assessment of any underlying problems. Once samples have been taken, the crop should be emptied using a crop tube, and lavaged with warmed fluids to remove older crop contents and reduce the microbial burden. Frequent small feeds should be given, using a crop tube if the feeding response is poor. Diluted feeding formula, or even simple electrolyte solution (supplemented with glucose if required) should be used for the first few feeds. Many breeders and veterinary surgeons add dilute fennel tea to the hand-rearing formula to assist digestion in the early stages of crop stasis. Drainage and lavage of crop contents should continue regularly, until crop motility begins to return. As this occurs, the hand-rearing formula concentration and feeding volume per feed can increase, and the frequency of feeding can reduce. The use of antimicrobials is described below, in the section on gastrointestinal infection.

> **WARNING**
>
> When dealing with a static crop, *never* turn the bird upside down and 'milk' out the crop contents, as this can lead to aspiration pneumonia and nasal infections

Infections

The gastrointestinal tract is the most common site for infection in the young bird. Poor hygiene and husbandry commonly contribute to this prevalence, and crop infections are particularly common. Crop stasis is a common clinical sign, as is weight loss, decreased begging for food and depression. Diagnosis is via wet smear and Gram stain (or Diff-Quik®, as a second option) evaluation of both crop wash and faecal samples. The normal microbial flora of birds is listed in Figure 31.7.

Group	Flora
Psittaciformes	Mainly Gram-positive, rods and cocci
Passeriformes	Often minimal (small passerines such as canaries) May be towards more mixed Gram-positive/ Gram-negative population in softbill passerines such as Mynah birds
Raptors	Mixed bacterial population with large numbers of Gram-negative bacteria Gram stain often unrewarding unless a homogenous population of bacteria is obtained

31.7   Common microbial flora of birds.

Bacterial and fungal infections

Treatment for bacterial infection is dictated by the Gram stain result, compared with the expected flora for that species. Co-amoxiclav is a common choice for infections involving Gram-positive bacteria, while enrofloxacin is a good initial choice for Gram-negative bacterial infections.

Chicks are very susceptible to post-antibiotic candidiasis (Figure 31.8). Any baby bird placed on antibiotics should commence prophylactic antifungal medication.

Candidiasis is a common sequel to antibiotic use in young chicks, and can cause severe clinical signs. Candidal infection is assessed according to Figure 31.9. Nystatin is not systemically absorbed through intact mucosa. It needs to be given on a relatively empty gastrointestinal tract in order to increase mucosal contact time and efficacy. Fluconazole should be used with caution in cases of hepatopathy.

Systemic bacterial and fungal infections can occur in baby birds. Haematological examination can provide evidence of a failing immune response, and should prompt aggressive treatment with both antibiosis and supportive care.

Chlamydia psittaci may cause problems in young birds, and should be on the list of differential diagnoses with sick chicks. Clinical signs can include, but are not limited to, conjunctivitis, oculonasal discharge, hepatopathy, depression, sepsis, weight loss and death. *Chlamydia* is an important disease to rule out, due to the zoonotic implications of infection (see Chapter 20). Treatment is with doxycycline, for 42 days. Secondary candidiasis is extremely common secondary to oral doxycycline treatment.

Viral infections

Viral infections are most common in psittacine nursery situations, especially when there are multiple sources of birds. Some commercial hand-rearers buy in a number of chicks from different breeders to boost their turnover, and as quarantine is usually not practised in these situations, epidemics can result. Polyomavirus and adenovirus are commonly implicated in these situations. Both viruses cause rapid deterioration, often death with full crops. Post-mortem examinations show ascites and subcutaneous oedema, haemorrhagic changes on intestinal serosa and other organs, and hepatic changes, including hepatomegaly and hepatic necrosis (Figure 31.10). It is not possible to differentiate

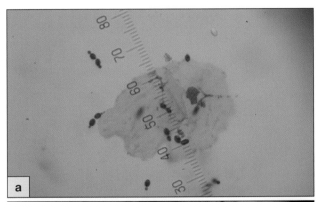

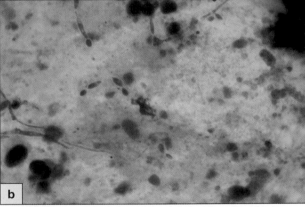

| 31.8 | Candidiasis in chicks. **(a)** Budding *Candida* in a crop wash from a young parrot on antibiotics. This type of yeast overgrowth can be treated with nystatin. **(b)** Budding *Candida* with pseudohyphae. This type of yeast overgrowth should be treated with systemic antifungal medication. (© Deborah Monks) |

Grade	Appearance	Treatment
0	No yeast present	Only required as prophylaxis if on antibiotics
1	Single yeast	Nystatin at 300,000 IU/kg twice to three times daily, given 20 minutes prior to feeding
2	Budding yeast (see Figure 31.8a)	Nystatin if low to moderate numbers, may consider fluconazole if high numbers
3	Pseudohyphal yeast (see Figure 31.8b)	Fluconazole at 5 mg/kg once daily or 10 mg/kg every second day

| 31.9 | Candidal infection grading system. |

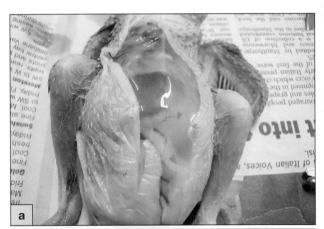

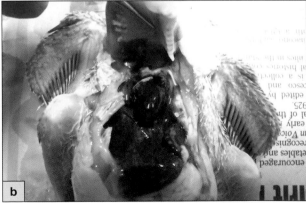

| 31.10 | **(a)** This young chick was one of several that died acutely in a hand-rearing nursery. The owner purchased birds from multiple sources. Subcutaneous oedema can clearly be observed. **(b)** Petechial haemorrhages, serosal oedema and liver pathology can be seen on post-mortem examination. Differential diagnosis was polyomavirus or adenovirus, later proven to be adenovirus by PCR. (© Deborah Monks) |

these two viruses histologically, so polymerase chain reaction (PCR) testing must be done. This is important, because there is much information about handling polyomavirus outbreaks (see Chapter 19) and very little information about the epidemiology of parrot adeno-virus infections.

Psittacine circovirus can also cause problems during the rearing process. Although acute death is possible, psittacine circovirus tends to cause ill-thrifty chicks with poor plumage. Powder down is lacking and feather dystrophy is present in other feathers. Clinically affected chicks will go on to die from their disease, usually after a period of repeated secondary infections (occurring due to the immunosuppressive effects of the virus). Chronic or recurrent infections in young birds should trigger an index of suspicion regarding this virus, and testing is recommended.

For these three viruses, as in most cases of viral disease, there is no treatment once birds are exhibiting clinical disease. Life may be prolonged by treating secondary infections (if the disease does not progress rapidly), but prognosis is poor. Surviving birds may be lifelong carriers. Owners should be counselled about biosecurity and quarantine.

In finches, polyomavirus can cause acute death (as in parrots) but also leads to birds with chronic ill-thrift. Long, tubular misshapen beaks (Figure 31.11) can be observed in surviving birds. In raptors, there are few viruses that specifically affect young birds.

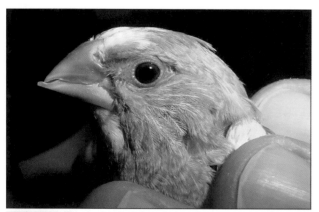

31.11 Tubular beak deformity in a finch from an aviary with endemic polyomavirus. (Courtesy of Dr S Echols)

Dehydration
Chicks that are dehydrated show reddened skin, with increased skin turgor. Their eyes may be sunken. Mucous membranes are tacky, and the passage of crop tubes is more difficult. Increased PCV and total solids may reflect dehydration, but be aware that young birds have lower normal values of these parameters than adult birds. If possible, consult an age-appropriate species-specific reference range for these values.

The daily fluid maintenance requirement of a chick is 50 ml/kg/day. Additional to daily fluid requirements, dehydrated chicks will need their fluid deficit replaced over 24–48 hours. In chicks with functional crop motility, this can be done orally. When crop stasis or delayed crop emptying is present, fluid may need to be given subcutaneously. This is usually done in the precrural fold (see Chapter 11). As soon as crop function is restored, fluid supplementation should be done orally.

Hypoglycaemia
The main clinical sign of hypoglycaemia is depression, which makes it difficult to diagnose without additional testing. In cases of severe hypoglycaemia or where the chick is severely obtunded, immediate parenteral supplementation of 100 mg/kg glucose is recommended. This should be diluted prior to administration, especially if being given subcutaneously. With mild to moderate hypoglycaemia, or suspected hypoglycaemia, glucose may be supplemented at a reduced level. If the crop is functional, supplementation into oral electrolytes, or simply using hand-rearing formula is sufficient. If the crop is static, then glucose may be added into parenteral fluids. If vitamin B$_1$ deficiency is suspected, then parenteral supplementation can be added.

Hypothermia
Chicks should feel warm to the touch. Cold, shivering or cyanotic chicks should be immediately warmed to the appropriate ambient temperature (see Figure 31.4). When warming chicks, always keep your hand between the animal and the heat source to avoid thermal burns. Care should be taken that forced warm air (hairdryers, some brooders) does not contribute to dehydration. To ensure an adequate ambient temperature, it is recommended to monitor with a thermometer that records maximum and minimum levels.

Crop burn
Hand-rearing formula needs to be fed at approximately 41°C. Too cold, and the chicks will likely refuse it, and it will also chill the chicks, predisposing them to crop stasis. Too hot, and crop burns can result (Figure 31.12). A single feed above 45–46°C, or multiple feeds at a slightly lower temperature, can be sufficient to damage the lining of the crop wall. It is not advisable that hand-feeding formula is heated in microwave ovens, as this can result in focal hot spots that exceed safe temperatures for birds.

Full-thickness burns will initially have an area of ery-thema and oedema, which may be noticed by an astute hand-rearer. As the tissues begin to slough, a scab will form, and finally a fistula (Figure 31.13). The full extent of damage can take up to 5 days to become apparent, so it is advised to delay surgery until that time. While waiting for surgery, the chick must be kept hydrated and have sufficient caloric intake. This may

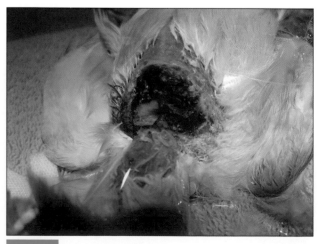

31.12 A severe crop burn.

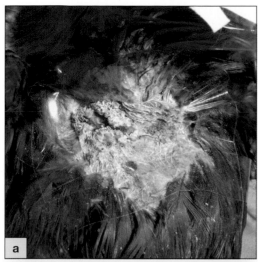

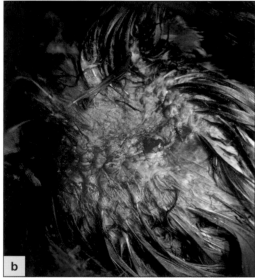

31.13 (a) A mild crop fistula in a female Eclectus Parrot. The reddened area is just visible centrally. **(b)** The same crop fistula, after repair. (© Deborah Monks)

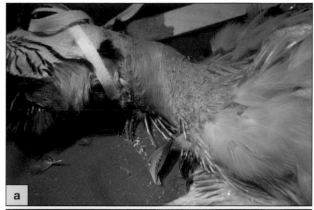

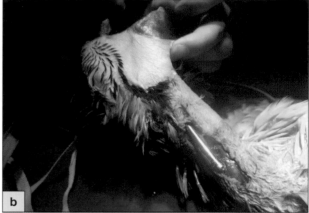

31.14 Crop perforation in a macaw chick. This bird had been sold unweaned to a young, inexperienced keeper, who was advised to hand feed it via crop tube. The bird perforated its oesophagus due to the exuberant head bobbing response. **(a)** Before the skin was opened. The external changes are subtle and include mild swelling and erythema. **(b)** View of the lesion after opening the skin. (© Deborah Monks)

necessitate frequent feedings and altered delivery of food (as much may leak out of the fistula). Affected birds need to be regularly cleaned to prevent hygiene problems secondary to food leakage.

Partial-thickness burns are more insidious because feeding formula can leak through devitalized crop wall to deposit subcutaneously, potentially resulting in sepsis. In the case of a suspected partial-thickness burn, surgery is immediately indicated. Antibiosis is always required, along with prophylactic antifungal medication. Co-amoxiclav (125 mg/kg orally q12h) is a good, broad-spectrum choice. Analgesia is, of course, required. See Chapter 17 for the surgical approach.

Gastrointestinal foreign bodies

Hand-reared chicks often have exuberant feeding responses (Figure 31.14), which can lead to ingestion of crop tubes and other feeding equipment (Figure 31.15). As the chicks begin to develop, they become very curious about their environment and can easily ingest substrate, toys and other objects.

Crop foreign bodies can often be palpated, and can be removed either orally or via ingluviotomy (see Chapter 17). When removing orally, anaesthesia may be useful as it reduces iatrogenic trauma and allows placement of an endotracheal tube to protect

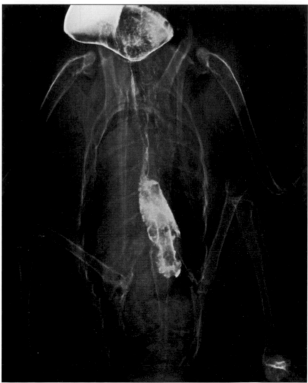

31.15 A barium study on an African Grey Parrot chick that had ingested a crop tube. The tube can be clearly seen outlined in this ventrodorsal view. (Courtesy of Dr A Gallagher)

the airway from food aspiration. If the item is too large, or has the potential to cause damage while being removed, ingluviotomy is a better removal option (see Chapter 17). Postoperative care involves smaller, more frequent feeds to avoid excessive pressure on the surgical site.

If foreign bodies are not removed promptly, then passage into the proventriculus or even the ventriculus can occur. An endoscopic approach to retrieval has fewer chances of complications than a proventriculotomy or ventriculotomy. Regardless, foreign bodies more distal than the crop should be referred to specialist facilities for retrieval. Diagnosis is usually via radiography. Contrast media may be indicated if the object is radiolucent (see Figure 31.15).

References and further reading

Flammer K and Clubb S (1994) Neonatology. In: *Avian Medicine: Principles and Application*, ed. B Ritchie, GJ Harrison and LR Harrison, pp. 805–838. Wingers Publishing, Lake Worth

Doneley RJ (1996) Control and therapy of diseases of birds. In: *TG Hungerford Vade Mecum Series for Domestic Animals. Series A, Number 21*, p. 97. Sydney Post-Graduate Foundation in Veterinary Science, Sydney

Case example 1: Cockatiel chick with bacterial crop infection

Presentation and history

A Cockatiel chick was presented with an enlarged crop. The owner noted that the crop had not been emptying overnight, and the chick was crying for food continuously. The chick was being kept without additional heating, but was being covered with towels for warmth. The owner had not been giving probiotics, and had been mixing the hand-rearing formula according to directions. He had been washing the hand-feeding implements with hot water only.
On examination, the chick was constantly vocalizing for feeding, and had a very distended crop. Minimal muscle contractions were observed during crop palpation. The chick weighed 50 g.

Diagnostic work-up

Examination of the crop wash showed large numbers of bacteria, which were heterogeneous Gram-positive rods on Gram stain. Gram-negative bacteria constituted less than 5%. The crop fluid had a fetid odour. Bacterial crop infection was diagnosed, probably secondary to poor husbandry (insufficient heating) and poor hygiene.

Therapy

The bird was hospitalized and the crop was emptied via crop tube immediately after admission, and lavaged with warmed saline. Hartmann's solution with additional glucose was given for the first two feeds. Antibiosis with co-amoxiclav and prophylactic nystatin was commenced. Crop muscle contractions were observed to increase in frequency and strength, and feeding with diluted hand-rearing formula was begun. The morning after admission, there was 2 ml of hand-rearing formula remaining in the crop, which was removed and the crop again lavaged. Feeding with diluted formula continued throughout the day. The next morning, the crop had almost completely emptied overnight, and the bird was discharged from hospital.

Outcome

The owner was instructed to purchase a heat lamp and thermostat and keep the chick at 28°C. Hand-feeding equipment was to be washed in hot soapy water, and then treated with disinfectant, copiously rinsed and left to dry.

Case example 2: Eclectus Parrot chick with crop fistula

Presentation and history

A 10-week-old Eclectus Parrot chick was presented with a chest wound. The owner believed that the bird had been scratched by their cat. The owner mixed up the bird's hand-feeding mixture once daily, and kept the remainder in the refrigerator. Prior to each feed, the required amount of formula was removed from the refrigerator and heated in the microwave prior to feeding. Hand-feeding equipment was washed with hot soapy water each evening after the last feed, and left to dry on the counter. The owner reported that the bird had seemed quiet for a few days, starting around a week ago, but was back to being bright again.

Diagnostic work-up

There was a damp patch on the chest, just cranial to the coracoid border. On examination, underlying the damp patch was a small fistula approximately 3 mm in diameter. The edges were scabbed and slightly erythematous. A crop needle was passed, and the metal of the crop tube could be visualized through the defect in the skin, confirming a crop fistula (see Figure 31.13).

Therapy

The bird was hospitalized and given subcutaneous fluids. Premedication with butorphanol and a mask induction with isoflurane and oxygen was performed. The bird was intubated, and the crop fistula was repaired.

Outcome

The chick's recovery was fine, and it was discharged from hospital the following day, on trimethoprim/sulphonamide antibiosis, prophylactic nystatin, and meloxicam for analgesia. The owner was instructed to prepare the food adequately, and feed smaller, more frequent amounts until the crop had healed.

Case example 3: Suspected polyomavirus in hand-reared chicks

Presentation and history

A dead 4-week-old Indian Ringnecked Parakeet chick was presented. The owner was rearing 20 baby birds, at least half of which had been purchased from other breeders. Species being reared included Moustached Parrots, Indian Ringnecks, Cockatiels and lovebirds. In the last week, six chicks had suddenly died. Chicks were kept in different boxes grouped according to size, but not separated by origin, age or species. The owner was syringe feeding, and the same hand-rearing equipment was used on multiple birds. After use, the equipment was cleaned with hot soapy water, disinfected, rinsed and left to dry after each feeding.

Diagnostic work-up

On post-mortem examination, the chick was in good body condition but had subcutaneous oedema overlying the chest. There was ascites and clear pericardial effusion visible when the coelom was opened (see Figure 31.10). Petechial haemorrhages were present on the heart, intestinal serosa and pectoral muscles. There was mild to moderate hepatosplenomegaly. The most likely differential diagnosis was thought to be polyomavirus.

Outcome

The owner was instructed to immediately cease purchasing new birds, and to cease sharing feeding equipment between birds. If that was not possible, then he was to use the same feeding equipment only for each 'box' of birds. Sterilization of feeding equipment was to continue.

Tissues were sent away for histopathological examination, which showed eosinophilic inclusion bodies, consistent with either polyomavirus or adenovirus. PCR testing was done on banked frozen tissue, which was negative for polyomavirus and positive for adenovirus. When the owner was notified of the results, he noted that only 4 more birds had died and the rest of the birds were looking healthy. He was advised to notify prospective purchasers that these birds could be carriers of adenovirus, but it was unknown if he followed that recommendation.

Weakness and seizures

Michael Pees

Many bird species try their best to hide signs of ill health, either to avoid being excluded from the social group or so as not to appear as easy prey for predators, therefore clinical signs in birds are often non-specific and disease processes might only appear in cases of decompensation. Weakness and seizures are often the result of a chronic disease process. In cases of weakness without accompanying specific clinical signs, it is not always easy to decide which diagnostic measure is appropriate, and this chapter can only give a guideline for a possible step-by-step diagnostic work-up. As weakness is often the result of emaciation, following a diagnostic protocol for this sign may be useful (see Chapter 28). See also Chapters 15, 30 and 31.

In cases of neurological signs, it is essential to perform a neurological examination, even though there are some limiting factors in birds: firstly, in contrast to mammals, birds often react to pain stimuli with inactivity, and, secondly, examination of the birds' sensorium might not give many results due to the overall stress of the handling procedure. However, although the signs normally do not allow a tentative diagnosis, it is important to specify the kind of seizure. Typical neurological alterations seen in birds include ataxia, head swinging, opisthotonos, torticollis and tremor seizures, as well as paresis or paralysis, and circular movements.

PRACTICAL TIP

It should be noted that although various established diagnostic procedures are available for birds, in many cases with neurological signs, the birds respond to the symptomatic therapy, but the initial cause for the signs remains unrevealed

Immediate life-saving measures

As mentioned above, weakness and seizures might be the result of a chronic disease process. Nevertheless, the birds are often presented in an acute emergency situation that requires therapeutic measures even before specific diagnostic tests can be performed. These measures all target stabilization of the circulatory system, and in cases of a suspected toxicosis, the prevention of further damage due to the suspected causative agent.

Stabilization of the circulatory system

The clinical examination allows a rough estimation of the hydration status of the bird, using the capillary filling time of the ulnar vein and, at least in some parrot species, the assessment of the periocular area, as this area might be sunken in cases of severe dehydration.

Fluid replacement can be performed subcutaneously, intravenously or intraosseously, using a warm isotonic fluid solution at a dose of 20 ml/kg. Fluid can be saline solution or Ringer's solution, with amino acid solutions or glucose solution added (each up to 25%). This procedure can be repeated several times each day, but in general a total of 40 ml/kg/day should normally not be exceeded. This recommendation is based on a normal food and water intake, to secure fluid maintenance. Higher dosages might be necessary in anorectic birds that are not force-fed. In these cases the hydration status of the bird should be carefully evaluated to prevent both dehydration and overhydration.

WARNING

In cases of suspected trauma, the administration of fluid can be contraindicated, to prevent the formation of oedema around the central nervous tissue (brain, spinal column)

Oxygen administration

In cases of a suspected respiratory or cardiovascular disease and hypoxia, the administration of pure oxygen before any further handling is done can be life-saving. The best way is to put the bird in a humid incubator in a calm place, but it is also possible to cover the cage with a plastic sheet and to direct the oxygen flow into the cage. Although pure oxygen might have toxic effects, this procedure is well tolerated over several hours.

Administration of food via crop tube

For passerines and parrots, specific formulas are available (e.g. Harrison's Recovery Formula) to assist-feed the debilitated patient. Whilst important, assist or force-feeding should not be performed if the bird is stressed from transport and examination or seizuring. There is a risk of regurgitation and potentially fatal aspiration pneumonia in both these cases.

Treatment of neurological disorders

In cases of seizures, diazepam (0.3–1 mg/kg i.m.) can be administered as an initial treatment. In birds with a suspected calcium deficiency (particularly Grey Parrots), calcium should be administered at a dosage of 40–100 mg/kg i.m. The use of ultra-short-acting glucocorticoids, however, is only advisable in cases of acute trauma in order to prevent inflammatory swellings in the central nervous system. In birds, the use of glucocorticoids has a severe side effect of long-lasting immunosuppression.

Anti-infective agents

The use of antifungal drugs can be taken into account in bird species that have a special predisposition to fungal infections of the respiratory system (see Chapter 22) and demonstrate clinical signs that support this tentative diagnosis. The use of antibiotics, however, is only advisable in cases with a strong indication of a bacterial (septicaemic) process, as well as cases of animal bites (peracute Pasteurella infections). It should, whenever possible, be combined with culture and sensitivity testing, even though a first-guess antibiosis (e.g. enrofloxacin) may be started.

Diagnostic work-up

Although any bird with clinical signs should be examined carefully, there are some points that need special attention in cases of weakness and/or seizures. The work-up given here is only a proposal that can serve as a guideline for diagnostic procedures. The most common causes mentioned in this work-up are discussed below.

History taking

- Species:
  - Predisposition for aspergillosis
  - Predisposition for obesity.
- Trauma/injury:
  - Cat/dog bite
  - Mate aggression
  - Hit by car
  - Time elapsed since injury.
- Intoxication:
  - Bird in household or aviary
  - Chemical agents including insecticides, plants, toys
  - Check environment.
- Husbandry conditions:
  - Food quality
  - Exercise
  - Vitamin/calcium supplementation.
- Faeces:
  - Maldigestion
  - Undigested seeds.

Clinical examination

- Overall activity:
  - Flight activity
  - Depression
  - Incoordination.
- Body condition:
  - Emaciation
  - Chronic processes
  - Adiposity.

- Respiratory tract:
  - Increased breathing
  - Breathlessness.
- Trauma/injuries:
  - Wounds (see Chapters 15 and 30)
  - Fractures
  - Choana, eyes, ears: bleeding.
- Neurological examination:
  - Coordination
  - Reflexes
  - Eye examination.
- Abdominal shape:
  - Swollen (palpable eggs).

Further diagnostics

- Abdominal swelling:
  - Ultrasonography (alternatively/additionally radiography):
    - Egg binding
    - Neoplasia
    - Organomegaly
    - Ascites/heart disease.
- Neurological signs:
  - Blood chemistry:
    - Calcium deficiency.
  - Radiography:
    - Organ function (liver)
    - Trauma
    - Atherosclerosis.
  - Ultrasonography:
    - Cardiac disease
    - Ascites.
- Respiratory signs:
  - Radiography:
    - Aspergillosis
    - Displacement of air sacs
    - Organomegaly.
- Intoxication:
  - Radiography:
    - Radiodense foreign bodies.
  - Blood chemistry:
    - Lead/zinc concentrations.
- Maldigestion/emaciation:
  - Radiography:
    - Proventricular dilatation (parrots).
  - Faeces examination:
    - Endoparasites.
  - Cloacal examination:
    - Yeasts/bacteria.
  - Swabs/blood:
    - Bornavirus (parrots).

Common causes of weakness and seizures

Although weakness and seizures can be caused by a broad variety of diseases, some are – even though not very specific – common causes, and often do not lead to more specific clinical signs. This list only presents a selection of important diseases that should be taken into account.

Chlamydiosis/bacterial infection

Many bacterial infections can cause weakness and some can also be responsible for neurological signs.

Accompanying clinical signs often include regurgitation, diarrhoea and apathy, but the specific clinical situation depends very much on the causative agent and the overall condition of the bird. Chlamydia psittaci is of special importance as this bacterium is widespread amongst wild and captive bird populations and can cause a variety of signs including neurological disorders. Weakness is seen in both acute and advanced stages of the disease. A radiographic examination often demonstrates an enlarged spleen as well as liver and kidney enlargement. *Chlamydia* spp. can only be detected using special media, paired serology, ELISA test kits or polymerase chain reaction (PCR), and is of importance also because of its zoonotic potential. Treatment is possible with some antibiotics, such as tetracycline or fluoroquinolones, but an effective disinfection procedure is necessary to avoid reinfection.

Mycobacterium spp. can also cause chronic emaciation and weakness. Mycobacteria are found worldwide in both wild and pet birds. Parrots and passerine birds in captivity might still have a history of being wild-caught. In raptors, falconry birds are often affected, due to possible infection via their prey. Mycobacteria normally cause chronic disease processes, with a progressive emaciation despite good or even increased appetite. They can be detected using special stains (Ziehl–Neelsen) for faecal smears or biopsy samples, and a culture or PCR can be used to confirm the tentative diagnosis. There is no effective therapy described, although in some cases, according to the experience in human medicine, the combination of different antibiotics has been attempted.

Further bacterial infections of relevance include Gram-negative bacteria, especially *Salmonella* spp. This is of special relevance in pigeons (*Salmonella* Typhimurium var. Copenhagen). Diagnosis is often difficult, as isolation from faeces/swabs does not allow a definite conclusion that they caused an encephalitis. Serology is also helpful in cases of suspected salmonellosis.

Aspergillosis/fungal infection

Fungal respiratory infections, commonly referred to as aspergillosis, are an important disease in birds kept in captivity. Most affected are parrots from tropical habitats (e.g. Grey Parrots, Amazons, macaws), falcons and some owl and eagle species. In wild birds, the disease can occur but is far less important. The clinical picture varies but can include respiratory signs due to fungal growth in the lower respiratory system, central nervous signs due to the fungal toxins and effects on other organs, and weakness due to the chronic disease process. Therefore, especially as the isolation of fungi from the upper respiratory system is only of limited diagnostic value, imaging techniques are of special importance. They include radiography, computed tomography (CT) and endoscopy, and allow the assessment of the fungal growth (directly via endoscopy, indirectly by radiography or CT due to the radiodense structures in the air sacs and the lung). Further diagnostic methods are described but are of limited value. Birds suffering from a severe aspergillosis are often in a very reduced body condition and need immediate therapy for stabilization of the circulatory and respiratory systems (see above). Specific therapy normally includes the use of anti-fungals, most often itraconazole or the more effective

(but also more expensive) agent voriconazole. In Grey Parrots, itraconazole has been shown to be not well tolerated. Another option is the oral use of terbinafine, but despite an often promising initial effect, long-term use can lead to the quick development of drug resistance. An accompanying vitamin A supplementation is essential for the regeneration of the respiratory and air sac epithelium. Fluid substitution is helpful to wash out fungal toxins, and to support liver and kidney function. Husbandry conditions should be optimized according to the physiological needs of the bird.

Macrorhabdus ornithogaster

Over the last years, this fungus has become more and more important in conures and (especially) in Budgerigars. It is found in the whole digestive tract, particularly the crop and the proventriculus. Clinical signs include weakness and emaciation, as well as regurgitation. Typically, the birds demonstrate an increased appetite but can be anorectic in later stages of the disease. The diagnosis is made using microscopic examination of droppings and crop washes/swabs (either fresh or after staining) for the pathogen. However, the presence of *Macrorhabdus ornithogaster* in a dropping means that the bird is infected, but not necessarily clinically diseased at that moment, as many healthy Budgerigars also harbour this fungus. Therapy can be attempted using oral solutions of amphotericin B over a period of 4 weeks. However, recurrence of the disease is seen quite often, and the disease is infectious.

Proventricular dilatation disease and bornavirus infection

Proventricular dilatation disease (PDD) is presumably caused by a bornavirus, and occurs in many bird species, with clinical signs predominantly in parrots. Even though many studies demonstrate the association between bornavirus and the disease signs, there are still some open questions on the pathogenesis of the infection. Clinical signs include emaciation and weakness as well as central nervous signs. A typical finding is the presence of undigested seeds in the droppings, however, this is not a pathognomonic sign. As the infection of nervous tissue leads to a dilatation of the proventriculus, radiography can be used to demonstrate the size of this organ. However, in some cases, the proventriculus might not be dilated. Bornavirus can be detected using PCR, and serological tests are also available. Final diagnosis is normally made using a biopsy sample from the proventriculus (often because it is safer and easier to obtain from the crop tissue) followed by histopathological examination. There is no causative therapy, but in some studies the use of anti-inflammatory drugs (COX-2 inhibitors such as celecoxib or meloxicam) seem to sometimes reduce the clinical signs.

Endoparasitic infection

Endoparasites are a common cause of emaciation and weakness, in both wild and pet birds. In the author's experience, all birds (at least at their first presentation to a veterinary surgeon (veterinarian)) should be checked for endoparasites by examining a simple faecal dropping sample after suitable flotation. The most frequently found endoparasitic worms are ascarids. However, flagellates, coccidia and other parasites can play a role, therefore further examinations (e.g. crop wash and microscopic examination for flagellates) might be necessary. Besides the specific therapy, accompanying tube-feeding can be necessary in advanced stages, as the birds can lose their appetite and are in urgent need of nutrition. Effective endoparasiticides are available, and appropriate cleaning and disinfection procedures are highly recommended (see also Chapter 19).

Intoxication (lead, chemical substances, plants, iatrogenic)

A broad variety of possible toxins in birds is described, including plants, fruits and chemical substances as well as therapeutic drugs. Due to their different physiology, many substances that are known to be toxic in mammals do not harm birds, but the contrary is also true. In addition to some pharmaceuticals, well known toxic substances for birds include avocado and polytetrafluoroethylene (PTFE, well known for its use for non-stick coatings in kitchenware). Both substances (avocado given orally, PTFE after inhalation following heating of pans) cause severe seizures and often lead to the death of the bird. The most common toxic substance in parrots (particularly Cockatiels) is lead, which is still found in many household articles, such as drawstrings and Tiffany lamps. Zinc and copper toxicosis, often due to aviary or electrical wire, is common. It can be challenging to determine the cause of the toxicosis, and a thorough history (including the owners checking the bird's environment) is necessary. Heavy metal particles such as lead (sometimes also metal particles with zinc) can be seen on radiographs, and can also be determined by checking the blood concentrations. Therapy includes the use of specific antidotes, such as chelating agents (e.g. EDTA at 200 mg/kg i.m. initially, followed by 20–40 mg/kg i.m. q24h; or diethylenetriaminepentaacetic acid (DTPA) at 35 mg/kg i.m. q24h, then every other day from day 3) against heavy metals, but also symptomatic therapy such as fluid administration and the use of vitamins (e.g. vitamin E in the case of heavy metal poisoning).

Trauma

Trauma is an important problem in wild and pet birds, often caused by windows, cars (wild birds), cage mates or other animals in the household. The diagnostic work-up should include a detailed history (Was the trauma observed? How much time has passed since?) and a thorough clinical examination. Birds are often very depressed and apathetic, and lameness can occur. Where cats or rats are involved the skin wounds can be rather discrete but the deep bite can cause a *Pasteurella* septicaemia, therefore a systemic antibiotic therapy is required as an emergency procedure. In nearly all cases of trauma, a radiograph is necessary to assess the bony structures, including the spinal column (see also Chapter 29).

Space-occupying processes

Any process that compresses the air sacs will automatically lead to a certain degree of weakness, as the air sacs are necessary to ventilate the lungs and provide adequate oxygen saturation. Therefore, neoplasia (but also egg binding and even the normal process of egg laying) can cause weakness, apathy, and nervous system clinical signs due to compression of the pelvic nerves. As these processes most often affect the inner organs and the abdominal region, this area should always be carefully palpated during the clinical examination. Any bird with a swollen abdomen (which can also be caused by liver or circulatory problems; see below) should be handled as a critically ill bird, as circulatory collapse can be a consequence of prolonged handling or examination procedures. Therefore, radiography, although of great value, might not be the first diagnostic step, because the bird has to be placed in a dorsal position, which can cause further circulatory problems. If possible, in all birds with a swollen abdomen, ultrasonography should be attempted to visualize the inner organs, with the bird held in an upright position.

Liver failure

Liver failure is often the result of inappropriate feeding conditions and often occurs in parrots (particularly Amazon parrots, Budgerigars and Galahs). The birds are often overweight, and a fatty liver syndrome develops, finally leading to anorexia and liver failure. Further causes are infections (e.g. herpesvirus, chlamydiosis). Clinical signs are weakness, apathy and sometimes seizures due to the decreased liver function. An increase in liver size can be demonstrated using radiography or ultrasonography, with ultrasonography also giving information on the liver tissue texture. Blood chemistry (glutamate dehydrogenase, cholesterol and bile acids; see Chapter 12) can further indicate liver failure. Basic treatments include fluid administration, force-feeding with highly digestible carbohydrates, vitamins and, if applicable, an anti-infective treatment. Although non-specific, liver stimulants such as silymarin have a clinically proven beneficial effect on liver function.

Nutritional deficiency

Companion bird diets are often deficient in calcium and various vitamins, and these deficiencies can lead to clinical signs including weakness and seizures. The most common deficiency causing neurological disease in parrots is calcium. In most seeds (especially sunflower), the calcium concentration is very low and the calcium:phosphorus ratio is poor. Amongst all parrot species, the African Grey Parrot is known to be most susceptible to seizures caused by a low serum calcium level. The calcium concentration in a blood sample can be determined, but initial treatment of suspicious cases should always include the parenteral administration of a calcium solution.

Circulatory/cardiac insufficiency (including atherosclerosis)

Heart disease in birds used to be considered very rare. However, many studies have shown the relevance of cardiac and vessel alterations in pet and aviary birds. It is suspected that the causes of heart and vessel diseases in birds are similar to those in humans, and include poor diet and a lack of exercise. A post-mortem study of parrots demonstrated that one-third suffered from macroscopic heart alterations (Krautwald-Junghanns *et al.*, 2004), and almost all birds demonstrated, at least microscopically, a pathological alteration of the heart. The most common cardiac alterations leading to clinical signs include heart hypertrophy and dilatation, and pericardial effusion. As a consequence of cardiac insufficiency the birds become apathetic, demonstrate reduced exercise tolerance and seizures can occur. Besides heart disease, major blood vessel disease also plays an important role, and is predominantly caused by atherosclerosis.

Atherosclerosis can occur in all bird species and has been found in both indoor and aviary birds. Seizures, other neurological signs and sudden death can occur. Diagnostic work-up includes the use of radiography (conventional and CT, assessment of heart size and vessel density), ultrasonography (cardiac function, blood flow) and blood chemistry (e.g. cholesterol levels). Medical therapy is normally symptomatic. Angiotensin-converting enzyme inhibitors such as enalapril have been proven to be effective and well tolerated, however the prognosis should be cautious once clinical signs occur.

References and further reading

Krautwald-Junghanns ME, Braun S, Pees M, Straub J and Valerius HP (2004) Research on the anatomy and pathology of the psittacine heart. *Journal of Avian Medicine and Surgery* **18(1)**, 2–11

Case example 1: Amazon parrot with lead toxicosis

Presentation and history

A 2-year-old male Amazon parrot was presented with a history of intermittent seizures over 24 hours, anorexia, apathy and bloody diarrhoea. The bird was allowed to move freely in the house, and a tentative diagnosis was intoxication. Although the owners denied the presence of heavy metal material in their home, they were asked to check the whole household for possible sources. Finally, they found an old glass lamp with lead bindings and fresh bite marks.

Diagnostic work-up

A radiograph was taken and radiodense material was found in the ventriculus. An initial treatment using a chelating agent was initiated and, to confirm the diagnosis, a blood sample was examined and a lead concentration of 0.7 ppm was determined (normal up to 0.2 ppm). Lead poisoning is a common finding and can cause both weakness and neurological clinical signs. These cases should be handled as emergencies, as early treatment is important to improve the prognosis.

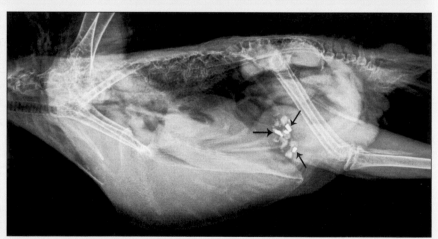

Lateral view of an Amazon parrot with weakness and apathy. In addition to some normal grit stones, radiodense material is also present in the ventriculus (arrowed). Parrots are highly susceptible to heavy metal intoxication.

Therapy

The bird was treated with calcium EDTA i.m. (initially 200 mg/kg i.m., followed by 40 mg/kg i.m. q24h), barium sulfate and paraffin via crop tube (each 10 ml/kg q24h), supported with fluids (20 ml/kg s.c. q12h) and force-fed using a commercial recovery formula. (Alternatively to calcium EDTA, DTPA can be used at 35 mg/kg i.m. q24h for 3 days, then q48h for a week.)

Outcome

The bird recovered quickly. Therapy was stopped after 10 days and a negative radiographic control examination. The owners were advised to make sure the environment of the bird was free of possible toxic agents.

Case example 2: Liver failure in an Indian Hill Mynah

Presentation and history

A 13-year-old single-kept female Indian Hill Mynah was presented because of sudden weakness and inability to fly. The bird was fed on commercial mynah food and a variety of fruits. Clinical examination revealed a reduced body condition and a massively swollen abdomen.

Diagnostic work-up

On radiography, a severe soft tissue swelling and displacement of the air sacs in the coelomic cavity was seen. A massive organ enlargement or fluid accumulation was suspected, and ultrasonography was conducted to get more information. In the ultrasound image, a severely enlarged liver was diagnosed. An ultrasound-guided biopsy sample was examined histologically and haemochromatosis of the liver was diagnosed.

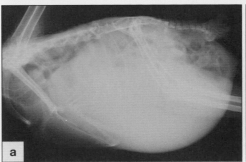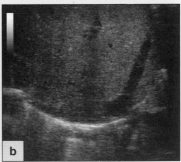

Indian Hill Mynah with weakness. (a) Lateral view showing a massive swelling.
(b) Ultrasonography via a ventromedial approach (10 MHz and 4 cm examination depth) confirmed the mass to be a soft tissue swelling, with an echotexture that corresponded to the liver tissue.

Therapy

The bird was hospitalized, and therapy for iron intoxication was started (DTPA at 35 mg/kg i.m. q24h) plus nutritional support with a low-iron diet.

Outcome

Haemochromatosis is a common problem in mynahs, as they require a specialized diet with low iron concentrations. Accumulation of iron leads to liver cell necrosis and liver failure in the long term. The birds often lose their ability to speak, and suffer from progressive weakness and dyspnoea. Long-term prognosis is poor; this patient died after a few days despite therapy.

Case example 3: Heart disease in an African Grey Parrot

Presentation and history

A 23-year-old wild-caught male African Grey Parrot showed signs of progressive weakness, anorexia and loss of speaking behaviour. For the last 2 days the owners had noticed the bird was having problems while perching and demonstrating progressive incoordination. The bird was susceptible to collapse during the clinical examination and was therefore first placed in an oxygen tent.

Diagnostic work-up

Radiography (post-stabilization) revealed an increased cardiac shadow, a soft tissue mass caudal to the heart and possible displacement of the ventriculus. Ultrasonographically, the heart was found to be dilated, and cardiac function (contractility) was reduced. Furthermore, fluid was found in the coelomic cavity and the liver was congested.

Therapy

Cardiac therapy was instituted using enalapril at 1.25 mg/kg given orally q12h.

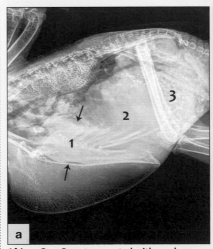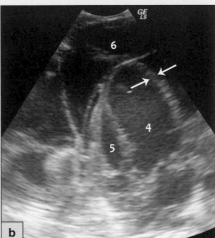

African Grey Parrot presented with weakness and incoordination. (a) Lateral view demonstrating an increased cardiac shadow (1), as well as a soft tissue mass (2) in front of the ventriculus/intestines (3). (b) Ultrasonography via a ventromedial approach (10 MHz and 6 cm examination depth). The left heart chamber (4) is severely distended, and the walls are thin (arrowed). The right chamber (5) appears unremarkable, and some fluid can be seen in the coelomic cavity (6).

Outcome

The clinical situation improved over the few next days, but the bird died a few weeks after presentation. Heart disease in companion birds has a poor prognosis as clinical signs are often only noticed in the advanced stage of disease, after decompensation. For the initial clinical signs calcium deficiency is a major differential diagnosis in African Grey Parrots and should be investigated by measurement of the (ionized) calcium level in blood serum.

Case example 4: Weakness in a wild Common Buzzard

Presentation and history

A male Common Buzzard was found close to a road. The bird was in a weak, depressed status. He did not react to handling and clinical examination; however, this might be a physiological reaction in stressful situations and should not be misinterpreted as a neurological clinical sign. The bird was in a poor body condition, and trauma was suspected.

Diagnostic work-up

In these cases, an ophthalmological examination is essential to check for possible intraocular bleeding. Some old wounds were found on the head, but the ears, the choana and the eyes were unremarkable. A radiograph was taken to assess the skeletal system and the inner organs. No abnormality of the skeletal system was diagnosed, but the digestive

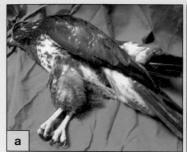 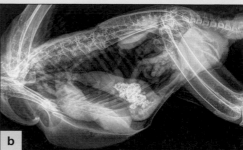

(a) Wild Common Buzzard presented weak and depressed. (b) A lateral view did not reveal any indication for a trauma as the cause of the bird's inability to fly, but the intestinal system is almost empty and stony material can be seen in the ventriculus.

system was almost empty and stony material could be seen in the stomach, indicating that the bird had been feeding on ground material for a while. The bird's weakness was most likely a consequence of a head trauma, and its condition was too reduced for normal hunting and feeding behaviour.

Therapy

Following hospitalization, fluid therapy, a parasite check and feeding (day-old chicks, mice), the bird recovered rapidly and was released back into the wild after 3 days.

Appendix

Common and scientific species names

Common name	Latin name
Psittaciformes	
Macaws	
Blue and Gold Macaw (*also* Blue and Yellow)	*Ara ararauna*
Blue-throated Macaw	*Ara glaucogularis*
Great Green Macaw (*also* Buffon's or Great Military)	*Ara ambiguus*
Green-winged Macaw	*Ara chloroptera*
Harlequin Macaw	*Ara ararauna* × *Ara chloroptera*
Hyacinth Macaw (*also* Hyacinthine)	*Anodorhynchus hyacinthus*
Lear's Macaw	*Anodorhynchus leari*
Military Macaw	*Ara militaris*
Noble Macaw	*Diopsittaca nobilis cumanensis*
Red-bellied Macaw (*also* Guacamaya Manilata)	*Orthopsittaca manilata*
Red-fronted Macaw	*Ara rubrogenys*
Red-shouldered Macaw (*also* Hahns Macaw)	*Diopsittaca nobilis*
Severe Macaw (*also* Chestnut-fronted)	*Ara severus*
Scarlet Macaw	*Ara macao*
Yellow-naped Macaw	*Primolius auricollis*
Amazon parrots	
Blue-fronted Amazon (*also* Turquoise-fronted)	*Amazona aestiva*
Cuban Amazon (*also* Rose-throated)	*Amazona leucocephala*
Double Yellow-headed Amazon (*also* Yellow-headed)	*Amazona oratrix* ssp.
Green-cheeked Amazon (*also* Red-crowned, Mexican Red-headed)	*Amazona viridigenalis*
Imperial Amazon	*Amazona imperialis*
Mealy Amazon	*Amazona farinosa*
Orange-winged Amazon (*also* Loro guaro)	*Amazona amazonica*

Common name	Latin name
Psittaciformes continued	
Amazon parrots continued	
Red-browed Amazon	*Amazona rhodocorytha*
Red-lored Amazon	*Amazona autumnalis*
Saint Vincent Amazon	*Amazona guildingii*
Tucumán Amazon (*also* Alder)	*Amazona tucumana*
White-fronted Amazon (*also* Spectacled)	*Amazona albifrons*
Yellow-fronted Amazon (*also* Yellow-crowned)	*Amazona ochrocephala*
Yellow-naped Amazon	*Amazona (oratrix) auropalliata*
Yucatan Amazon (*also* Yellow-lored)	*Amazona xantholora*
Cockatoos/corellas	
Ducorps' Cockatoo (*also* Solomons)	*Cacatua ducorpsii*
Galah (*also* Rose-breasted, Roseate, Pink and Grey)	*Eolophus roseicapilla*
Gang-gang Cockatoo	*Callocephalon fimbriatum*
Glossy Black Cockatoo (*also* Casuarina Black)	*Calyptorhynchus lathami*
Goffin's Cockatoo (*also* Tanimbar Corella)	*Cacatua goffini*
Greater Sulphur-crested Cockatoo	*Cacatua galerita galerita*
Lesser Sulphur-crested Cockatoo (*also* Yellow-crested Cockatoo)	*Cacatua sulphurea*
Little Corella (*also* Bare-eyed Cockatoo)	*Cacatua sanguinea*
Long-billed Corella (*also* Slender-billed)	*Cacatua tenuirostris*
Major Mitchell's Cockatoo (*also* Pink, Leadbeater's)	*Lophochroa leadbeateri*
Moluccan Cockatoo (*also* Salmon-crested)	*Cacatua moluccensis*
Palm Cockatoo (*also* Goliath, Great Black)	*Probosciger aterrimus*

▶

Common name	Latin name
Psittaciformes continued	
Cockatoos/corellas continued	
Red-tailed Black Cockatoo (_also_ Banks' Black)	_Calyptorhynchus banksii_
Sulphur-crested Cockatoo	_Cacatua galerita_
Umbrella Cockatoo (_also_ White)	_Cacatua alba_
Yellow-tailed Black Cockatoo	_Calyptorhynchus funereus_
Conures/parakeets	
Blue-crowned Conure (_also_ Sharp-tailed)	_Thectocercus (formerly Aratinga) acuticaudatus_
Blue-throated Conure (_also_ Ochre-marked)	_Pyrrhura cruentata_
Crimson-bellied Conure	_Pyrrhura perlata_
Dusky-headed Conure (_also_ Weddell's)	_Aratinga weddellii_
Golden Conure (_also_ Queen of Bavaria's Conure)	_Guaruba guaruba_
Greater Patagonian Conure (_also_ Burrowing Parrot)	_Cyanoliseus patagonus byroni_
Green-cheeked Conure	_Pyrrhura molinae_
Jenday Conure (_also_ Jandaya)	_Aratinga jandaya_
Mitred Conure	_Psittacara mitratus_
Painted Conure	_Pyrrhura picta_
Pearly Conure	_Pyrrhura lepida_
Red-masked Conure	_Psittacara (formerly Aratinga) erythrogenys_
Rose-crowned Conure (_also_ Rose-headed)	_Pyrrhura rhodocephala_
Sun Conure	_Aratinga solstitialis_
Small parrots	
Abyssinian Lovebird (_also_ Black-winged)	_Agapornis taranta_
Black-masked Lovebird (_also_ Yellow-collared, Eye Ring)	_Agapornis personatus_
Budgerigar (common pet parakeet)	_Melopsittacus undulatus_
Cockatiel	_Nymphicus hollandicus_
Madagascar Lovebird (_also_ Grey-headed)	_Agapornis canus_
Peach-faced Lovebird (_also_ Rosy-faced)	_Agapornis roseicollis_
Red-faced Lovebird (_also_ Red-headed)	_Agapornis pullarius_
Lories and lorikeets	
Black-capped Lory	_Lorius lory_
Chattering Lory	_Lorius garrulous_
Iris Lorikeet	_Psitteuteles iris_
Rainbow Lorikeet	_Trichoglossus moluccanus_
Red Lory (_also_ Moluccan)	_Eos bornea (formerly E. rubra)_
Little Lorikeet	_Glossopsitta pusilla_
Musk Lorikeet	_Glossopsitta concinna_

Common name	Latin name
Psittaciformes continued	
Lories and lorikeets continued	
Musschenbroek's Lorikeet (_also_ Yellow-beaked Lory)	_Neopsittacus musschenbroekii_
Scaly-breasted Lorikeet	_Trichoglossus chlorolepidotus_
Yellow-bibbed Lory	_Lorius chlorocercus_
Other psittacine groups	
African Grey Parrot	_Psittacus erithacus_
Alexandrine Parakeet	_Psittacula eupatria_
Australian Ringnecked Parakeet	_Barnardius zonarius_
Black-capped Caique (_also_ Black-headed, Pallid Parrot)	_Pionites melanocephalus_
Blue-headed Pionus	_Pionus menstruus_
Derbyan Parakeet	_Psittacula derbiana_
Eastern Rosella	_Platycercus eximius_
Eclectus Parrot	_Eclectus roratus_
Emerald-collared Parakeet (_also_ Layard's)	_Psittacula calthorpe_
Hawk-headed Parrot	_Deroptyus accipitrinus_
Indian Ringnecked Parakeet (_also_ Rose-ringed)	_Psittacula krameri_
Jardine's Parrot (_also_ Red-fronted)	_Poicephalus gulielmi_
Australian King Parrot	_Alisterus scapularis_
Malayan Long-tailed Parakeet	_Psittacula longicauda_
Malabar Parakeet (_also_ Blue-winged)	_Psittacula columboides_
Maximilian Pionus (_also_ Scaly Parrot)	_Pionus maximiliani_
Meyer's Parrot	_Poicephalus meyeri_
Monk Parakeet (_also_ Quaker)	_Myiopsitta monachus_
Moustached Parakeet	_Psittacula alexandri_
Plum-headed Parakeet	_Psittacula cyanocephala_
Princess Parrot	_Polytelis alexandrae_
Red-bellied Parrot	_Poicephalus rufiventris_
Red-winged Parakeet (_also_ Crimson-winged)	_Aprosmictus erythropterus_
Regent Parrot (_also_ Rock Pebbler)	_Polytelis anthopeplus_
Rosa Bourke's Parakeet	_Neopsephotus bourkii_
Senegal Parrot	_Poicephalus senegalus_
Splendid Parakeet	_Neophema splendida_
Superb Parrot (_also_ Barraband's. Green Leek)	_Polytelis swainsonii_
Timneh African Grey Parrot	_Psittacus erithacus timneh_
Turquosine Parakeet (_also_ Turquoise Parrot)	_Neophema pulchella_
White-bellied Caique (_also_ Green-thighed Parrot)	_Pionites leucogaster_

Common name	Latin name
Passeriformes	
Mynah	
Bali Mynah (*also* Bali Starling, Rothschild's Mynah)	*Leucopsar rothschildi*
Common Hill Mynah	*Gracula religiosa*
Common Mynah (*also* Indian Mynah)	*Acridotheres tristis*
Canaries and finches	
Bengalese Mannikin	*Lonchura striata domestica*
Black-throated Finch	*Poephila cincta*
Bullfinch	*Pyrrhula pyrrhula*
Atlantic Canary	*Serinus canaria*
Domestic Canary	*Serinus canaria domestica*
Greenfinch	*Chloris chloris*
Goldfinch	*Carduelis carduelis*
Gouldian Finch (*also* Rainbow)	*Erythrura gouldiae*
Hawfinch	*Coccothraustes coccothraustes*
Linnet Finch	*Carduelis cannabina*
Orange Bishop Weaver (*also* Northern Red)	*Euplectes franciscanus*
Painted Finch	*Emblema pictum*
Red Crossbill	*Loxia curvirostra*
St Helena Waxbill	*Estrilda astrild*
Siskin Finch	*Carduelis spinus*
Tri-coloured Munia	*Lonchura malacca*
Zebra Finch	*Taeniopygia guttata*
Softbills	
Metallic Starling (*also* Shining)	*Aplonis metallica*
Northern Cardinal	*Cardinalis cardinalis*
Pekin Robin (*also* Red-billed Leiothrix)	*Leiothrix lutea*
White-rumped Shama	*Copsychus malabarious*
Raptors	
Hawks	
Black Kite	*Milvus migrans*
Common Buzzard	*Buteo buteo*
Cooper's Hawk	*Accipiter cooperii*
Eurasian Sparrowhawk (*also* Northern)	*Accipiter nisus*
Ferruginous Hawk	*Buteo regalis*
Marsh Harrier	*Circus approximans*
Harris' Hawk	*Parabuteo unicinctus*
Northern Goshawk	*Accipiter gentilis*
Red Kite	*Milvus milvus*
Red-tailed Hawk	*Buteo jamaicensis*
Falcons	
Gyrfalcon	*Falco rusticolus*
Kestrel	*Falco tinnunculus*
Lanner Falcon	*Falco biarmicus*

Common name	Latin name
Raptors continued	
Falcons continued	
Laggar Falcon	*Falco jugger*
Merlin	*Falco columbarius*
Peregrine Falcon	*Falco peregrinus*
Saker Falcon	*Falco cherrug*
Eagles	
African Fish Eagle	*Haliaeetus vocifer*
Booted Eagle	*Aquila pennata*
Golden Eagle	*Aquila chrysaetos*
Martial Eagle	*Polemaetus bellicosus*
Philippine Eagle (*also* Monkey-eating)	*Pithecophaga jefferyi*
South Nicobar Serpent Eagle (*also* Great Nicobar)	*Spilornis klossi*
Steller's Sea Eagle	*Haliaeetus pelagicus*
Tawny Eagle	*Aquila rapax*
White-tailed Eagle (*also* Sea, Erne)	*Haliaeetus albicilla*
Owls	
African Spotted Eagle Owl	*Bubo africanus*
American Bald Eagle	*Haliaeetus leucocephalus*
Barn Owl	*Tyto alba*
Blakiston's Fish Owl	*Bubo blakistoni*
Brown Wood Owl	*Strix leptogrammica*
Elf Owl	*Micrathene whitneyi*
Eurasian Eagle Owl	*Bubo bubo*
Great Grey Owl	*Strix nebulosa*
Great Horned Owl	*Bubo virginianus*
Indian Eagle Owl (*also* Rock, Bengalese)	*Bubo bengalensis*
Little Owl	*Athene noctua*
Long-eared Owl	*Asio otus*
Short-eared Owl	*Asio flammeus*
Snowy Owl	*Bubo scandiacus*
Southern White-faced Scops Owl	*Ptilopsis granti*
Other	
Osprey	*Pandion haliaetus*

Appendix

Sex identification of selected species

Species	Sex identification
Psittaciformes	
Macaws	
All species	Monomorphic; require DNA/surgical sexing
Amazon parrots	
Most species	Monomorphic; require DNA/surgical sexing
Cockatoos	
Most white cockatoos species have sexual dimorphism (although this is not 100% accurate) with the male being larger, with black/very dark brown irides. Females tend to have red irides, although dark-eyed females have been reported	
Galah	Delayed dimorphism: most (not all) hens develop a red iris at 12–18 months of age
Gang Gang Cockatoo	Dimorphic: the hen lacks the red-coloured head of the cock. Immature birds look like hens except for some red scalloping of the head feathers in young males, which may be seen even in the nest
Greater Sulphur-crested Cockatoo	Delayed dimorphism: most (not all) hens develop a pink iris at 2–4 years of age
Little Corella	Monomorphic; requires DNA/surgical sexing
Long-billed Corella	Monomorphic; requires DNA/surgical sexing
Moluccan Cockatoo	Dimorphic: males are much larger and have black irides. Females tend to have red irides
Palm Cockatoo	Monomorphic, although cocks may have a larger head and beak than hens
Red-tailed Black Cockatoo	Delayed dimorphism: at 4–5 years of age cocks develop red ventral tail feathers and a black beak; the hen's tail feathers are barred and orange-red in colour, the upper beak is ivory, and there is yellow spotting on the black contour feathers
Umbrella Cockatoo	Delayed dimorphism: most (not all) hens develop a pink iris at 2–4 years of age
Conures	
Green-cheeked Conure	Monomorphic; requires DNA/surgical sexing
Sun Conure	Monomorphic; requires DNA/surgical sexing

Species	Sex identification
Psittaciformes continued	
Cockatiels, Budgerigars and lovebirds	
Budgerigar	Dimorphic: cocks have a blue cere while hens have a brown cere (Note, this dimorphism is not present in some colour mutations esp lutinos)
Cockatiel	Delayed dimorphism: at 6 months of age normal-coloured cocks develop a bright yellow head and bright orange cheek patches. The hen has a grey head with duller orange cheek patches, ventral wing stripe and horizontal barring on the ventral tail. Colour mutations may vary (Note, this dimorphism is not present in some colour mutations esp lutinos)
Lovebirds (*Agapornis* spp.)	Monomorphic; require DNA/surgical sexing
Lories and lorikeets	
Most species	Monomorphic; require DNA/surgical sexing
Other psittacine groups	
African and Timneh Grey Parrot	Monomorphic; requires DNA/surgical sexing
Alexandrine Parakeet	Delayed dimorphism: cocks develop a purple and black neck ring at 18–24 months of age
Caiques (*Pionites* spp.)	Monomorphic; requires DNA/surgical sexing
Eclectus Parrot	Dimorphic from hatch: hens are red and purple with a black beak; cocks are green with an orange-yellow beak
Indian Ringnecked Parakeet	Delayed dimorphism: cocks develop a purple and black neck ring at 18– 24 months of age
Jardine's Parrot	Monomorphic; requires DNA/surgical sexing
Meyer's Parrot	Monomorphic; requires DNA/surgical sexing
Monk Parakeet	Monomorphic; requires DNA/surgical sexing
Neophema spp.	Most are monomorphic, requiring DNA/surgical sexing

▶

BSAVA Manual of Avian Practice: A Foundation Manual. Edited by John Chitty and Deborah Monks. ©BSAVA 2018

Species	Sex identification
Psittaciformes continued	
Other psittacine groups continued	
Princess Parrot	Delayed dimorphism: cocks over 12 months of age are more intensely coloured, have a longer tail, and have a spatulate extension of the third primary feather on each wing
Psephotus spp.	Most are dimorphic, with the cocks noticeably brighter than the hens. The exception is the Blue Bonnet Parrot, where the sexes are very similar
Regent Parrot	The cock is a bright olive-yellow bird with an olive-green back and patches of red on the inner-wing coverts. The hen is a more olive-green colour, similar in other colour aspects but has pinkish striations to the under-tail feathers
Rosellas (Platycercus spp.)	Often monomorphic; requires DNA/surgical sexing. In some species e.g. Pale-Headed Rosellas, mature hens have a ventral wing stripe
Senegal Parrot	Monomorphic; requires DNA/surgical sexing

Species	Sex identification
Passeriformes	
Domestic Canary	Visually monomorphic; cues such as voice and the seminal glomus is cocks can be used to help distinguish the sex
Mynahs	Monomorphic; requires DNA/surgical sexing
Raptors	
Hawks	
Cooper's Hawk	Reverse size dimorphism: the hen is larger (440–570 g) than the cock (280–350 g)
Harris' Hawk	Reverse size dimorphism: the hen (825–1200 g) is larger than the cock (550–880 g)
Northern Goshawk	Reverse size dimorphism: the hen (800–1200 g) is larger than the cock (530–750 g), but geographical variations can make this difficult to determine
Red-tailed Hawk	Reverse size dimorphism: the hen (1–1.4 kg) is larger than the cock (900–1100 g)
Falcons	
Gyrfalcon	Reverse size dimorphism: the hen (1.13–2.1 kg) is larger than the cock (800–1320 g)
Lanner Falcon	Reverse size dimorphism: the hen is larger (700–900 g) than the cock (500–600 g)
Peregrine Falcon	All ages can be sexed by size; male (500–800 g) with wing shorter than 300 mm; female (900–1000 g) with wing longer than 320 mm
Saker Falcon	Reverse size dimorphism: the hen (970–1300 g) is larger than the cock (730–950 g)
Eagles	
Golden Eagle	In adult birds, the cock usually has a darker throat, nape and underparts than the hen. The cock is smaller (2.8–4.6 kg), with wings shorter than 595 mm compared to the hen (3.8–6.7 kg) with wings longer than 630 mm. Juvenile of both sexes alike appear alike
Owls	
Barn Owl	Dimorphic: females have a rounder, less heart-shaped face and flecking of the breast feathers
Eurasian Eagle Owl	Monomorphic; requires DNA/surgical sexing as juveniles although mature hens (2.28–4.2 kg) are larger than cocks (1.62–3 kg)

Appendix

Haematology and biochemistry

Haematology

The following tables present normal haematology reference values for selected species of birds.

Psittaciformes				
Parameter	Macaw	Amazon	Cockatiel	Grey Parrot
WBC (x 10⁹/l)	10–20	5–17	5–11	6–13
Haematocrit (l/l)	42–54	42–53	41–59	41–54
Heterophils (%)	50–75	31–71	46–72	45–73
Lymphocytes (%)	23–53	20–67	26–60	19–50
Monocytes (%)	0–1	0–2	0–1	0–2
Eosinophils (%)	0	0	0–2	0–1
Basophils (%)	0–1	0–2	0–1	0–1

Haematology values for selected species/species groups of Psittaciformes. (Fudge, 2000)

Pigeons and Passeriformes				
Parameter	Pigeon	Canary	Finch	Hill Mynah
RBC (x 10¹²/l)	3.1–4.5[a]	2.5–4.5[b]	2.5–4.6[b]	2.4–4[b]
PCV (l/l)	0.425[a]	0.45–0.6[b]	0.45–0.62[b]	0.44–0.55[b]
Hb (g/l)	81–99[a]	NDA	NDA	NDA
WBC (x 10⁹/l)	13–22.3[a]	4–9[b]	3–8[b]	6–11[b]
Heterophils (%)	NDA	20–50	20–65	25–65
Heterophils (x 10⁹/l)	4.3–6.2[a]	NDA	NDA	NDA
Lymphocytes (%)	NDA	40–75[b]	20–65[b]	25–65[b]
Lymphocytes (x 10⁹/l)	10.9–12.2[a]	NDA	NDA	NDA
Monocytes (%)	NDA	0–1[b]	0–1[b]	0–3[b]
Monocytes (x 10⁹/l)	0.4–1.1[a]	NDA	NDA	NDA
Eosinophils (%)	NDA	0–1[b]	0–1[b]	0–1[b]
Eosinophils (x 10⁹/l)	0.1–0.3[a]	NDA	NDA	NDA
Basophils (%)	NDA	0–5[b]	0–5[b]	0–7[b]
Basophils (x 10⁹/l)	0.1–0.5[a]	NDA	NDA	NDA
Thrombocytes (x 10⁹/l)	7–27[a]	NDA	NDA	NDA

Haematology values for pigeons and selected Passeriformes. NDA = no data available. ([a]Beynon *et al.*, 1996; [b]Chitty and Lierz, 2008)

Falcons

Parameter	Saker	Gyr	Peregrine	Lanner	Laggar	Merlin	Gyr hybrid
RBC (x 10¹²/l)	2.54–3.96[a]	NDA	2.95–3.94[a]	2.63–3.98[a]	2.65–3.63[a]	2.84–4.1[a]	NDA
PCV (l/l)	0.38–0.49[a]	NDA	0.37–0.53[a]	0.37–0.53[a]	0.39–0.51[a]	0.39–0.51[a]	NDA
Hb (g/l)	115–165[a]	NDA	118–188[a]	122–171[a]	128–163[a]	132–179[a]	NDA
MCV (fl)	124–147[a]	NDA	118–146[a]	127–150[a]	123–145[a]	105–130[a]	NDA
MCH (pg)	41.4–45.4[a]	NDA	40–48.4[a]	42.3–48.8[a]	38–47.7[a]	36–45.9[a]	NDA
MCHC m(g/l)	304–349[a]	NDA	319–352[a]	317–353[a]	312–350[a]	340–360[a]	NDA
WBC (x 10⁹/l)	3.8–11.5[a]	NDA	3.3–11[a]	3.5–11[a]	5–9[a]	4–9.5[a]	NDA
Heterophils (%)	61.68 ± 11.16[b]	60.42 ± 14.68[b]	60.95 ± 12.01[b]	NDA	NDA	NDA	60.42 ± 146[b]
Heterophils (x 10⁹/l)	2.6–5.85[a]	2.31–8.85[c]	1.4–8.55[a]	1.65–8.8[a]	3.5–6.57[a]	3.2–4.03[a]	NDA
Lymphocytes (%)	31.11 ± 11.46[b]	34.37 ± 14.23[b]	32 ± 11.81[b]	NDA	NDA	NDA	34.37 ± 14.23[b]
Lymphocytes (x 10⁹/l)	0.8–4.25[a]	0.48–2.36[c]	1.1–3.3[a]	1.1–5.13[a]	1.7–4[a]	1.2–1.56[a]	NDA
Monocytes (%)	4.72 ± 3.02[b]	4.73 ± 3.67[b]	6.23 ± 3.65[b]	NDA	NDA	NDA	4.73 ± 3.67[b]
Monocytes (x 10⁹/l)	0–0.8[a]	0.03–0.9[c]	0.1–0.86[a]	0–0.9[a]	0–0.85[a]	0–0.5[a]	NDA
Eosinophils (%)	1.12[b]	0.31[b]	0.52[b]	NDA	NDA	NDA	0.31[b]
Eosinophils (x 10⁹/l)	0–0.2[a]	0–0.68[c]	0–0.3[a]	0–0.2[a]	0–0.2[a]	0–0.15[a]	NDA
Basophils (%)	0.4[b]	0.04[b]	0.26[b]	NDA	NDA	NDA	0.04[b]
Basophils (x 10⁹/l)	0–0.45[a]	0–0.29[c]	0–0.6[a]	0–0.45[a]	0.17–0.83[a]	0–0.15[a]	NDA
Thrombocytes (x 10⁹/l)	12–25[a]	NDA	6–46[a]	5–40[a]	12–35[a]	NDA	NDA
Fibrinogen (g/l)	<3.5[a]	NDA	<4.2[a]	<4[a]	<4[a]	<4[a]	NDA

Haematology values for selected species of falcons. NDA = no data available. ([a]Beynon et al., 1996; [b]Wernery et al., 2004; [c]Chitty and Lierz, 2008)

Hawks and eagles

Parameter	Common Buzzard	Northern Goshawk	Ferruginous Hawk	Red-tailed Hawk	Harris' Hawk	Golden Eagle	Tawny Eagle
RBC (x 10¹²/l)	2.13–2.76	2.6–3.48	2.41–3.59	2.3–3.5	2.63–3.5	1.69–3.21	2.32–2.83
PCV (l/l)	0.32–0.44	0.43–0.53	0.37–0.48	0.35–0.53	0.4–0.55	0.31–0.53	0.37–0.47
Hb (g/l)	101–167	121–177	107–166	123–175	121–171	112–173	108–175
MCV (fl)	151–165	141–156	150–178	157–168	147–163	165–186	163–188
MCH (pg)	48–53	44.5–51.6	46–57.4	43–50.4	45.4–51.1	53.8–67.7	54–62
MCHC m(g/l)	307–339	305–343	297–345	312–350	301–330	326–364	296–360
WBC (x 10⁹/l)	5–13	4–11	4.5–6.8	3.4–7.5	4.8–10	6.2–17	5–9.5
Heterophils (x 10⁹/l)	3.2–11	3.5–6.97	1.89–3.76	1.9–3.5	2.3–6.71	4.5–15.2	3.58–6.45
Lymphocytes (x 10⁹/l)	0.3–3.1	1.38–1.93	0.78–1.74	1.3–1.1	0.6–2.36	0.75–3.37	0.51–2.72
Monocytes (x 10⁹/l)	0.2–0.68	0–0.1	0.24–1.5	0.12–1.2	0.2–1.49	0–0.63	0.2–1.07
Eosinophils (x 10⁹/l)	0.1–0.8	0–0.65	0.3–0.7	0.1–0.9	0–0.75	0.1–0.6	0.3–2.1
Basophils (x 10⁹/l)	0–0.9	0–0.35	0.15–0.6	0–0.5	0–1.55	0–0.16	0–0.4
Thrombocytes (x 10⁹/l)	8–46	15–35	8–47	4–33	10–59	7–45	19–25
Fibrinogen (g/l)	<3.6	<3.5	<3.5	<3	<4.3	<4.5	<3.5

Haematology values for selected species of hawks and eagles. (Beynon et al., 1996)

Owls

Parameter	Northern Eagle Owl	Parameter	Northern Eagle Owl
RBC (x 10^{12}/l)	1.65–2.35	Lymphocytes (x 10^9/l)	1.5–5.07
PCV (l/l)	0.36–0.52	Monocytes (%)	NDA
Hb (g/l)	107–180	Monocytes (x 10^9/l)	0–0.48
MCV (fl)	189–204	Eosinophils (%)	NDA
MCH (pg)	64.6–76	Eosinophils (x 10^9/l)	0–0.48
MCHC m(g/l)	325–376	Basophils (%)	NDA
WBC (x 10^9/l)	3.5–12.1	Basophils (x 10^9/l)	0–0.35
Heterophils (%)	NDA	Thrombocytes (x 10^9/l)	1–29
Heterophils (x 10^9/l)	2.2–9.23	Fibrinogen (g/l)	<4.5
Lymphocytes (%)	NDA		

Haematology values for selected species of owls. NDA = no data available. (Beynon *et al*.1996)

Biochemistry

The following tables present normal biochemistry reference values for selected species of birds.

Psittaciformes

Parameter	Macaw[a]	Amazon[a]	Cockatiel[b]	Grey Parrot[a]
Uric acid (mmol/l)	109–231	72–312	202–648	93–414
Urea (mmol/l)	0.3–3.3	0.9–4.6	NDA	0.7–2.4
Bile acid (mmol/l)	25–71	19–144	44–108	18–71
Aspartate aminotransferase (AST) (IU/l)	58–206	57–194	128–396	54–155
Creatine kinase (IU/l)	61–531	45–265	160–420	123–875
Gamma glutamyl transferase (GGT) (IU/l)	1–5	1–10	NDA	1–4
Glutamate dehydrogenase (GDH) (IU/l)	<8	<8	NDA	<8
Calcium (mmol/l)	2.2–2.8	2–2.8	2.05–2.71	2.1–2.6
Glucose (mmol/l)	12–17.9	12.6–16.9	12.66–24.42	11.4–16.1
Total protein (g/l)	33–53	33–50	21–48	32–44
Albumin:globulin ratio	1.4–3.9	2.6–7	NDA	1.4–4.7

Biochemistry values for selected species of Psittaciformes. NDA = no data available. ([a]Lumeij and Overduin, 1990; [b]Fudge, 2000)

Pigeons and Passeriformes

Parameter	Pigeon[a]	Canary[b]	Finch[b]	Hill Mynah[b]
A:G ratio	1.5–3.6	NDA	NDA	NDA
Alanine aminotransferase (ALT) (IU/l)	19–48	NDA	NDA	NDA
Alkaline phosphatase (ALP) (IU/l)	NDA	146–397	NDA	NDA
Aspartate aminotransferase (AST) (IU/l)	45–123	45–170	150–350	150–350
Bile acids (µmol/l)	22–60	NDA	NDA	NDA
Calcium (mmol/l)	1.9–2.6	1.28–3.35	NDA	2.25–3.25
Cholesterol (mmol/l)	NDA	NDA	NDA	NDA
Creatinine kinase (IU/l)	110–480	NDA	NDA	NDA
Creatinine (µmol/l)	23–36	8.85–88.5	NDA	8.85–53.1
Glucose (mmol/l)	12.9–20.5	16.15–21.7	11.1–24.97	10.54–19.44
Gamma-glutamyl transferase (GGT) (IU/l)	0–2.9	NDA	NDA	NDA
Lactate dehydrogenase (LDH) (IU/l)	30–205	1300–1816	NDA	600–1000
Phosphorus (mmol/l)	NDA	0.52–1.8	NDA	NDA

Biochemistry values for pigeons and selected species of Passeriformes. NDA = no data available. ([a]Beynon *et al.*, 1996; [b]Chitty and Lierz, 2008) (continues) ▶

Pigeons and Passeriformes

Parameter	Pigeon[a]	Canary[b]	Finch[b]	Hill Mynah[b]
Potassium (mmol/l)	3.9–4.7	2.7–4.8	NDA	0.3–5.1
Sodium (mmol/l)	141–149	125–154	NDA	136–152
Total protein (g/l)	21–35	20–44	30–50	23–45
Urea (mmol/l)	0.4–0.7	NDA	NDA	NDA
Uric acid (µmol/l)	150–765	4.3–14.8 mg/dl	4–12 mg/dl	4–10 mg/dl

(continued) Biochemistry values for pigeons and selected species of Passeriformes. NDA = no data available. ([a]Beynon et al., 1996; [b]Chitty and Lierz, 2008)

Falcons

Parameter	Saker	Gyr	Peregrine	Lanner	Merlin	Kestrel	Gyr–Saker	Gyr–Peregrine
Albumin (g/l)	9–12.3[a] 5.2–15[b]	6.6–16.8[c]	6.9–14.8[d] 12.7–22.4[e]	9.6–16[a]	8.6–16.1[a]	NDA	NDA	6.8–14.3[d]
A:G ratio	0.45–0.57[a]	NDA	NDA	0.44–0.57[a]	0.47–0.58[a]	NDA	NDA	NDA
Alanine aminotransferase (ALT) (IU/l)	36–55[a] 29–362[b]	32–589[c]	38–303[d] 29–90[e]	NDA	NDA	35–60[e]	28–393[d]	29–429[d]
Alkaline phosphatase (ALP) (IU/l)	285–450[a]	NDA	31–121[e]	180–510[a]	54–310[a]	20–100[e]	NDA	NDA
Aspartate aminotransferase (AST) (IU/l)	45–95[a] 40–358[b]	44–471[c]	35–327[d] 34–162[e]	30–118[a]	50–125[a]	100–200[e]	40–544[d]	44–469[d]
Bile acids (µmol/l)	20–90[a] 1.7–13.3[e]	NDA	5–69[e]	NDA	NDA	NDA	NDA	NDA
Calcium (mmol/l)	2.15–2.61[a] 1.97–2.77[b]	1.98–3.48[c]	1.94–2.54[d]	2.07–2.45[a]	2–2.45[a]	2.1–2.4[e]	1.95–3.12[d]	1.88–2.58[d]
Cholesterol (mmol/l)	4.5–8.6[a] 3.43–7.54[b]	3.42–7.12[c]	3.18–9.97[d]	3–8.8[a]	3–7.8[a]	NDA	2.77–10.05[d]	3.06–7.71[d]
Chloride (mmol/l)	114–125[a]	NDA	NDA	NDA	NDA	NDA	NDA	NDA
Creatinine kinase (IU/l)	355–651[a]	NDA	120–442[f]	350–650[a]	521–807[a]	NDA	NDA	NDA
Creatinine (µmol/l)	23–75[a] 11–64[b]	14–73[c]	12–64[d]	37–75[a]	16–50[a]	NDA	13–75[d]	16–73[d]
Glutamate dehydrogenase (GLDH) (IU/l)	NDA	NDA	<8[f]	NDA	NDA	NDA	NDA	NDA
Globulin (g/l)	18–28[a]	NDA	NDA	21.2–28.8[a]	17.2–25[a]	NDA	NDA	NDA
Glucose (mmol/l)	12–14[a]	NDA	NDA	11–15[a]	9–12[a]	NDA	NDA	NDA
Gamma-glutamyl transferase (GGT) (IU/l)	0.8–5.9[a]	NDA	0–3[f]	NDA	NDA	NDA	NDA	NDA
Lactate dehydrogenase (LDH) (IU/l)	551–765[a] 664–3852[b]	870–3871[c]	721–3799[d]	434–897[a]	320–630[a]	NDA	662–3720[d]	544–3595[d]
Phosphate, inorganic (mmol/l)	0.72–2.16	NDA	NDA	0.68–2[a]	0.95–1.79[a]	NDA	NDA	NDA
Phosphorus (mmol/l)	0.81–2.08[b]	0.45–2.89[c]	0.87–1.88[d] 0.55–1.53[e]	NDA	NDA	NDA	0.78–2.38[d]	0.66–2.21[d]
Potassium (mmol/l)	0.8–2.3[a] 1.6–4.7[b]	1.9–4.9[c]	1.8–5.1[d]	1–2.1[a]	1–1.8[a]	NDA	1.8–4.9[d]	1.6–4.7[d]
Sodium (mmol/l)	154–161[a]	NDA	NDA	152–164[a]	155–170[a]	NDA	NDA	NDA
Total protein (g/l)	27–36[a] 85–44.6[b]	4.5–46.2[c]	16–38.9[d] 24–41	33–42[a]	27.5–39[a]	25–34[e]	5–46.7[d]	4.7–40.2[d]
Urea (mmol/l)	0.5–2.6[a] 0–8.3[b]	0–9.5[c]	0.3–9[d]	1.3–2.7[a]	NDA	NDA	0–9.5[d]	0.3–7.8[d]
Uric acid (µmol/l)	320–785[a] 110–1260[b]	80–690[c]	170–1250[d]	318–709[a]	174–800[a]	NDA	100–1180[d]	120–1740[d]

Biochemistry reference values for selected species of falcons. NDA = no data available. ([a]Beynon et al., 1996; [b]Lierz, 2002; [c]Lierz, 2003; [d]Lierz and Hafez, 2006; [e]Chitty and Lierz, 2008; [f]Lumeij et al., 1998)

Hawks and eagles

Parameter	Common Buzzard	Northern Goshawk	Sparrowhawk	Harris' Hawk	Black Kite	Marsh Harrier	White-tailed Sea Eagle	Tawny Eagle
Albumin (g/l)	5–14[a]	8.8–12.4[b]	NDA	13.9–17[b]	6–23[a]	NDA	NDA	11.5–18[b]
A:G ratio	NDA	0.4–0.57[b]	NDA	0.46–0.55[b]	NDA	NDA	NDA	0.44–0.55[b]
Alanine aminotransferase (ALT) (IU/l)	0.5–58[a]	0–44	2.5–30.5[a]	NDA	35–60 (GPT)[a]	18–58 (GPT[a]	0–30 (GPT)[a]	NDA
Alkaline phosphatase (ALP) (IU/l)	35–86[a]	15.6–87.5[b] 42–63[a]	103–118[a]	20–96[b]	20–100[a]	NDA	7–76[a]	17.1–69.7[b]
Aspartate aminotransferase (AST) (IU/l)	0.5–27 (GOT)[a]	176–409[b] 0–31 (GOT)[a]	140–151 (GOT)[a]	160–348[b]	100–200 (GOT)[a]	140–440 (GOT)[a]	30–160 (GOT)[a]	124–226[b]
Calcium (mmol/l)	2–2.8[a]	2.15–2.69[b]	NDA	2.1–2.66[b]	1.8–2.7[a]	NDA	NDA	2.21–2.66[b]
Cholesterol (mmol/l)	NDA	4–11.5[b]	NDA	6.6–13.1[b]	NDA	NDA	NDA	7.9–10.7[b]
Chloride (mmol/l)	NDA	NDA	NDA	113–119[b]	NDA	NDA	NDA	114–123[b]
Creatinine kinase (IU/l)	NDA	218–775[b]	NDA	224–650[b]	NDA	NDA	NDA	NDA
Creatinine (µmol/l)	NDA	41–94[b]	NDA	20–59[b]	NDA	NDA	NDA	31–59[b]
Globulin (g/l)	NDA	18–29.2[b]	NDA	21–29.4[b]	NDA	NDA	NDA	25.3–28.4[b]
Glucose (mmol/l)	NDA	11.5–15.9[b]	NDA	12.2–15.7[b]	NDA	NDA	NDA	10.2–14.5[b]
Gamma-glutamyl transferase (GGT) (IU/l)	NDA	3–7.6[b]	NDA	2–6.9[b]	NDA	NDA	NDA	1–2.7[b]
Lactate dehydrogenase (LDH) (IU/l)	NDA	120–906[b]	NDA	160–563[b]	NDA	NDA	NDA	211–369[b]
Phosphate, inorganic (mmol/l)	NDA	0.8–1.97[b]	NDA	0.8–2.14[b]	NDA	NDA	NDA	1.2–1.78[b]
Potassium (mmol/l)	NDA	NDA	NDA	0.8–2.3[b]	NDA	NDA	NDA	1.5–3.1[b]
Sodium (mmol/l)	NDA	NDA	NDA	155–171[b]	NDA	NDA	NDA	153–157[b]
Total protein (g/l)	33–50[a]	26.3–42[b]	NDA	31–45.7[b]	30–41[a]	31–58[a]	28–45[a]	29–41.4[b]
Urea (mmol/l)	NDA	NDA	NDA	0.7–1.9[b]	NDA	NDA	NDA	0.8–2.7[b]
Uric acid (µmol/l)	NDA	511–854[b]	NDA	535–785[b]	NDA	NDA	NDA	413–576[b]

Biochemistry reference values for selected species of hawks and eagles. NDA = no data available. ([a]Chitty and Lierz, 2008; [b]Beynon et al., 1996)

Owls

Parameter	Northern Eagle Owl[a]	Barn Owl[b]	Tawny Owl[b]
Albumin (g/l)	11.1–13.5	NDA	NDA
A:G ratio	NDA	NDA	NDA
Alanine aminotransferase (ALT) (IU/l)	NDA	NDA	32.5–40 (GPT)
Alkaline phosphatase (ALP) (IU/l)	NDA	NDA	42.2–215
Aspartate aminotransferase (AST) (IU/l)	NDA	NDA	23.5–103.5
Bile acids (µmol/l)	NDA	NDA	NDA
Calcium (mmol/l)	2.16–2.61	2.2–2.6	NDA
Cholesterol (mmol/l)	3.9–7.1	NDA	NDA
Creatinine kinase (IU/l)	NDA	NDA	NDA
Creatinine (µmol/l)	31–49	NDA	NDA
Globulin (g/l)	18.7–22.4	NDA	NDA
Glucose (mmol/l)	13.5–21.7	NDA	NDA
Gamma-glutamyl transferase (GGT) (IU/l)	NDA	NDA	NDA
Lactate dehydrogenase (LDH) (IU/l)	NDA	NDA	NDA
Phosphate, inorganic (mmol/l)	1.15–1.94	NDA	NDA

Biochemistry reference values for selected species of owls. NDA = no data available. ([a]Beynon et al., 1996; [b]Chitty and Lierz, 2008) (continues) ▶

Owls *continued*			
Parameter	**Northern Eagle Owl[a]**	**Barn Owl[b]**	**Tawny Owl[b]**
Phosphorus (mmol/l)	NDA	NDA	NDA
Potassium (mmol/l)	NDA	NDA	NDA
Sodium (mmol/l)	NDA	NDA	NDA
Total protein (g/l)	30.1–34.5	32	NDA
Urea (mmol/l)	0.9–2.9	NDA	NDA
Uric acid (µmol/l)	475–832	NDA	NDA

(continued) Biochemistry reference values for selected species of owls. NDA = no data available. ([a]Beynon *et al.*, 1996; [b]Chitty and Lierz, 2008)

References and further reading

Beynon PH, Forbes NA and Harcourt-Brown NH (1996) *BSAVA Manual of Raptors, Pigeons and Waterfowl*, pp. 75–78. BSAVA Publications, Gloucester

Chitty J and Lierz M (2008) *BSAVA Manual of Raptors, Pigeons and Passerine Birds*, pp. 394–397. BSAVA Publications, Gloucester

Fudge AM (2000) Avian clinical pathology – haematology and chemistry. In: *Avian Medicine and Surgery*, ed. RB Altman, SL Clubb, G Dorrestein and K Queensberry, p. 151. WB Saunders, Philadelphia

Lierz M (2002) Blood chemistry values of the Saker Falcon (*Falco cherrug*). *Tierärztliche Praxis* **30**, 386–388

Lierz M (2003) Plasma chemistry reference values for gyrfalcons (*Falco rusticolus*). *Veterinary Record* **153**, 182–183

Lumeij JT and Overduin LM (1990) Plasma chemistry reference values in psittaciformes. *Avian Pathology* **19**, 234–244

Lumeij JT, Remple JD, Remple CJ and Riddle KE (1998) Plasma chemistry in peregrine falcons (*Falco peregrinus*): reference values and physiological variations of importance for interpretation. *Avian Pathology* **27**, 129–132

Wernery U, Kinne J and Wernery R (2004) *Colour Atlas of Falcon Medicine*. Schlutersche, Hanover

Appendix

Droppings

The droppings of a bird can provide a wealth of information to the observant practitioner. Knowing the normal appearance of droppings for each species can allow the practitioner to infer abnormalities of hepatic, renal or digestive function, which allows a more targeted exploration of disease.

Condition	Psittacines	Passerines	Raptors
Normal	African Grey Parrot Budgerigar		
Anorexia			(© John Chitty)
Biliverdinuria			

BSAVA Manual of Avian Practice: A Foundation Manual. Edited by John Chitty and Deborah Monks. ©BSAVA 2018

Condition	Psittacines	Passerines	Raptors
Diarrhoea			
Melaena			 (© John Chitty)
Polyuria			
Seed-contaminated			
Miscellaneous presentations	 Parrot fed on red grapes Proventricular dilatation disease due to maldigestion Steatorrhea resulting from pancreatic insufficiency (© John Chitty)		

Appendix

Falconry terminology

The following table lists terms commonly used in falconry that may be unfamiliar to non-specialist staff at the veterinary practice.

Term	Definition
Anklets (or aylmeri)	Leather loops around the legs to which the jesses (see below) attach
Baiting	Attempting to fly off the fist whilst being restrained with jesses
Breeding chamber	Sometimes termed a seclusion chamber, where pairs of birds are placed in order that they might breed It is usually completely enclosed on all four sides but with a mesh roof The birds are fed and/or observed by means of a hatch so that they are not disturbed by human contact
Block and bow perches	Most common perch designs
Box	An entirely enclosed carrying box with a perch in it so that the bird can sit quietly in the dark Used for travelling
Cadge	An open system of perches used for transporting a number of birds, usually for hooded falcons (i.e. not in a darkened box)
Castings	The undigested parts of the diet (e.g. feathers) that are regurgitated sometime after feeding, usually the following morning for captive birds The consistency is usually fairly dry and they are firm Slimy malodorous castings are not normal
Cast off	To release the bird to hunt (flying in a cast is to fly more than one bird together at the same quarry)
Coping	Filing beak or talons
Creance	A length of cord /fine rope used during training so that the bird cannot fly away from the falconer
DOC	Day-old chicks, a common raptor food
Flicking food	An expression that is used to describe a bird that is picking at its food but not ingesting most of it
Flying weight	The ideal weight at which a raptor is keen to hunt and return to its keeper, as opposed to fat weight when the bird is allowed to gain weight when not working (i.e. breeding or moulting)
Free lofted	Birds kept in aviaries
Furniture/equipment	These include jesses and anklets used to attach leashes to so that the birds van be restrained on the fist or tethered
Gauntlet	The glove worn by the falconer
Going light	Used to describe a bird that is losing weight due to any cause
Hooded	Falcons that have been 'manned' are usually hooded (a leather hood used over the eyes) and are then much quieter to handle Hawks aren't hooded normally; eagles sometimes are
Imping	Replacing a broken feather
Jessed/jesses	If the birds are 'jessed' then they can be restrained on a glove by holding the leather 'jesses' which are attached to anklets around the lower part of the legs
Manned/unmanned	Birds that have had no human contact or have not been 'trained' are 'unmanned' and usually relatively wild to handle
Mutes	Droppings, consisting of faecal component, urates and urine
Not putting food 'over'	Delayed emptying of crop
Put down to moult	The bird is given more food so that its weight increases and moulting takes place over a few months
Sour crop	Distended crop which has not emptied and contains rotten food Can be very serious if not treated promptly and correctly
Tail guard	A cover to protect the tail feathers from damage
Tethered	Birds not in aviaries, are likely to be tethered to 'bow' perches or 'blocks'

BSAVA Manual of Avian Practice: A Foundation Manual. Edited by John Chitty and Deborah Monks. ©BSAVA 2018

Appendix

Formulary

Dose rates described in the table below relate to those found in this Manual, as well as those in common usage in avian medicine. For a more complete formulary, the reader is referred to the *BSAVA Small Animal Formulary, 9th edition: Part B – Exotic Pets or Exotic Animal Formulary, 4th edition* (Carpenter, 2012). It should be noted that few of these drugs are licensed for use in avian species in the UK. Where licensed, the stated drug dose may differ from that detailed in the table below (where drug doses recommended by authors within this Manual have been included). It is recommended that clinicians follow the relevant prescribing legislation in their own country and use licenced products at the licensed dose rate before considering using alternative drugs or alternative dose rates.

Drug	Parrots	Raptors	Passerines
Antibacterial drugs			
Amoxicillin	150–175 mg/kg orally q12h 150 mg/kg i.m. q24h long-acting injection	150 mg/kg orally q12h 150 mg/kg i.m. q24h long-acting injection	1.5 g/l drinking water for 5–7 days
Azithromycin	40 mg/kg orally q24–48h Treatment for 45 days is required for chlamydiosis	50 mg/kg orally q24h Treatment for 5 days is required for chlamydiosis	
Cefalexin	35–100 mg/kg orally, i.m. q6–8h	40–100 mg/kg orally, i.m. q8–12h	40–100 mg/kg orally, i.m. q8–12h
Ceftazidime	100 mg/kg i.m., i.v. q8–12h	100 mg/kg i.m., i.v. q8–12h	
Clindamycin	25 mg/kg orally q8h 50 mg/kg orally q12h 100 mg/kg orally q24h	100 mg/kg orally q24h Halve dose if used with marbofloxacin	
Co-amoxiclav (amoxicillin/clavulanate)	125 mg/kg orally q12h 125 mg/kg i.m. q24h	150 mg/kg orally, i.v. q12h or i.m. q24h May cause regurgitation if used orally	150 mg/kg orally, i.v. q12h or i.m. q24h
Doxycycline	15–50 mg/kg orally q24h 1000 mg/kg in dehulled seed/soft food 75–100 mg/kg i.m. once a week (Vibravenos) Vibravenos is recommended for psittacosis in larger parrots. Macaws may be more sensitive to this drug than other psittacine species. Side-effects include vomiting/regurgitation. Injection may cause significant irritant reactions. If large injection volume required, then dose should be divided between several injection sites. If injected subcutaneously then skin slough may result. In Germany, Vibravenos is one of the statutory therapies recommended for psittacosis, where it should be given at 75 mg/kg i.m. every 5 days for six occasions, then every 4 days for three occasions. Many texts suggest 75–100 mg/kg weekly for six occasions is sufficient to achieve clearance of *Chlamydia psittaci* from the body, although this is not totally reliable	50 mg/kg orally q12h 100 mg/kg i.m. every 5–7 days (Vibravenos – specific treatment certificate required in the UK)	40 mg/kg orally q12–24h 200–500 mg/l daily in water

▶

Drug	Parrots	Raptors	Passerines
Antibacterial drugs continued			
Enrofloxacin	10–15 mg/kg orally, i.m. q12h 100–200 mg/l in drinking water Preparations licensed for use in birds in the UK. Licensed dose rate = 10 mg/kg orally, i.m. q12h, although many authors recommend a higher dose rate. Injection may cause irritant reactions, so it is advised that dosing should be switched from systemic to oral as soon as possible. Injectable preparations >2.5% concentration should **not** be used. May cause vomiting. Enrofloxacin is one of the statutory treatments for psittacosis in Germany, where the recommended dose is 10 mg/kg i.m. q24h for 21 days or in food at 1000 mg/kg corn (or nectar food for lories/lorikeets) fed as sole diet for 21 days or at 500 ppm drinking water for 21 days for Budgerigars. Many texts recommend enrofloxacin at 15 mg/kg orally, i.m. q12h for 45 days in cases of psittacosis	15 mg/kg orally, i.m. q12h Licensed in companion birds Irritant injection Use with care in working birds due to muscle damage May cause regurgitation	15 mg/kg orally, i.m. q12h 100–150 mg/l in water
Lincomycin		50–75 mg/kg orally, i.m. q12h	
Marbofloxacin	10 mg/kg orally, i.m., i.v. q24h	10 mg/kg orally, i.m., i.v. q24h	10 mg/kg orally, i.m., i.v. q24h
Oxytetracycline	50 mg/kg i.m. q24h Use long-acting preparation. Some preparations may cause irritant reactions	200 mg/kg i.m. q24h long-acting preparation 25–50 mg/kg orally q8h	100 mg/kg orally q24h 4–12 mg/l drinking water for 7 days
Piperacillin	100–200 mg/kg i.m., i.v. q8–12h Often combined with tazobactam; use as above and base dosage on piperacillin dose Above preparation should be reconstituted with glucose/saline for improved stability	100–200 mg/kg i.m., i.v. q8–12h Often combined with tazobactam; use as above and base dosage on piperacillin dose Above preparation should be reconstituted with glucose/saline for improved stability Prepared solution also suitable as a topical flushing agent	
Trimethoprim/Sulphonamide	8 mg/kg i.m. q12h 20–100 mg/kg orally q8–12h Reduce dose if regurgitation occurs	30 mg/kg i.m. q12h 12–60 mg/kg orally q12h	
Tylosin			1 g/l drinking water daily for 7–10 days
Antifungal drugs			
Amphotericin-B	1.5 mg/kg i.v. q8h for 3 days 1 mg/kg intratracheally q8–12h 100–300 mg/kg orally q12–24h for *Macrorhabdus* infection Nephrotoxic: use with care. Concurrent fluid therapy advised Useful adjunctive therapy to azole drugs in cases of aspergillosis owing to the slow onset of action of azoles	1.5 mg/kg i.v. q12h for 3–5 days Give with 10–15 ml/kg saline	100,000 IU/kg orally q8–12h 1–5 g/l drinking water for 10 days Note that the cheaper suspension of this drug is now unavailable in the UK. Suspension can be imported from within the EU on a Special Treatment Certificate (STC). Intravenous forms are available but are very expensive. A form for flock treatment (Megabac-S) is licensed in Australia and can be imported using an STC
Enilconazole		Dilute 10% solution 10:1 and give 0.5 ml/kg/day intratracheally for 7–14 days	
Fluconazole	5 mg/kg orally q24h May be hepatotoxic May cause vomiting	2–5 mg/kg orally q24h	
Itraconazole	5–10 mg/kg orally q12h Less hepatotoxic than ketoconazole. However, many Grey Parrots have an idiosyncratic reaction to this drug that may prove lethal. Some will tolerate the lower dose rate	10–20 mg/kg orally q24h (prophylactic) 10–15 mg/kg orally q12h (therapeutic)	

Drug	Parrots	Raptors	Passerines
Antifungal drugs continued			
Ketoconazole	30 mg/kg orally q12h May be hepatotoxic May cause vomiting	25 mg/kg orally, i.m. q12h	
Nystatin	300,000 IU/kg orally q12h Not absorbed from the gastrointestinal tract	300,000 IU/kg orally q12h Not absorbed from the gastrointestinal tract	5000–300,000 IU/bird orally q12h for 10 days for *Macrorhabdus* infection (although there are some doubts as to its efficacy)
Sodium benzoate	1 tsp/l drinking water for 5 weeks for *Macrorhabdus* infection Reports of toxicity		
Terbinafine	15 mg/kg orally q12h Less toxic than itraconazole to Grey Parrots. May have faster onset of action compared to azole drugs	10–15 mg/kg orally q12h	
Voriconazole	12.5 mg/kg orally q12h for 30–60 days	12.5 mg/kg orally q12h for 30–60 days	
Antiprotozoal drugs			
Amprolium			50–100 mg/l drinking water for 5 days or longer
Carnidazole	30–50 mg/kg orally; repeat after 14 days for trichomoniasis	25–30 mg/kg orally once; may repeat the next day if required	
Chloroquine	25 mg/kg orally at 0h, then 15 mg/kg orally at 12h, 24h and 48h for *Plasmodium* infection		2 g/l drinking water daily for 14 days
Chloroquine/ Primaquine		Crush 1 x 500 mg chloroquine tablet + 1 x 26 mg primaquine tablet and add 10 ml water 0.5 ml of this solution gives 15 mg chloroquine + 0.75 mg primaquine 25 mg/kg chloroquine + 1.3 mg/kg primaquine at 0h, then 15 mg/kg chloroquine at 12h, 24h and 48h for avian malaria 26.3 mg/kg orally weekly from 1 month before until 1 month after mosquito season as prophylaxis	
Clazuril		30 mg/kg orally once	
Diclazuril		10 mg/kg orally q24h on days 1, 3 and 10	
Mefloquin		50 mg/kg orally q24h for 7 days for avian malaria	
Melarsamine		0.25 mg/kg i.m. q24h for 4 days for leucocytozoonosis	
Metronidazole	30 mg/kg orally q12h Active against *Giardia*	50 mg/kg orally q24h for 5 days for trichomoniasis	50 mg/kg orally q12h 200 mg/l drinking water daily for 7 days
Paromomycin		100 mg/kg orally q12h for 7 days; repeat after 1 week	
Pyrimethamine	0.5 mg/kg orally q12h for 2 weeks for leucocytozoonosis	0.5 mg/kg orally q12h for 28 days for leucocytozoonosis	
Ronidazole			50–400 mg/l drinking water for 5 days
Sulfachloropyridazine			150–300 mg/l for 5 days a week for 2–3 weeks
Toltrazuril	7 mg/kg orally q24h for 3 days for coccidiosis	25 mg/kg orally weekly for 3 weeks for coccidiosis	75 mg/l for 2 days a week for 4 weeks
Trimethoprim (40 mg/ml) + sulfamethoxazole (200 mg/ml)		0.15 ml/kg i.m. q24h for 7 days for leucocytozoonosis	30 mg/kg orally q12–24h

▶

Drug	Parrots	Raptors	Passerines
Antiparasitic drugs			
Doramectin		1000 µg/kg s.c. twice 1–2 weeks apart for *Serratospiculum* infection	
Fenbendazole	20–100 mg/kg orally once; may need to repeat in 14 days for gut nematodes 50 mg/kg orally q24h for 3 days for Giardia	25–100 mg/kg orally once for nematodes and some cestodes 25 mg/kg orally q24h for 5 days for capillariasis Blood dyscrasias have been reported at higher doses in vultures and some other raptors	20 mg/kg by gavage q24h for 3 days
Fipronil	For the treatment of ectoparasites, spray should be applied to cotton wool and dabbed behind the head, under the wings and at the base of the tail. Do not soak the bird. May cause hypothermia. Spot-on preparations are not recommended	For the treatment of ectoparasites, spray should be applied to a pad and dabbed at the base of the neck, under the wings and at the base of the tail. Do not soak the bird	For the treatment of ectoparasites, spray should be applied lightly under each wing on to the skin
Flubendazole			60 mg/kg food for 7–14 days
Ivermectin	200 µg/kg orally, s.c. Licensed spot-on preparation (0.1% or 1% ivermectin) available	200 µg/kg orally, i.m.	200 µg/kg orally, s.c.
Levamisole	20 mg/kg orally once for gut nematodes 40 mg/kg for capillariasis May cause vomiting		150 mg/l daily in drinking water for 3 days
Mebendazole	25 mg/kg orally q12h for 5 days	20 mg/kg orally q24h for 10–14 days	10 mg/kg orally q12h for 5 days Do not use in breeding season
Moxidectin		500–1000 µg/kg orally once for capillariasis	
Niclosamide		220 mg/kg orally; repeat after 10–14 days	500 mg/kg orally weekly for 4 weeks
Piperazine	3.7 g/l drinking water for 12 hours; repeat in 2–3 weeks		3.7 g/l drinking water for 12 hours; repeat in 2–3 weeks
Piperonal powder		Shake over entire bird	Shake over entire bird
Praziquantel	10 mg/kg orally, i.m.; repeat after 10 days for trematodes and cestodes	10 mg/kg i.m.; repeat after 1 week for trematodes and cestodes	
Pyrethrum (powder/spray)			0.8% spray from 60 cm; use 2–3 x 1 second bursts
Rafoxanide		10 mg/kg orally	
Anti-inflammatory drugs			
Carprofen	1–5 mg/kg orally, i.m. q24h	1–5 mg/kg orally, i.m. q12–24h Use with care in cases of dehydration, shock and renal dysfunction Higher dose rate appears effective for 24 hours	1–5 mg/kg orally, i.m. q12–24h
Celecoxib	10 mg/kg orally q24h		
Ketoprofen	2 mg/kg i.m., s.c. q8–24h	1–5 mg/kg i.m. q8–24h	1–5 mg/kg i.m. q8–24h
Meloxicam	0.5–1 mg/kg orally, i.m. q12–24h up to 1.6 mg/kg orally q12–24h	0.1–0.5 mg/kg orally, i.m. q24h Use with care in cases of dehydration, shock and renal dysfunction	0.1–0.5 mg/kg orally, i.m. q24h
Piroxicam	0.5 mg/kg orally q12h	0.5 mg/kg orally q24h	0.5 mg/kg orally q24h
Anaesthetic, analgesic and emergency drugs			
Adrenaline	0.1 g/kg i.v., intraosseously, intracardially, intratracheally	0.5–1 mg/kg i.v., intraosseously, intratracheally	0.5–1 mg/kg i.v., intraosseously, intratracheally
Atropine		0.04–0.5 mg/kg i.m.	Not indicated
Bupivacaine	<2 mg/kg topical as local nerve block	<2 mg/kg topical Mix with DMSO for topical analgesia	

▶

Drug	Parrots	Raptors	Passerines
Anaesthetic, analgesic and emergency drugs continued			
Buprenorphine		0.01–0.05 mg/kg i.m., i.v. q8–12h	0.01–0.05 mg/kg i.m., i.v. q8–12h
Butorphanol	1–4 mg/kg i.m. q2–6h	0.3–4 mg/kg i.m. q6–12h	0.3–4 mg/kg i.m. q6–12h
Dexamethasone sodium phosphate	1–2 mg/kg i.m., i.v. Corticosteroids should be used with care in birds; immunosuppression and other side-effects common	2–6 mg/kg i.m., i.v. Corticosteroids should be used with care in birds; immunosuppression and other side-effects common	2–6 mg/kg i.m., i.v.
Diazepam	0.1–1.0 mg/kg i.v., i.m. for seizures 0.2–0.5 mg/kg i.m. or 0.05–0.15 mg/kg i.v. as premedicant	0.2–1 mg/kg i.v., i.m. q12–24h for control of fitting Lower dose orally q24h may be useful as an appetite stimulant	0.5 mg/kg orally
Doxapram	5–10 mg/kg i.v.	5–20 mg/kg i.v., intraosseously, intratracheally	5–20 mg/kg i.v., intraosseously, intratracheally
Fentanyl	0.2 mg/kg s.c.		
Glycopyrrolate	0.01 mg/kg i.m., i.v.	0.01–0.03 mg/kg i.m.	Not indicated
Lidocaine	1–4 mg/kg (maximum dose) topical as local nerve block Must not contain adrenaline Dilute to at least 1:10 with saline	<2.5 mg/kg topical local perfusion	Unlikely to be able to dose safely
Prednisolone sodium succinate		10–30 mg/kg i.v., i.m.	10–30 mg/kg i.v., i.m.
Tramadol	30 mg/kg orally q8–12h Hispaniolan Amazon: doses of 5–30 mg/kg orally q8–12h described with large species variations		
Topical agents			
Bacitracin–neomycin–polymyxin (Vetropolycin) ophthalmic ointment		Ophthalmic use or for topical use at orthopaedic pin–skin interfaces	
DMSO		Anti-inflammatory; may be combined with other drugs	
Prostaglandin E2 gel	0.1 mg/kg per cloaca		Dystocia
Miscellaneous drugs			
Aciclovir		333 mg/kg orally q12h for 7–14 days for herpesvirus	
Allopurinol	10 mg/30 ml drinking water daily	10 mg/kg orally q12h Toxicity reported in Red-tailed Hawks at 50 mg/kg	
Bismuth salts (Pepto-Bismol)	1–2 ml/kg orally q12h		1–2 ml/kg orally q12h
Cabergoline	10–20 µg/kg orally q24h for 1 week, then once weekly (or more frequently if required) for chronic egg laying		
Calcium gluconate	10 mg/kg i.m., s.c. q1h prn 100 mg/kg s.c. with fluids	10 mg/kg i.m., s.c. q1h prn	10 mg/kg i.m., s.c. q1h prn
Colchicine	0.04 mg/kg orally q12h for gout and hepatic cirrhosis/fibrosis	0.04 mg/kg orally q12h	
Deslorelin	4.7 mg implant i.m., s.c. for reproductive-related disease	4.7 mg implant i.m., s.c. for reproductive-related disease	
Digoxin	10–20 µg/kg orally q12h 0.02 mg/kg orally q24h	0.02–0.05 mg/kg orally q12h for 2–3 days, then reduce to 0.01 mg/kg q12–24h	
Dimercaprol/British Anti-Lewisite		2.5 mg/kg i.m. q4h for 2 days, then q12h until signs resolve	
Enalapril	0.5–2.5 mg/kg orally q12–24h	5 mg/kg orally q24h until signs improve, then decrease to 1 mg/kg	
Furosemide	0.5–2 mg/kg orally, i.m. q12h	0.1–6.0 mg/kg orally, i.m., i.v. q6–24h Do not use in dehydrated or hyperuricaemic birds	

▶

Drug	Parrots	Raptors	Passerines
Miscellaneous drugs continued			
Human chorionic gonadotropin	500 IU/kg i.m. on days 1, 3, 7, 14 and 21 for ovarian cysts 500–1000 IU/kg i.m. every 2–4 weeks for chronic egg laying		
Isoxsuprine		Small pinch powder/kg orally q12h	
Kaolin/pectin mixture	2 ml/kg orally	15 ml/kg orally	2 ml/kg orally
Lactulose	0.2–1.0 ml/kg orally q8h	0.5 ml/kg orally q12h	
Leuprolide acetate	100–750 µg/kg i.m. every 2 weeks for 3 doses for ovarian cysts 100–700 µg/kg i.m. every 2–4 weeks for 3–4 doses, then as required for chronic egg laying		
Medroxyprogesterone acetate	5–25 mg/kg i.m. every 6 weeks Severe side-effects (diabetes mellitus, obesity, hepatopathies and sudden death) limit its use and great care should be exercised		
Metoclopramide	0.3–2.0 mg/kg i.m. q8–24h	0.3–2.0 mg/kg orally, i.m. q12–24h	
Oxprenolol		2 mg/kg orally q24h	
Oxytocin	3–5 mg/kg i.m. for egg retention There are doubts about efficacy		
Penicillamine	55 mg/kg orally q12h Chelating agent for use in heavy metal toxicosis. Low therapeutic index	55 mg/kg orally q12h for 10 days	
Pimobendan	0.15–0.3 mg/kg orally q12h		
Pralidoxime	10–100 mg/kg i.v. q24h for organophosphate or carbamate toxicity	10 mg/kg i.m.	
Propentofylline		5 mg/kg orally q12h	
Silybin (milk thistle extract)	5 mg/kg orally q8h for liver disease		
Sodium calcium edetate	35–40 mg/kg i.m. q12h for heavy metal toxicosis An initial dose of 200 mg/kg i.m. may be given In chronic zinc toxicosis 100 mg/kg i.m. weekly has been described as effective	35–50 mg/kg i.m. q12h for 5 days, then stop for 2 days; repeat courses until lead levels normal	35–50 mg/kg i.m. q12h for 5 days, then stop for 2 days; repeat courses until lead levels normal
Terbutaline	0.01 mg/kg i.m. as a bronchodilator		
Vitamin B1 (thiamine)	3 mg/kg i.m. weekly	10–30 mg/kg i.m. q24h	
Vitamin E/Selenium		0.5 mg selenium + 1.34 IU vitamin E/kg s.c.; repeat after 72 hours	
Vitamin K1	0.2–2.5 mg/kg orally, i.m. q6–24h	0.2–2.5 mg/kg orally, i.m. q6–24h	0.2–2.5 mg/kg orally, i.m. q6–24h

References and further reading

Carpenter JW (2012) *Exotic Animal Formulary, 4th edn*. Saunders, Philadelphia

Meredith A (2015) *BSAVA Small Animal Formulary, 9th edn: Part B – Exotic Pets*. BSAVA Publications, Gloucester

Phalen DN (2014) Update on the diagnosis and management of *Macrorhabdus ornithogaster* (formerly megabacteria) in avian patients. *Veterinary Clinics of North America: Exotic Animal Practice* **17(2)**, 203–210

Index

Page numbers in *italics* indicate figures

Page numbers in **bold** indicate QRGs